INTRAOCULAR LENSES
in CATARACT *and*
REFRACTIVE SURGERY

Dimitri T. Azar, M.D.

Director of Corneal and Refractive Surgery Services and
Associate Chief of Ophthalmology, Massachusetts Eye and Ear Infirmary

Associate Scientist, Schepens Eye Research Institute

Associate Professor of Ophthalmology, Harvard Medical School
Boston, Massachusetts

W.B. SAUNDERS COMPANY
A Harcourt Health Sciences Company
Philadelphia   London   New York   St. Louis   Sydney   Toronto

W.B. SAUNDERS COMPANY
A Harcourt Health Sciences Company

The Curtis Center
Independence Square West
Philadelphia, Pennsylvania 19106

Library of Congress Cataloging-in-Publication Data

Intraocular lenses in cataract and refractive surgery / edited by Dimitri T. Azar;
associate editors, Walter J. Stark . . . [et al.].

p. cm

Includes bibliographical references.

ISBN 0–7216–8699–0

1. Intraocular lenses.   2. Eye—Surgery.   3. Crystalline lens—Diseases—
Treatment—Complications.   4. Aphakia—Surgery.   I. Azar, Dimitri T.
[DNLM: 1. Lenses, Intraocular.   2. Cataract Extraction.   3. Pseudophakia.
WW 260 I622 2001]

RE988 J584 2001

617.7′1—dc2l   00-049227

Last digit is the print number: 9   8   7   6   5   4   3   2   1

To my parents for helping me set higher goals.

To Drs. B. Ang, L. Glazer, and T. Hoang-Xuan, without whom this project would have remained unfinished.

To Drs. M. Abdu, N. Aswad, I. Maloof, E. Shaya, and N. Zalzal, for encouragement along the way.

To Dr. Walter Stark, for transmitting his skills and expertise with passion and enthusiasm.
To Drs. Sonia Yoo and Roberto Pineda, for rekindling my fascination with IOL surgery.
And to Dr. Nathalie Azar, my loving life partner, for sharing my journey and making it worthwhile.

Associate Editors

Walter J. Stark, M.D.

Professor, Department of Ophthalmology, Johns Hopkins University; Director of Corneal Service, Wilmer Ophthalmological Institute, Johns Hopkins Hospital, Baltimore, Maryland

Nathalie F. Azar, M.D.

Director, Pediatric Ophthalmology and Strabismus Service, Massachusetts Eye and Ear Infirmary and Harvard Medical School, Boston, Massachusetts

Roberto Pineda, M.D.

Assistant Professor, Department of Ophthalmology, Harvard Medical School; Chief of Ophthalmology, Brigham and Women's Hospital; Corneal Service, Massachusetts Eye and Ear Infirmary, Boston, Massachusetts

Sonia H. Yoo, M.D.

Assistant Professor, Department of Clinical Ophthalmology, Bascom Palmer Eye Institute, University of Miami, Miami, Florida

INTRAOCULAR LENSES
in CATARACT and
REFRACTIVE SURGERY

Contributors

Anthony P. Adamis, M.D.
Associate Professor, Harvard Medical School; Director, Eye Residency Training, Massachusetts Eye and Ear Infirmary, Boston, Massachusetts

Nasrin A. Afshari, M.D.
Corneal and Refractive Surgery Service, Massachusetts Eye and Ear Infirmary and Harvard Medical School, Boston, Massachusetts

Balamurali K. Ambati, M.D.
Massachusetts Eye and Ear Infirmary and Harvard Medical School, Boston, Massachusetts

Jayakrishna Ambati, M.D.
Retina Service, Massachusetts Eye and Ear Infirmary and Harvard Medical School, Boston, Massachusetts

Robert T. Ang, M.D.
Corneal and Refractive Surgery Service, Massachusetts Eye and Ear Infirmary, Boston, Massachusetts; Attending Surgeon, Asian Eye Institute, Makati, Philippines

Jean-Louis Arné, M.D.
Professor, Department of Ophthalmology, Faculty of Medicine, Universite P. Sabatier; Head, Department of Ophthalmology, Hospital Purpan, Toulouse, France

M. Farooq Ashraf, M.D.
Corneal Service, Wilmer Ophthalmological Institute, Johns Hopkins Hospital, Baltimore, Maryland

Dimitri T. Azar, M.D.
Director of Corneal and Refractive Surgery Services and Associate Chief of Ophthalmology, Massachusetts Eye and Ear Infirmary; Associate Scientist, Schepens Eye Research Instititute; Associate Professor of Ophthalmology, Harvard Medical School, Boston, Massachusetts

Nathalie F. Azar, M.D.
Director, Pediatric Ophthalmology and Strabismus Service, Massachusetts Eye and Ear Infirmary and Harvard Medical School, Boston, Massachusetts

George Baikoff, M.D.
Professor, Clinique Monticelli, Marseille, France

Teresa C. Chen, M.D.
Instructor, Department of Ophthalmology, Harvard Medical School; Massachusetts Eye and Ear Infirmary; Clinical Associate in Surgery, Massachusetts General Hospital; Clinical Associate in Surgery, Brigham and Women's Hospital, Boston, Massachusetts

Béatrice Cochener, M.D.
Professor and Chair, Department of Ophthalmology, University of Brest, Brest, France

Glenn C. Cockerham, M.D.
Glaucoma–Cataract Consultants, Inc., St. Clair Professional Building, Pittsburgh, Pennsylvania

Joseph Colin, M.D.
Professor, Department of Ophthalmology, University of Bordeaux; Chair, Department of Ophthalmology, CHU Pellegrin, Bordeaux, France

Elizabeth A. Davis, M.D., Ph.D.
Assistant Clinical Professor, University of Minnesota, St. Paul Minnesota; Associate, Minnesota Eye Consultants, P. A., Minneapolis, Minnesota

C. Stephen Foster, M.D., FACS
Professor, Department of Ophthalmology, Harvard Medical School; Director, Immunology Service, Massachusetts Eye and Ear Infirmary, Boston, Massachusetts

Liane Clamen Glazer, M.D.
Massachusetts Eye and Ear Infirmary and Harvard Medical School, Boston, Massachusetts

Bonnie An Henderson, M.D.
Clinical Instructor, Harvard Medical School; Associate Director of General Eye Service, Massachusetts Eye and Ear Infirmary, Boston, Massachusetts

Thanh Hoang-Xuan, M.D.
Professor and Chair, Department of Ophthalmology, Hospital Bichat and Foundation Ophthalmologique A. de Rothschild, Paris, France

Brien A. Holden, BAppSc, LOSC, Ph.D., DSc
Professor, School of Optometry, CRC for Eye Research and Technology, University of New South Wales, Sydney, NSW, Australia

Sandeep Jain, M.D.
Corneal and Refractive Surgery Service, Massachusetts Eye and Ear Infirmary and Harvard Medical School, Boston, Massachusetts

Herbert E. Kaufman, M.D.
Boyd Professor of Ophthalmology, Pharmacology, and Neuroscience; Head, Department of Ophthalmology; Director, Louisiana State University Eye Center, Louisiana State University Health Sciences Center, New Orleans, Louisiana

Ivana Kim, M.D.
Massachusetts Eye and Ear Infirmary and Harvard Medical School, Boston, Massachusetts

Mary Gilbert Lawrence, M.D., M.P.H.
Associate Professor, Department of Ophthalmology, University of Minnesota; Associate Chief of Ophthalmology, Minneapolis Veterans Affairs Medical Center, Minneapolis, Minnesota

Francois Melçaze, M.D., Ph.D.
Professor, Hospital Purpan, Toulouse, France

Samir A. Melki, M.D., Ph.D.
Clinical Instructor, Harvard Medical School, Massachusetts Eye and Ear Infirmary, Boston, Massachusetts

David J. Galaretta Mira, M.D.
Massachusetts Eye and Ear Infirmary, Boston, Massachusetts

Edward Murphy, M.D.
Instructor, Department of Ophthalmology, Harvard Medical School; Director, General Eye Service, Massachusetts Eye and Ear Infirmary, Boston, Massachusetts

Georgios P. Paleokastritis, M.D.
Massachusetts Eye and Ear Infirmary, Boston, Massachusetts; Surgeon, Department of Ophthalmology, Hellenic Air Force VA General Hospital, Athens, Greece

George P. Papadopoulos, M.D.
Ophthalmologist, Private Practice, Athens, Greece

Jean-Marie Parel, Ph.D.
Associate Professor, Bascom Palmer Eye Institute; Departments of Ophthalmology and Biomedical Engineering; Director, Ophthalmic Biophysics Center, University of Miami School of Medicine and College of Engineering, Miami, Florida; Professeur Associe, University of Paris, Paris, France; Professeur Visiteur, University of Liege, Liege, Belgium

Victor L. Perez, M.D.
Corneal and Uveitis Services, Massachusetts Eye and Ear Infirmary and Harvard Medical School, Boston, Massachusetts

Roberto Pineda, M.D.
Assistant Professor, Department of Ophthalmology, Harvard Medical School; Chief of Ophthalmology, Brigham and Women's Hospital; Corneal Service, Massachusetts Eye and Ear Infirmary, Boston, Massachusetts

Shimon Rumelt, M.D.
Department of Ophthalmology, Western Galilee Medical Center–Nahariya, Holon, Israel

H. John Shammas, M.D.
Clinical Professor, Department of Ophthalmology, University of Southern California School of Medicine, Los Angeles, California; Medical Director, Shammas Eye Medical Center, Lynwood, California

Tueng T. Shen, M.D., PLD
Massachusetts Eye and Ear Infirmary and Harvard Medical School, Boston, Massachusetts

Yichieh Shiuey, M.D.
Corneal and Refractive Surgery Specialist, Ophthalmic Surgical Associates, Waterbury, Connecticut

Walter J. Stark, M.D.
Professor, Department of Ophthalmology, Johns Hopkins University; Director of Corneal Service, Wilmer Ophthalmological Institute, Johns Hopkins Hospital, Baltimore, Maryland

Panagiota Stavrou, M.D., FACS
Uveitis Service, Massachusetts Eye and Ear Infirmary and Harvard Medical School, Boston, Massachusetts

Stephen U. Stechschulte, M.D.
Corneal and Refractive Surgery Service, Massachusetts Eye and Ear Infirmary and Harvard Medical School, Boston, Massachusetts

Rasik B. Vajpayee, M.D.
Professor of Ophthalmology, Director of Cornea Service, Rajendra Prasad Centre for Ophthalmic Sciences, All India Institute of Medical Sciences, New Delhi, India

Sonia H. Yoo, M.D.
Assistant Professor, Department of Clinical Ophthalmology, Bascom Palmer Eye Institute, University of Miami, Miami, Florida

Jeffriane S. Young, M.D.
Department of Ophthalmology and Visual Science, Yale University School of Medicine, New Haven, Connecticut

Foreword

The publication of this book is most timely. One could argue that, in this 52nd year since Sir Harold Ridley implanted the first intraocular lens (IOL), the field of intraocular lenses dominates ophthalmology for reasons that include the following:

- IOLs are used in the most common ophthalmic procedure, cataract surgery, and IOLs are increasingly used in the field of refractive surgery both as phakic IOLs and in clear lens extraction.
- The science of IOL biomaterials has exploded. The first IOL material was discovered serendipitously by Ridley as he noted the excellent tolerance of PMMA in the eyes of RAF pilots. The second group of IOL materials (certain silicones and hydrogels) was selected from preexisting polymers. Now we are in an era in which new biomaterials are being made specifically to meet the optical and biological needs of the human eye.
- The science of IOL design is reaching new levels of sophistication as we tackle our greatest IOL challenges to date: developing safe and effective phakic IOLs and designing true accommodative IOLs.

The editors have brought together an outstanding group of authors who balance clinical and basic science aspects and cover all major topics, ranging from IOL design, to surgical techniques, to complications, to special indications and situations. *Intraocular Lenses in Cataract and Refractive Surgery* is a practical but scientific reference that belongs at every clinician's fingertips and in every researcher's library. One year after the knighting of Sir Harold Ridley, this book comprehensively captures the diversity and complexity of the field that he began.

Douglas D. Koch, M.D.
The Allen, Mosbacher, and Law Chair in Ophthalmology
Cullen Eye Institute
Baylor College of Medicine
Houston, Texas

Foreword

General and ophthalmic surgery have both undergone revolutionary transformations over the past forty years. From the ophthalmic point of view, the sacred and inviolate vitreous has been found to be surgically dispensable, an intact posterior capsule of a cataractous lens is now preserved habitually, submacular surgery is now widely performed, and all manner of surgical manipulations are performed on the cornea to help resolve refractive problems.

In the vanguard of ophthalmic surgery during the second half of the twentieth century have been developments in cataract surgery and visual rehabilitation therefrom. Mr. Harold Ridley in England experienced savage criticism when he introduced his glass intraocular lens. Over the ensuing 30 years, serial refinements in the design and surgical placement of intraocular lenses were accomplished; it is now one of the most successful forms of invasive surgery performed anywhere in the body.

It is noteworthy that all of these developments in cataract surgery with the placement of intraocular lenses were pioneered and initally advanced outside of the groves of ophthalmic academe. There was a regnant orthodoxy and stodginess that led to the stigmatization of intraocular lenses, which were often described by senior professors as "ticking time bombs." How times have changed! Most of these fustian leaders of erstwhile ophthalmic academic opinion are now in their early dotage, and virtually all of them have undergone cataract surgery with intraocular lens placement.

We have at last come full circle back to the academic parapets. Dr. Dimitri Azar and many of his colleagues and trainees have assembled an extremely valuable textbook covering virtually every aspect of the placement and design of lenses within the cornea and the intraocular chambers. Having now nearly perfected the mechanics of cataract and corneal surgery, as well as the manufacture of appropriate lenses, the task of further improving the success of intraocular lenses has returned to the ophthalmic scientist and cell biologist. We will be hearing more and more about the immunomodulation of inflammation, as well as the molecular genetics of wound healing, as we attempt to provide medical supplements to the elegant contemporary praxis of surgery.

Dr. Dimitri Azar leads one of the most outstanding and eclectic groups addressing the cell biological problems. At the Massachusetts Eye and Ear Infirmary and the Schepens Eye Research Institute he has developed a clinical service and laboratory capability including seven clinical fellows and seven research fellows who work with him, and a half a dozen of the top anterior segment scientists at the Schepens, among whom are Drs. Ilene Gipson, Darlene Dartt, Nancy Joyce and James Zieske. He also has as faculty members and colleagues on his corneal service Drs. Claes Dohlman, Deborah Langston, Anthony Adamis, M. Reza Dana, Roberto Pineda, and Kathryn Colby. This textbook summarizes our contemporary knowledge on intraocular lenses in a cogent and practical way, but more importantly, identifies problems that will have to be solved in the years ahead with a consortium of talented investigators such as Dr. Azar has assembled in the clinic and the laboratory. The desiderata of objectivity and standardized prospective studies will continue to raise confidence in cataract and refractive surgery, which now can be accomplished almost ideally in academic environments.

Frederick A. Jakobiec, M.D., D.Sc. (Med)
Henry Willard Williams Professor of Ophthalmology
Professor of Pathology, and Chairman of Ophthalmology
Harvard Medical School; Chief of Ophthalmology
Massachusetts Eye and Ear Infirmary

Preface

Developments in intraocular lens (IOL) technology in the latter half of the 20th century may have their seeds in a passing comment of a precocious British medical student who, upon observing Harold Ridley perform cataract surgery, expressed his disappointment that the removed cataractous lens was not replaced. The advances in intraocular lens (IOL) surgery since the first Transpex PMMA lens, which Ridley was compelled to develop, have revolutionized ophthalmology beyond the expectations of Pike, Ridley, and their most enthusiastic contemporaries.

Despite multiple attempts to use phakic IOLs in the past 50 years, this approach did not receive wide acceptance until the last decade. In this book, dedicated to the basic principles and practical applications of IOLs, we emphasize current and forthcoming improvements in refractive IOL technology. Several studies have established the relative safety and efficacy of phakic IOLs for patients with extreme refractive errors, and the future will undoubtedly bring further advances in this field.

We also describe the indications, surgical techniques, and complications of IOLs in cataract and refractive surgery. In addition to the history of IOLs and their development, there are chapters on cataract surgery, IOL surgery, secondary IOLs in aphakia, phakic IOLs, management of IOL complications, and recent advances in astigmatic, multifocal, and specialized IOLs.

We use three-dimensional diagrams to illustrate IOL designs and preferred and alternative surgical techniques for IOL implantation, suturing, and repositioning. We include up-to-date reviews of the indications, surgical innovations, and clinical outcomes of anterior chamber-, posterior chamber-, and iris-fixated refractive IOLs, as well as extensive coverage of phakic IOL complications and their prevention and management.

This book represents the amalgamation of the care and attention of the editors Kim Cox and Richard Lambert at W. B. Saunders with the expertise of the contributors and associate editors. I am indebted to Rhonda Harris, my capable assistant, for her dedication to this project, to Leona Greenhill, and to all who helped shape my cataract and refractive surgical experience. I would like to acknowledge the Boston ophthalmologists who helped to shape my IOL experience (Drs. M. Abelson, A. Adamis, M. Antigua, M. Aswad, A. Bajart, A. Boruchoff, C. Dohlman, B. Faris, R. Floyd, C. S. Foster, G. Frangieh, G. Garcia, R. Gorn, P. Harris, F. Jakobiec, N. Jarudi, K. Kenyon, R. Lacy, D. Langston, M. Mead, T. Murphy, J. Rosenberg, and R. Steinert), my friends who were there for my first cataract surgical procedures (Drs. K. Itani, L. Maroof, S. Salamoun, and I. Shammas), and several of the Wilmer surgeons who helped launch my career as a refractive surgeon (Drs. E. DeJuan, M. Goldberg, J. Gottsch, D. Guyton, I. Maumenee, T. O'Brien, O. Schein, W. Stark, and E. Traboulsi).

Many other ophthalmologists have improved my understanding of IOLs through their innovations, research, and publications. The extensive chapter bibliographies attest to their seminal contributions. They will continue to inspire generations of ophthalmologists to push the field of IOL surgery forward.

This textbook, *Intraocular Lenses in Cataract and Refractive Surgery,* serves as a testament to their contributions and summarizes the major achievements of the pioneers, innovators, and students of the field of IOL surgery. We hope that it conveys the diversity of techniques of IOL surgery and provides valuable information not only to the beginning resident but also to more seasoned cataract and refractive surgeons. As was the case with Sir Harold Ridley, it is our hope that one of our readers will have the good fortune of being fertile ground for transforming a critical comment of a young medical student into the next frontier in ophthalmology.

Dimitri T. Azar, M.D.

Contents

Part I

Introduction

Chapter 1

History of Cataract Surgery and Intraocular Lenses

Georgios P. Paleokastritis, Liane Clamen Glazer, George P. Papadopoulos, Dimitri T. Azar, and Anthony P. Adamis

Two of the most significant achievements in ophthalmology were the improvement and refinement of cataract extraction surgery and the development of the intraocular lens (IOL). More than 50 million people worldwide suffer from cataract-related visual impairment, and millions of people around the world have benefited from cataract extraction and IOL implantation.[1] As D. W. Greene so eloquently noted at a 1910 American Academy of Ophthalmology meeting, "Other surgeries relieve suffering, some prolong life, and some correct deformity, but the extraction of the opaque lens does all of these and more."[2] With the introduction of the IOL many years after that statement, outcomes after cataract surgery are even more impressive than in Greene's day.

■ The History of Cataract Surgery

Over the centuries, there have been a variety of creative surgical as well as medical treatment attempts for cataracts. Bronze cataract needles of Roman origin have been discovered in France (Fig. 1.1). These needles, dating from the first or second century A.D., are evidence that both suction aspiration and couching of the cataract were performed in ancient times.[3] Couching (from the French *coucher*, to lay down, to put to bed) refers to displacement of the lens into the vitreous cavity and out of the line of vision.

Nonsurgical treatments for cataract extraction have also been attempted throughout history. Many unfortunate patients were disappointed over the years by promises that exercises, drops, or even staring at colored lights could help improve their cataract-impaired vision.[3] Other nonsurgical treatments for cataracts included the instillation of sodium iodide or mercury cyanide, and ionization.[4] None of these treatments worked.

More than 250 years ago, in 1747, Jacques Daviel performed the first reported extracapsular cataract extraction (ECCE) when a couching procedure failed. By 1752, Daviel had presented a paper to the Royal Academy of Surgery in Paris in which he reported on 206 extractions with an impressive success rate of 88%.[5] For more than a hundred years after this surgery was reported, a cataract debate raged among ophthalmologists: extraction or couching? Both intracapsular and extracapsular extraction were favored in Europe, whereas U.S. ophthalmologists tended to prefer couching. Finally, the prestigious ophthalmic surgeon Albrecht von Graefe introduced his linear cataract extraction procedure in 1866, and with it extraction became the treatment of choice for cataracts.[6] For the next century, a new debate raged: intracapsular or extracapsular extraction?

In 1967, Kelman introduced the technique of phacoemulsification, whereby the cataract is fragmented to allow ease of aspiration (Fig. 1.2). This elegant form of ECCE allowed the surgeon to remove a cataract through a 3.0-mm incision. Phacoemulsification eliminated many of the potential problems of cataract surgery, including wound healing complications secondary to a large incision and the lengthy postoperative recuperative period.[7] Today, ECCE with phacoemulsification is the technique most commonly used for cataract extraction.

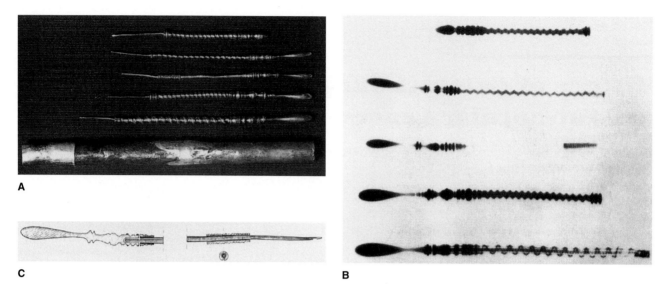

A

C

B

FIGURE 1.1. Ancient cataract needles. *A,* Bronze cataract needles of Roman origin, dating to the first or second century A.D., were found in Montbelle/Burgundy, France. *B,* A radiograph of the Roman needles shows that needles 1, 2, and 4 are couching needles. Needles 3 and 5 are hollow with holes at the tip and with trocars in the center; these needles were used to aspirate the cataractous lens. *C,* During surgery, the trocar was removed and the surgeon aspirated the cataract with suction. *(From Apple DJ, Mamalis N, Olson RJ, Kincaid MC. Intraocular Lenses: Evolution, Designs, Complications, and Pathology. Baltimore, MD: Williams & Wilkins; 1989, with permission.)*

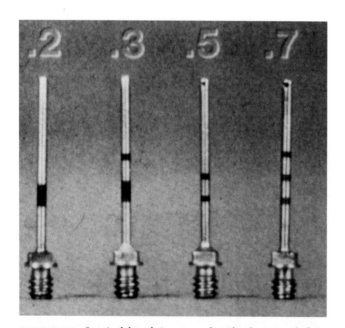

FIGURE 1.2. Surgical handpieces used with phacoemulsification. These more sophisticated handpieces are used in modern cataract extraction procedures. The hollow devices allow simultaneous irrigation and aspiration so that residual cortical material can be removed after fragmentation of the nucleus by phacoemulsification. *(From Jaffe NS, Jaffe MS, Jaffe GF. Cataract Surgery and Its Complications. 5th ed. Philadelphia: CV Mosby; 1990, with permission.)*

■ The Early History of Intraocular Lenses

For those who underwent surgical removal of cataracts in the pre-IOL era, adjusting to aphakia was a necessary side effect. Patients traded in their cataractous lenses for "Coke bottle bottom" spectacles. The prismatic effect of these thick lenses causes a ring scotoma between 40 and 60 degrees. Associated difficulties include a markedly constricted visual field, lack of stereopsis, spherical aberrations, problems of false orientation, and difficulty with coordination. Not surprisingly, the idea of an IOL did occur to some creative thinkers.

As early as the 1760s, ophthalmologists had explored the idea of an artificial replacement for the cataractous lens. The 18th century Italian adventurer and paramour Casanova described in his memoirs a conversation he had had in 1766 with an oculist named Tadini. Tadini purportedly showed Casanova a box of lenses he intended to implant "under the cornea in the place of the crystalline lens." It is unclear whether or not Tadini actually performed such a procedure; however, legend has it that Casanova mentioned the idea to one of his contemporaries, Casaamata, the Court Eye Doctor of Dresden. Around 1795, Casaamata inserted a glass lens into an eye at the time of cataract surgery, and it immediately sank back toward the posterior pole.[3,8–10]

■ Ridley's Posterior Chamber Lens

After such a disappointing early attempt at lens implantation, lens replacement was apparently not attempted again until the British ophthalmologist Harold Ridley ushered in the age of modern lens implantation in 1949 (Fig. 1.3). Ridley "felt compelled" to develop his artificial lens after a precocious medical student, Steve Parry, observed a cataract operation and conveyed his disappointment to Ridley that the removed lens was not replaced in any way.[7] Ridley was inspired, and he learned from World War II experiences as he searched for an appropriate material for his artificial lens. During the war, British Air Force planes' cockpits and gunnery canopies were fabricated from an acrylic plastic, poly-

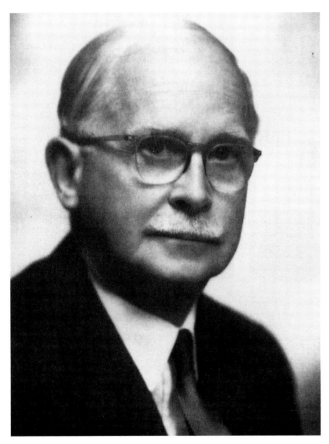

FIGURE 1.3. Harold Ridley, originator of the intraocular lens. *(From Apple DJ, Mamalis N, Olson RJ, Kincaid MC.* Intraocular Lenses: Evolution, Designs, Complications, and Pathology. *Baltimore, MD: Williams & Wilkins; 1989, with permission.)*

methyl methacrylate (PMMA). When a canopy was shattered by gunfire, fragments of this material sometimes penetrated the eyes of the flight crew. These PMMA splinters did not irritate the eye, and seemed to be inert.

As he considered which material would be best suited for an IOL, Ridley conferred with his friend John Pike, an optical scientist at Rayners of London. Aware that commercial PMMA was not sufficiently pure to be inserted into an eye, Pike consulted his friend John Holt at Imperial Chemical Industries. They succeeded in synthesizing a suitable PMMA, first named Transpex I, later Perspex CQ (Clinical Quality), which is still in common use today. Transpex I had a refractive index of 1.49 and a specific gravity of 1.19.[11–15] For the optical properties of the new lens, they studied the work of the Swedish ophthalmologist Allval Gullstrand.[16]

The first IOL was made by Rayners of London. In its final form it measured 8.35 mm in diameter and 2.40 mm in thickness. Its weight in air was 112 mg. The radius of the anterior curve was 17.8 mm and the radius of the posterior curve was 10.7 mm; its dimensions were about 1 mm less than those of the human lens. At the periphery, on both sides, a circumferential groove was cut before polishing to permit grasping with forceps. The refractive power of the lens was + 24 diopters. The compound system of cornea and acrylic lens closely approximated the physiologic state. The lens was designed to be inserted with the flatter surface facing the cornea (Fig. 1.4A).

Thus, in Ridley's first IOL operation, he implanted a lens made of PMMA into the capsular bag following ECCE. The procedure was performed on a 45-year-old woman at St. Thomas Hospital in London on November 29, 1949.[7] Because Ridley feared the IOL would not stay in place, he removed it just after implanting it. He implanted it again as a secondary procedure on February 8, 1950, when the eye had stabilized.[16–19] The surgery was an anatomic success, but the patient was left highly myopic. Her postoperative visual acuity was 6/18, requiring a refractive correction of −18.0 −6.0 × 120. There was clearly an error in the optical calculation.[20,21]

Ridley implanted a second lens on August 23, 1950, at Moorfield's Hospital.[16,20,22] Once again, the patient was left myopic (visual acuity of 6/60 with a correction of −14.00 −2.00 × 60). With the use of new methods for calculating the dioptric power of the IOL, the postoperative visual acuity in subsequent patients significantly improved and the level of myopia decreased to −1.0 diopter.

Ridley first described his new procedure at the Oxford Ophthalmological Conference on July 9, 1951. At that time, the eye with the very first implant had 20

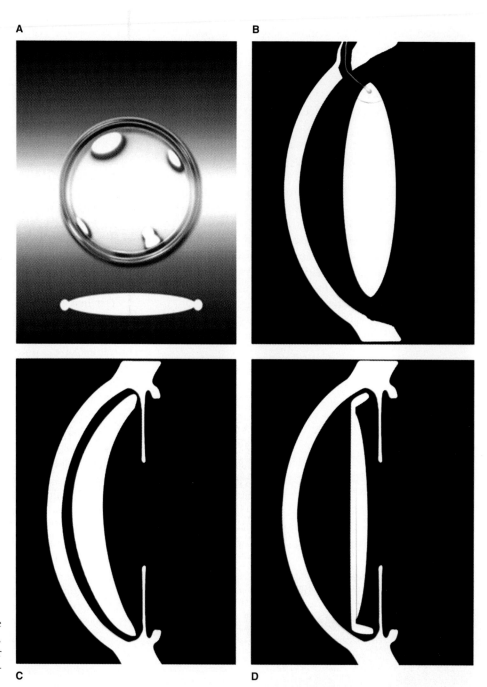

FIGURE 1.4. The evolution of the intraocular lens. *A,* Ridley lens. *B,* Parry lens. *C,* Baron's anterior chamber lens. *D,* Baron's modification of his original lens.

months of follow-up.[16,20] After his report, many ophthalmic surgeons performed the procedure. Some of those initial patients still had good vision 42 years later (Fig. 1.5).[23]

It is difficult to find accurate statistics on these early patients. One case series reported a 10-year success rate of approximately 70%. Failures were caused by dislocations (20%) and secondary glaucoma (10%). The latter was usually associated with an iritis in the early postoperative period. In 15% of cases the IOL had to be explanted. Other complications Ridley mentioned were pupillary occlusion by a dense inflammatory membrane, late thickening of the posterior capsule in young patients, loss of the anterior chamber, and iris atrophy from pressure incurred by the rim of a poorly centered lens.[11,20,22,24–26]

Ridley's first article describing IOL implantation was published in 1951 in *Transactions of the Ophthalmological Societies of the United Kingdom*. He wrote that the cataract "must be perfectly removed, leaving

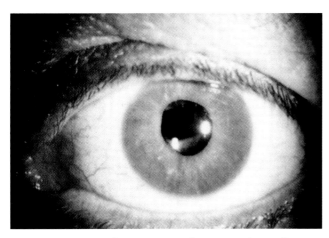

FIGURE 1.5. External appearance of an eye with a Ridley IOL 44 years after surgery. *(From Letocha CE, Pavlin CJ. Follow-up of 3 patients with Ridley intraocular lens implantation.* J Cataract Refract Surg. *1999;25:588, with permission.)*

intact the posterior layer of the lens capsule to prevent dislocation of the prosthesis into the vitreous cavity. The lens might be inserted either immediately after the extraction of the cataract or at a separate operation some weeks later."[11,16,19]

In the United States, the first IOL implantation was done by Warren Reese at the Wills Eye Hospital on March 17, 1952. Reese performed this surgery one day after Ridley gave his first lecture in the United States, at the annual meeting of the Chicago Ophthalmological Society.[13,16] When Ridley later presented his procedure at the 57th session of the American Academy of Ophthalmology and Otolaryngology in Chicago on October 12, 1952, it met with great hostility from several ophthalmologists.[16,21] Some of them referred to the IOL as a "time bomb."[19] Ridley implanted lenses in about 750 eyes and developed many different types of lenses. However, he grew discouraged by the frequency of complications and perhaps by his many detractors, and by 1959 he had given up lens implantation altogether.[7,8] In 1954, Parry tried to anchor the Ridley lens by means of a tantalum thread with the ends left loose beneath the conjunctiva (Fig. 1.4B).

■ Anterior Chamber Lenses

One of the most common complications of the Ridley lens was its tendency to dislocate into the vitreous. Noting that the frequency of dislocation with the Ridley lens was approximately 13%, ophthalmologists considered a new implantation site: the anterior chamber, with fixation of the lens in the angle recess.[27] The purported advantages of the anterior chamber IOL

(ACIOL) included the following: (1) Implantation could be performed after both ECCE and ICCE. (2) Dislocation might occur less frequently. (3) If necessary, the lens could be more easily removed. (4) The ACIOL could potentially be used for the correction of high refractive errors and anisometropia in phakic eyes.[12,20,24,28,29] Although the anterior chamber placement avoided the problem of dislocation and was technically easier than posterior chamber placement, the AC lens often damaged the corneal endothelium.

Baron, in France, designed and implanted the first ACIOL on May 13, 1952.[20,22] Baron's IOL, made of PMMA, had a very steep anterior curve and a short radius of curvature. The lens, which looked like a curved disc, floated in the anterior chamber (Fig. 1.4C). The curve was so steep that corneal endothelial contact and the resultant pseudophakos-induced corneal disease was inevitable.[3] The original Baron lens was associated with a number of complications, including late endothelial cell loss, corneal decompensation, pseudophakic bullous keratopathy (PBK), and corneal opacification. Many other rigid ACIOL designs caused similar problems, which often did not manifest until years after implantation. Baron tried to avoid corneal injury using various models, including a square lens (Fig. 1.4D). None of these models was successful.

Baron's 1952 implantation unleashed a flurry of innovations of the ACIOL. On September 26, 1953, Scharf implanted an ACIOL of his own design in Germany. It had the shape of a shark's egg (Fig. 1.6A). Two days later, on September 28, 1953, Benedetto Strampelli of Italy implanted a different type of ACIOL. It was an acrylic plate 4.5 mm in width and 11–13 mm in length, and bowed anteriorly to leave 1 mm between it and the anterior surface of the iris (Fig. 1.6B). The inferior edge of the lens was rounded so that it adapted itself to the shape of the anterior chamber angle. The upper end of the lens was shaped like a dove's tail. The thickness of the lens and its curvatures were altered according to the required refractive power.[29]

Strampelli presented his IOL at the Congress of the Societas Lombardo di Optalmologica in Pavia on December 8, 1953. This was the first public report describing an ACIOL. At the same meeting, Apollonio from Italy presented his results with a tripod-type IOL of his own design (Fig. 1.6C). From July 1954 to June 1956, Barraquer from Spain implanted 62 Strampelli ACIOLs, with minor modifications. His indications were aphakia, nonprogressive high myopia, and high hyperopia. The results were described as satisfactory, with "insignificant complications."[28,29]

From then on, the pace of design and implantation accelerated. Schreck constructed a bipod lens that had

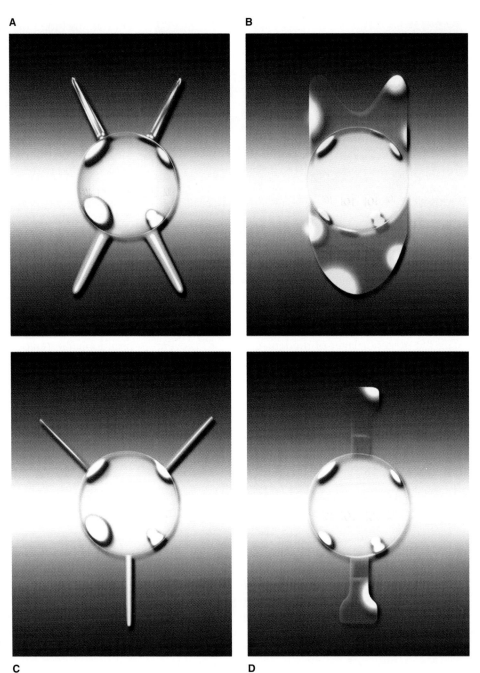

FIGURE 1.6. The further evolution of the intraocular lens. *A,* Scharf anterior chamber lens. *B,* Strampelli acrylic plate anterior chamber IOL. *C,* Apollonio lens. *D,* Schreck's bipod lens.

wider ends and a 10-mm radius (Fig. 1.6D). Bietti modified Strampelli's IOL in an effort to reduce the points of contact with the anterior chamber angle and to allow easier insertion into the eye. In its final form, the IOL was a rectangular curved plate with a triangular cut at its upper end and a lens of 6 mm diameter in its central part (Fig. 1.7A). The size of the optic had been increased to achieve good vision at the periphery and when the pupil was dilated. This lens could be implanted after either ICCE or ECCE, or to correct high myopia and hyperopia.[28,29]

Most of the ACIOLs of that era were made of one rigid plane and were thick, with imperfectly finished edges and an anterior curvature that brought the lens close to the endothelium. Because it was difficult to precisely measure the width of the anterior chamber in individual patients, many surgeons devised nonrigid implants with flexible bases. Danheim tried to solve the problem of centration by using elastic supporting loops of 0.1-mm Supramid (Fig. 1.7B). This IOL failed because of eventual hydrolysis of the Supramid and subsequent lens dislocation. Lieb and Guerry used a

A

B

C

D

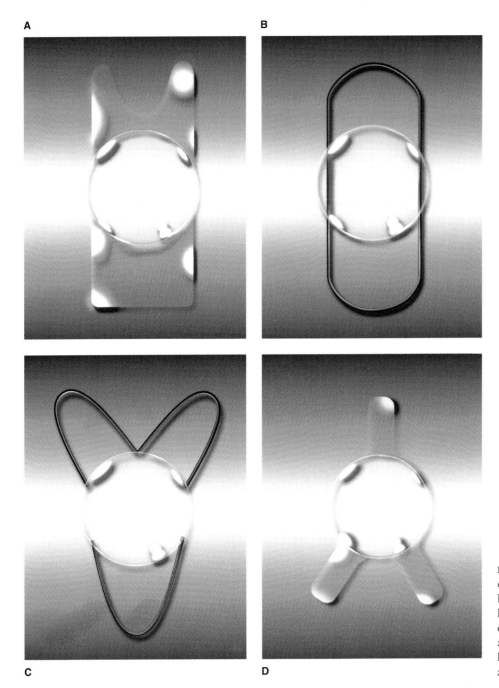

FIGURE 1.7. The further evolution of the intraocular lens. *A,* Bietti lens with 6 mm optic. *B,* Danheim lens, which used Supramid elastic supporting loops. *C,* Lieb and Querry lens. *D,* Ridley Mark I lens, which aimed to minimize angle pressure.

lens that was similar to Danheim's, but the Supramid loops were affixed tangentially by means of peripheral grooves, thus increasing the refracting surface of the IOL (Fig. 1.7C).[20,22] Ridley also participated in ACIOL lens design, producing a lens called the Mark I. His goal was to achieve maximal stability with minimal pressure on the angle. His ACIOL consisted of a central optic supported by three legs that curved posteriorly, arranged to provide wide triangular support. The posterior curvature and the diameter of the haptics varied

(Fig. 1.7D).[11,30,31] Barraquer modified the Danheim IOL either by cutting away half of the loops, giving a J shape to the lens (an important landmark in the evolution of IOLs), or by enlarging the optical portion and reducing the size of the loops. The design changes were made to decrease the danger of forward displacement of the optical portion (Figs. 1.8A and B).

In 1956, at the Congress of Ophthalmology, in Madrid, Strampelli proposed that the best way to implant a lens was to suspend it in the center of the

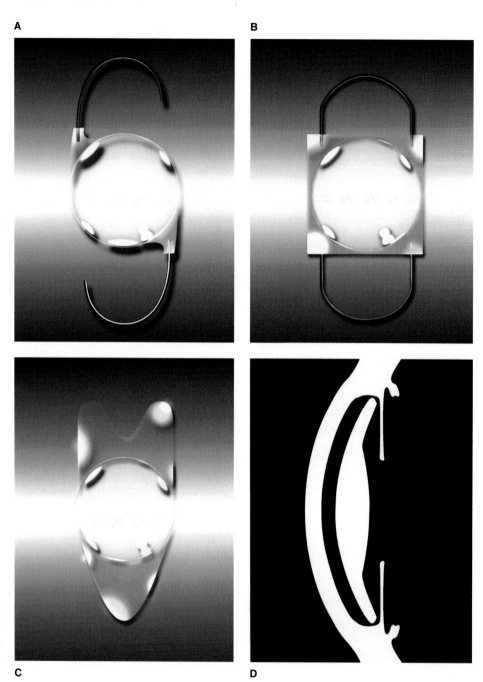

FIGURE 1.8. The further evolution of the intraocular lens. *A* and *B,* Two IOLs designed by Barraquer gave the lens more stability with the J-loop. *C* and *D,* Choyce Mark I lens.

anterior chamber without letting it touch any part of the chamber wall. He achieved this goal by passing sutures through the corneal-scleral wall and fixing the lenses to the external surface of the eye.

Peter Choyce, who had watched Ridley perform a cataract extraction in 1949, designed the Choyce Mark I (1956) through the Mark IX (1967) lenses. The many modifications to these lenses included the curvature of the optics, the form of the footplates, and the tips of the haptics (Figs. 1.8C and D and 1.9A–C). The Choyce IOLs were more vaulted and thinner than Strampelli's

lenses to avoid damaging the corneal endothelium. The most successful model was the Mark VIII (Figs. 1.9A and B). Initially implanted on June 28, 1963, it was the first ACIOL with four haptics. The lens was supplied in diameters from 11 to 14 mm in 0.5-mm increments. The biconvex optic part was 6 mm in diameter and ranged from 10 to 27 diopters in 0.5-diopter steps. The outer 2 mm of each haptic was flattened in the horizontal plane, keeping it away from the endothelium. Among the purported advantages of this IOL were (1) it could be used as a primary or secondary implant, (2) there was

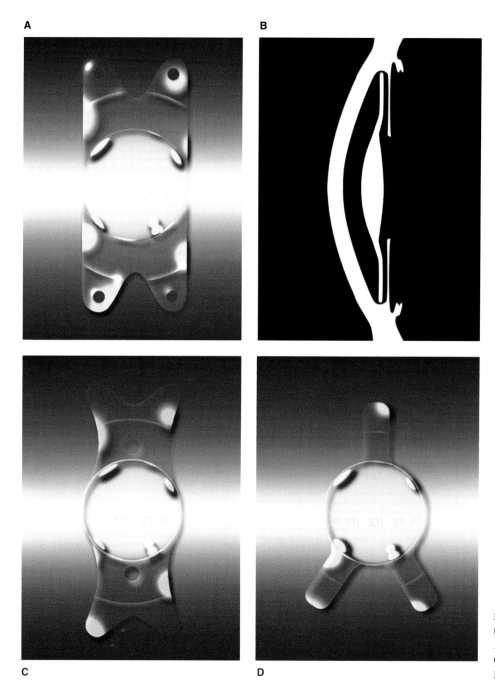

FIGURE 1.9. The further evolution of the intraocular lens. *A* and *B*, Choyce Mark VIII lens. *C*, Choyce Mark IX lens. *D*, Ridley Mark II lens.

minimal contact with the iris and cornea, (3) posterior dislocation was rare, (4) the lens was more easily explanted, (5) secondary capsulotomy was easier, (6) no sutures were required for fixation, and (7) it was easy to use in conjunction with penetrating keratoplasty. Of note, the lens worked better in larger eyes and was not stable in children's eyes. Complications included pupillary block and dislocation.[20,27,32–36]

In the meantime, Ridley had modified his ACIOL, producing the Mark II model. The new model was thinner and the tips of the haptics were flattened, to lessen the danger of pressure on the corneal periphery and to keep the IOL close to but clear of the iris (Fig. 1.9D). This lens position was close to the nodal point of the eye and minimized aniseikonia. The implant was easy to insert, and if properly fitted it would not tilt. Ridley used this IOL in 59 cases between January 1960 and 1969, with only one case of corneal decompensation.[12,20] Boberg-Ans of Denmark created an ACIOL that was a one-piece, three-point fixation lens that was fenestrated in order to minimize the incidence of pupillary block (Fig. 1.10A).

A

B

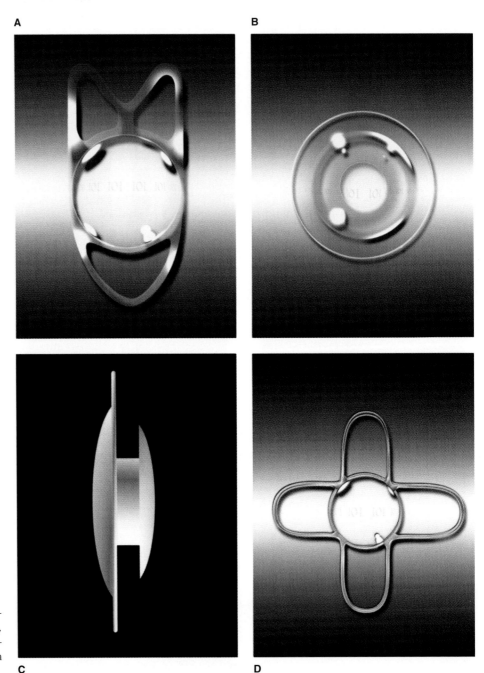

C   D

FIGURE 1.10. The further evolution of the intraocular lens. *A,* Boberg-Ans lens. *B* and *C,* Epstein collar-stud lens. *D,* Epstein Maltese cross iris lens.

■ Iris-Fixated Lenses

In the 1950s, in an attempt to create lenses that had lower rates of complications than the ACIOLs, some innovative ophthalmologists designed iris-fixated lenses. Cornelious Binkhorst designed an iris clip lens, Epstein created a Maltese cross–shaped lens, Worst used a suture or a metal clip for fixation, and Fyodorov developed the popular "Sputnik" lenses.[27] Unfortunately, iris-fixated lenses were associated with a high rate of

cystoid macular edema (CME), corneal decompensation, and dislocation.

In 1951, Epstein implanted his first Ridley posterior chamber IOL (PCIOL) in a child, with excellent results. After his initial experience with the Ridley IOL, he designed a modification in 1953, the "collar-stud" IOL (Figs. 1.10B and C).[37–39] A deep equatorial groove 0.6 mm wide was cut. The IOL was placed so that the iris fit into the equatorial groove after an ICCE. After the first 24 cases, Epstein's design evolved to the one-piece Maltese cross IOL, which consisted of a central optic supported by four arms in the form of a cross (Figs. 1.10D and 1.11A).[20] Eventually Epstein's IOL had two arms placed posterior to the iris and the remaining two anterior to the iris (Fig. 1.11A).[7,20,24] Epstein did not report on his work until 1959.[37] In 1957, at a meeting of the Italian Society of Ophthalmology, in Milan, he described his results. Stampelli's implant had a disc-shaped optic measuring 5 mm in diameter (Fig. 1.11B). It was made of acrylic and had two lateral canals, through which a Supramid suture passed and formed an ellipse with an average total length of about 14 mm. The two loops perforated the sclera at the 12 and 6 o'clock positions and were buried under the conjunctiva.[20,22,30]

Cornelius Binkhorst of Holland developed his iris clip IOL in 1957 and used it for the first time on August 11, 1958. In December 1958, at the 142nd meeting of the Netherlands Ophthalmological Society, he presented the results of his first 28 cases. At the

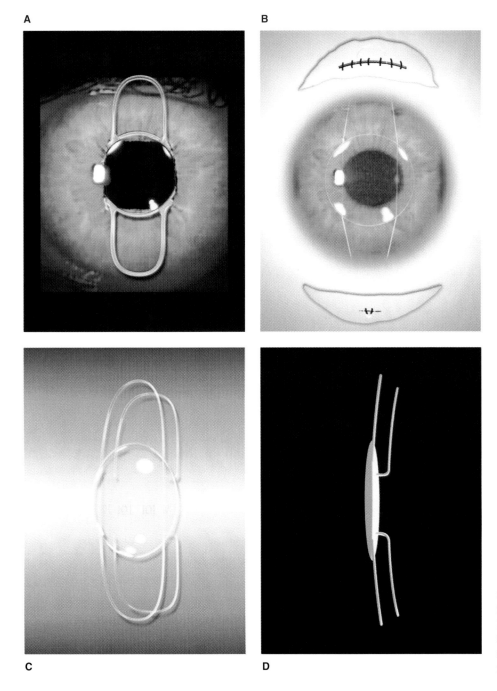

FIGURE 1.11. The further evolution of the intraocular lens. *A,* Epstein Maltese cross iris lens inserted in the eye. *B,* Strampelli sutured lens. *C* and *D,* Binkhorst iris clip lens.

Oxford Ophthalmological Congress in 1959 he used the term "artificial pseudophakia" to indicate the presence of an artificial lens implant.[29] His implant was supported entirely by the iris and did not touch either the angle or other vital structures (Figs. 1.11C and D). The contact between the IOL and both the anterior and posterior surfaces of the iris was very well tolerated.[40–43] In order to be located immediately in front of the pupil and to be kept in place, the lens was provided with two wire loops attached to its posterior sur-

face, close to the equator and bent at right angles. These wire loops were inserted through the pupil and positioned at the posterior surface of the iris, without reaching the ciliary body. The distance between the ends of these loops was about 7 mm, and their role was to prevent anterior dislocation. To prevent posterior dislocation from occurring with dilated pupils, two flat wire loops were mounted to the equator of the IOL, increasing the greatest diameter of the part in front of the pupil to 8 mm. These anterior loops were

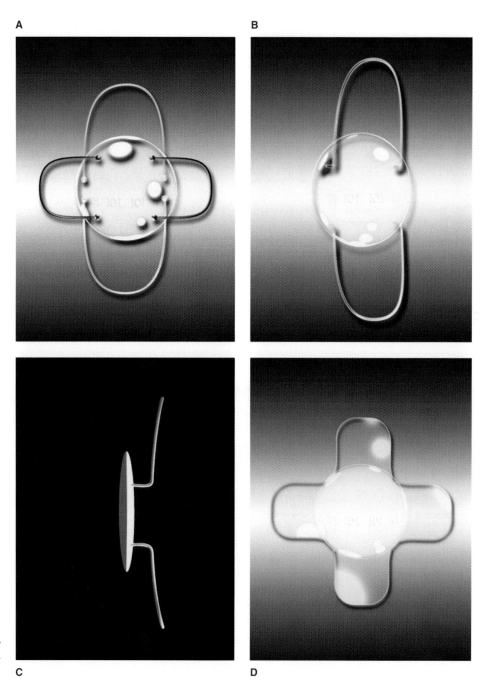

A

B

C

D

FIGURE 1.12. The further evolution of the intraocular lens. *A,* Fyodorov's modification of the Binkhorst and Epstein lens. *B* and *C,* Binkhorst iridocapsular lens. *D,* Copeland-Binkhorst lens.

adjacent to the anterior surface of the iris, maintaining a safe distance from the anterior chamber angle. The clearance between the anterior and posterior loops was 0.5–0.75 mm, just enough to enable iris to slide in between.

Fyodorov, of the Soviet Union, modified Binkhorst's iris clip IOL in 1964, rotating the posterior loops so that they were 90 degrees to the anterior loops (Fig. 1.12A). This made a lens as easy to insert as Epstein's Maltese cross lens and purportedly lessened the likelihood of pupillary block.[7,35] The visual results with the iris clip IOL were generally good, but Binkhorst made additional modifications. In 1963, he performed his first ECCE operation and inserted an iris clip IOL. The iridocapsular adhesions that formed prevented the IOL from dislocating anteriorly. The intact posterior capsule prevented posterior dislocation. Recognizing this, he began to cut off the anterior loops, forming the two-loop Binkhorst IOL (Figs. 1.12B and C). On September 16, 1965, an iridocapsular IOL in the form of an iris clip IOL without its anterior loops was inserted for the first time.[20,42]

Binkhorst's iridocapsular IOL was designed for use in children after ECCE. The optic was the same as in the iris clip IOL and was located in the anterior chamber, immediately in front of the pupil and lightly touching the iris. It permitted the free flow of aqueous through the pupillary aperture. One pair of wire loops made of 0.15-mm platinum-iridium, bent slightly backward, was laid behind the optical part and buried in the iridocapsular cleft. This fixation mechanism required a relatively strong posterior capsule and adhesions between the capsule and the iris. The implantation was generally easier to perform and was independent of the anterior chamber dimensions. Moreover, the absence of the anterior loops limited contact with the cornea. The relative disadvantages were that insertion was possible only after ECCE and that total removal of the IOL was difficult in the event of good fixation. There was also the possibility of posterior dislocation because of the relatively heavy weight of the lens.[20,42]

In 1968, Peter Choyce developed the Mark IX, a one-piece, single-material (Perspex CQ), four-point-fixation ACIOL (Fig. 1.9C). The Mark IX was a lighter version of the Mark VIII, with a couple of holes drilled between the optic and the footplates to allow better circulation of aqueous after the operation. Both models were extremely successful and were used throughout the world. The initial reported incidence of corneal decompensation over a 10-year period was 1%.[32] Improved manufacturing, which was quite crude in many of the early IOL designs, was thought to contribute to the improving results.[20,31]

A modification of Epstein's Maltese cross IOL became known as the Copeland-Binkhorst IOL and later as the iris-plane IOL.[22,44] This lens received extensive use in Miami, Flordia, where the first was implanted by Norman Jaffe on May 13, 1968. The lens was in the shape of a symmetric cross and looked like an airplane propeller (Fig. 1.12D). It was an all-PMMA IOL with four solid arms.[7,45] Because of the high incidence of chronic iris chafing, secondary CME, and bullous keratopathy, use of this IOL declined despite its easy insertion.[44]

Fyodorov's 1968 modification of the iris clip IOL led to the Sputnik IOL (Fig. 1.13A). This lens consisted of three posterior loops and three anterior prongs at 120 degrees to one another. The prongs were situated between the three posterior loops of a triple-loop design, with a bulbous tip that rested against the iris surface. The posterior loops angled 10–15 degrees posteriorly. The design of this IOL freed it from the requirement for fixation sutures. It had little tendency to dislocate.[7,20,35]

In 1969, Worst, working in Holland, modified the iris clip IOL by adding either a suture or a metal clip. This led to the design of the iris medallion lens, or MW (Medical Workshop) iris clip lens (Fig. 1.13B). The lens consisted of an optic portion of 5 mm diameter surrounded by an eccentric haptic portion of 8 mm diameter. The whole lens was made of one piece of material. There were only the usual posterior loops and two holes (one nasal and one temporal) in the eccentric haptic portion for suturing the implant to the iris at the 12 o'clock position. It was inserted for the first time on December 18, 1970.

The main advantages of the Worst lens over the iridocapsular lens were that it could be inserted after ICCE and it could be removed easily. Its disadvantage was that it depended on the Perlon suture and its proper fixation to the iris. Worst eventually changed the holes into notches in the upper part of the haptic support so that a stainless steel wire suture could be used. He also modified the medallion lens to utilize transiridectomy fixation. The platinum clip lens (or Worst platina) was the original medallion lens with a short loop at the 12 o'clock position, just reaching the upper edge of the haptic (Fig. 1.13C). It had a significantly longer loop at the 6 o'clock position that was placed in the capsular bag. The platinum clip was engaged to the superior loop, and total dislocation could not occur. A subsequent modification of this lens was the single-loop transiridectomy clip lens. With this lens, inferior loop displacement no longer occurred because the lower loop was eliminated. The placement of the iridectomy became critical because the lens rested at the inferior edge of the iridectomy.[4,7,20,22,27,35]

A   B

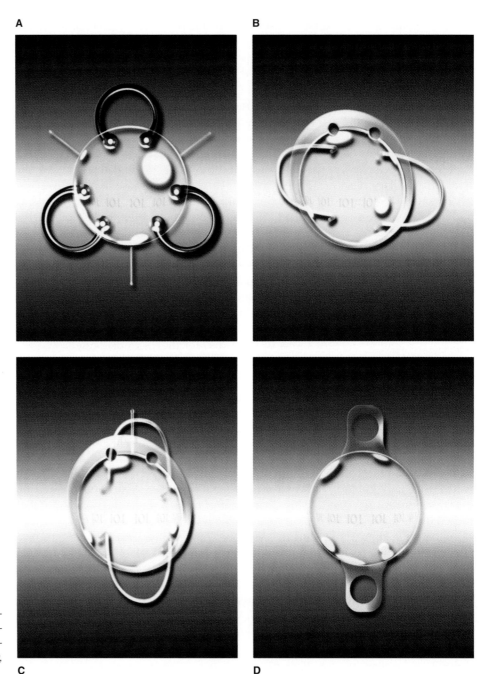

FIGURE 1.13. The further evolution of the intraocular lens. *A,* "Sputnik" lens. *B,* Worst iris medallion lens. *C,* Worst platina lens. *D,* Pearce bipod lens.

C   D

■ Overcoming Skepticism

Even as the design and quality of IOLs were improving, many ophthalmologists had strong memories of earlier failures and resisted using IOLs. Two important events helped to allay fears about and build confidence in IOLs. First, 1968 saw the creation of the American Intra-Ocular Implant Society, later called the American Society of Cataract and Refractive Surgery. As the largest organization devoted to cataract and lens implant surgery, this society provided a forum for information exchange, including a hotline for alerting ophthalmologists to quality control issues.[4]

Second, community ophthalmologists in Miami, Florida, declared a moratorium on lens implantations from 1969 to 1971 while they studied the results of the 243 operations performed before that time. The results of the study were favorable enough to permit resumption of IOL use. A registry of all patients undergoing lens implantation was also begun, and the Miami surgeons continued to review the results in hundreds of patients who had received lens implants. The data reassured American ophthalmologists of the benefits of IOLs.[4] Finally, in 1973, intravitreous antibiotics were introduced as a successful treatment for the dreaded complication of postoperative bacterial endophthalmitis.[45] From the early 1970s, the practice of ECCE with phacoemulsification and PCIOL implantation grew more and more popular.

▪ Posterior Chamber Intraocular Lenses in the 1970s

The 1970s saw the evolution of ECCE, the reappearance of PCIOLs, numerous modifications to ACIOLs, and major improvements in surgical techniques and IOL material and design. Binkhorst had recognized the benefits of ECCE since 1963. His iridocapsular IOL had proved very successful because the frequency and severity of CME, dislocation, and corneal decompensation was significantly lower with the capsular-fixated IOLs.[30] According to Shearing, the evolution of ECCE surgery was marked by four milestones: (1) microscopic surgical techniques, (2) phacoemulsification, (3) iridocapsular fixation, and (4) flexible PCIOLs.[38]

The introduction of phacoemulsification by Kelman in 1967 set the stage for a return to the PCIOL. The leader in the PCIOL movement was John Pearce, of Birmingham. In 1975, Pearce removed the posterior loops of an iris clip Binkhorst IOL, placed it in the posterior chamber, and sutured the superior anterior loop to the iris.[46,47] Shortly thereafter, he designed PCIOLs with several bipod (Fig. 1.13D) and tripod (Fig. 1.14A) variations. His tripod PCIOL was a rigid IOL with two inferior feet in the bag and a superior foot sutured to the iris.[24,46] It was similar to Ridley's Mark II ACIOL but modified in size and of better manufacture. In a later modification of this IOL, Pearce extended the superior haptic by 1.5 mm so that the lens could be fixated in the ciliary sulcus without an iris suture (Fig. 1.14B).[48,49] Pearce's lenses were successful and helped provide the impetus for a return to the posterior chamber as the preferred IOL implantation site.

At about the same time, iris-supported PCIOLs of the Boberg-Ans and Little-Arnot styles were introduced (Fig. 1.14C). Harris was the first American surgeon to consistently champion PCIOLs. He designed his own unique PCIOL (Fig. 1.14D).

The initial results suggested that the ideal location for the fixation of IOLs was the posterior chamber. In the posterior chamber, the optic was placed far from the anterior chamber angle and cornea and much closer to the nodal point of the original lens of the eye. This posi-

tion allowed better image resolution and size. The glare of the IOL was reduced as well. In addition, there was a decrease in pseudophakodonesis, which had been a problem with the pupil-supported IOLs.[24,34,44,46]

In March 1977, Shearing in Las Vegas began using compressible, nonsutured IOLs that stretched out completely to the ciliary sulcus.[34] His IOL was a plano-convex lenticular disc, 5–6 mm in diameter and 13 mm in length (Fig. 1.15A). The lens had two incomplete (J-shaped) haptic loops of 4–0 polypropylene suture extending from the disc. Shearing's lens resembled the Barraquer ACIOL made in the 1950s. However, the loops were made of a different material and were treated to keep their original shape and to spring back to that shape after being compressed.[44]

A primary concern with Shearing's IOL was the possibility of tissue damage from loop–ciliary body contact. Initially Shearing intended to place his IOL entirely in the capsular bag, but he soon realized that it was very hard to know whether the haptics were both in the bag or both in the sulcus, or whether one was in the bag and the other in the sulcus. In 1978, this type of IOL held a 4% market share. By 1983, 75% of cataract surgeries were ECCE in nature and 70% involved the use of a PCIOL.[44]

In 1977, a syndrome characterized by uveitis, glaucoma, and hyphema was recognized and described by Thomas Ellingson. Poor-quality anterior chamber lenses with rough edges were often the culprit, and the condition resolved on removal of the offending IOL. This complication accelerated research and interest in PCIOLs. Many innovative surgeons developed modifications to improve the open-loop PCIOLs. The first and most significant modification of Shearing's IOL was to angle the loops forward. This single alteration provided three benefits: it reduced the incidence of iris contact, avoided the complication of pupil capture, and allowed the optic to be closer to the nodal point of the eye. This modification was suggested by Mazzoco and introduced by Kratz. Simcoe of Tulsa introduced a C-loop PCIOL shortly after Shearing's J-loop design appeared (Fig. 1.15B). The C-loop IOLs were designed for uniform compressibility and capsule tension.[50] In 1975, Simcoe implanted an unsutured, open-end, compressible-loop PCIOL made by modifying the loops of the four-loop Binkhorst iris clip IOL. These prototype C-loop PCIOLs were placed either in the capsular bag or in the ciliary sulcus. Simcoe believed that when C-loops were placed in the capsular bag, they spread the bag uniformly and with fewer wrinkles.[50]

Sinskey of Santa Monica and Kratz of Newport Beach introduced various modified J-loop designs (Fig. 1.15C).[38] Sheets of Odessa and Anis of Lincoln introduced early closed-loop PCIOLs.[46] Arnott of London

A   B

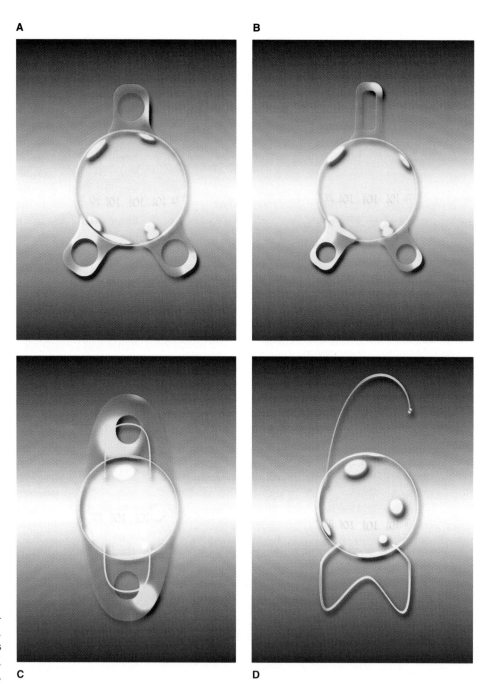

FIGURE 1.14. The further evolution of the intraocular lens. *A,* Pearce tripod lens. *B,* Pearce's modification of his tripod lens. *C,* Boberg-Ans lens. *D,* Harris lens.

C   D

and Jaffe of Miami were early advocates of one-piece all-PMMA PCIOLs.[14,38] Lindstrom of Minneapolis introduced a modified J-loop IOL with haptics made from PMMA (Fig. 1.15D).[38]

In the 1970s, angle-supported ACIOLs were very popular, and many surgeons used this mode of fixation in designs of their own. Azar and Tennant modified the Mark VIII IOL. Azar designed both rigid and flexible tripod, plano-convex IOLs that were narrower than the Mark VIII (Fig. 1.16B). Tennant's final modification was the Tennant anchor IOL, which had broad foot-

plates to reduce globe tenderness, iris tucking, and lens rotation—three complications seen with the previous models (Fig. 1.16C).[34,44]

Although ECCE was gaining favor, surgeons more familiar with ICCE worked with closed-loop ACIOLs with more flexible properties.[30] In 1978 the Lieske lens was created (Fig. 1.16D). This lens, a modification of the Danheim IOL, had less tucking than its predecessor. In addition, it required only one iridectomy, which was easily performed in the center of the lens loop. Unfortunately, it was difficult to find the proper size lens,

A   B

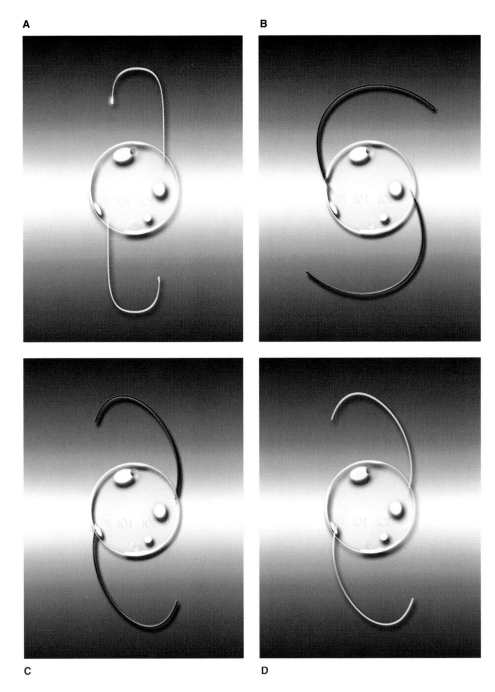

C   D

FIGURE 1.15. The further evolution of the intraocular lens. *A,* Shearing lens. *B,* Simcoe lens. *C,* Sinskey lens. *D,* Lindstrom lens.

since no one lens seemed to fit perfectly.[34] It is no surprise, then, that this lens was associated with many complications, including CME, secondary glaucoma, uveitis, hyphema, and corneal decompensation. In the 1980s, pseudophakic bullous keratopathy became the number one indication for keratoplasty. To make matters worse, the IOL's round, small, closed loops became "cocooned" in the trabecular meshwork and were difficult to remove. A 360-degree fibrous encapsulation formed around the small-diameter loops. They were eventually removed from the market in the United States after a Food and Drug Administration (FDA) investigation in 1987.[38,51]

Kelman introduced his one-piece, PMMA, open-loop ACIOL. Kelman's lenses had flexible three-point (Figs. 1.17A and B) or four-point fixation (Figs. 1.17C and D). These lenses had two opposing right-angled arms emanating from a central optic. The arms were flexible over only a narrow range, with flexion occurring at the "knees" of the right-angled arms.[34] The Kelman lenses remain the ACIOLs of choice today. They do not have the complications associated with

A   B

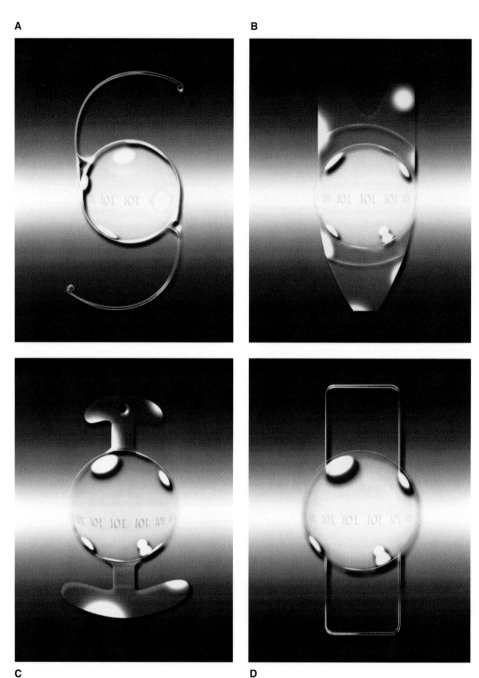

FIGURE 1.16. The further evolution of the intraocular lens. *A,* Graether lens. *B,* Azar lens. *C,* Tenant anchor lens. *D,* Lieske lens.

C   D

previous ACIOL designs. The flexible open-loop designs (J-loop, modified J-loop, C-loop, and modified C-loop) are still in use today throughout the world.[38]

■ Modern Posterior Chamber and Foldable Intraocular Lenses

Since the early 1980s, new IOLs have been designed for capsular bag fixation. In 1981, Graether designed a one-piece, all-PMMA IOL of 12 mm total length for capsular bag fixation. However, this IOL was not widely implanted.[52] With the advent of phacoemulsification performed through a small incision, there was increasing interest in soft, foldable lenses, which require a much smaller incision than the PMMA lenses require. By the mid-1980s, Davison and Mambless had become early advocates of smaller-sized PCIOLs. They used three-piece polypropylene loop PCIOLs 12–12.5 mm in length.[52]

The idea of using soft materials for IOL manufacture was conceived in the late 1950s by Dreifus,

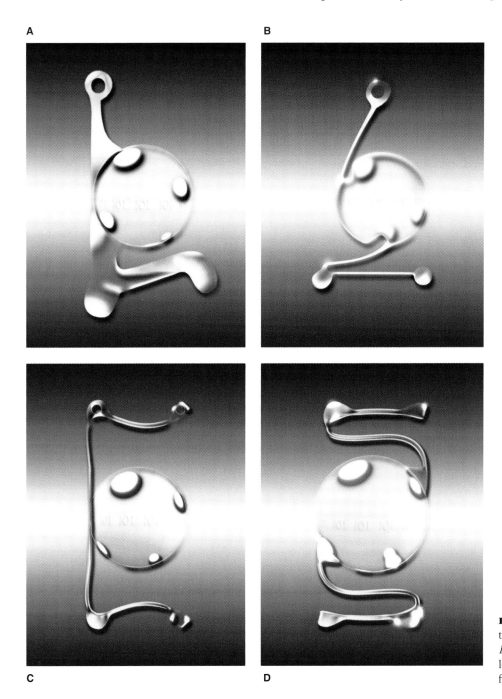

FIGURE 1.17. The further evolution of the intraocular lens. *A* and *B,* Kelman three-point fixation lens. *C* and *D,* Kelman four-point fixation lens.

Wichterle, and Lim.[14,53] They performed the first animal experiments in 1960 by implanting hydrogel ACIOLs in rabbits. In 1965, Epstein began to consider the possibility of implanting soft lenses. Silicone was an attractive material, but none of the silicone manufacturers he approached expressed interest in his concept.[36] Nearly 10 years later he performed experiments in monkeys and noticed that polyhydroxyethyl methacrylate (poly-HEMA) was better tolerated than PMMA. His clinical investigations of poly-HEMA started in 1976, and the material found its way into the "hydrogel" IOLs.[36]

In the early 1980s, a design in widespread clinical use was the plate lens design of Mazzoco, known as the "Mazzoco taco" (Fig. 1.18). This lens earned its nickname from its appearance when folded in the longitudinal dimension. In 1984, Shearing wrote, "Now there is excitement about the possibility of a soft silicone optic material advanced by Mazzoco because of the possibility of lens insertion through a small phaco-emulsification wound."[47]

Today, the most popular materials for foldable lenses include silicone (Fig. 1.19), acrylic (Fig. 1.20), and hydrogel. Some claim that the wave of the future

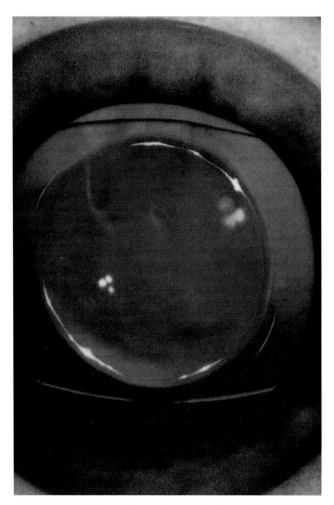

FIGURE 1.18. Plate silicone intraocular lens. *(From Steinert RF, ed. Cataract Surgery: Technique, Complications, and Management. Philadelphia: WB Saunders; 1995, with permission.)*

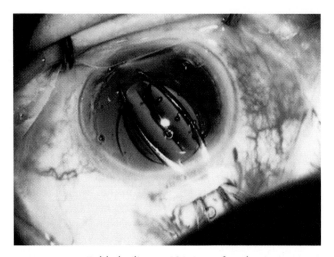

FIGURE 1.19. Folded silicone IOL just after the insertion in the eye. *(From Steinert RF, ed. Cataract Surgery: Technique, Complications, and Management. Philadelphia: WB Saunders; 1995, with permission.)*

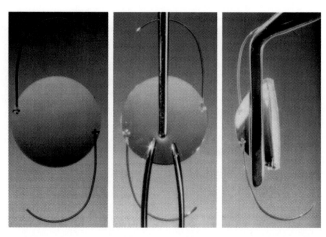

FIGURE 1.20. The Acrysof IOL unfolded (*left*), gripped by the special introducing folding forceps (*middle*), and folded in the special introducing folding forceps (*right*). *(From Pearce JL. Intraocular lenses.* Curr Opin Ophthalmol. *1992;3:34, with permission.)*

is injectable lenses: lenses formed by injecting a liquid polymer gel directly into the capsular bag after a small-incision ECCE. Direct light exposure polymerizes the gel inside the capsular bag. With this gel, the diopteric power can be adjusted by varying the quantity of gel that is injected into the capsular bag. In vitro and in vivo animal studies have yielded promising results.[53,54] Of course, injectable lenses can only be used for primary IOLs implantation directly following an ECCE, and only when the capsular bag remains intact.

■ Multifocal Intraocular Lenses

The loss of accommodation after cataract surgery can be quite significant. The desire to correct IOL-induced presbyopia has driven the development of bifocal and multifocal IOLs.[55] The goal of all multifocal IOLs is to provide two or more focal points. The multifocal IOLs are designed based on the principle of simultaneous vision, in contrast to the well-known multifocal contact lenses, which are based on the principle of alternating vision. Depending on the eye's gaze, one image is in focus at the retina and the second image is highly defocused. Distant objects are placed in focus by the distance power of the lens and defocused by the near power. Near objects are focused by the near power of the lens and defocused by the distance power. This splitting produces a final image of reduced contrast. Thus, a loss of contrast sensitivity is associated with these lenses.

There are a variety of multifocal IOLs. The IOLAB IOL (Nuvue) is a two-zone lens that has a 1.5–2 mm diameter near zone in the center of a 5.5 mm optic.

The peripheral zone is for distance correction and is lower in power by 4 diopters. The Storz (True Vista), Alcon, and Pharmacia (BI-89) models contain central and peripheral zones for distance vision and midperipheral zones for near vision. The Alcon design places the bifocal surface posteriorly.

Another variant of the multifocal IOL uses a combination of one posterior and multiple anterior spheric refractive surfaces for distance, intermediate, and near correction (Array, Allergan Medical Optics [AMO]). This was the first multifocal IOL approved by the FDA for commercial distribution in the United States.[56] The front surface of the AMO Array lens has five zones, each of which progressively adds from 0 to 3.5 diopters to the overall lens power (Fig. 1.21). In a large study, this zonal-progressive multifocal IOL provided a high level of uncorrected and corrected distance vision, improved uncorrected and distance-corrected near vision, reduced spectacle dependency, and was associated with a high level of patient satisfaction. There was, however, some loss of low-contrast visual acuity and increased reports of halos and glare.[56]

Before implanting a multifocal IOL, surgeons should consider patient selection criteria. For example, a patient with a monofocal IOL in the other eye may not tolerate the multifocal lens as well. Patients should also be informed that they may still need glasses for either distance or near correction. In addition, the possibility of glare and decreased contrast sensitivity should be discussed.[13,55]

■ Secondary Intraocular Lenses

As detailed in the chapters on secondary IOL implantation (see Part III), there are four main options for secondary IOLs: ACIOLs, iris-fixated IOLs, standard PCIOLs and sutured PCIOLs. The decision regarding the type of IOL for secondary implantation depends largely on the presence or absence of the capsular support. With capsular support, standard PCIOL placement in either the ciliary sulcus or the capsular bag is the procedure of choice. However, reopening the capsular bag can pose a significant obstacle to surgery. If the bag cannot be reopened, ciliary sulcus fixation is an alternative. This requires at least peripheral capsular and intact zonular support. If there is no capsular support, the surgeon can use flexible open-loop ACIOLs, transcleral-sutured PCIOLs, or iris-sutured PCIOLs. If the iris and the posterior capsule are both absent or insufficient, the transcleral-sutured PCIOL is the only option.

Parry implanted the first suture-fixated IOL in 1954. He anchored the Ridley IOL by means of a tantalum thread with the ends left loose under the conjunctiva. In the mid-1970s, Worst pioneered use of the iris-fixated IOL. McCannel in 1976 reported on the use of iris-fixated sutures to stabilize dislocated IOLs. Since then many techniques that use sutures to secure PCIOLs to the iris or sclera have been described. Some surgeons describe both two-point and four-point iris fixation for PCIOLs. Scleral-sutured IOLs can be sutured from the inside out (ab interno), which is quick, and easier with penetrating keratoplasty, or from the outside in (ab externo), also known as the Lewis technique.[13,57]

Other techniques for secondary IOL implantation include a combination of scleral and iris sutures. There are some key points to remember during suturing of a secondary PCIOL: extensive anterior vitrectomy is necessary before the IOL placement, viscoelastics should be used to push the vitreous posteriorly, and the haptics should reside in the sulcus. Some surgeons recommend scleral flaps so that the polypropylene (prolene) suture knot is buried; this avoids exposed suture ends and inadvertent cutting of the fixation sutures. It also prevents erosion of the knot through the conjunctiva. The current scleral-sutured PCIOLs have eyelets on the haptics to help suture fixation and 7.00 mm diameter optics to avoid decentration.

Visual results after secondary IOL placement with modern ACIOLs, scleral-sutured PCIOLs, or iris-sutured PCIOLs are similar. However, there is an increased risk

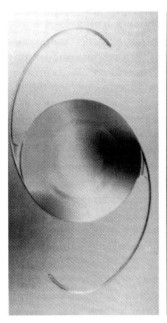
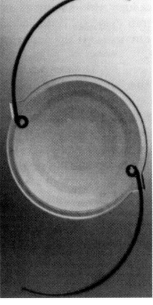

FIGURE 1.21. Multizone, multifocal lens of silicone that can be folded for placement through a small phacoemulsification incision (*left*). The single-piece, PMMA multizone AMO Array lens (*right*). *(From Pearce JL. Intraocular lenses. Curr Opin Ophthalmol. 1992;3:35, with permission.)*

of complications with scleral-sutured PCIOLs. These complications include persistent CME, endothelial cell loss, retinal detachment, hemorrhagic choroidal detachment, and late lens dislocation. Until more data are available, some authors recommend limiting the use of sutured PCIOLs to situations in which an anterior chamber lens cannot be implanted, such as eyes with extensive peripheral anterior synechiae and insufficiency of iris tissue.[13,57]

■ History and Classification of Phakic Intraocular Lenses

Since the end of the 19th century, several techniques have been developed to correct myopia and try to eliminate the need for contact lenses or eyeglasses. In 1890, Fukala extracted the entire transparent crystalline lens in patients with high myopia. This practice was criticized by many ophthalmologists because of the high complication rate.[58–60]

In 1953, Strampelli introduced the concept of phakic IOLs when he began to implant concave lenses in front of the crystalline lens to correct myopia. The radius of curvature of the nonoptical portion was 13 mm, which ensured lens separation from the iris and the corneal endothelium. However, the lens was thick and rigid and frequently caused hyphema, iritis, endothelial cell damage, and glaucoma.[59–61]

Danheim and Barraquer modified the design of Strampelli's lenses. In 1959, Barraquer reported that 239 phakic IOL implantations corrected anisometropia in monocular cases of high myopia or hypermetropia and improved visual conditions in binocular cases.[26,59–62] Unfortunately, almost 50% of the lenses had to be removed because of complications attributed to poor manufacturing quality.[59,60]

In the mid-1980s, Dvali revived the concept of minus-power IOL implantation in phakic myopes.[59,63] At the same time, Fechner, Praeger, Momose, Baikoff, and Fyodorov were developing new models of lens fixation, including (1) the anterior chamber biconcave or convex-concave iris claw lenses with iris fixation, (2) the Praeger-Momose glass-optic anterior chamber lens with angle fixation, (3) the Baikoff-type lens with angle fixation, and (4) the Fyodorov phakic posterior chamber lens with anterior crystalline lens support.[59] In 1986, Worst and Fechner developed their own phakic lens, which was based on Worst's 1977 iris-fixated IOL.[60] This phakic lens was an anterior chamber, biconcave, one-piece PMMA "iris claw" lens (Fig. 1.22).[59,61] The haptic in the Worst iris claw lens consisted of two flexible pincerlike arms (claws) contigu-

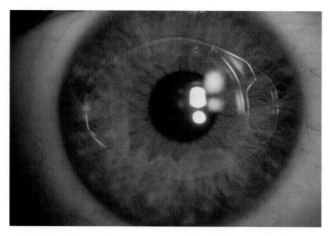

FIGURE 1.22. Iris claw phakic IOL. *(From Fechner PU. Die Zrisklaven tinge. Klin Monatsbl Augenheilkd.* 1987;191:27, *with permission.)*

ous to the optic. Fixation of the lens was achieved when a fold of the midperiphery of the iris was pulled through the slit in each of the two claws.[64] A later phakic model, developed in 1991, had a convex-concave profile (convex toward the endothelial surface and concave toward the anterior surface of the crystalline lens). This model is currently under investigation for the correction of high myopia.[64,65]

In May 1987, Momose in Japan implanted the Praeger-Momose phakic lens. It had a glass optical part with a high index of refraction (1.62). The haptics were made of polyamide, and the wetting angle was low. The iridocorneal angle was used for support.[59]

In August 1988, during the 6th Congress of the European Intraocular Implant-Lens Council in Copenhagen, Baikoff of France presented his phakic lens.[61] This lens was derived from Kelman's multiflex IOL design.[58,59] The lens had a biconcave optic that was 4.5 mm in diameter. The haptics permitted only localized contact with the anterior chamber angle, and the surface was large enough to avoid causing peripheral anterior synechiae. The anterior vaulting of this model was 25 degrees.[58,59] To limit the rate of complications, Baikoff modified his lens and called the new model the ZB5M. The angulation in this model was 20 degrees. The optic edge was thinned, thereby gaining 0.6 mm in the lens-cornea spacing. The power was also limited to −18.00 diopters.[59]

Since 1987, the Moscow Research Institute of Eye Microsurgery has reported favorably on PCIOL implantation in phakic eyes to correct high myopia. Moscow's implanted IOLs were initially the collar-button type, with the optic located in the anterior chamber and the haptics in the posterior chamber, just behind the iris.

Optic and haptics were connected by a bridge through the pupil.[62,66] As the study of biomaterials developed, Fyodorov designed a lens that was centered on the pupil and could be placed in the posterior chamber, between the iris diaphragm and the crystalline lens, thus retaining the accommodation of the latter. This lens is known as the implantable contact lens (ICL).[65]

The ICL, manufactured by Staar Surgical AG, is referred to as a collamer because it is made of a proprietary hydrophilic collagen-HEMA copolymer. The lens can be folded and inserted through a sutureless corneal incision smaller than 3.00 mm. Its thickness is 60 μm and its optical zone varies between 4.8 and 5.8 mm, depending on the power required. The width of the lens is 6.0 mm, and the length is adjusted to each eye by relating lens length to the horizontal corneal diameter. In hyperopic eyes, the estimated corneal diameter is reduced by 0.5 mm. In myopic eyes, the estimated diameter is increased by 0.5 mm.[67–69]

The 6-month outcome of the first ten ICLs implanted for myopia in the United States showed excellent results. However, time and more cases will determine whether ICL implantation is a feasible refractive treatment option. Kelman has also been collaborating with Chiron to develop foldable phakic IOLs for use in the anterior and posterior chambers in patients with high myopia.[70]

Some of the potential benefits of phakic IOL implantation include good refractive predictability and stability. Risks associated with phakic anterior chamber implants include damage to the corneal endothelium, which might not become evident until years after the operation. For this reason, if the endothelial density clearly starts to decrease, removal of the implant is recommended.[61,63]

Contraindications to the use of phakic posterior chamber implants include glaucoma and pigment dispersion syndrome, pseudoexfoliation syndrome, diabetic eye disease, a history of unhealthy corneal endothelium, dystrophies that cause an abnormal shape of the cornea (i.e., keratoconus), and a history of iritis.[66] Only time and further studies will determine whether the allure of phakic IOL implantation is greater than that of other refractive procedures, such as LASIK.

■ References

1. International Agency for the Prevention of Blindness. *World Blindness and Its Prevention*. New York: Oxford University Press; 1980.
2. Greene DW. Smith's cataract operation. *Trans Am Acad Ophthalmol Otolaryngol*. 1910;15:98–106.
3. Apple DJ, Mamalis N, Olson RJ, et al. *Intraocular Lenses: Evolution, Designs, Complications, and Pathology*. Baltimore, MD: Williams & Wilkins; 1989.
4. Jaffe NS. History of cataract surgery. *Ophthalmology*. 1996;103(8):S5–S16.
5. Daviel J. Sur une nouvelle methode de guerir la cataracte par l'extraction du crystallin. *Mem Acad R Chir*. 1753; 2:337–352.
6. Latocha CE. A bicenquinquagenary worth noting: Daviel's introduction of the modern cataract operation. *Arch Ophthalmol*. 1997;15:526–528.
7. Jaffe NS, Jaffe MS, Jaffe GF. *Cataract Surgery and Its Complications*. 5th ed. Philadelphia: CV Mosby; 1990.
8. Alpar JJ, Fechner PU. *Fechner's Intraocular Lenses*. New York: Thieme; 1985.
9. Choyce DP. Recollections of the early days of intraocular lens implantation. *J Cataract Refract Surg*. 1990;16:505–508.
10. Clayman HM. *The Surgeon's Guide to Intraocular Lens Implantation*. Thorofare, NJ: Slack; 1985.
11. Ridley H. Intra-ocular acrylic lenses. *Trans Ophthalmol Soc UK*. 1951;71:617–621.
12. Vail D. Intraocular acrylic lenses: recent development in surgery of cataract. In: *The 1952 Year Book of the Eye, Ear, Nose and Throat (October 1951–September 1952)*. Chicago: Year Book Medical Publishers; 1952:85–86.
13. Jaffe NS, Jaffe MS, Jaffe GF. *Cataract Surgery and Its Complications*. 6th ed. St. Louis, MO: CV Mosby; 1997:147–156, 189–197.
14. Jaffe NS. Thirty years of intraocular lens implantation: the way it was and the way it is. [Guest Editorial]. *J Cataract Refract Surg*. 1999;25:455–459.
15. Ridley H. Intra-ocular acrylic lenses: a recent development in the surgery of cataract. *Br J Ophthalmol*. 1952; 36:113–122.
16. Apple DJ, Sims J. Harold Ridley and the invention of the intraocular lens. *Surv Ophthalmol*. 1996;40:279–292.
17. Spalton DJ. Harold Ridley's first patient [letter]. *J Cataract Refract Surg*. 1999;25:156.
18. Choyce P. Harold Ridley's first patient [letter]. *J Cataract Refract Surg*. 1999;25:731.
19. Apple DJ. Harold Ridley, MA, MD, FRCS: A golden anniversary celebration and a golden age. *Arch Ophthalmol*. 1999;117:827–828.
20. Nordlohne ME. The intraocular implant lens development and results: with special reference to the Binkhorst lens. *Doc Ophthalmol*. 1974;2(38):14–37.
21. Rosen E. History in the making: father of the intraocular lens. *J Cataract Refract Surg*. 1997;23:4–5.
22. Anis AY. Principles and evolution of intraocular lens implantation. *Int Ophthalmol Clin*. 1982;22(2):1–9.
23. Letocha CE, Pavlin CJ. Follow-up of 3 patients with Ridley intraocular lens implantation. *J Cataract Refract Surg*. 1999;25:587–591.
24. Shearing SP. The history of ciliary fixated intraocular lenses. *Contact Intraocular Lens Med J*. 1980;6:295–301.
25. Ridley H. Intra-ocular acrylic lenses: 10 years' development. *Br J Ophthalmol*. 1960;44:705–712.

26. Barraquer J. The use of plastic lenses in the anterior chamber: Indications—technique—personal results. *Trans Ophthalmol Soc UK*. 1956;76:537–552.

27. Lindstrom RL. The polymethylmethacrylate (PMMA) intraocular lenses. In: Steinert RF, ed. *Cataract Surgery: Technique, Complications, and Management*. Philadelphia: WB Saunders; 1995.

28. Bietti GB. The present state of the use of plastics in eye surgery. *Acta Ophthalmol*. 1955;33(suppl 43):356–364.

29. King H Jr, Skeehan RA. Acrylic lenses in the anterior chamber. *Arch Ophthalmol*. 1957;58:392–393.

30. Strampelli B. Anterior chamber lenses: present technique. *Arch Ophthalmol*. 1961;66:12.

31. Ridley H. An anterior chamber lenticular implant. *Br J Ophthalmol*. 1957;41:355–358.

32. History in the making: full life with the intraocular lens. *J Cataract Refract Surg*. 1997;23:812–813.

33. Choyce P. The evolution of the anterior chamber implant. *Ophthalmology*. 1979;86:197–206.

34. Shepard DD. Anterior chamber lens implantation today. *Int Ophthalmol Clin*. 1982;22(2):77–85.

35. Hirschman H. Advantages and disadvantages of the types of intraocular lenses available. *Trans Am Acad Ophthalmol Otolaryngol*. 1976;81:89–92.

36. History in the making: it began with a traumatic cataract. *J Cataract Refract Surg*. 1998;24:428–429.

37. Epstein E. Modifed Ridley lenses. *Br J Ophthalmol*. 1959;43:29–33.

38. Apple DJ, Rabb MF. *Ocular Pathology: Clinical Applications and Self Assessment*. 5th ed. St. Louis, MO: CV Mosby; 1998:141–161.

39. Apple DJ, Mamalis N, Loftfield K, et al. Complications of IOLs: a historical and histopathological review. *Surv Ophthalmol*. 1984;29:1–54.

40. Binkhorst CD. Iris-supported artificial pseudophakia: a new development in intra-ocular artificial lens surgery (iris clip lens). *Trans Ophthalmol Soc UK*. 1959;74:569–584.

41. Binkhorst CD. Iris-clip and irido-capsular lens implants (pseudophakoia): personal techniques of pseudophakia. *Br J Ophthalmol*. 1967;51:767–770.

42. Hurite FG, Lempert SL. Iridocapsular intraocular lenses and extracapsular cataract surgery. *Int Ophthalmol Clin*. 1982;22(2):103–105.

43. Binkhorst CD. The iridocapsular (two loop) lens and the iris-clip (four loop) lens in pseudophakia. *Trans Am Acad Ophthalmol Otolaryngol*. 1973;77:589–590.

44. Perrit RA. Intraocular lens implantation from Ridley to the present: my 25 years' experience. *Int Ophthalmol Clin*. 1979;19(3):11–25.

45. Peyman GA, Vastine DW, Crouch ER, et al. Clinical use of intravitreal antibiotics to treat bacterial endophthalmitis. *Trans Am Acad Ophthalmol Otolaryngol*. 1974;78:862–875.

46. Shearing SP. Evolution of the posterior chamber intraocular lens. *Am Intraocular Implant Soc J*. 1984;10:343–346.

47. Shearing SP. Posterior chamber lens implantation. *Int Ophthalmol Clin*. 1982;22(2):135–137.

48. Pearce JL. New lightweight sutured posterior chamber lens implant. *Trans Ophthalmol Soc UK*. 1976;96:6–10.

49. Pearce JL. Pearce-style posterior chamber lenses. *Am Intraocular Implant Soc J*. 1980;6:33–36.

50. Simcoe WC. Simcoe posterior chamber lens: theory, techniques and results. *Am Intraocular Implant Soc J*. 1981;7:154–157.

51. Isaacs RT, Apple DJ. Lens replacement: evolution and pathology of intraocular lens implantation. In: Yannof M, Dunker JS, eds. *Ophthalmology*. St. Louis, MO: CV Mosby; 1999:13.1–13.8.

52. Auffarth GU, Wesendahl TA, Assia EI, et al. Pathophysiology of modern capsular surgery. In: Steinert RF, ed. *Cataract Surgery: Technique, Complications, and Management*. Philadelphia: WB Saunders; 1995:318–321.

53. Lindstrom RL. Foldable intraocular lenses. In: Steinert RF, ed. *Cataract Surgery: Technique, Complications, and Management*. Philadelphia: WB Saunders; 1995:279.

54. Hettlich HJ, Lucke K, Asiyo-Vogel MN, et al. Lens refilling and endocapsular polymerization of an injectable intraocular lens: in vitro and in vivo study of potential risks and benefits. *J Cataract Refract Surg*. 1994;20:124–128.

55. Lindstrom RL. Multifocal Intraocular Lenses. In: Steinert RF, ed. *Cataract Surgery: Technique, Complications, and Management*. Philadelphia: WB Saunders; 1995:24.

56. Steinert RF, Aker BL, Trentacost DJ, et al. A prospective comparative study of the AMO Array zonal-progressive multifocal silicone intraocular lens and a monofocal intraocular lens. *Ophthalmology*. 1999;106:1243–1255.

57. Arkin MS, Steinert RF. Secondary intraocular lenses. In: Steinert RF, ed. *Cataract Surgery: Technique, Complications, and Management*. Philadelphia: WB Saunders; 1995:302–313.

58. Baikoff G, Jolly P. Comparison of minus power anterior chamber intraocular lenses and myopic epiceratoplasty in phakic eyes. *Refract Corneal Surg*. 1990;6:252–260.

59. Baikoff G, Samaha A. Phakic intraocular lenses. In: Azar D, ed. *Refractive Surgery*. Stamford, CT: Appleton & Lange; 1997:545–559.

60. Menezo JL, Cisneros A, Hueso JR, et al. Long-term results of surgical treatment of high myopia with Worst-Fechner intraocular lenses. *J Cataract Refract Surg*. 1995;21:93.

61. Fechner PU, Strobel J, Wichmann W. Correction of myopia by implantation of a concave Worst-iris claw lens into phakic eyes. *Refract Corneal Surg*. 1991;7:286–298.

62. Waring GO III. Phakic intraocular lenses for the correction of myopia: where do we go from here? *Refract Corneal Surg*. 1991;7:275–276.

63. Fechner PU, Wichmann W. Correction of myopia by implantation of minus optic (Worst iris claw) lenses into the anterior chamber of phakic eyes. *Eur J Implant Refract Surg*. 1993;5:55–59.

64. Menezo JL, Cisneros AL, Rodriguez-Salvador V. Endothelial study of iris-claw phakic lens: four year follow up. *J Cataract Refract Surg*. 1998;24:1040.

65. Landesz M, Worst JGF, Van Rij G, et al. Opaque iris claw lens in a phakic eye to correct acquired diplopia. *J Cataract Refract Surg*. 1997;23:137–138.

66. Fechner PU, Haigis W, Wichmann W. Posterior chamber myopia lenses in phakic eyes. *J Cataract Refract Surg.* 1996;22:178–181.

67. Rosen E, Gore C. Staar collamer posterior chamber phakic intraocular lens to correct myopia and hyperopia. *J Cataract Refract Surg.* 1998;24:596–606.

68. Sanders DR, Brown DC, Martin RG, et al. Implantable contact lens for moderate to high myopia: Phase 1 FDA clinical study with 6 month follow-up. *J Cataract Refract Surg.* 1998;24:607–611.

69. Assetto V, Benedetti S, Pesando P. Collamer intraocular contact lens to correct high myopia. *J Cataract Refract Surg.* 1996;22:551–555.

70. History in the making: In tune with the father of phacoemulsification. *J Cataract Refract Surg.* 1997;23:1128–1129.

Chapter 2

Anatomic Considerations

Yichieh Shiuey and Dimitri T. Azar

■ Anterior Chamber

The anterior chamber is bounded anteriorly by the cornea and posteriorly by the iris. The average central anterior chamber depth in the normal adult emmetropic eye is approximately 3 mm and becomes most narrow at the midperipheral iris.[1] However, the depth of the anterior chamber varies. Patients who are aphakic or myopic tend to have deeper anterior chambers and those who are hyperopic tend to have shallower anterior chambers. The anterior chamber deepens to approximately 4.5 mm after cataract extraction.[1] The anterior chamber angle is delineated by the junction of the cornea and the iris and consists of four structures: Schwalbe's line, a trabecular meshwork, the scleral spur, and the anterior ciliary body.

The diameter of the anterior chamber angle is very important clinically for proper sizing of an angle-fixated anterior chamber intraocular lens (ACIOL). Lenses that are too large tend to erode into the ocular tissues. Lenses that are too small can move and chafe against the ciliary body, iris, trabecular meshwork, or corneal endothelium. A commonly used clinical rule is that the corneal diameter (white-to-white distance) plus 1 mm is approximately equal to the diameter of the anterior chamber angle. One study compared white-to-white plus 1 mm estimates with direct measurements of the diameter of the ring made by the scleral spur in 20 cadaver eyes.[2] The white-to-white plus 1 mm measurement underestimated the internal diameter of the scleral spur by an average of 0.26 mm, although in one case the estimated diameter was less than the measured diameter by 1.2 mm. The same report offered a comparison between white-to-white plus 1 mm estimates and dipstick measurements in 50 pa-

tients using a spatula with 0.5-mm gradations to measure the anterior chamber diameter. By this method the investigators also found that the white-to-white plus 1 mm measurement underestimated the anterior chamber diameter by an average of 0.40 mm. Based on these findings the authors advocated routine measurement of the anterior chamber diameter by the dipstick method prior to insertion of an angle-fixated lens.[2] Exact measurement of the anterior chamber angle diameter may be less crucial for the flexible open-loop lenses in common use today than for the older-style rigid and closed-loop angle-fixated lenses.[3]

Angle-Fixated Lenses

ACIOLs that are fixated in the angle are, by definition, touching the delicate angle structures. In the past it was frequently assumed that angle-fixated lenses rested on the scleral spur. It was presumed that there would be few adverse effects with the implant resting against this relatively nonreactive collagenous tissue. However, clinicopathologic studies have disproved this assumption. The loops of angle-fixated lenses usually rest in the angle recess posterior to the scleral spur.[4] In this location the loops or footplates of the anterior chamber lens touch the anterior ciliary body or the peripheral iris (Fig. 2.1). Direct contact with these delicate structures may cause irritation, with erosion of tissue and chronic inflammation. Glaucoma may result from direct contact of the loops or footplates with the trabecular meshwork, but it may also occur secondary to chronic inflammation and the formation of peripheral anterior synechiae (Fig. 2.2).

When the loops or footplates of the angle-fixated lens are misplaced anteriorly, the resulting direct

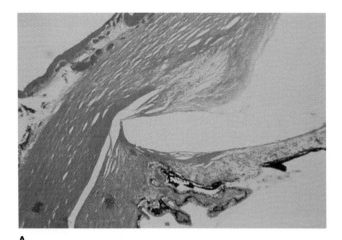

A

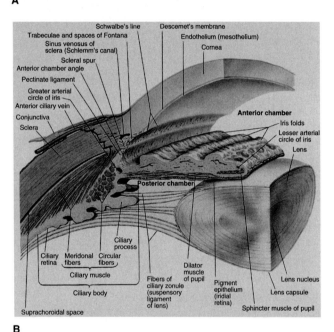

Schwalbe's line
Trabeculae and spaces of Fontana
Sinus venosus of
sclera (Schlemm's canal)
Scleral spur
Anterior chamber angle
Pectinate ligament
Greater arterial
circle of iris
Anterior ciliary vein
Conjunctiva
Sclera

Descemet's membrane
Endothelium (mesothelium)
Cornea

Anterior chamber

Iris folds
Lesser arterial
circle of iris
Lens

Posterior chamber

Ciliary
process
Ciliary   Meridonal   Circular
retina   fibers   fibers
Ciliary muscle
Ciliary body
Suprachoroidal space

Dilator
muscle
of pupil
Fibers of
ciliary zonule
(suspensory
ligament
of lens)
Pigment
epithelium
(iridial
retina)
Sphincter muscle of pupil

Lens nucleus
Lens capsule

B

FIGURE 2.1. *A,* Pathology specimen demonstrating iris tucking in a patient with a Choyce-style ACIOL. *B,* Corresponding diagram of the anterior and posterior chamber of a normal eye. For clarity only single plane of zonular fibers shown; actually fibers surround entire circumference of lens. *(A, Courtesy of Dr. N. Mamalis. B, Copyright © 1999. Icon Learning Systems. Reprinted from Icon Learning Systems, illustrated by Frank H. Netter, MD. All rights reserved.)*

contact with the peripheral corneal endothelium causes the death of these cells. Human corneal endothelial cells cannot divide; they can only enlarge and migrate to fill in the spaces left by the dead cells. As the central corneal endothelial cells spread and migrate to the periphery, the corneal endothelial cell count drops to a critically low level. At this point these cells are no longer able to adequately dehydrate the central stroma, and corneal edema and clouding result. Endothelial cell

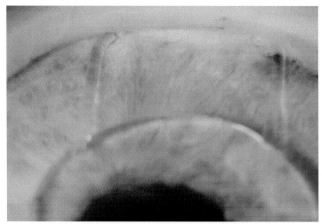

FIGURE 2.2. Pathology specimen demonstrating peripheral anterior synechiae (PAS) formation in a patient with a Leiske-style closed-loop ACIOL. *(Courtesy of Dr. N. Mamalis.)*

loss may also occur as a result of chronic anterior chamber inflammation due to the erosion of uveal tissues, even when there is no direct contact of the anterior chamber lens with the corneal endothelium.

Closed-loop design lenses, such as those of the Leiske style, have been noted to exert a cheese-cutter effect in the angle recess. The loops may erode deeply into the ciliary body, such that the location of the haptic may be indistinguishable from that of a ciliary sulcus-fixated posterior chamber lens.[4] Because the loops of these lenses become deeply embedded in the uveal tissue, the lenses may be very difficult to explant. Not infrequently the loops must be cut to remove the optic of the lens (Fig. 2.3). An attempt may be made to rotate the cut haptics out of their fibrotic cocoons.

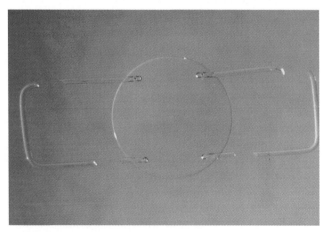

FIGURE 2.3. Explanted Leiske-style ACIOL. The haptics were cut and then rotated out of their cocoon of fibrosis. This was necessary to avoid excessive bleeding and inflammation. *(Courtesy of Dr. N. Mamalis.)*

However, sometimes it is simply not possible to remove the loops themselves without causing excessive bleeding. Closed-loop designs have been clearly associated with the development of pseudophakic bullous keratopathy (PBK) and many other complications.[4,5]

Kelman-style flexible open-loop ACIOLs were designed to minimize some of the complications associated with rigid and closed-loop anterior chamber lenses. The open loops increased the flexibility of the lens, so that it would not require as precise sizing as rigid anterior chamber lenses or closed-loop lenses. The footplates were also designed to rest against a smaller area of the anterior chamber angle to minimize damage to the angle structures (Fig. 2.4). The increased flexibility and smaller footplates of the Kelman-style lenses have been reported to decrease the likelihood of tenderness and ciliary body erosion. Despite these design improvements, in a study of 16 explanted Kelman flexible ACIOLs, Kincaid and colleagues showed that it is still possible to develop the complications of iris tuck, ciliary body erosion, tenderness, anterior uveitis, and corneal decompensation with these lenses.[3] However, the complication rate is clearly lower for open-loop than for closed-loop lenses with respect to corneal pathology, inflammation, cystoid macular edema, decentration, glaucoma, and hemorrhage.[6]

■ Iris

The iris acts as a dynamic diaphragm that controls the amount of light entering the eye by regulating the size of its aperture, the pupil. The diameter of the iris is approximately 12 mm and its circumference is about 37.5 mm. The iris thickness is greatest at the collarette (2 mm from the edge of the pupil), where it is 0.5 mm in anteroposterior dimension. The iris is thinnest at its root where it is attached to the anterior surface of the ciliary body. The average thickness of the iris is approximately 0.3 mm. The iris can be anatomically divided into anterior and posterior portions. The anterior portion consists of the iris stroma; the posterior portion consists of pigmented and nonpigmented epithelial layers.

The stroma is composed of vascularized connective tissue that contains collagen fibers, fibroblasts, melanocytes, and matrix. The two muscular layers of the iris, the sphincter pupillae and the dilator pupillae, the blood supply, and the nerves are all located within the stroma. The anterior surface of the stroma is bare of epithelium and has a velvet appearance. The stroma has a spokelike configuration that is produced by a radial configuration of blood vessels and connective tissue. Between the spokes lie oval crypts (crypts

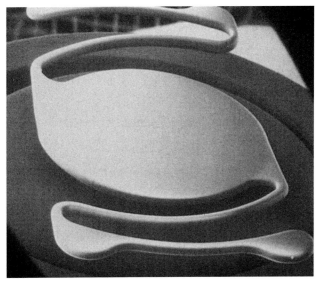

A

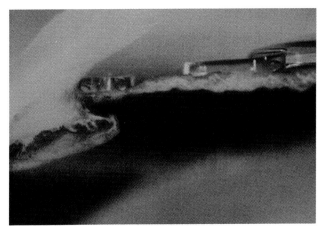

B

FIGURE 2.4. *A,* Scanning electron micrograph of a Kelman-style ACIOL. Note the small contact area of the haptics, the open-loop flexible design, and the smooth finish. *B,* Gross histopathologic appearance of a properly placed Kelman ACIOL showing the relationship of the haptic and optic to the iris and angle. *(A, Courtesy of Dr. N. Mamalis. B, From Apple BJ, Mamalis N, Olson RJ, et al. Intraocular Lenses: Evolution, Designs, Complications, and Pathology. Baltimore, MD: Williams & Wilkins; 1989, with permission.)*

of Fuchs). Near the edge of the pupil there is a ring of smooth muscle fibers about 1 mm wide, the sphincter pupillae. When the sphincter pupillae contracts, the pupil constricts. Peripheral to the sphincter pupillae is the dilator pupillae. The fibers of this muscle are oriented radially and extend to the most peripheral point of the iris root.[4] When the dilator fibers contract, the pupil dilates.

The arterial supply of the iris is derived from the major arterial circle of the ciliary body, which in turn is derived from the two long posterior ciliary arteries and the seven anterior ciliary arteries. Radial vessels branch from the major arterial circle through the anterior stroma and converge near the pupillary border. On reaching the collarette, these radial arteries form an incomplete minor arterial circle. The veins form a corresponding minor venous circle and radial venous system. However, the radial veins do not drain into a major venous circle. Instead, the radial veins converge and drain into the vortex system and the ciliary plexus. The endothelial lining of all the arteries and veins of the iris, including the capillaries, is nonfenestrated. An important feature of the iris vasculature is that there are no tight junctions between the endothelial cells. This is clinically significant, because when the iris becomes inflamed, the lack of tight junctions allows proteins and other large molecules to leak into the anterior chamber. This leakage is easily appreciated on slit lamp examination as flare.

Iris-Supported Lenses

The optic in many of the implant designs used between 1953 and 1982 was located in the anterior chamber and the lens was supported by the peripupillary iris (Fig. 2.5). Generally speaking, these lenses were "clipped" onto the iris immediately surrounding the pupil by various methods (Fig. 2.6). Although several of these lenses were initially well tolerated, there was an unacceptably high long-term complication rate, and these lenses were largely abandoned by the early 1980s.

Some of the long-term problems associated with these lenses could be predicted from knowing the anatomy and physiology of the iris. Because they were fixated on the highly mobile iris of the pupillary border, the pupil's natural movements in response to light and near vision would cause movement of the lens implant. This movement produced chafing of the iris with resulting inflammation or hemorrhage, or both. Frequently the effects of the chafing were exacerbated by the rough surfaces of these early lens implants.

A second anatomic consideration relevant to the pupillary clip lenses involves the iris vasculature. The iris tissue, which lacks tight junctions in its vasculature, responds to even minor irritation by releasing inflammatory mediators, proteins, and cells. The pupillary border and collarette, which is particularly rich in blood supply, is an especially sensitive location for the fixation of a lens implant. Inflammatory glaucoma is a common complication of pupillary clip lenses, and the full syndrome of uveitis-glaucoma-hyphema can be seen.[4]

One type of iris-supported ACIOL, the iris claw lens developed by Jan Worst, differed from other

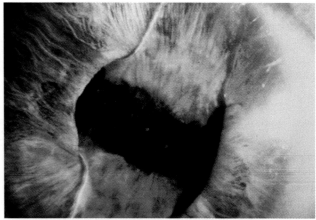

A

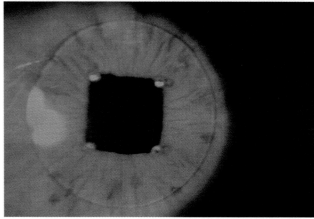

B

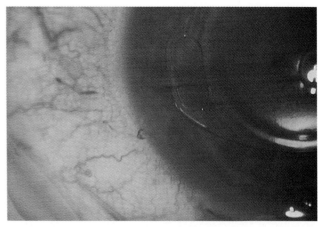

C

FIGURE 2.5. *A,* Copland-style iris-supported IOL. *B,* Iris clip lens supported by posterior haptics. *C,* Worst iris claw lens showing haptics tucking the peripheral iris. (*A, Courtesy of Dr. N. Mamalis. B, From Apple BJ, Mamalis N, Olson RJ, et al.* Intraocular Lenses: Evolution, Designs, Complications, and Pathology. *Baltimore, MD: Williams & Wilkins; 1989, with permission. C, Courtesy of Dr. Thanh Hoang-Xuan.)*

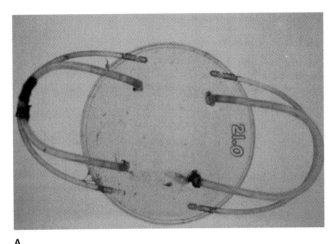

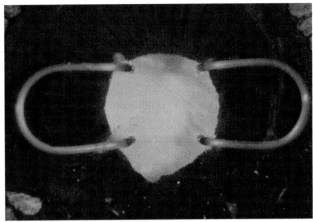

A   **B**

FIGURE 2.6. Explanted iris clip lenses. *A,* Four-loop Binkhorst lens. The iris was intentionally incarcerated between the anterior and posterior loops of the lens to provide fixation. *B,* Posterior view of iris clip lens. *(A, Courtesy of Dr. N. Mamalis. B, From Apple BJ, Mamalis N, Olson RJ, et al.* Intraocular Lenses: Evolution, Designs, Complications, and Pathology. *Baltimore, MD: Williams & Wilkins; 1989, with permission.)*

iris-supported designs in that the fixation point of the lens was not at the highly mobile pupillary border (Fig. 2.5C).[4] Instead, the lens was fixated near the peripheral iris, which is relatively immobile.[4] Worst believed that the peripheral fixation of his lens implant allowed it to be better tolerated than other iris-supported lenses. However, there is probably still some movement of the peripheral iris, since histologic studies show that the pupil dilator muscle extends all the way to the iris root. The Worst iris claw lens is now essentially the only iris-supported lens still implanted worldwide, although it is not generally available in the United States. Recently there has been renewed interest in this lens design for use in phakic IOL implantation for the correction of refractive errors (see Chapter 20).

Anatomic Considerations in Phakic ACIOL Implantation

The placement of an anterior chamber lens in a phakic eye for the treatment of high myopia was first performed in the 1950s by Strampeli[7] and Barraquer.[8] These procedures were largely unsuccessful because of problems common to anterior chamber lenses of that time, such as uveitis, glaucoma, and corneal decompensation. Phakic intraocular lens (IOL) implantation in the anterior chamber has all of the potential problems associated with aphakic anterior chamber lens implantation. In addition, certain anatomic considerations make phakic implantation more difficult than aphakic implantation.

The presence of a healthy, clear crystalline lens presents a number of problems to the implantation of an ACIOL. Many of the problems relate to the fact that the anterior chamber depth is substantially shallower in the phakic (3 mm) than in the aphakic (4.5 mm) situation. At surgery, this increases the difficulty of the procedure because in the relatively cramped space it is possible to inadvertently damage the healthy crystalline lens and produce a cataract, or to damage the corneal endothelium. The former complication is not an issue in aphakic implantation.

Another problem is that since the anterior chamber is shallower, there is less distance between the lens optic and the corneal endothelium. This may cause corneal decompensation if there is intermittent endothelial implant touch. The natural increase in the crystalline lens size throughout life may also produce further shallowing of the anterior chamber. It has been estimated that a −15.00 diopter Worst iris claw phakic IOL would have a clearance of approximately 2 mm between the optic and the corneal endothelium.[9] However, the distance between the endothelium and the lens may be decreased further in some situations such as eye rubbing. Implantation of an anterior chamber lens for the treatment of hyperopia would generally be more difficult than for myopia because the anterior chamber depth would be even shallower.

The loops and footplates of angle-fixated anterior chamber phakic IOLs may also need to be modified to account for the more convex configuration of the iris in the phakic eye as compared with the aphakic eye.[10]

Otherwise there may be a risk of chafing of the iris against the phakic IOL. The size of the lens may also be more crucial in phakic than in aphakic patients, because patients receiving phakic IOLs for refractive error surgery will typically be younger and more likely to be affected by long-term complications of incorrect sizing such as chronic inflammation and endothelial cell loss. The Worst iris claw style of lens (marketed as the Artisan lens in the United States) has a potential advantage in that it does not have to be sized because it is fixated not in the angle but on the peripheral iris. A disadvantage is that fewer surgeons are familiar with the enclavation method of fixation that is used for this lens.

Despite the various anatomic challenges to anterior chamber phakic IOL implantation for the treatment of refractive errors, some early studies show encouraging results with this new modality.[9,10]

■ Posterior Chamber

The posterior chamber is bounded anteriorly by the iris and posteriorly by the anterior hyaloid face of the vitreous. The circumference of the posterior chamber consists of the ciliary sulcus and the ciliary body. Within the posterior chamber sits the crystalline lens, which is attached to the ciliary body by zonules.

Lens Anatomy

Using a uveoscleral window technique and a modified posterior view Miyake technique, Assia and Apple measured the mean diameter of the lens to be 9.5 mm and the mean thickness to be 4.5 mm.[11] The lens equator is typically adjacent to the midpoint of the ciliary body. There is a space of 0.2–0.3 mm between the ciliary body and the lens equator. Physiologically this space is necessary for accommodation because it allows the ciliary ring to contract and reduce the tension on the lens zonules. Without this space, accommodation would not be possible.

Using the same technique, Assia and Apple also demonstrated the dimensions of the capsular bag following cataract removal. After evacuation of the bag, the bag volume collapses to essentially zero as the anterior capsule comes into apposition with the posterior capsule. The equator of the evacuated bag extends laterally, causing the bag diameter to enlarge from the normal 9.5 mm to approximately 10.5 mm. At this larger diameter, the lens equator directly contacts the ciliary body and the normal physiologic space is lost. The equator of the evacuated capsular bag also moves to a location posterior to the ciliary processes.[11]

Intracapsular Fixation

The shape and dimensions of the capsular bag following intracapsular IOL implantation vary depending on the style and material of the IOL. When a 12-mm all-PMMA posterior chamber intraocular lens (PCIOL) with C-loops is implanted into the capsular bag, the bag becomes oval, with dimensions of 11.2 mm × 9.2 mm.[12] J-loop haptics tend to ovalize the capsular bag even more than C-loop designs.[12] More rigid materials such as polymethyl methacrylate (PMMA) tend to distort the shape of the bag more than do more flexible materials such as polypropylene.[12] The optics of almost all intracapsular IOLs will be positioned at a plane posterior to the ciliary body. One reason for this is that the angulation of the haptics in most IOLs produces direct contact of the optic with the posterior capsule and stretching of the posterior capsule. The thickness and volume of the capsular bag are greatly reduced after IOL implantation. The thickness of a normal lens in a 70-year-old is approximately 4.5 mm and the thickness of an IOL is typically 1 mm. The normal volume of the crystalline lens is 250–300 mm^3 and the volume of an IOL implant is only 30–40 mm^3.[12] This decrease in thickness and volume results in an increase in the diameter of the capsular bag. In the axis of the haptics the capsular bag will stretch to an even larger diameter, and in the axis opposite the haptics the zonules will be maximally relaxed. These observations indicate that physiologic accommodation is effectively impossible with any thin IOL (looped, one-piece plate, or disc shaped). For an IOL to allow physiologic accommodation, a precondition would be that it fill the entire capsular bag and retain the physiologic position and stretch of the zonules.[12]

When the capsular bag is intact, in-the-bag fixation of both haptics is clearly the most optimal method of IOL fixation. Bag-bag fixation avoids direct contact between the haptics and uveal tissue and is associated with a lower likelihood of decentration and central posterior capsule opacification (Fig. 2.7).[13] However, an intact capsular bag with a continuous anterior capsular rim and stable zonules is not always achievable in cataract surgery. Not infrequently the capsular-zonular supports are completely removed as a part of pars plana lensectomy or destroyed as a result of trauma. In these situations, alternative methods of fixation must be considered.

Sulcus Fixation

The ciliary sulcus, also known as the posterior chamber angle, is formed by the junction of the posterior iris with the ciliary body. The average diameter of the

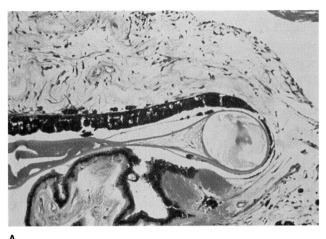

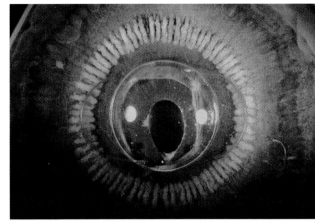

A
B

FIGURE 2.7. *A,* Pathology specimen demonstrating the loop of an intracapsular PCIOL. Note that the loop is completely surrounded by the lens capsule and has no direct contact with uveal tissues. *B,* Miyake view of PCIOL in-the-bag. *(A, Courtesy of Dr. N. Mamalis. B, From Apple BJ, Mamalis N, Olson RJ, et al. Intraocular Lenses: Evolution, Designs, Complications, and Pathology. Baltimore, MD: Williams & Wilkins; 1989, with permission.)*

ciliary sulcus is 11.0 mm.[1] The ciliary sulcus is a common location for PCIOL implantation when the posterior capsule does not provide sufficient support for the placement of an intracapsular lens and the anterior capsule is intact. When a continuous curvilinear capsulorrhexis has been performed and remains intact, the ciliary sulcus can be a very stable site of fixation for a posterior chamber lens. Because the fixation of the lens implant will be slightly more anterior than with intracapsular fixation, an adjustment of approximately 0.5 diopter less power will be needed for most lens implants to achieve the same intended refraction.[14]

However, sulcus fixation of an IOL has the inherent disadvantage of direct contact between the implant and the uveal tissues, which may result in several complications. Pigment dispersion and glaucoma may occur if there is contact between the posterior iris and the implant (Fig. 2.8). Erosion of the haptics into the ciliary sulcus may also occur, with resulting chronic inflammation (Fig. 2.9). The complications of chronic intraocular inflammation were described earlier in this

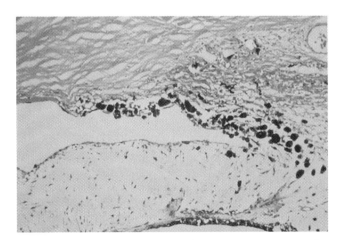

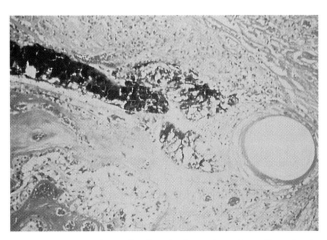

FIGURE 2.8. Pathology specimen demonstrating pigment dispersion due to a sulcus-fixated PCIOL. Note the pigment granules within the trabecular meshwork. *(Courtesy of Dr. N. Mamalis.)*

FIGURE 2.9. Erosion of a haptic loop into the ciliary body due to a sulcus-fixated PCIOL. This anatomic appearance may be indistinguishable from that of a closed-loop ACIOL. *(Courtesy of Dr. N. Mamalis.)*

chapter. In most cases, long-term sequelae do not occur with sulcus implantation of modern, smoothly finished PCIOLs.

Sutured Scleral Fixation

The haptics of sutured scleral-fixated PCIOLs ideally are meant to reside in the ciliary sulcus. However, ultrasound biomicroscopic studies have shown that these haptics are frequently not located in the ciliary sulcus and may instead be fixated to the ciliary body or the pars plana.[15] An understanding of the relationship between surgical anatomic landmarks and the ciliary sulcus is essential for the proper fixation of these lenses.

Duffey and associates studied the anatomic relationships relevant to sutured scleral-fixated PCIOLs in 21 cadaver eyes.[16] First, straight surgical needles were passed perpendicular to the globe in the vertical meridian at the surgical limbus and 1, 2, 3, 4, and 5 mm posterior to the surgical limbus. The surgical limbus was defined as the location where the white sclera meets the blue-gray zone of the corneoscleral limbus. A needle passed through the surgical limbus pierced the peripheral iris. A needle passed 1 mm posterior to the surgical limbus closely corresponded to the ciliary sulcus, passed 2 mm posterior, pierced the pars plicata of the ciliary body, and passed 3, 4, and 5 mm posterior to exit from the pars plana.

In the same study sutures were passed perpendicularly from inside the eye at the ciliary sulcus and the exit sites on the sclera were measured. This was done for the vertical axis (6 and 12 o'clock), the oblique axis (1 and 7 o'clock), and the horizontal axis (3 and 9 o'clock). The locations where the sutures exited were on average 0.94 mm posterior to the surgical limbus in the vertical axis, 0.87 mm posterior in the oblique axis, and 0.5 mm posterior in the horizontal axis.

In the anterior ciliary body the branches of the anterior ciliary arteries anastomose to form the major arterial circle of the iris. This is the most highly vascularized area of the ciliary body.[16] Avoiding the ciliary body, and the major arterial circle in particular, is therefore a worthwhile goal when attempting the placement of a scleral-fixated PCIOL. The long posterior ciliary arteries and nerves enter the ciliary body at the 3 and 9 o'clock meridians. The anterior ciliary arteries enter the ciliary body at the 3, 6, 9, and 12 o'clock positions. Because of these anatomic considerations, it is most prudent to avoid suture fixation in the vertical and horizontal axes. Vitreoretinal surgeons also avoid these locations for sclerotomies for the same reasons. We may conclude that a scleral-fixated sutured PCIOL will most likely be safely and correctly placed in the ciliary sulcus when the needles are passed approximately 0.87 mm posterior to the surgical limbus in the oblique meridians.

The haptics of properly positioned scleral-fixated PCIOLs will rest in the ciliary sulcus. This location is more anterior than that of a PCIOL placed within the capsular bag. On average, the anterior chamber depth of an eye with an intracapsular PCIOL is 4.27 mm, and for an eye with a scleral-fixated PCIOL it is 3.59 mm.[14] This difference in depth should be taken into account when calculating IOL powers for scleral fixation. It has been recommended that the power of the lens implant used for scleral fixation be decreased by 0.5 diopter from that calculated for intracapsular placement.[14] However, the exact amount of the adjustment probably depends on the surgical technique and lens implant used by an individual surgeon.

Iris Fixation Within the Posterior Chamber

In the absence of capsular support, PCIOLs may also be fixated in the posterior chamber by sutures to the iris. Typically the suture is either threaded through the positioning holes of the optic or tied to the proximal portion of the IOL loop. These sutures are then fixated to the peripupillary iris. When this technique was first developed, it was assumed that the haptics of the PCIOL would rest in the ciliary sulcus.[17,18] However, postmortem studies have shown that it is unusual for the haptics to be positioned in the ciliary sulcus (Fig. 2.10).[19] In four patients who received iris-fixated PCIOLs, only (12%) one of the eight loops was found to be situated in the ciliary sulcus. These lenses are actually suspended behind the iris and ciliary body by the sutures themselves, with minimal contact of the IOL with the uveal tissues.

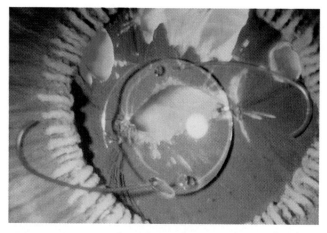

FIGURE 2.10. An iris-fixated posterior chamber lens. The optic has been sutured to the peripupillary iris through two positioning holes. The haptics of the IOL are clearly outside of the ciliary sulcus. *(Courtesy of Dr. N. Mamalis.)*

A theoretical advantage of this type of fixation over scleral fixation is that there is no suture tract passing from the surface of the eye to the inside of the eye. This may potentially reduce the risk of late endophthalmitis. However, suture fixation of the lens to the relatively mobile and highly vascularized peripupillary iris may lead to the long-term complications of chronic uveitis, glaucoma, and corneal decompensation that have been seen with pupillary clip lenses. Dependence on iris sutures alone for fixation also poses a risk of late dislocation of the PCIOL consequent on suture breakage or iris erosion.

Anatomic Considerations in Posterior Chamber Phakic IOLs

Posterior chamber lens implantation in phakic eyes is currently being investigated for the treatment of refractive errors. Sometimes a posterior chamber phakic IOL is referred to as an intraocular contact lens (ICL). These lenses are placed between the iris and the crystalline lens. Placement of a lens implant in this space would be expected to decrease the depth of the anterior chamber. This has been confirmed by ultrasound biomicroscopy (UBM) (Fig. 2.11). Trindade and Pereira performed UBM on a patient preoperatively and 1 month following ICL implantation and found that the anterior chamber depth was 2.419 mm preoperatively and 2.245 mm postoperatively.[20]

The space between the iris and lens is very narrow, with the potential for the lens implant to contact both the iris and the crystalline lens. Contact of the lens with the iris raises the possibility of several complications. Pupillary block and angle-closure glaucoma are likely if the optic occludes the pupil. Usually these complications can be prevented by performing a laser iridotomy prior to ICL implantation. Implant to iris touch may also potentially lead to pigment dispersion and glaucoma as well as chronic inflammation. A UBM study has confirmed that there can be contact between an ICL and the iris.[20]

UBM studies have shown that the minimum distance between the ICL and the crystalline lens surface varies with the lighting situation and near work. In situations of accommodation or pupillary constriction in response to light, the minimum ICL to crystalline lens surface distance is less than in the dark.[21] Actual contact between the crystalline lens and an ICL has also been demonstrated in at least one study by UBM.[20] Cataract formation is the most worrisome sequela associated with contact of the ICL with the crystalline lens, a complication reported by several authors.[20,22,23]

One study of a silicone ICL that was explanted because of cataract formation gives some insight into de-

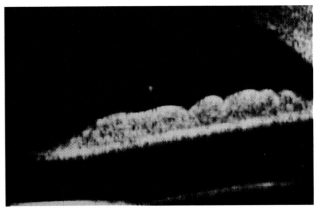

A

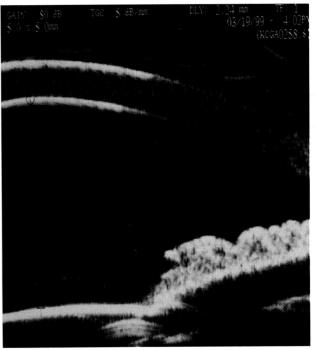

B

FIGURE 2.11. *A,* Ultrasound biomicroscopy (UBM) of a PCIOL in-the-bag. *B,* UBM of sulcus-fixated PCIOL. Note the anterior location of the lens and the close proximity of the iris to the lens in *B* as compared with *A.*

sirable and undesirable characteristics of ICLs.[24] The explanted ICL was reimplanted into a human cadaver eye. The lens was too long and could not be fixated into the ciliary sulcus as intended. Instead the lens passed through the zonules onto the surface of the pars plicata and decentered easily. The lens was also too thick and demonstrated significant contact with the iris anteriorly and the crystalline lens posteriorly. One good feature of this lens was a polished surface, which should have decreased its chafing against the iris. It appears that ICLs need at least the minimum following characteristics to be well tolerated: a relatively thin design, proper sizing and configuration of the haptics to allow stable fixation, good clearance from the crystalline lens, and good surface finish and polish.

■ Summary

Knowledge of ocular anatomy and its relationship to IOLs helps the surgeon choose the appropriate lens implant and optimize the surgical technique of lens implantation. Anatomic studies should be used as a guide in the development of new lens implants and as a method of assessing implant complications. Newer methods of anatomic study such as UBM allow precise anatomic descriptions of lens implants with the ocular structures in vivo. In the future, UBM may also be used as a method to size precisely an IOL for an individual patient prior to surgery.

■ References

1. Auffarth GU, Wesendahl TA, Assia EI, et al. Pathophysiology of modern capsular surgery. In: Steinert RF, ed. *Cataract Surgery: Technique, Complications, and Management*. Philadelphia: WB Saunders; 1995:314–324.

2. Heslin KB. Is "white-to-white" right? *Am Intraocular Implant Soc J.* 1979;5:50–51.

3. Kincaid MC, Apple DJ, Mamalis N, et al. Histopathologic correlative study of Kelman-style flexible anterior chamber intraocular lenses. *Am J Ophthalmol.* 1985;99:159–169.

4. Apple DJ, Mamalis N, Olson RJ, et al. *Intraocular Lenses: Evolution, Designs, Complications, and Pathology*. Baltimore, MD: Williams & Wilkins; 1989:533.

5. Apple DJ, Mamalis N, Loftfield K, et al. Complications of intraocular lenses: a historical and histopathological review. *Surv Ophthalmol.* 1984;29:1–54.

6. Auffarth GU, Wesendahl TA, Brown SJ, et al. Are there acceptable anterior chamber intraocular lenses for clinical use in the 1990s? An analysis of 4104 explanted anterior chamber intraocular lenses [see comments]. *Ophthalmology.* 1994;101:1913–1922.

7. Strampelli B. Anterior chamber lenses: present technique. *Arch Ophthalmol.* 1961;66:12–17.

8. Barraquer J. Anterior chamber plastic lenses: results of and conclusions from five years' experience. *Trans Ophthalmol Soc UK.* 1959;79:393–424.

9. Menezo JL, Aviño JA, Cisneros A, et al. Iris claw phakic intraocular lens for high myopia. *J Refract Surg.* 1997; 13:545–555.

10. Baikoff G, Arne JL, Bokobza Y, et al. Angle-fixated anterior chamber phakic intraocular lens for myopia of −7 to −19 diopters [see comments]. *J Refract Surg.* 1998; 14:282–293.

11. Assia EI, Apple DJ. Side-view analysis of the lens. I. The crystalline lens and the evacuated bag. *Arch Ophthalmol.* 1992;110:89–93.

12. Assia EI, Apple DJ. Side-view analysis of the lens. II. Positioning of intraocular lenses. *Arch Ophthalmol.* 1992; 110:94–97.

13. Ram J, Apple DJ, Peng Q, et al. Update on fixation of rigid and foldable posterior chamber intraocular lenses. Part II. Choosing the correct haptic fixation and intraocular lens design to help eradicate posterior capsule opacification. *Ophthalmology.* 1999;106:891–900.

14. Hayashi K, Hayashi H, Nakao F, et al. Intraocular lens tilt and decentration, anterior chamber depth, and refractive error after trans-scleral suture fixation surgery. *Ophthalmology.* 1999;106:878–882.

15. Pavlin CJ, Rootman D, Arshinoff S, et al. Determination of haptic position of transsclerally fixated posterior chamber intraocular lenses by ultrasound biomicroscopy [see comments]. *J Cataract Refract Surg.* 1993;19:573–577.

16. Duffey RJ, Holland EJ, Agapitos PJ, et al. Anatomic study of transsclerally sutured intraocular lens implantation. *Am J Ophthalmol.* 1989;108:300–309.

17. Wong SK, Stark WJ, Gottsch JD, et al. Use of posterior chamber lenses in pseudophakic bullous keratopathy. *Arch Ophthalmol.* 1987;105:856–858.

18. Stark WJ, Gottsch JD, Goodman DF, et al. Posterior chamber intraocular lens implantation in the absence of capsular support [see comments]. *Arch Ophthalmol.* 1989; 107:1078–1083.

19. Apple DJ, Price FW, Gwin T, et al. Sutured retropupillary posterior chamber intraocular lenses for exchange or secondary implantation: the 12th Annual Binkhorst Lecture, 1988. *Ophthalmology.* 1989;96:1241–1247.

20. Trindade F, Pereira F. Cataract formation after posterior chamber phakic intraocular lens implantation. *J Cataract Refract Surg.* 1998;24:1661–1663.

21. Kim DY, Reinstein DZ, Silverman RH, et al. Very high frequency ultrasound analysis of a new phakic posterior chamber intraocular lens in situ. *Am J Ophthalmol.* 1998; 125:725–729.

22. Wiechens B, Winter M, Haigis W, et al. Bilateral cataract after phakic posterior chamber top hat-style silicone intraocular lens. *J Refract Surg.* 1997;13:392–397.

23. Fechner PU, Haigis W, Wichmann W. Posterior chamber myopia lenses in phakic eyes [see comments]. *J Cataract Refract Surg.* 1996;22:178–182.

24. Visessook N, Peng Q, Apple DJ, et al. Pathological examination of an explanted phakic posterior chamber intraocular lens. *J Cataract Refract Surg.* 1999;25:216–222.

Chapter 3

Intraocular Lens Material

Liane Clamen Glazer, Tueng T. Shen, Dimitri T. Azar,
and Edward Murphy

Intraocular lens (IOL) implantation has revolutionized visual rehabilitation following cataract surgery. Advances in IOL technology have depended on growth in the field of synthetic polymer chemistry and manufacturing. This chapter describes the chemical and physical properties of IOL materials currently or formerly in use, and considers new designs for the future.

Natural polymeric materials (such as silk, cellulose, and natural rubber) have been a part of human civilization for centuries. It was not until 1919, however, that the chemical nature of plastic polymers was elucidated by the German chemist Hermann Staudinger.[1] By covalently linking multiple small molecular units, Staudinger synthesized a series of model polymers. For example, he linked styrene units to create polystyrene. These initial investigations established the foundation of modern polymer chemistry and initiated an intense systematic study of polymer properties in relationship to their chemical structure.

During World War II, the industries of many countries were hindered by the short supply of vital natural materials (such as rubber). This spurred an intense worldwide effort to synthesize new polymers to replace such staples; the plastic industry flourished as a result. A variety of valuable new synthetic materials were produced during the war. For example, polymethyl methacrylate (PMMA), a hard, transparent, moldable polymer, became the material of choice for airplane canopies. During the air war over England, many British airmen sustained penetrating injuries from PMMA canopy fragments. Although these fragments caused injury on penetration, they incited little or no inflammatory response in situ, even in the eye. Harold Ridley, a British ophthalmologist, cared for many of downed airmen who had sustained eye injuries and was able to observe this phenomenon closely. As a direct result, Ridley in 1949 selected PMMA as the material for his pioneering artificial IOLs implant.[2] In terms of optical clarity, biocompatibility, and long-term intraocular stability, PMMA is still the benchmark material against which all other materials are judged.

The evolution of lens implantation surgery has been driven by a need to marry the best and safest cataract removal surgery with the most appropriate lens implant optic and haptic design. Changes in surgical technique stimulated changes in IOL design, and vice versa. Kelman phacoemulsification together with the Shearing posterior chamber IOL heralded the move to extracapsular cataract extraction (ECCE) with posterior chamber lens implantation, a technique that remains predominant today. Throughout the 1980s, this innovation stimulated intense efforts by many ophthalmic surgeons to refine phaco techniques and lens designs. It was the development of small-incision technology, not any perceived inadequacies of PMMA, that triggered a search for new IOL materials. There was now a need for a flexible, foldable implant that would easily, safely, and predictably enter the eye through an ever smaller self-sealing incision. Scleral tunnel and clear corneal incisions that measure 2.5–3.5 mm are the current standard. The search for new IOL materials continues, as surgical technology strives for even smaller incisions. A clear corneal incision of 1.0–1.5 mm, coupled with a microcapsulotomy and endocapsular cataract removal, could support an initially fluid pseudophakic material that, when "set" intracapsularly, would give stable distance vision plus useful accommodation.

■ Classification of Current Intraocular Lens Materials

The Basics of Polymer Chemistry

Commonly used IOL materials are generally either acrylic-based polymers or silicone-based elastomers.[3] A basic knowledge of polymer chemistry and its terminology is essential for understanding the chemical and physical properties of current IOL materials and for the development of future IOLs.

The primary building blocks, the repeating units that form a polymer, are known as monomers. For example, methyl methacrylate is the monomer of PMMA (Fig. 3.1). Polymerization is the process by which these monomers are linked by covalent bonds. When different monomers are polymerized together, the process is called copolymerization. These polymeric chains can be further linked three-dimensionally by intermolecular bonds, a process known as cross-linking (Fig. 3.2). The degree of cross-linking is determined by the monomeric structure, and specifically by the structure of the side chains. The elasticity of the polymer is determined by the degree of cross-linking. Materials that exhibit elastic behavior, such as silicone polymers, are called elastomers. The chemical and physical properties of polymeric materials are determined by three basic attributes: the monomeric structure, the molecular weight of the polymeric chain, and the extent of cross-linking. Among the many physical properties, glass transition temperature is of particular interest for IOL materials. This temperature determines the thermoplastic properties of the polymers. Above this temperature the polymer exhibits flexible properties, and below this temperature the material remains rigid. Polymers can be custom designed to have specific properties. For instance, when ophthalmologists needed a foldable IOL, the polymer chemists were able to modify materials to create these foldable lenses. Continued future collaborations between ophthalmologists and chemists will undoubtedly create new polymers to suit the changing needs of ophthalmic surgery.

General Requirements for Lens Materials

The basic requirements for IOL materials are similar to those for other biomaterials. The material must be chemically inert, noncarcinogenic, nonallergenic, durable, and easily manufactured and sterilized. It should cause minimal inflammatory reaction in the body.[4] For

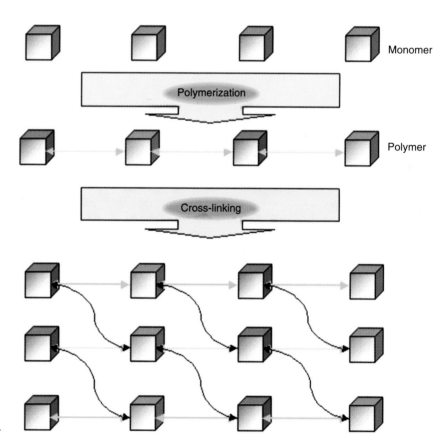

FIGURE 3.1. Schematics of polymerization.

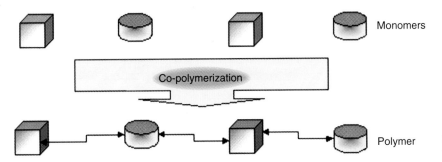

FIGURE 3.2. Schematics of copolymerization.

IOL implantation, the material should also have excellent optical properties: high transmission of visible light, absorption of ultraviolet (UV) light, and a high index of refraction. In addition, the ideal material should be lightweight and have a high degree of flexibility so that it can be used for small-incision cataract surgeries. Finally, it should be easy to insert and remove.

Acrylate-Methacrylate-Based Lens Materials

This category includes PMMA, hydrogels, and the acrylate-methacrylate copolymers (foldable acrylic). The earliest polymer was PMMA, a homopolymer of methyl methacrylate. Methyl methacrylate polymer was first synthesized from methylacrylic acid methylester in a mold formed by two layers of glass. It was found to have near-perfect transmission of light of 300 to 1,000 nm wavelength. The commercial value of these sheets was readily apparent, and PMMA soon became the most valuable member of the acrylate-methacrylate polymer series. The original developments were carried out by Rohm and Haas Co. and E. I. du Pont de Nemours & Co.[5,6] By 1936, methyl methacrylate was being used to produce organic glass (Plexiglas) by a cast polymerization process. Because of its lighter weight compared to glass (specific gravity 1.19), high

transparency to light, and ease of molding, the first significant market for PMMA sheets was in windows and canopies for military aircraft. By 1938, compression and injection molding processes of methacrylate powder had been introduced. These processes significantly facilitated the manufacturing of more complex shapes.[7] Current PMMA IOLs are manufactured by similar methods.

Acrylate and methacrylate polymers are asymmetrically substituted ethylene esters. Methacrylates differ from acrylates in that the α-hydrogen of the acrylate is replaced by a methyl group. This methyl group imparts stability, hardness, and stiffness to the methacrylate polymers (Table 3.1). Methacrylate polymers have greater resistance to both acidic and alkaline hydrolysis than acrylate polymers. Foldable acrylic IOLs, such as Alcon's Acrysof lens, are composed of an acrylate-methacrylate copolymer. This composition provides a temperature-dependent viscoelasticity while imparting good three-dimensional stability.

Methacrylate monomers are extremely versatile building blocks and can be copolymerized with a variety of other monomers, such as PMMA and poly-2-hydroxethyl methacrylate (poly-HEMA) (Figs. 3.3 and 3.4). All of the methacrylates copolymerize with each other as well as with acrylate monomers to form polymers with a wide range of properties, from soft

Table 3.1
Comparison of the Mechanical Properties of Polymethacrylate and Polyacrylate

	Tensile Strength (Mpa)		Elongation at Break (%)	
	Polymethacrylate	*Polyacrylate*	*Polymethacrylate*	*Polyacrylate*
Methyl	62.0	6.90	4	750
Ethyl	34.0	0.20	7	1,800
Butyl	06.9	0.02	230	2,000

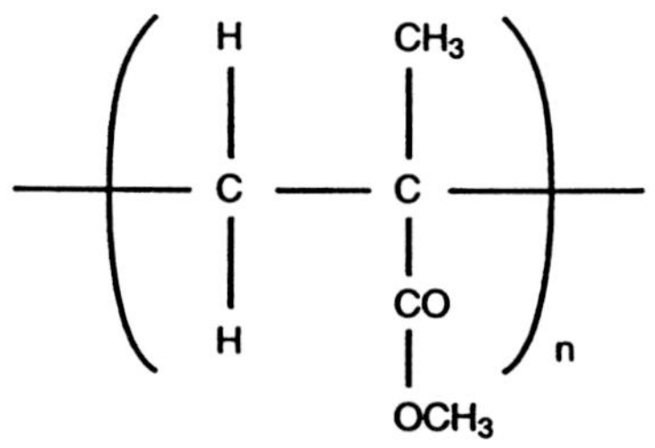

FIGURE 3.3. The chemical structure of PMMA.

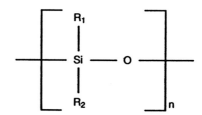

FIGURE 3.5. The chemical structure of the silicone backbone polyorganosiloxane. *(From Steinert R, ed.* Cataract Surgery: Technique, Complications, and Management. *Philadelphia: WB Saunders; 1995, with permission.)*

adhesives to rubbers to tough plastics. The length of the polymer can be measured by its molecular weight. In general, the higher the polymeric molecular weight, the more solid the polymer. In addition to the mechanical properties, the glass transition temperature (Tg) of these polymers can also be varied based on the polymeric composition. For example, PMMA has a Tg of 105°C and the MemoryLens (60% poly-HEMA and 16% PMMA) has a Tg of 27°C. This transition temperature allows the latter hydrogel lens to be prerolled for small-incision IOL implantation, with subsequent controlled unfolding in vivo at body temperature during cataract surgery.

Silicone-Based Lens Materials

Silicones are a large family of polymers with a common silicone and oxygen polymeric backbone, polyorganosiloxane (Fig. 3.5). Silicones were discovered in the late 1930s by scientists at General Electric and were rapidly commercialized for a variety of applications. They are synthesized in polymerization processes similar to those used for carbon-based polymers (PMMA). The characteristics of the silicone polymers include excellent heat stability, great resistance to degradation in vivo, and minimum foreign body reaction in vivo. A great variety of silicone polymers are available, differing mainly in the side chains. The most common of these in practical use are elastomers based on dimethylsiloxane.[8] One of the earliest surveys of silicone as implants in clinical medicine

was published by Barondes and colleagues in 1950.[9] Figure 3.6 outlines the chemical composition of many popular IOLs.

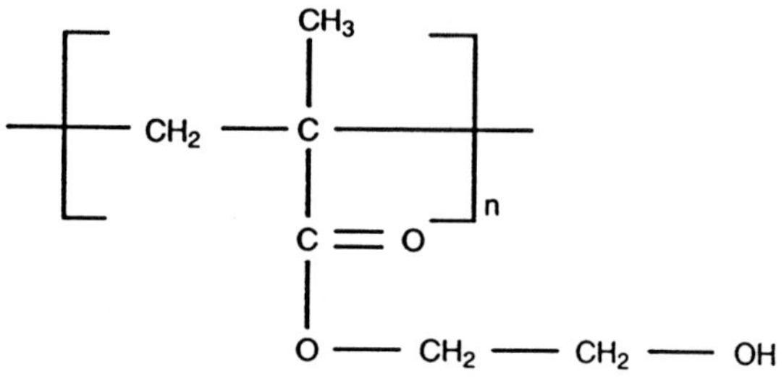

■ Specific Optic Materials

Polymethyl Methacrylate

PMMA is one of the most widely used materials in lens optics because of its light weight, durability, clarity, refractive index (1.49), and inertness. This material is produced by free radical polymerization of methacrylic acid methylester. PMMA is durable, with a high resistance to aging and to changes in the climate.[2]

Lens manufacturers use two different types of PMMA in IOLs. Perspex CQ, the type used by Ridley in 1949, has a high molecular weight ranging from 2.5 to 3.0 million daltons.[10-12] Manufacturers can easily lathe cut, compression cast, cast mold, and tumble polish this commonly used form of PMMA. The second type of PMMA has a lower molecular weight, ranging from 80,000 to 140,000 daltons.[2] Injection-molded lens optics and extruded loops are made from this form of PMMA. PMMA cannot be autoclaved and is commonly sterilized using ethylene oxide gas sterilization, which may cause the plastic to become brittle. Because ethylene oxide residues can be toxic, it is important to rinse the PMMA lens carefully before implantation.

PMMA is relatively inert and does not degrade within the eye or induce leukocyte chemotaxis. However, even in clinically well-tolerated implants, a cellular reaction occurs on the surface of the PMMA.[12] A PMMA IOL can activate the alternative complement system in vitro and generate peptides capable of stimulating inflammation.[13] In some instances, an initial inflammation may persist, but almost all such reactions will resolve with corticosteroid therapy.[2]

IOLs of earlier design had unpolished rough edges, causing an increased rate of inflammatory re-

FIGURE 3.4. The chemical structure of poly-HEMA.

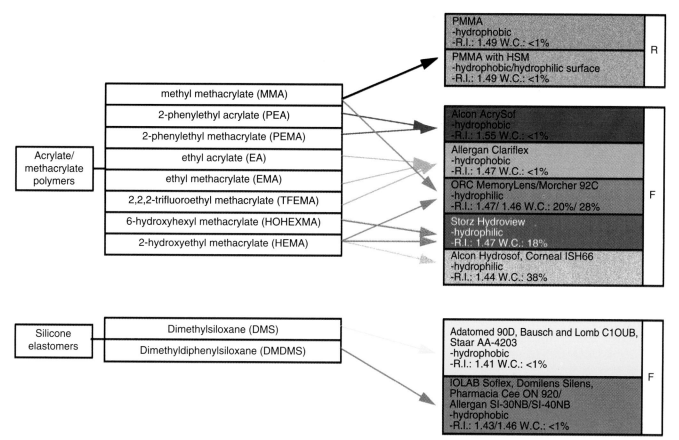

FIGURE 3.6. Schematic drawing of the major components of rigid and foldable IOL optics. Some currently available IOLs are depicted in the figure. The hydrophilicity of the IOL depends on the water contact angle in air: the lower this value, the more hydrophilic the IOL surface. PMMA, polymethyl methacrylate; HSM, heparin surface modification; R, rigid; F, foldable; R.I., refractive index; W.C., water content. *(From Kohnen T. The variety of foldable intraocular lens materials.* J Cataract Refract Surg. *1996;22(suppl 2):1255–1258, with permission. Figure developed with the assistance of Douglas D. Koch, F. Richard Christ, Graham D. Barrett, Joseph I. Weinschenk III, Anil Patel, George F. Green, and Olaf K. Morcher.)*

sponses in vivo. Careful polishing of the IOLs reduced the rate of inflammation. Posterior capsular opacification (PCO) is still a common problem for all IOLs. Recent studies seem to indicate that the development of PCO is related less to the material itself than to the lens design.[14]

Early in the development of IOLs, an issue of concern was that UV radiation, which enters the eye through the PMMA lens, could damage the retina.[11] The human cornea blocks UV wavelengths below 300 nm, and the crystalline lens prevents the transmittance of UV light above 400 nm. However, the Perspex CQ PMMA IOL blocks only wavelengths below 330 nm. Therefore, an eye with a PMMA lens was more susceptible to retinal damage from UV radiation.[11,15] To solve this problem, polymeric materials have been cus-

tomized to absorb UV light by inserting specific additives ("UV chromophores"). The most common additives in IOL materials are benzotri-azole and the benophenones.[16,17] PMMA IOLs with UV-absorbing molecules absorb light up to 400 nm.[18]

Soft IOL Materials

Although PMMA is a very good material for IOLs, it is a hard, rigid material that can cause mechanical irritation to sensitive uveal tissues, creating chronic low-grade inflammation. In addition, PMMA is hydrophobic and can cause corneal endothelial cells to adhere to its surface.[19] Finally, the larger incision required for a PMMA lens may cause more intraoperative complications and delay postoperative healing and recovery of function. With the advances in small-incision surgery and phaco-emulsification techniques, less rigid IOL materials have necessarily been developed. Some of the most commonly used soft polymers are the acrylate-methacrylate copolymers (foldable acrylic), poly-HEMA hydrogels, and silicone.[19]

Acrylic Polymers

Pure acrylic polymers are soft hydrophobic materials with weak mechanical properties. However, when these polymers are combined with methacrylates (by copolymerization of methacrylates and acrylates), the new materials have both the flexibility of pure acrylate polymers and the durability of methacrylate polymers. Many of the current soft acrylic lenses are based on this chemical formulation. For instance, Alcon's Acrysof lens is composed of 2-phenylethyl acrylate (PEA) and 2-phenylethyl methacrylate (PEMA).

Hydrogels

Hydrogels are a unique group of water-containing polymers. They are characterized by hydrophilic properties as well as insolubility in water. The dehydrated material can be formed and cut to the desired shape, swell to an equilibrium volume in water, and still maintain its designed shape. The hydrophilicity is due to the presence of hydrophilic side chains on the polymeric backbone, such as $-OH$, $-COOH$, $-CONH_2$, $CONH-$, SO_3H. The hydrophilicity can be measured by the water content of a particular hydrogel. The extensive cross-linking determines the insolubility and stability of the hydrogel. Hydrogels can be synthesized by copolymerizing a variety of monomers with a cross-linking agent, most commonly ethylene dimethacrylate (EDMA), formerly known as ethylene glycol dimethacrylate (EGDMA). Methacrylate- and acrylate-based hydrogels are the most commonly used IOL materials. An example of a popular hydrogel lens is the Memory Lens.

Silicone

In ophthalmology, medical-grade silicone polymers have been used for drains in glaucoma surgeries, scleral buckles in retinal surgeries, and for nasolacrimal intubation tubes in oculoplastics surgeries. Silicone elastomers are commonly used in IOLs. Extensive cross-linking and the high molecular weight reduce the biodegradability of the IOL in vivo.

Silicone has the advantages of being extremely inert, nonadherent to tissues, flexible at a range of temperatures, and yet stable at high temperatures. In addition, silicone elastomers have a high refractive index (1.41–1.46), and are lightweight (specific gravity 1.03–1.16 g/mL).[12] Popular models of silicone lenses include silicone plate haptic lenses and three-piece silicone IOLs.

Advantages and Disadvantages of Soft IOL Materials

Compared to PMMA, soft IOL materials have a variety of advantages: (1) soft IOL can be folded and inserted through incisions 3.0 mm in width or smaller; (2) a small surgical incision is associated with better surgical control and safety as well as faster postoperative wound healing and less astigmatism; (3) the softer lenses may do less damage to the corneal endothelium and other ocular structures; and (4) silicone and hydrogel lenses can be autoclaved, a much more convenient method of sterilization than the ethylene oxide sterilization that is required for PMMA lenses.[20,21] In a 1997 survey of the practice styles of members of the American Society of Cataract and Refractive Surgery (ASCRS), the foldable IOL was the preferred type of IOL. Foldable materials were favored by 58% of ASCRS respondents (silicone elastomers, 20%; acrylate-methacrylate polymers, 38%). Only 40% preferred rigid PMMA materials.[22]

The verdict is still out as to the biocompatibility of soft lenses. For example, although Carlson and colleagues observed that silicone and hydrogel were as well tolerated as PMMA lens materials when placed in the capsular bag of rabbit's eyes following ECCE, they also noted a chronic nongranulomatous reaction at the limbus in eyes with silicone and hydrogel lenses compared to no inflammatory reaction in eyes with PMMA lenses.[21] In a study on cats' eyes, Yalon and colleagues found that although no fibroblasts grew on the surface of hydrogel implants, microvilli formed on the corneal endothelium. The authors suspected that the microvilli indicated a mild adverse reaction to the hydrogel material, possibly due to impurities.[23] More studies are needed to determine the incidence of capsular opacification with soft lenses as well as the frequency of soft IOL absorption of topical and systemic medications.

The mechanical disadvantages of foldable lenses include decentration and lens tilting, which may occur after capsular bag fixation with plate lens designs.[19] Damage to the IOL during implantation is another possible disadvantage of foldable lenses. There have been reports of grooves on soft lenses corresponding to the forceps used during implantation.[19] Theoretically, folded lenses that are released abruptly in the eye during implantation can scrape and injure the corneal endothelium. However, Hayashi and colleagues recently determined that silicone lenses implanted in the capsular bag cause only minimal corneal endothelial cell loss, a loss that was not statistically significant compared to results in groups of patients with either

**Table 3.2
Advantages and Disadvantages of Different Intraocular
Lens Materials**

IOL Materials	Advantages	Disadvantages
PMMA	High optic quality Large optic center Proven biocompatibility Surface modification Good laser resistance	Large incision wound Monomeric release Mild foreign body reaction Not autoclavable

Soft acrylic	Foldable
	Controlled unfolding
	Good laser resistance
	Good biocompatibility
	Good optical quality
		Limited long-term experience
		Possible damage during
		    implantation
		Sticky surface can adhere
		    to instruments

Hydrogel	Good biocompatability Good optic quality Good laser resistance Easy handling	Lack of long-term experience

Silicone	Good biocompatability
	Less cystoid macular
	    edema
		Irreversible adherence to
		    silicone oil
		Can tear
		Slippery when wet
		Limited control in implantation
		Discoloration

PMMA in-the-bag lens implants or patients who underwent phacoemulsification with no subsequent IOL placement.[20]

Finally, brown discoloration of silicone lenses has been documented. Milauskas reported brown discoloration in 15 silicone IOLs he had implanted.[24] Koch and Leit reported two cases of brown discoloration in the central region of implanted silicone lenses, which they believed was due to a manufacturing defect.[25] Although thousands of silicone IOLs have been implanted and no other similar problems have been reported,[26,27] these reports warrant consideration. Table 3.2 summarizes the advantages and disadvantages of the major types of IOL materials.

Multifocal Intraocular Lenses

Multifocal lenses potentially correct both distance and near visual acuity, thereby obviating spectacle correction. Multifocal IOLs are relatively new lenses, developed to correct for loss of accommodation. These lenses achieve their goal by refractive or diffractive optical principles (or both) in order to distribute light to different focal points and provide two or more planes of focus.[28] The three main types of multifocal lenses are (1) the bull's-eye or ring configuration, which has two or more zones of distinct optical powers (Figs. 3.7A and B); (2) the zonal-progressive aspherical design, which incorporates multiple rings on the anterior surface of the lens (Fig. 3.7C); and (3) a style that utilizes diffractive optics on the posterior lens surface and conventional refractive spherical optics on the anterior surface (Fig. 3.7D).[29] Currently, the Allergan aspherical lens is the only multifocal lens on the market.

The major disadvantage of the multifocal IOL is that one must sacrifice contrast sensitivity to gain depth of focus.[30] Another disadvantage is its dependence on pupil size and visual axis centration of the lens. For example, a decentration of 2 mm or more could cause a loss of near visual acuity; at the other extreme, pupillary apertures less than 2 mm could cause a loss of distance visual acuity. Either loss could require corrective spectacles, thus defeating the purpose of the multifocal lens.[28] Another possible cause for spectacles would be an incorrect IOL power. Because an accurate IOL power is essential for good results with a multifocal IOL, both preoperative measurements and formula calculations must be precise. Finally, some patients with multifocal IOLs report disturbing visual phenomena such as glare, halos, and blurred vision.[31] Current models of multifocal lenses are being revised, and clinical trials are under way to determine whether these lenses

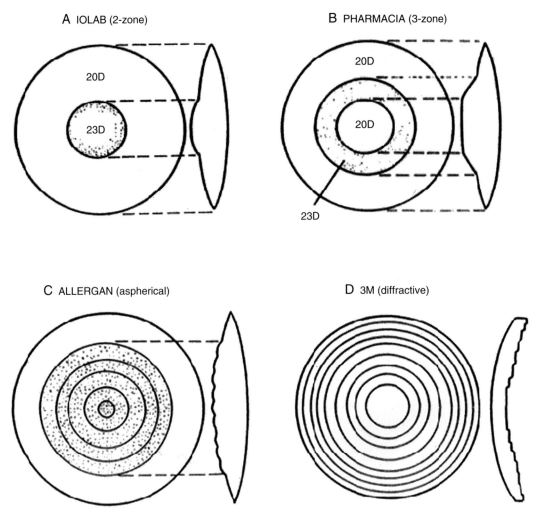

FIGURE 3.7. Multifocal IOL designs. Examples of the bull's-eye configuration include the IOLAB two-zone lens (*A*) and the Pharmacia three-zone lens (*B*). *C,* The zonal-progressive aspherical lens incorporates rings on the anterior surface of the lens. *D,* The diffractive design utilizes diffractive optics on the posterior lens surface and conventional refractive spherical optics on the anterior surface. *(From Mead MD, Sieck EA, Steinert RF. Optical rehabilitation of aphakia. In: Albert DM, Jakobiec FA, eds.* Principles and Practice of Ophthalmology: Clinical Practice. *Vol 1. Philadelphia: WB Saunders; 1994, with permission.)*

will be a viable alternative to spectacles for the correction of pseudophakic presbyopia.

Glass

The first documented IOL implant, inserted in 1795, was a glass lens, which immediately sank into the vitreous. Although this Icarus-like beginning did not bode well for glass implants, Emmrich, Strampelli, Binkhorst, Weinstein, and Troutman all experimented with glass IOLs in the 1950s and 1960s. Barasch and Poler revived the concept in 1979 with their design of a 6 mg, glass and polyimide iris clip IOL.[32] They em-

phasized the major advantages of glass: inertness within the eye, autoclavability, and resistance to degradation. These ophthalmologists also noted that the use of glass IOLs had been limited both by the weight of the glass and by the difficulty of drilling holes in the glass for loop supports.[32] In the early 1980s, Biedner and Sachs implanted glass lenses in ten eyes, with good effect and no complications. They recommended continued trials of iris-fixated glass IOL implantation.[33] Unfortunately, YAG lasers, used for posterior capsulotomies, were found to crack glass IOLs, and glass IOLs were withdrawn from the American market in 1984.[2,34,35]

▪ Haptic Materials

Modern lens design features one-piece IOLs (haptics made as one piece with the optic center) or three-piece IOLs (with the haptics and optics as two distinct parts). Many of today's haptics are polypropylene (prolene), a synthetic polymer first marketed in the late 1950s. Prolene's advantages include good tolerance by the eye, strength, nonabsorbency, relative inertness and stability, elasticity, and resistance to bacterial con-tamination. Polypropylene's characteristics of high compressibility, flexibility, and memory loss, although previously thought to offer significant advantages over other biomaterials, should now be reconsidered because of the increasing trend toward capsular bag implantation, in which loop polymer memory retention (as is found with all-PMMA lenses) has become desirable because the lens capsule can be returned to its original shape.[2] Of note, early prolene haptics were 5-0, while some of the modern prolene haptics, like those used in the MemoryLens, are 4-0. The 5-0 haptics more readily developed cracks, while the 4-0 haptics provide more stability while retaining ease of implantation.

Although prolene has stood the test of time, in vitro studies reveal potential problems with this material. First, polypropylene materials can attract circulating inflammatory cells via activation of complement.[36] Second, studies have shown that both in vitro and in vivo, bacteria adhere in greater concentration to prolene haptics than to PMMA haptics.[37] Finally, a recent study by Menikoff and colleagues found that polypropylene haptics are an independent risk factor for postoperative endophthalmitis.[38] The study predicted that there would be approximately 700 fewer cases of postoperative endophthalmitis each year in the United States if ophthalmologists used IOLs with haptics made of PMMA rather than polypropylene.[38]

PMMA is quite commonly used to make haptics. The late 1970s saw substandard quality control resulting in marked quality variation in PMMA haptics, sometimes even causing in vivo fracture of the haptics. Some manufacturers have attempted to produce small-diameter, flexible PMMA loops that would resist fracture but would still be rigid enough to retain their shape after compression. However, the brittle nature of the PMMA haptic persists in many of the lenses commonly used today. Both low and high molecular weight PMMA is used to make haptics. One-piece, all-PMMA posterior chamber lenses made from high molecular weight PMMA are becoming more popular.[2]

Polyimide is another material that can be used to make lens haptics. This synthetic material contains an imino (NH) group and a benzoyl ring. Polyimide can be heat sterilized because it is able to withstand high temperatures as well as high-energy radiation. Currently, polyimide works well as a support loop in some silicone IOLs, such as the Bausch and Lomb three-piece silicone IOL.[12]

Although polyamide is often referred to simply as nylon, it is a polymer whose category also includes materials such as Terlon and Supramid. While polyamide is flexible and can be manufactured in many different shapes and sizes, the material is not stable in the eye. Nylon undergoes hydrolytic biodegradation in the eye; as time goes by, it implants into tissue. There have been many published reports of nylon loops and sutures breaking and degrading within the eye.[2] Because of this tendency to degrade within the eye, polyamide materials are no longer used as haptics.

Metals such as platinum, platinum-iridium, titanium, and stainless steel were once a popular material for loops in iris-supported lenses. It soon became clear, however, that the excessive weight and the cutting effect of the sharp metal edges in contact with uveal tissue caused many complications.[2] Because of these problems, metal loops were removed from the market.

▪ Future Directions

Future advances in IOL materials include injectable IOL materials.[39,40] Lenses made of liquid polymer gel can be injected into the capsular bag after a small-incision cataract extraction. The gel remains clear after the solidification process. The dioptric power can be varied by changing the injectable material (i.e., the refractive index) and the amount injected into the capsular bag. Preliminary animal studies also indicate the presence of accommodative power with this type of IOL. The major setback in developing injectable lenses has been the difficulty of controlling the refractive power of the lens after it has formed in the posterior capsular bag. It is clear that the postoperative refraction is determined both by the refractive index of the material and by the degree of filling of the capsular bag. However, the goal of accurately controlling postoperative refractive power remains elusive with injectable IOLs.[41] In addition, PCO occurs soon after cataract surgery with injectable IOL implantation, presumably secondary to migration of lens epithelial cells.[41,42] A potential advantage of the injectable IOL is that it may preserve accommodation postoperatively. Unfortunately, Nd:YAG laser capsulotomy may annul any accommodation obtained.

Therefore, PCO after lens refilling must be prevented before the benefit of accommodation will be attainable.[43]

■ References

1. Straudinger H. *Schweiz Chem Z.* 1919;1(28):60.

2. Apple D, Mamalis N, Olson R. *Intraocular Lenses: Evolution, Designs, Complications, and Pathology.* Baltimore, MD: Williams & Wilkins; 1989.

3. Kohnen T. The variety of foldable intraocular lens materials. *J Cataract Refract Surg.* 1996;22(suppl 2):1255–1259.

4. Scales J. Discussion on metals and synthetic materials in relation to tissues: tissue reaction to synthetic materials. *Proc R Soc Med.* 1953;46:647–652.

5. Riddle E. *Monomeric Acrylic Esters.* New York: Reinhold Publishing Corp; 1959.

6. Salkind M, Riddle E, Keefer R. *Ind Eng Chem.* 1959; 51:1232.

7. Novak R, Lesko P. Methacylate polymers. In: Kroschwitz J, Howe-Grant M, eds. *Encyclopedia of Chemical Technology.* 4th ed, vol 16. New York: John Wiley & Sons; 1990:506–537.

8. Hardman B, Torkelson A. Silicon compounds (silicones). In: *Encyclopedia of Chemical Technology,* vol 20. New York: John Wiley & Sons; 1982:922–962.

9. Barondes RDR, Judge W, Towne C, Baxter M. The silicones in medicine: new organic derivatives and some of their unique properties. *Milit Surg.* 1950;106:379–387.

10. Auffarth G, Wesendahl T, Brown S, Apple D. Are there acceptable anterior chamber intraocular lenses for clinical use in the 1990s? An analysis of 4104 explanted anterior chamber intraocular lenses. *Ophthalmology.* 1994;101: 1913–1922.

11. Mainster M. Spectral transmittance of intraocular lenses and retinal damage from intense light sources. *Am J Ophthalmol.* 1978;85:167–170.

12. Lindstrom R. The polymethyl methacrylate (PMMA) intraocular lenses. In: Steinert R, ed. *Cataract Surgery: Technique, Complications, and Management.* Philadelphia: WB Saunders; 1995.

13. Tuberville A, Wood T. Aqueous humor protein and complement in pseudophakic eyes. *Cornea.* 1990;3:249–253.

14. Nishi O, Nishi K. Preventing posterior capsule opacification by creating a discontinuous sharp bend in the capsule. *J Cataract Refract Surg.* 1998;25:521–526.

15. Lerman S. Ultraviolet radiation protection. *CLAO J.* 1985; 11:39–45.

16. Clayman HM. Ultraviolet absorbing intraocular lens. *Am Intraocular Implant Soc J.* 1984;10:429–432.

17. Clayman HM. Intraocular lenses. In: Duane T, Jaeger E, eds. *Clinical Ophthalmology.* Philadelphia: JB Lippincott; 1991.

18. Gupta A. Long-term aging behavior of ultraviolet absorbing intraocular lenses. *Am Intraocular Implant Soc J.* 1984;10:309–314.

19. Lindstrom R. Foldable intraocular lenses. In: Steinert R, ed. *Cataract Surgery: Technique, Complications, and Management.* Philadelphia: WB Saunders; 1995.

20. Hayashi K, Hayashi H, Nakao F, et al. Corneal endothelial cell loss in phacoemulsification surgery with silicone intraocular lens implantation. *J Cataract Refract Surg.* 1996;22:743–747.

21. Carlson K, Cameron J, Lindstrom R. Assessment of the blood-aqueous barrier by fluorophotometry following poly(methylmethacrylate), silicone, and hydrogel lens implantation in rabbit eyes. *J Cataract Refract Surg.* 1993; 19:9–15.

22. Leaming DV. Practice styles and preferences of ASCRS members: 1997 survey. *J Cataract Refract Surg.* 1998; 24:552–561.

23. Yalon M, Blumenthal M, Goldberg E. Preliminary study of hydrophilic hydrogel intraocular lens implants in cats. *Am Intraocular Implant Soc J.* 1984;10:315–317.

24. Milauskas A. Silicone intraocular lens discoloration in humans. *Arch Ophthalmol.* 1991;109:913.

25. Koch D, Heit L. Discoloration of silicone intraocular lenses. *Arch Ophthalmol.* 1992;110:319–320.

26. Kerschner R. In reply to: Milauskas AT. Silicone intraocular lens discoloration in humans. *Arch Ophthalmol.* 1991; 109:913.

27. Ziemba S. In reply to: Milauskas AT. Silicone intraocular lens discoloration in humans. *Arch Ophthalmol.* 1991; 109:913.

28. Duffey R, Zabel R, Lindstrom R. Multifocal intraocular lenses. *J Cataract Refract Surg.* 1990;16:423–429.

29. Mead M, Sieck E, Steinert R. Optical rehabilitation of aphakia. In: Albert D, Jakobiec F, eds. *Principles and Practice of Ophthalmology: Clinical Practice.* Philadelphia: WB Saunders; 1994.

30. Holladay J, Van Dijk H, Lang A. Optical performance of multifocal intraocular lenses. *J Cataract Refract Surg.* 1990;16:413–422.

31. Rossetti L, Carraro R, Rovati M. Performance of diffractive multifocal intraocular lenses in extracapsular cataract surgery. *J Cataract Refract Surg.* 1994;20:124–128.

32. Barasch K, Poler M. A glass intraocular lens. *Am J Ophthalmol.* 1979;88:556–559.

33. Biedner B, Sachs U. Results of glass intraocular lens insertion. *Ann Ophthalmol.* 1982;14:456–457.

34. Fritch C. Neodymium:YAG laser damage to glass intraocular lens. *Ann Ophthalmol.* 1984;16:1177.

35. Fritch C. Neodymium:YAG laser damage to glass intraocular lens. *Am Intraocular Implant Soc J.* 1984; 10:225.

36. Apple D, Mamalis N, Loftfield K. Complications of IOLs: a historical and histopathological review. *Surv Ophthalmol.* 1984;1:54.

37. Dilly P, Holmes, Sellors P. Bacterial adhesion to intraocular lenses. *J Cataract Refract Surg.* 1989;15:317–320.

38. Menikoff J, Speake M, Marmor M, Raskin E. A case-control study of risk factors for postoperative endophthalmitis. *Ophthalmology.* 1991;98:1761–1768.

39. Banker D, Sodero E, Mazzocco T, et al. Lenses of the future: Gel substitute, compressible silicone, expansile hydrogel. In: Abrahamson I, ed. *Cataract Surgery.* New York: McGraw-Hill; 1986;266–280.

40. Chapman J, Cheek L, Green K. Drug interaction with

intraocular lenses of different materials. *J Cataract Refract Surg.* 1992;18:456–459.

41. Nishi O, Nishi K, Mano C, et al. Lens refilling with injectable silicone in rabbit eyes. *J Cataract Refract Surg.* 1998;24:975–982.

42. Hettlich H, Lucke K, Asiyo-Vogel M. Lens refilling and endocapsular polymerization of an injectable intraocular lens: in vitro and in vivo study of potential risks and benefits. *J Cataract Refract Surg.* 1994;20: 124–128.

43. Nishi O, Nishi K. Accommodation amplitude after lens refilling with injectable silicone by sealing the capsule with a plug in primates. *Arch Ophthalmol.* 1998; 16:1358–1361.

Chapter 4

Intraocular Lens Power Calculations

H. John Shammas

■ Historic Overview

Before 1975 the power of an intraocular lens (IOL) to be inserted after a cataract extraction was calculated with the use of an equation based on the clinical history:[1]

$$P = 18 + (1.25 \times Ref)$$

where P is the power of an iris-supported IOL for emmetropia and Ref is the preoperative refractive error in diopters before the development of the cataract. Errors exceeding 1 diopter occurred in over 50% of cases in which this clinical history method was used, and some errors were so large that they were referred to as the "9 diopter surprise." These large errors were caused by the difficulty of determining the patient's refractive error before the development of the cataract and the large variations in the crystalline lens power.

A number of formulas for IOL power calculations have since been published; all of these formulas are based on an accurate measurement of the corneal power and the axial length. The original formulas were developed prior to 1980. They included theoretical formulas and regression formulas. These formulas were then modified in the mid-1980s to correct some of the errors in short and long eyes. Although these formulas are rarely used now, they are at the base of all modern formulas.

Original Theoretical Formulas

All theoretical formulas for IOL power calculations are based on a two-lens system, the cornea and the pseudophakos lens, focusing images on the retina.[1]

Thijssen's,[2] Colenbrander's,[3] Fyodorov's,[4] and van der Heijde's[5] formulas yield approximately the same IOL power for emmetropia. Binkhorst's formula[6] differed by 0.50 diopter because it was based on a corneal index of refraction of 4/3 instead of 1.3375.

The resultant postoperative refractive error measured at the cornea after the insertion of an IOL with a certain power can be predicted before surgery by Binkhorst's formula[6] or Hoffer's modification of Colenbrander's formula.[7]

Original Regression Formulas

Regression formulas are derived empirically from retrospective computer analysis of data accrued on a great many patients who have undergone surgery.

A regression formula for emmetropia is based on the following equation:

$$P = A + BL - CK$$

where P is the IOL power for emmetropia, L is the axial length in millimeters, and K is the corneal power in diopters. A, B, and C are constants.

In the SRK formula,[8,9] the most popular original regression formula, B is 2.5 and C is 0.9. The formula becomes:

$$P = A - 2.5L - 0.9K$$

The constant A varies with the IOL style and manufacture.

Modified Formulas for Emmetropia

These formulas are modifications of the original theoretical and regression formulas to correct for errors occurring in long and short eyes.

Hoffer's formula[10] is based on a modification of Colenbrander's formula. The expected postoperative error at the cornea (R) is added to the corneal power. When calculations are made for emmetopia, R becomes nil. Also, the anterior chamber depth (ACD) value is changed in accordance with the axial length.

Shammas's formula[11] is also a modified Colenbrander's formula. The first modification involves the corneal index of refraction; it is changed from 1.3375 to 4/3, as suggested by Binkhorst. The corneal power, such as read on the Bausch and Lomb keratometer, is decreased by a factor of 1.0125. The second modification is the incorporation of a fudge factor linked to the axial length.

Binkhorst used his own original formula for emmetropia and varied the postoperative ACD value according to the axial length.[12] The ACD value is decreased by 0.17 mm for each millimeter the axial length is shorter than 23.45 mm and is increased by 0.17 mm for each millimeter the axial length is longer than 23.45 mm.

The SRK II formula[13] is a modification of the original SRK formula with the addition of a correction factor that increases the lens power in short eyes and decreases it in long eyes.

■ Calculating for Emmetropia

Modern theoretical formulas are more complex than the original and modified formulas. The most striking difference is the manner in which the estimated ACD value is calculated:

- In the original formulas, ACD value is a constant value.
- In the modified formulas, ACD value varies with the axial length. It decreases in the shorter eye and increases in the longer eye.
- In the modern formulas, ACD value varies not only with axial length, but with the corneal curvature as well. The anterior chamber is deeper in the presence of a steep cornea and shallower in the presence of a flat cornea.

The best-known modern formulas are the Holladay formula,[14] the SRK-T formula,[15] and the Hoffer-Q formula.[16]

Holladay's Formula

Holladay's formula is a modification of the theoretical formula.[14] It is based on a three-part system that includes data screening criteria to identify improbable axial length and keratometry measurements, a more accurate postoperative ACD estimate that increases the accuracy in short, medium, and long eyes, and a personalized "surgeon factor" that adjusts for any consistent bias in the surgeon's formula.

The data screening identifies measurements that are unusual and might require remeasurement, such as

- Axial length less than 22.0 mm or greater than 25.0 mm
- Average corneal power less then 40 diopters or greater than 47 diopters
- Calculated emmetropic IOL power of more than 3 diopters from specific lens style
- A difference between the two eyes of more than 1 diopter in the average corneal power, more than 0.3 mm in the axial length, and more than 1 diopter in the emmetropic IOL power

The postoperative ACD is estimated more accurately. The concept is that the effective lens position of any IOL is the sum of the anatomic ACD and the distance from the anterior plane of the iris to the optical plane of the IOL, called the surgeon factor (S).

The surgeon factor is personalized for the surgeon, the surgical technique, and the type of implant used. It is calculated by solving the formula in reverse, using as input variables the postoperative corneal and axial length measurements, the IOL power implanted, and the stabilized postoperative refraction.

The SRK-T Formula

The SRK-T formula,[15] in contradistinction to the SRK I and SRK II formulas, is a theoretical formula based on Fyodorov's formula and uses empirical regression methodology for optimization of

- The postoperative ACD prediction
- The axial length (by adding a retinal thickness correction factor)
- The corneal refractive index

The estimated postoperative ACD is calculated:

$$ACD\ (estimate) = corneal\ dome\ height\ (H) + offset$$

$$Offset = ACD\ value - 3.336$$

It is based on the hypothesis that the IOL lies at a constant distance from the calculated iris plane. The height of the corneal dome (H) is the distance between the cornea and the iris plane and is calculated mathematically within the formula.

The optical axial length is measured by adding retinal thickness to the axial length. The corneal radius of curvature (r) in millimeters is measured using the formula:

$$r = 337.5/K$$

where K is the average keratometric reading in diopters.

Hoffer-Q Formula

The Hoffer-Q formula uses the basic Hoffer modification of Colenbrander's formula with a new ACD prediction formula.[16] Hoffer studied the relationship between the ACD value and axial length and found it to be a tangent curve instead of a straight line. He then tried, by trial and error, many mathematical formula variations until the desired curve was reached. The anterior chamber prediction formula consists of:

- A personalized ACD value developed from any series of one IOL style
- A factor that increases the ACD with increasing axial length
- A factor that increases the ACD with increasing corneal curvature
- A factor that moderates the change in ACD for extremely long (more than 26 mm) and short (less than 22 mm) eyes
- A constant added to the ACD

Comparing the Formulas

Figure 4.1 shows that the results of the modified modern formulas fall between the results of the original theoretical (Colenbrander) and regression (SRK) formulas.

■ Measuring the Normal Phakic Eye

Prior to any IOL power calculations, the technician needs to take axial length measurements and corneal power readings. These values are then entered into the formula to be used.

Measuring the Axial Length

The axial length can be measured by an immersion technique or a contact technique using an ultrasound biometer. No matter which technique is used, both eyes should be measured for comparison purposes.

With the *immersion technique*[17,18] the patient is placed supine on a flat examination table or seated in a reclining examination chair. A drop of local anesthetic is instilled in each eye. The proper scleral shell is chosen (Fig. 4.2). Although the 20-mm shell fits most eyes, the larger cup provides a better fit in bigger eyes with large palpebral fissures and the small cup fits

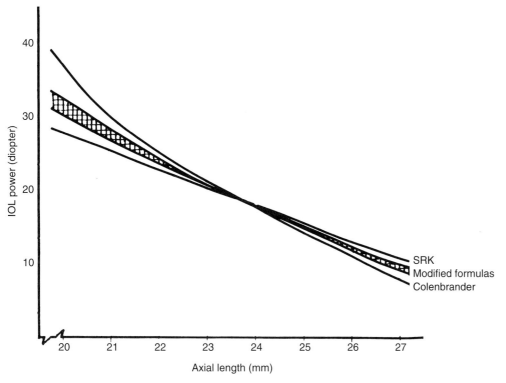

FIGURE 4.1. IOL power calculated by the modified modern formulas (shaded interval) compared to powers calculated by the SRK and Colenbrander's formulas.

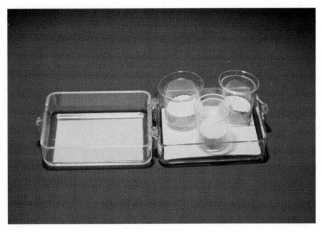

A

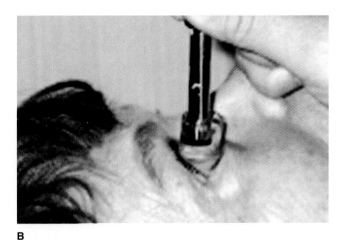

B

FIGURE 4.2. *A,* Ossoinig scleral shells used in the immersion technique of measuring axial length. *B,* The solid probe is immersed in the solution but kept 5–10 mm away from the cornea.

better in an eye with a narrow palpebral fissure. The flared edges of the scleral shell are placed between the lids, with the technician making sure that the cup is stable on the eye. The cup is filled with gonioscopic solution and the ultrasound probe is immersed in the solution but kept 5–10 mm away from the cornea (Fig. 4.2B). The patient is asked to look with the fellow eye at a fixation point on the ceiling. Attention is then focused on the screen. The probe is gently moved until it is properly aligned with the optical axis and an acceptable A-scan echogram is displayed on the screen. A Polaroid picture or a printout is obtained.

With the *contact technique,* a drop of local anesthetic is instilled in each eye.[19,20] The patient is examined in the seated position with the chin correctly positioned on a freestanding chin rest. The probe is positioned in front of the eye and the patient is asked to fixate on the red light in the probe. The probe is then brought forward to gently touch the cornea without indenting it (Fig. 4.3). The probe is moved slightly up and down or to the side to optimize the echospikes displayed on the oscilloscope. A Polaroid picture or a printout is obtained.

Other probes are mounted on a Goldmann tonometer holder and are used with a slit-lamp. The examination is conducted in the same manner as previously described.

Differences between the two examination techniques do exist.[21,22] The contact technique yields a shorter measurement than the immersion technique. The differences between the two methods of examina-

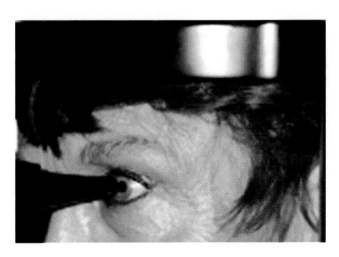

FIGURE 4.3. Contact axial length measured using the solid probe.

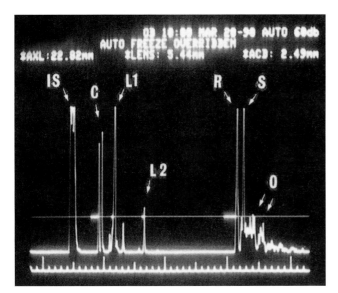

FIGURE 4.4. Ultrasound display of the different echospikes during axial length measurement. Identified are the initial spike (IS) and spikes from the cornea (C), the lens surfaces (L1 and L2), the retina (R), the sclera (S), and orbital tissues (O).

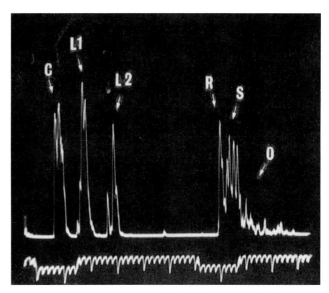

FIGURE 4.5. A-scan pattern of a phakic eye with the initial spike removed from the screen display.

tion include the patient's position and possible corneal applanation by the ultrasound probe.

The A-scan pattern of a phakic eye examined with an immersion technique displays the following echospikes from left to right (Figs. 4.4 and 4.5):

IS: The initial spike (IS) represents reverberations at the tip of the probe and has no clinical significance. Many units allow the technician to move the whole A-scan pattern to the left and remove the IS from the picture.

C: The corneal spike is double-peaked, representing the anterior and posterior surfaces of the cornea.

L1: The anterior lens spike is generated from the anterior surface of the lens.

L2: The posterior lens spike is generated from the posterior surface of the lens and is usually smaller than L1.

R: The retinal spike is generated from the anterior surface of the retina. It is straight, highly reflective, and tall whenever the ultrasound beam is perpendicular to the retina, as it should be during axial length measurement.

S: The scleral spike is another high-reflective spike generated from the scleral surface, right behind the retinal spike, and should not be confused with it.

O: The orbital spikes are low-reflective spikes located behind the scleral spike.

The A-scan pattern of a phakic eye examined with the contact technique demonstrates similar echospikes except that the corneal spike is merged with the initial spike because the cornea is in touch with the tip of the probe.

Some biometers give the reading directly in millimeters using an average sound velocity. This velocity is reported in meters per second (m/s), with a recommended value of 1,553 m/s.

Many modern biometers use separate sound velocities for the different eye components to obtain the total axial length. The eye is divided ultrasonically into four compartments (Fig. 4.6):

• The corneal thickness is measured between the anterior (C1) and posterior (C2) surfaces of the cornea using a velocity of 1,620 m/s. The thickness of a normal cornea is approximately 0.5 mm.

• The true ACD is measured between the posterior corneal surface (C2) and the anterior lens surface (L1) using a velocity of 1,532 m/s. This measurement is not to be confused with the anterior chamber constant (ACD constant) used in the IOL power calculation formulas, which is the sum of the corneal thickness and the true ACD.

• The lens thickness is measured between the anterior lens surface (L1) and the posterior lens surface (L2) using a velocity of 1,641 m/s. The sound velocity is lower in the intumescent cataracts

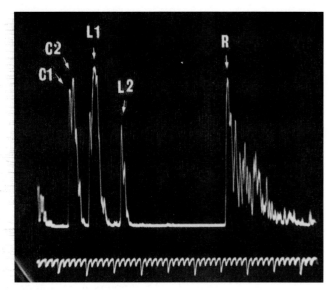

FIGURE 4.6. A-scan pattern of a phakic eye taken with the Kertz 7200 MA unit and with the initial spike removed from the screen display. Identified are the two corneal peaks (C1 and C2), the anterior lens spike (L1), the posterior lens spike (L2), and the retinal spike (R).

because of their high water content; it averages 1,590 m/s.

- The vitreous cavity's depth is measured between the posterior lens surface (L2) and the anterior surface of the retina (R) using a velocity of 1,532 m/s.

A new device, the IOL Master, yields accurate axial length measurements using optical coherence biometry. The instrument directs a beam from an eye-safe laser into the eye. It then separates the portion of the beam that is reflected by the cornea from the portion reflected by the retina. The distance between the two reflecting surfaces is determined by interferometry. This technique is very helpful when long eyes with posterior staphylomas. However, it is difficult to obtain a measurement in the presence of a dense cataract, which limits the use of this unit.

Measuring the Corneal Power

Manual keratometry is the method most commonly used to measure the corneal curvature.[4] It is fast, easy, cheap, and very accurate in most cases.

The patient is seated behind the keratometer with the chin well positioned in the chin rest and the forehead touching the headrest. The keratometer is directed toward the eye to be examined while the occluding shield is placed in front of the opposite eye. The keratometer is focused on the central portion of the cornea using the focusing knobs. At this time, the

central ring appears as one circle. The instrument is rotated to align the (−) signs in the same vertical meridian and the (+) signs in the same horizontal meridian. This will determine the axis of any preexisting astigmatism. The left drum is rotated to superimpose the (+) signs and a horizontal measurement is taken. The right drum is then rotated to superimpose the (−) signs and a vertical measurement is taken.

IOL power formulas rarely use the horizontal (K1) and vertical (K2) readings. They usually call for the average value K = 0.5 (K1 + K2).

It is important to remember that the keratometer has to be calibrated every 6 months. A set of calibrations balls with a known radius of curvature can be used. The horizontal and vertical drums are then set at the same value.

Automatic keratometry is designed to give accurate, objective, and reproducible measurements of the corneal curvature.

Corneal topography is used to evaluate central and peripheral corneal curvature. The patient is seated behind a corneoscope that projects a 16-ring conical placido disc on the cornea. A camera captures the image reflection (first Purkinjee image) and transmits it to a computer that converts the data into a series of color graphic displays. Although a regular keratometer gives accurate and reproducible measurements in most cases, corneal topography can be helpful in certain cases:

- When the cornea is flatter than 40 diopters or steeper than 46 diopters
- When the surgeon wants to better evaluate the preexisting astigmatism
- When the cornea is irregular, for example after trauma or in the presence of a concomitant keratoconus
- When certain corneal procedures have already been performed, such as radial keratotomy or laser photorefractive keratectomy

■ The Anterior Chamber Constant

All original theoretical formulas take into consideration the ACD, defined as the distance between the corneal vertex and the anterior surface of the IOL.[1–7] The advent of the SRK regression formula[8,9] brought with it the concept of the "A constant." The A constant varied not only with the ACD but also with a variety of factors that had not been taken into consideration in the original theoretical formulas, namely, variations in axial length measurement due to different biometers, different velocities and different measurement techniques; variations in IOL design; and variations in surgical technique.

The concept of individualizing the A constant revolutionized IOL power calculations. Three constants are used in modern IOL formulas:

- The ACD value, representing the postoperative ACD estimate in the Binkhorst and Hoffer formulas
- The A constant in the SRK II and SRK-T formulas
- The S factor constant in the Holladay formula

The ACD Value

The ACD value is the distance between the corneal vertex and the optical center of the IOL. It is important to note that the postoperative ACD does not correlate with the preoperative ACD. Instead, it correlates with the placement of the IOL—whether it is in the anterior chamber, in the sulcus, or in the capsular bag. The ACD value also varies with the implant's configuration and the location of its optical center. The use of a meniscus lens with its anteriorly located center calls for a smaller ACD value than a biconvex IOL, in which the optical center is more posteriorly located.

The ACD values differ in each of the formulas in which they are used because of the different characteristics of these formulas. When referring to a specific ACD value, it becomes important to refer to it as the Binkhorst ACD, the Hoffer ACD, or the Shammas ACD.

The commonly used ACD values for the different IOL styles are as follows:

Anterior chamber lens	2.8 to 3.1 mm
Posterior chamber lens in the sulcus	3.7 to 4.1 mm
Posterior chamber lens in the bag	4.3 to 5.1 mm

An error of 1 mm in the ACD value affects the postoperative refraction by approximately 1.0 diopter in a myopic eye, 1.5 diopters in an emmetropic eye, and up to 2.5 diopters in a hyperopic eye.

The A Constant

The A constant was originally designed for the SRK linear equation. The A constant encompasses multiple variables, including the implant manufacturer, implant style, the surgeon's technique, implant placement within the eye, and measuring equipment. Because of its simplicity, the A constant became the value used to characterize intraocular implants. The same A constant is used in the SRK II regression formula and in the SRK-T theoretical formula.

The most commonly used A constants are as follows:

Anterior chamber lens	115.0 to 115.3
Posterior chamber lens in the sulcus	115.9 to 117.2
Posterior chamber lens in the bag	117.5 to 118.8

Clinical Application

Surgery is planned and IOL calculations call for a 21-diopter posterior chamber implant for emmetropia. During surgery, the capsule breaks and vitreous is lost. The surgeon now has to insert an anterior chamber lens, and no calculations for this implant have been made. A decision on the implant power has to be made on the spot. This is where the A constant comes in handy, no matter what formula has been used.

A constant of the posterior chamber lens = 117.8
A constant of the anterior chamber lens = 115.3

In most cases, the power of the IOL lens for emmetropia varies in a 1:1 relationship with the A constant: if A decreases by 1 diopter, P decreases by 1 diopter also. This straight relationship adds to the simplicity and popularity of the A constant. In our case, the A constant is lower by 2.5 diopters if an anterior chamber lens is used; the implant power is then decreased by the same amount to avoid any unwanted postoperative myopia. An 18.5-diopter anterior chamber lens should be inserted to keep the eye in the emmetropic range.

The S Factor

The postoperative ACD represents the distance between the corneal vertex and the optical plane of the IOL. It is the sum of two components:

1. The anatomic ACD, which is the distance from the corneal vertex to the anterior iris plane after surgery; this distance is more accurately predicted with a mathematical formula based on the corneal curvature and the axial length
2. The distance between the anterior iris plane and the effective optical plane of the implanted IOL; this distance has been labeled the surgeon factor (S factor)

Although theoretically the S factor is a measurable distance, it should be personalized by solving the formula in reverse. Like the A constant, the S factor represents variations due to lens style, lens manufacturer, surgeon's technique, and measurement devices.

Because of the close relationship between the S factor and ACD value (almost 1:1), a change of 1 unit in the S factor is identical to a change of 1 mm in the ACD and affects the postoperative refraction in an average eye by around 1.5 diopters.

The most commonly used S factors are as follows:

Anterior chamber lens	− 0.75 to − 0.40
Posterior chamber lens in the sulcus	+ 0.10 to + 0.70
Posterior chamber lens in the bag	+ 0.90 to + 1.60

Individualizing the Constants

All three constants (ACD, A, and S) have to be personalized to accommodate any consistent shift that might affect the IOL power calculations, namely, the surgical technique, the biometer used, the implant style and manufacturer.

Each constant has to be back calculated for a series of 20 or more cases. It is important for the series under review to have the same parameters:

- Same surgeon
- Same surgical technique
- Same biometry unit and same technician taking the measurement
- Same keratometer and same technician taking the readings
- Same IOL style from the same manufacturer

The constant (ACD, A, or S) is back calculated for each case using available computer programs and calculators. The constant values are averaged to obtain the personalized constant.

■ Unusual Cases

The Intumescent Cataract

In the presence of an intumescent cataract,[23] the water content of the lens increases and the lens becomes thicker (>5.0 mm). Concomitantly, the sound velocity within the lens decreases to around 1,590 m/s from the usual 1,641 m/s.

When the axial length is measured using separate sound velocities, the erroneous use of a 1,641 m/s sound velocity will yield a 0.15-mm longer measurement, calling for a weaker IOL and resulting in a +0.40 to +0.50 more hyperopic final refraction.

Recommendations

- Use a lens velocity of 1,590 m/s instead of 1,641 m/s if your ultrasound unit measures each eye component separately.
- Or use the average sound velocity of 1,553 m/s to measure the whole eye as in a normal phakic eye. The decrease in the sound velocity within the lens and the increase in the lens thickness leave the average sound velocity between 1,549 m/s and 1,553 m/s, which are very similar to the average velocity within an eye with nuclear sclerosis.

The Aphakic Eye

In an aphakic eye,[24] the A-scan pattern displays the following echospikes from left to right (Figs. 4.7 and 4.8):

IS: The initial spike; it can be moved out of the screen in an immersion technique and will merge with the corneal spike (C) on the A-scan in a contact technique
C: The double-peaked corneal spike
I: A medium-reflective echospike from the iris surface and/or anterior vitreous face
R: The retinal spike from the anterior surface of the retina

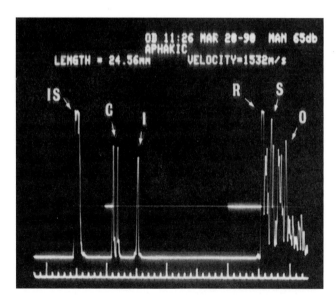

FIGURE 4.7. A-scan pattern of an aphakic eye. Identified are the initial spike (IS) and spikes from the cornea (C), the iris and/or anterior vitreous face (I), the retina (R), the sclera (S), and orbital tissues (O).

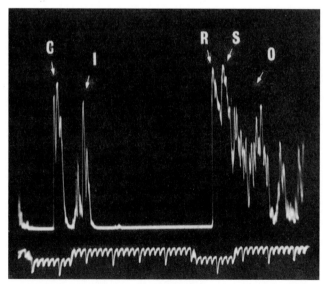

FIGURE 4.8. A-scan pattern of an aphakic eye with the initial spike removed from the screen display.

S: The scleral spike
O: The orbital spikes

The initial spike can also be removed from the screen (Fig. 4.8), leaving only the echospikes generated from the eye.

The axial length is measured between the anterior corneal surface (C) and the anterior retinal surface (R) using an average sound velocity of 1,534 m/s. This sound velocity is slightly higher than the 1,532 m/s velocity in aqueous and vitreous to account for the faster speed of sound within the cornea. If the ultrasound unit uses only a fixed 1,550 m/s velocity and does not allow for the use of a 1,534 m/s velocity, the axial length of the aphakic eye can then be calculated:

Aphakic AL = (1,534/1,550)
$\qquad$ × AL measured with 1,550 m/s

Recommendations

- Use an average sound velocity of 1,534 m/s to measure the whole eye.
- Remember to use the correct A constant when you are calculating the IOL power for emmetropia, especially if you are planning to use an ACIOL; the power of such an implant will be 2–3 diopters weaker than the calculated power for a PCIOL.

The Pseudophakic Eye

In a pseudophakic eye,[25,26] the A-scan pattern displays the following echospikes from left to right (Fig. 4.9):

IS: The initial spike; it can be moved out of the screen in an immersion technique and merges with the corneal spike (C) in a contact technique
C: The double-peaked corneal spike
P: A high-reflective spike from the anterior surface of the pseudophakic lens; it is usually followed by multiple smaller echospikes (M) that represent reverberations of the ultrasound beam between the anterior and posterior surfaces of the implant
R: The high-reflective retinal spike
S: The scleral spike
O: The orbital spikes

The axial length of a pseudophakic eye is calculated:

AL = MAL 1,532 + T (1 − 1,532/Vel)

where MAL 1,532 is the axial length measurement taken at a velocity of 1,532 m/s and T is the central

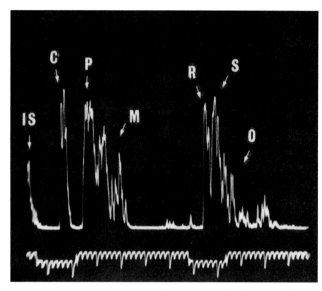

FIGURE 4.9. A-scan pattern of the pseudophakic eye. Identified are the initial spike (IS) and the spikes from the cornea (C), the pseudophakic lens (P), multiple reverberations (M), the retina (R), the sclera (S), and the orbital tissue (O).

thickness of the pseudophakic lens. If the measurement of the axial length is taken at a velocity of 1,550 m/s (MAL 1,550), it can easily be converted:

MAL 1,532 = (1,532/1,550) × MAL 1,550

The average sound velocities (VEL) and central thickness (T) of the different implants are as follows:

Implant	Sound Velocity	Central Thickness
PMMA	2,660 m/s	0.6 to 0.8 mm
Silicone	980 m/s	1.2 to 1.5 mm
Glass	6,040 m/s	0.3 to 0.4 mm
Acrylic	2,200 m/s	0.7 to 0.9 mm

Recommendations

If the eye is to be measured with an average sound velocity instead of using the preceding formula, the following values are recommended:

- 1,555 m/s for an eye with a PMMA IOL
- 1,476 m/s for an eye with a silicone IOL
- 1,549 m/s for an eye with a glass IOL
- 1,554 m/s for an eye with an acrylic IOL

If a pseudophakic eye is measured at the average phakic velocity of 1,553 m/s, the error is less than 0.1 mm for the eye with a PMMA, glass, or acrylic IOL. However, this error exceeds 1.0 mm for the eye with a silicone IOL.[26]

The Eye with Silicone-Filled Vitreous

In an eye where the vitreous is filled with liquid silicone,[27] the retinal echospike is small and difficult to display due to sound attenuation within the liquid silicone. The system sensitivity should be increased to better identify the retinal spike.

The measurement of such an eye is more difficult. The sound velocity in liquid silicone varies between 970 and 1,100 m/s, depending on the type and amount of silicone used. An average value of 990 m/s is used for calculation purposes. It would be best to measure each component of the eye separately for a more accurate result. This will require a measurement with an instrument that allows you to do so.

An average velocity for an eye where the vitreous cavity is filled with liquid silicone has been calculated to be 1,133 m/s. If the usual average velocity of 1,553 m/s is used instead of the calculated 1,133 m/s, the 23.5-mm eye will be measured as 33.2 mm—an error of over 8 mm.

Measuring the correct vitreous cavity's depth (VCD) needs some calculations because all ultrasound units measure it with a velocity of 1,532 m/s, and this measurement is not usually displayed on the screen. This value is calculated by subtracting the ACD and the lens thickness from the measured axial length (AL). However, since the vitreous cavity is filled with silicone oil, the true measurement of VCD has to be calculated using a velocity of 990 m/s:

$$\text{True VCD} = 990/1,532 \\ \times \text{VCD measured with 1,532 m/s}$$

The true VCD is then added to the lens thickness and the ACD to derive the true axial length.

This method can be used only if silicone fills the totality of the vitreous cavity. If silicone fills only part of the vitreous cavity, then separate measurements are needed.

Recommendations

- Compress the ultrasound scale for better visualization of the retinal echospike.
- Increase the system sensitivity if the retinal echospike is difficult to identify.
- Measure each eye component separately using the correct sound velocities.
- If these calculations are overwhelming, refer the patient to a center that is capable of doing them.

Calculating the Corneal Power for a Concurrent Keratotomy

Concurrent astigmatic keratotomy and implant surgery are being performed successfully to reduce the preex-isting astigmatism. Corneal topography will detect the correct amount of astigmatism and its axis prior to surgery.

Astigmatic keratotomy or peripheral relaxing incisions flatten the steep corneal meridian. This flattening is associated with a slight to moderate steepening of the cornea 90 degrees away. This is known as the coupling effect. If the amount of flattening is equal to the amount of steepening 90 degrees away, then the average K readings remain the same, and the power of the IOL remains the same. In fact, the amount of flattening slightly exceeds the amount of steepening, ending in a flatter cornea, which affects the IOL power calculations.

Ideally, the cornea is remeasured after the keratotomy and the IOL power is recalculated. However, if the microscope is not equipped with a keratometer or if the surgeon does not want to redo the calculations in the operating room, then the expected corneal curvature has to be calculated.

Recommendation

Subtract 0.25 diopter from the average preoperative K readings for every diopter of astigmatism to be corrected.

Clinical Application

Preoperative K readings: 41.00/45.00 diopters
Average preoperative K: 43.00 diopters
Plan: Astigmatic keratotomy to correct 4.00 diopters
Expected postoperative K: $43.00 - (0.25 \times 4) =$ 42.00 diopters

This last value of 42.00 diopters is used in the IOL power calculations.

Measuring of the Corneal Power after Corneal Refractive Surgery

Calculating the IOL power after corneal refractive surgery is more difficult than in normal eyes because of the changes that have occurred to the cornea and because the K readings do not accurately reflect the true power of the cornea.[28,29] Often, there is a discrepancy between the myopic correction achieved and the change in the keratometric readings.

Clinical Example

An eye with K readings of 45.00 diopters before RK had 5 diopters of myopia corrected at the cornea. After RK, one would expect readings of 40 diopters. Instead the keratometer gives an average reading of 41.5 diopters. The question becomes, which "K readings" have to be entered into the IOL power formula prior to the cataract surgery? Different methods are available to measure the corneal curvature.

The *"refractive history" method* is probably the easiest one. First, it is important to calculate the amount of correction at the cornea (Rc) from the correction obtained in the spectacle prescription (Rs). This is easily achieved with the formula: Rc = Rs/(1 − 0.012 Rs). If there is any astigmatism, the myopic correction is replaced by the spherical equivalent value. Find the K reading of the eye prior to the refractive surgery and subtract from it the correction obtained at the cornea by that surgery. This method requires obtaining the information from the surgeon who performed the surgery. Also, it is important not to include in the calculations any myopic changes caused by the cataract itself. Another drawback to this method is that the myopic correction achieved by the refractive surgery can change with time, and it is not unusual to notice a hyperopic shift a few years later.

The *"contact lens method"* is a more elaborate and more difficult way of measuring the corneal curvature. It consists in applying a hard contact lens with a known base curve to obtain the true corneal base curve. The patient is then overrefracted to obtain the true corneal power. Errors occur owing to refractive changes caused by the tear film layer (between the contact lens and the cornea) and by the cataract itself.

Recommendation

- The corneal power (K) to be used in the IOL power formula equals: (Prerefractive surgery K) − (Correction obtained by the refractive surgery at the corneal plane).
- The corneal power (K) to be used in the IOL power formula can be estimated if the prerefractive surgery K values are not available. It equals: (Measured postrefractive surgery K) − (0.25 × amount of myopia corrected by the refractive surgery). The patient can often produce the old glasses that he or she had used prior to the refractive surgery, or the information can be obtained from the patient's optometrist.

■ IOL Power Calculations in High Myopia

Highly myopic eyes present a certain challenge with IOL power calculations because of difficulties in axial length measurement, IOL power calculations, and the selection of the proper IOL.[30–32]

Difficulties in Axial Length Measurement

In axial myopia, the eye is quite elongated, with a possible staphyloma. The increase in the retinal curvature

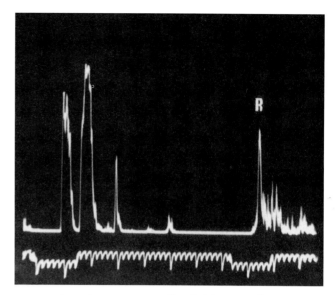

FIGURE 4.10. A-scan pattern of a phakic eye with a posterior pole staphyloma, yielding a measurement of 28.80 mm. Note the presence of a weak retinal spike (R) due to the increased curvature of the posterior pole.

in the posterior pole makes identification of the area relatively difficult. The retinal echospike has lower amplitude and is more difficult to display on the screen (Fig. 4.10). A B-scan ultrasound examination is recommended to rule out any vitreoretinal pathology (Fig. 4.11).

In the unsuspected case of unilateral axial myopia in which the cataractous eye is much longer than the opposite eye (by more than 3 mm), the technician will have difficulties in the measurements and might settle for an oblique measurement or, out of frustration, report a measurement equal to the normal fellow eye.

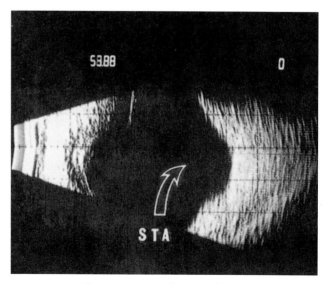

FIGURE 4.11. B-scan pattern showing the increased curvature of the posterior pole caused by the staphyloma (STA).

Difficulties in IOL Power Calculations

All available formulas are less accurate in long eyes than in normal eyes. It is always advisable to aim for − 0.50 diopter of myopia to keep a comfortable margin of error between plano and − 1.00 sphere, and to avoid any induced hypermetropia.

Difficulties in Selecting the Proper IOL

Myopes with a refraction ranging between − 1.00 and − 3.00 Sph usually use their prescription for distance vision and remove their glasses for reading, contrary to higher myopes and to hyperopes who are used to wearing their glasses for distance and reading.

Older sedentary patients usually prefer to remain near-sighted, while young, active myopes are more likely to request emmetropia. Surgeons should not aim for "bull's-eye" emmetropia, because they can push the patient into hyperopia in case of a minor error in IOL calculations. Instead, they should aim toward a − 0.50 to − 1.00 Sph, a refraction that most myopes seem to enjoy for distance vision and reading of large print.

In the presence of bilateral cataracts: Many surgeons will aim toward emmetropia or slight myopia.

In the presence of a monocular cataract in a myopic eye when the other eye is also myopic: Leaving the operate eye as myopic as before the surgery will avoid a significant degree of anisometropia and aniseikonia; however, the chance of correcting the preexisting myopia will be missed.

It is the dream of most young myopes to have clear uncorrected distance vision, and the surgeon should aim for emmetropia or slight myopia; however, this strategy will certainly create anisometropia in the fellow eye. This can be avoided by decreasing the myopia in the other eye with a contact lens, corneal surgery or by lensectomy.

In the presence of a monocular cataract in a myopic eye (− 2.00 to − 3.00 diopters) when the other eye is emmetropic: Bilateral axial length and corneal measurements will immediately establish whether the myopia is induced by the cataract; if so, the surgeon should aim for emmetropia. However, if the myopia is due to a longer axial length or steeper cornea, the patient could have been functioning with monocular vision using the emmetropic eye for distance and the myopic eye for reading. In such instances it might be wise not to aim for emmetropia but to leave the operate eye myopic. This will keep the status quo and a happy patient.

In the presence of unilateral axial myopia: Unilateral axial myopia is a rare congenital anomaly causing anisometropia and amblyopia in the affected eye. [33] It remains undetected throughout childhood; patients go to the ophthalmologist when they lose vision in the affected eye because of the cataract's progression. When the patient is examined for the first time, the myopia often is not detected, for two reasons: (1) the patient is not wearing the myopic correction because of associated anisometropia and amblyopia, and (2) the preoperative refraction is unreliable because of the opaque media.

Unilateral axial myopia causes unilateral visual deprivation during the critical first year of life. This will result in early amblyopia with a visual acuity of around 20/200. Surgery is recommended when the cataract becomes mature and visual acuity drops to light perception. It restores isometropia and partial vision, and increases the field of vision. One should not attempt to restore iseikonia; in these long eyes, iseikonia would have required a stronger IOL to be inserted during surgery, resulting in a high myopic correction postoperatively. The induced aniseikonia is not a problem because of the associated amblyopia.

■ IOL Power Calculations in Hyperopia

Hyperopic patients look forward to emmetropia after the cataract surgery. Older sedentary patients might even enjoy a certain degree of myopia.

In case of a unilateral cataract, the surgeon should definitely aim toward less hypermetropia and even emmetropia. The hypermetropia in the fellow eye could then be corrected with a contact lens, corneal surgery, or lensectomy.

In case of a very short or microphthalmic eye,[34] the axial length could be more difficult to measure. Also, in these short eyes, a l-mm error in axial length measurement causes a 3.0−3.5 diopters error, compared to 2.5 diopters in a normal eye. Compounding errors could be produced with the use of an SRK I or SRK II formula. The use of such linear formulas will cause errors up to 10 diopters, depending on how short the eye is.

■ IOL Measurements for Piggyback Implants

Piggyback implants are used whenever the first cataract surgery resulted in a significant refractive error or the IOL power calculations call for a stronger IOL power than what is actually available. The second implant is usually inserted in the bag or in the sulcus in front of the first implant.

The author has written new formulas to measure the power of the piggyback implant based on the nature of the refractive error (hyperopic or myopic) and on the A constant of the implant to be used.

In presence of a hyperopic (+) refractive error, the formula is:

$$P = \frac{Error\ (+)}{0.03\ (138.3 - A)} - 0.50$$

In presence of a myopic (−) refractive error, the formula is:

$$P = \frac{Error\ (-)}{0.04\ (138.3 - A)} - 0.50$$

These formulas will calculate the exact power of the piggyback implant needed for emmetropia.

■ IOL Power Selection in Children

At birth, the child's eye measures approximately 15 mm and increases rapidly to reach 21 mm by the age of 2 years. Thereafter growth continues at a much slower rate, with the eye reaching an average 23.5 mm in adulthood. Similarly, the cornea flattens from an average of 51 diopters to an average of 44 diopters between birth and age 2 years; the cornea flattens an additional 0.50 diopter by adulthood.

If surgery is done within the first 2 years of life and an implant is inserted, a large myopic shift is to be expected a few years later. This has led many surgeons to remove the cataract and fit the eye with a contact lens instead of inserting an IOL.

When surgery is performed after age 2 years, the expected myopic shift ranges from 4 to 6 diopters, as the axial length increases with time. Many surgeons recommend undercorrecting the IOL power by around 3 diopters to partially compensate for the myopic shift; any greater undercorrection would lead to an isometropia and would conflict with amblyopia treatment. The residual myopia in adulthood can be treated with spectacles, contact lenses, or corneal surgery.[35,36]

Axial length measurement might be a challenge in very young patients. If this is the case, the corneal power and the axial length should be measured under general anesthesia.

■ Summary

The selection of the proper IOL power prior to surgery is an important process and should not be rushed. It is best performed a few days before surgery and not at the last minute in the operating room.

Careful discussion with the patient will enlighten the surgeon as to the patient's expectations. Many patients know exactly what they want. On the other hand, some patients wish to leave the decision up to their ophthalmologist, and it becomes incumbent on the surgeon to make the proper decision.

Some ophthalmologists advocate emmetropia for all their patients, others routinely advocate slight myopia. Studies have shown that a small amount of myopic astigmatism can enhance the depth of focus of the pseudophakic eye, with adequate 20/30 visual acuity for both near and distance fixation, thus providing spectacle independence. However, not all eyes are the same, and certainly not all patients are. The surgeon should review the patient's needs and expectations, check whether the eye to be operated on is the dominant eye or not and the status of the fellow eye, determine the IOL power for emmetropia, isometropia, and iseikonia, and then choose the IOL power accordingly.

Patients' expectations usually coincide with their needs, and they should be accommodated accordingly. Active patients normally prefer emmetropia, while sedentary patients might prefer slight myopia. A patient with hyperopia will most certainly enjoy emmetropia, while a patient with high myopia might prefer to remain slightly myopic.

A patient's expectation can differ occasionally from his or her needs owing to a possible anisometropia or aniseikonia. This will happen if the fellow eye has normal vision with a certain degree of myopia or hyperopia. The situation is thoroughly discussed with the patient prior to surgery until an acceptable solution is reached.

■ References

1. Shammas HJ. *Atlas of Ophthalmic Ultrasonography and Biometry*. St. Louis, Mo: CV Mosby; 1984.
2. Thijssen JM. The emmetropic and iseikonic implant lens: computer calculation of the refractive power and its accuracy. *Ophthalmologica*. 1975;171:467–486.
3. Colenbrander MC. Calculations of the power of an iris clip lens for distance vision. *Br J Ophthalmol*. 1973; 57:735–740.
4. Fyodorov SN, Galin MA, Linksz A. Calculation of the optical power of intraocular lens. *Invest Ophthalmol*. 1975; 14:625–628.

5. van der Heijde GL. The optical correction of unilateral aphakia. *Trans Am Acad Ophthalmol Otolaryngol.* 1976; 81:80–88.

6. Binkhorst RD. The optical design of intraocular lens implants. *Ophthalmic Surg.* 1975;6:17–31.

7. Hoffer KJ. Accuracy of ultrasound intraocular lens calculation. *Arch Ophthalmol.* 1981;99:1819–1823.

8. Sanders DR, Kraff MC. Improvement of intraocular lens power calculation using empirical data. *Am Intraocular Implant Soc J.* 1980;6:263–267.

9. Sanders DR, Retzlaff J, Kraff MC. Comparison of empirically derived and theoretical aphakic refraction formulas. *Arch Ophthalmol.* 1983;101:965–967.

10. Hoffer KJ. Intraocular lens calculations: the problem of the short eye. *Ophthalmic Surg.* 1981;12:269–272.

11. Shammas HJF. The fudged formula for intraocular lens power calculation. *Am Intraocular Implant Soc J.* 1982; 8:350–352.

12. Binkhorst RD. *Intraocular Lens Power Calculation Manual: A Guide to the Author's TICC-40 Programs.* 3rd ed. New York: RD Binkhorst; 1984.

13. Sanders DR, Retzlaff J, Kraff MC. Comparison of the SRK II formula and the second-generation formulas. *J Cataract Refract Surg.* 1988;14:136–141.

14. Holladay JT, Prager TC, Chandler TY, et al. A three-part system for refining intraocular lens power calculations. *J Cataract Refract Surg.* 1988;14:17–24.

15. Retzlaff J, Sanders DR, Kraff MC. Development of the SRK/T intraocular lens implant power calculation formula. *J Cataract Refract Surg.* 1990;16:333–340.

16. Hoffer KJ. The Hoffer-Q formula: a comparison of theoretical and regression formulas. *J Cataract Refract Surg.* 1993;19:700–712.

17. Ossoinig KC. Standardized echography: basic principles, clinical applications and results. *Int Ophthalmol Clin.* 1979;19:127–210.

18. Shammas HJF. Axial length measurement and its relation to intraocular lens power calculations. *Am Intraocular Implant Soc J.* 1982;8:346–349.

19. Binkhorst RD. Biometric A-scan ultrasonography and intraocular lens power calculation. In: *Current Concepts in Cataract Surgery: Selected Proceedings of the Fifth Biennial Cataract Surgical Congress.* St. Louis, Mo: CV Mosby; 1987:175–182.

20. Coleman DJ, Carlin B. A new system for visual axis measurements in the human eye using ultrasound. *Arch Ophthalmol.* 1967;77:124–127.

21. Olsen T, Nielsen PJ. Immersion versus contact technique in the measurements of axial length by ultrasound. *Acta Ophthalmol.* 1989;67:101–102.

22. Shammas HJF. A comparison of immersion and contact techniques for axial length measurement. *Am Intraocular Implant Soc J.* 1984;10:444–447.

23. Pallikaris I, Gruber H. Determination of sound velocity in different forms of cataracts. *Doc Ophthalmol.* 1981; 29: 165–169.

24. Olsen T. Calculating axial length in the aphakic and pseudophakic eye. *J Cataract Refract Surg.* 1988;14:413–416.

25. Holladay JT, Prager TC. Accurate ultrasonic biometry in pseudophakia. *Am J Ophthalmol.* 1989;107:189–190.

26. Milauskas AT, Marney S. Pseudo axial length increase after silicone lens implantation as determined by ultrasonic scans. *J Cataract Refract Surg.* 1988;14:400–402.

27. Hoffer KJ. Ultrasound velocities for axial length measurement. *J Cataract Refract Surg.* 1994;20:554–562.

28. Holladay JT. IOL calculations following radial keratotomy surgery. *Refract Corneal Surg.* 1989;5:36.

29. Koch DD, Liu JF, Hyde LL, et al. Refractive complications of cataract surgery after radial keratotomy. *Am J Ophthalmol.* 1989;108:676–682.

30. Menezo JL, Cisneros A, Harto M. Extracapsular cataract extraction and implantation of a low power lens for high myopia. *J Cataract Refract Surg.* 1988;14: 409–412.

31. Shammas HJ. Spectacle correction desired after cataract removal. *J Cataract Refract Surg.* 1991;17:101–102.

32. Kora Y, Yagushi S, Inatomi M, et al. Preferred postoperative refraction after cataract surgery for high myopia. *J Cataract Refract Surg.* 1995;21:35–38.

33. Shammas HJ, Milkie CF. Mature cataracts in eyes with unilateral axial myopia. *J Cataract Refract Surg.* 1989; 15:308–311.

34. Shammas HJ. Axial length measurements and IOL power calculations in microphthalmic eyes. In: Sampaolesi R, ed. *Opththalmic Ultrasonography: Proceedings of the 12th SIDUO Congress. Doc Ophthalmol.* 1990;53:145–148.

35. Sinskey RM, Patel J. Posterior chamber intraocular lens implants in children: report of a series. *Am Intraocular Implant Soc J.* 1983;9:157–160.

36. Vasavada A, Chauhan H. Intraocular lens implantation in infants with congenital cataracts. *J Cataract Refract Surg.* 1994;20:592–598.

Part II

Cataract Surgery and Intraocular Lenses

Chapter 5

Techniques of Phacoemulsification Surgery*

Dimitri T. Azar and Shimon Rumelt

One of the most important advances in cataract surgery is the phacoemulsification technique. Extracapsular cataract extraction (ECCE) requires a relatively large wound and results in a long healing process and slow visual recovery. In contrast, phacoemulsification requires a smaller surgical wound, allowing a shorter healing process, less against-the-rule astigmatism, and more rapid visual recovery. Thus, it is not surprising that phacoemulsification was the preferred method for cataract extraction among the members of the American Society of Cataract and Refractive Surgery (86% in 1994).[1]

Cataract removal using phacoemulsification is achieved by ultrasonic fragmentation and aspiration of the lens material. The tip of the phacoemulsification handpiece is a hollow, roughly ~1-mm titanium needle that transmits vibrations at a high speed (30,000–60,000 cps) to emulsify the cataract.[2,3] The vibrations are transferred from piezoelectric or magnetostrictive crystals. The piezoelectric crystal is a solid crystal that contracts periodically in uniform fashion in response to a periodic electric field; the magnetostrictive crystal is formed of metallic material that expands and contracts in response to a magnetic field. The tip of the ultrasonic handpiece may have different bevel angles of 0 to 60 degrees or a double bevel-turbo. A 0-degree tip is easily occluded by the nucleus but is relatively difficult to pass through a small incision and to view during the emulsification. Soft nuclear material may be emulsified using small-angle tips (e.g., 15 degrees) that facilitate aspiration,[4] but larger bevels

(60 degrees) may be necessary for hard nuclei at the cost of easy occludibility.

The tip is vibrated forward repeatedly. The power by which emulsification occurs is determined by the amplitude of the tip movement. The frequency of the movement is predetermined. High amplitude can push the nucleus to such an extent that zonular integrity is endangered. The mechanisms of cataract destruction include acoustic shock waves, mechanical effects from the impact of the tip, the propagated fluid around it, and creation of a microvacuum around the tip (cavitation).[5] Nuclear fragments are aspirated through the hollow tip.[2] When the tip engages the lens material, a vacuum is created that facilitates aspiration of the lens material.

Three types of aspirating pumps are available in current phacoemulsification units: (1) The peristaltic pump employs rollers to squeeze a fluid column and move it from the handpiece to create the desired vacuum. (2) The Venturi pump creates a vacuum by blowing a gas stream across a port. (3) The diaphragmatic pump creates a vacuum by pulling a plunger (diaphragm) in a closed compartment attached to the aspiration tip. During the procedure, the aspiration should be sufficient to safely engage the nucleus to the tip without engaging the iris or the posterior capsule.

The tip of the ultrasonic handpiece is surrounded by a metal or plastic (polysulfone, polytetrafluoroethylene, or silicone) sleeve (Fig. 5.1). Irrigation fluid passes through the sleeve and exits through holes in its distal end. An irrigation bottle contains cold balanced salt solution (BSS) or BSS Plus (enriched with bicarbonate, dextrose, and glutathione, to better preserve the endothelium). Epinephrine, 0.3–0.5 mL of 1:1,000 solution, may be added to the 500-mL irrigation bottle to maintain mydriasis during the procedure. Antibiotics

*Modified from Azar DT, Rumelt S. Phacoemulsification. In: Albert DM, Jakobiec FA, eds. *Principles and Practice of Ophthalmology*. 2nd ed. Philadelphia: WB Saunders; 2000:1499–1514, with permission.

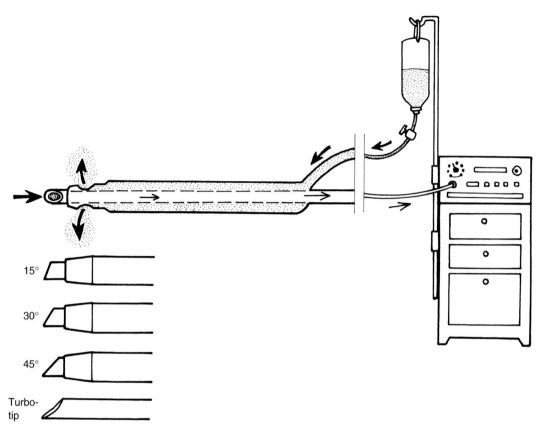

15°

30°

45°

Turbo-
tip

FIGURE 5.1. Schematic diagram of the phacoemulsification handpiece. *(From Azar DT, Rumelt S. Phacoemulsification. In: Albert DM, Jakobiec FA, eds.* Principles and Practice of Ophthalmology. *2nd ed. Philadelphia: WB Saunders; 2000:1501, with permission.)*

may also be added (4 mg/mL gentamicin or 10 mg/500 mL vancomycin). In most machines, a foot pedal controls irrigation (positions 0 and 1), aspiration (position 2), and power (position 3).

■ Indications and Contraindications

The indications for phacoemulsification are similar to those for other forms of cataract surgery. A history of a progressive decrease in visual acuity that interferes with the patient's activities is typical. Although recovery is faster after phacoemulsification, the risks of endothelial decompensation and posterior capsular tears may be greater, especially for the inexperienced surgeon. The ideal candidate is a patient with a mild to moderate nuclear cataract in an otherwise normal eye and with a well-dilated pupil (>6 mm). Relative contraindications to the procedure are dense nuclei (advanced nuclear sclerosis, brown or black cataract), endothelial dystrophies (Fuchs' and posterior polymorphous), and corneal grafts, which may lead to corneal endothelial decompensation. Corneal opacities may in-

terfere with adequate visualization, and a shallow anterior chamber may endanger the corneal endothelium if phacoemulsification is performed in the anterior chamber. Deep-set eyes may be associated with surgical difficulties. Phacoemulsification in these eyes may be facilitated by making a clear corneal incision. Iatrogenic tears in the posterior capsule may force the surgeon to convert to an ECCE. More experienced surgeons may still be able to continue phacoemulsification in such challenging situations.

Patient evaluation should include determination of best corrected visual acuity, assessment for other possible causes for decreased visual acuity, and a dilated fundus examination. The assessment should recognize disorders associated with weakness of the zonules, including trauma, pseudoexfoliation, and Marfan's and Weill Marchesani syndromes. Lens subluxation, pseudoexfoliation, iridodonesis, and phacodonesis should be documented. The size of the dilated pupil and the brightness of the fundus red reflex may also be helpful.

Patient satisfaction correlates with improvement in visual acuity and the elimination of preoperative glare.[6]

Patients with bilaterally similar preoperative visual acuities and postoperative improvement often report high satisfaction with the results of the first procedure. During the informed consent discussion, the patient is advised about other surgical alternatives and the need to minimize head movement during surgery.

■ Anesthesia

Several modes of anesthesia are available, including topical, subconjunctival, sub-Tenon's capsule, peribulbar, retrobulbar, and general (Table 5.1). The current trend is toward a technique associated with minimal complications, such as subconjunctival or topical anesthesia. Subconjunctival, sub-Tenon's capsule, and topical anesthesia are reserved for highly cooperative patients, since akinesia usually is not achieved. Topical anesthesia eliminates the complications associated with injection. The patient may not be patched at the completion of the surgery, and visual recovery is instant. The adverse reactions to topical anesthesia include some toxic effects on the corneal epithelium and the absence of akinesia. The least toxic agent is probably lidocaine.[7] The preferred anesthetic method is still retrobulbar anesthesia, followed by peribulbar anesthesia.[1] Patients undergoing cataract surgery should have an open vein line and cardiac monitoring; sedation is an additional option.

Topical anesthesia with proper sedation may be used alone or combined with intracameral injection.[8] The topical anesthetic agents include 0.5% proparacaine, 0.4% benoxinate, 4% cocaine, and 0.5% amethocaine (tetracaine). Their activity is usually limited to 15 minutes. Bupivacaine (0.75%) has longer activity. Usually 3–4 drops are instilled prior to surgery at 5-minute intervals, followed by 2–4 drops during surgery. Alternatively, a sponge soaked with 4% preservative-free lidocaine or 0.75% bupivacaine may be placed under the fornices and external pressure applied on the eyelids.[8] The sponge may be left in place for the entire procedure. Preservative-free lidocaine 1%, 0.5 mL, may be injected intracamerally with a 20-gauge needle.[9] Visual recovery and contrast sensitivity return to normal approximately 4 hours after the intracameral injection instead of almost immediately, as after topical anesthesia alone. Transient visual loss has been reported after posterior capsular tear in cases of intracameral lidocaine use. When topical anesthesia is being used, it is important to explain to the patient each step of the

Table 5.1
Modes of Anesthesia

	Advantages	Disadvantages	Indications	Contraindications
Topical	No perforation Rapid visual recovery No injection pain	No akinesia Some discomfort (pain)	Cooperative patient Adequate sedation Small-incision surgery	Uncooperative patient
Intracameral	Iris manipulation Less patient discomfort	No akinesia	Adjunctive to topical	Posterior capsular tear Corneal epitheliopathy
Subconjunctival	Supplemental anesthesia	No akinesia; chemosis	Cooperative patient; supplemental	Uncooperative patient
Peribulbar	Akinesia Avoids some retrobulbar complications	Complications: globe penetration, muscle injury		
Retrobulbar	Akinesia	Major complications: orbital hemorrhage, optic nerve/muscle injury	Bleeding dyscrasia	
General	Sparing patient cooperation	Anesthesia risks (e.g., malignant hyperthermia)	Pediatric and uncooperative patients	Systemic contraindications

procedure and the anticipated feeling. The microscope light should be increased gradually, and the irrigation fluid should be at room temperature. Manipulations of the globe should be avoided.

Subconjunctival or sub-Tenon's capsule anesthesia is performed with a 27-gauge needle.[10] Alternatively, a 19- to 23-gauge cannula may be used following dissection through the conjunctiva and Tenon's capsule about 6 mm from the limbus with Vannas scissors.[11] A sleeve of a vein line may replace a cannula for this purpose. The cannula allows continuous injection of anesthetic agent during the procedure. Circumferential perilimbal injection of diluted 4% lidocaine with a 30-gauge needle approximately 4 mm posterior to the limbus also results in excellent anesthesia during phacoemulsification.[12]

Peribulbar (periconal) anesthesia and akinesia are achieved by injecting 5–10 mL of anesthetic agent(s) in the periocular area with a 25- or 27-gauge needle.[13] A 1-inch (2.5-cm) needle is passed transcutaneously or transconjunctivally immediately above the inferior orbital rim at the juncture of the lateral third and medial two-thirds, and through the corresponding location of the superior orbital rim (Fig. 5.2). The needle is directed parallel to the adjacent orbital wall and should pass the

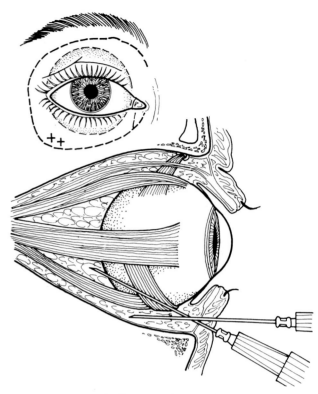

FIGURE 5.3. Retrobulbar anesthesia. The needle is introduced immediately superior to the lateral third of the inferior orbital rim. The needle is passed parallel to the orbital floor and angled superomedially immediately beyond the globe equator. *(From Azar DT, Rumelt S. Phacoemulsification. In: Albert DM, Jakobiec FA, eds.* Principles and Practice of Ophthalmology. *2nd ed. Philadelphia: WB Saunders; 2000:1502, with permission.)*

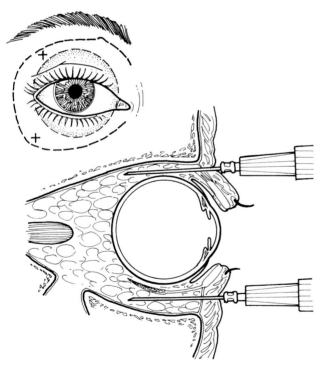

FIGURE 5.2. Peribulbar anesthesia. The needles are directed parallel to the orbital walls in the location corresponding to the superior and inferior lateral thirds of the orbital rim. The tip passes the globe equator. *(From Azar DT, Rumelt S. Phacoemulsification. In: Albert DM, Jakobiec FA, eds.* Principles and Practice of Ophthalmology. *2nd ed. Philadelphia: WB Saunders; 2000:1502, with permission.)*

plane of the globe equator. In some cases, injection in one quadrant is sufficient.[14] The temporal quadrants are preferred because of their relatively sparse blood and nerve supply. Some complications of retrobulbar anesthesia can be prevented, but globe penetration, peribulbar hemorrhage, and muscle injury can occur.

Retrobulbar anesthesia and muscle akinesia are achieved by injecting 4–5 mL of 2% lidocaine, 0.75% bupivacaine, or their equal mixture with a 25-gauge, 1.5-inch (37-mm) retrobulbar needle. Epinephrine, 0.1 mL of 1:1,000 solution, may be added to 20 mL of the anesthetic agent (final concentration, 1:200,000) to constrict local blood vessels and delay absorption of the anesthetics. Prior to injection, a topical anesthetic agent is applied and the patient is asked to look away from the needle. The injection is performed through the skin or the conjunctiva immediately above the inferior orbital rim at the juncture of the lateral third and middle two-thirds of the rim (Fig. 5.3).[15] The needle should be directed parallel to the bony orbit and, after it has passed the equator of the globe, toward the muscle cone. Anesthesia and akinesia are usually rapidly achieved, but possible complications include inadvertent penetration of the globe (especially in myopic eyes) or the optic nerve, injection of the optic nerve sheath, muscle injury, retrobulbar hemorrhage, oculocardiac reflex, and possible systemic toxic effects and allergic reaction. Before injecting, it is essential to pull the plunger to ascertain that there has been no penetration of a blood vessel.

In addition to these modes, general anesthesia may be used in children and in uncooperative patients (for example, patients with deafness, Parkinson's disease, or attention deficit disorder).

■ Surgical Techniques

Paracentesis

A paracentesis is performed to inject viscoelastic material or to insert an anterior chamber maintainer.[16] To place the maintainer, a paracentesis at the limbus is performed with an MVR (Stilleto) knife. The paracentesis is directed slightly posterior and obliquely to avoid flow toward the endothelium or the capsulorrhexis margins. The maintainer is open throughout the surgery. The height of the irrigation bottle is usually about 14 inches (35 cm), which corresponds to an intraocular pressure of 26 mm Hg. The bottle can be elevated if the anterior chamber shallows. Paracentesis is usually performed between 2 and 3 clock hours from the main incision to allow injection of viscoelastic agent or the introduction of a second instrument in a bimanual cataract extraction.

Planning the Scleral Tunnel Incision

The location, size, and configuration of the incision have important refractive consequences. The advantage of phacoemulsification is that small incisions can be used. Small incisions promote faster healing, minimize astigmatism, reduce potential infections, and allow rapid visual rehabilitation. Placing the incision on the steep meridian may reduce significant astigmatism. A temporal incision is usually used if against-the-rule astigmatism is noted before surgery. Access to the anterior chamber is more easily gained through a temporal incision because of the shallow lateral orbital wall. Additionally, fluid is easily drained via the lateral canthal angle. However, endothelial cell loss is higher with temporal incisions than with superior incisions.

Three types of external openings are possible: traditional curvilinear, straight, and frown incisions.[17] The curvilinear scleral and limbal incisions (circumlimbal) are parallel to the limbus. They offer the least support

to the wound. The opposite-shaped frown incision theoretically affords the greatest support and results in the least induced astigmatism. The ends of such incisions are swept away from the limbus. The straight incision shows some tendency to gape. The corneal induced astigmatism is in direct proportion to the cubic length of such incisions.[18] The astigmatism is also inversely proportional to the distance of a scleral incision from the limbus.

The internal opening into the anterior chamber also influences the induced astigmatism. A larger internal opening will increase the induced astigmatism. When the internal opening is in the cornea, anterior to the limbus, and the external opening is further posterior, the intraocular pressure may seal the opening. A self-sealed ("valve") internal opening improves wound stability, prevents aqueous leakage, and may obviate suturing the wound.

The scleral (or sclerocorneal) tunnel connecting the external and internal openings may have different configurations. A tunnel directed toward the anterior chamber will create a biplanar incision; a tunnel directed parallel to the surface will create a triplanar incision (Figs. 5.4 and 5.5).

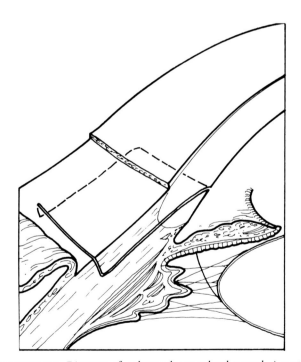

FIGURE 5.4. Diagram of a three-planar scleral tunnel. A vertical 300–500 μm incision is created and extended as a scleral tunnel parallel to the surface. The anterior chamber is penetrated by directing the blade posteriorly, creating the third plane. *(From Azar DT, Rumelt S. Phacoemulsification. In: Albert DM, Jakobiec FA, eds. Principles and Practice of Ophthalmology. 2nd ed. Philadelphia: WB Saunders; 2000:1503, with permission.)*

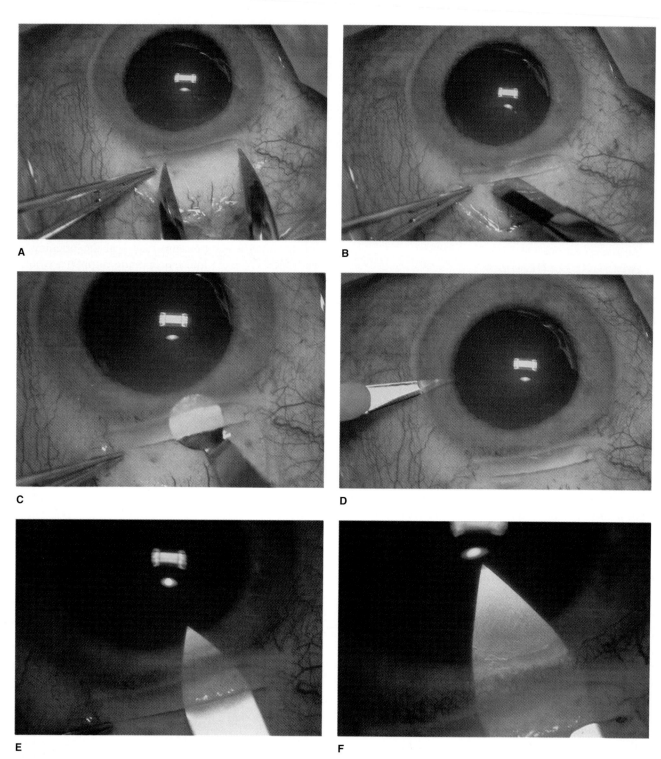

FIGURE 5.5. Scleral tunnel incision. *A,* The limbal incision is measured to accommodate the IOL. *B,* A limbal incision is made; this is considered the first plane. *C,* The second plane is dissected to clear the cornea without entering the anterior chamber. *D,* A paracentesis is created for injection of the viscoelastic and later the entry of the second instrument. This step is often performed prior to the limbal incision if a foldable lens is used. *E,* A keratome is used to enter the anterior chamber. By angling the keratome downward into the anterior chamber, the operator creates the third plane. *F,* Higher magnification view of the keratome entering the anterior chamber. *(Courtesy of Drs. R. Braunstein and W. J. Stark.)*

When a scleral tunnel is to be created, the incision usually requires raising a conjunctival fornix-based flap.[19] An external incision 1–4 mm posterior to the limbus is made with a no. 64 Beaver blade or a preset diamond blade perpendicular to the sclera up to a depth of one-third to one-half the scleral thickness. If the incision is too deep, the scleral tunnel should be continued more superficially, parallel to the surface. Although some surgeons may suture the incision and proceed with a new one, it is preferable to continue the tunnel in the same location, allowing for an adequately sealed incision. When the incision is too superficial, a buttonhole may result. The tunnel in this situation should be deepened, or a new location for incision may be selected. A bevel-up crescent knife is used to create the scleral tunnel parallel to the ocular surface. The tunnel is extended at least 1 mm in front of the corneal vascular arcade. The internal opening through the scleral tunnel is made with a keratome blade. The external lip of the wound can be grasped with forceps while the blade is wiggled in the tunnel and advanced 0.5–1 mm anterior to the limbal vascular arcade. The tip is turned posteriorly to dimple Descemet's membrane. The membrane folds, pointing to the tip, will be evident. These folds allow precise localization of the tip just before the anterior chamber is penetrated. The tip is advanced slowly with minimal posterior angulation in order to create a horizontal opening with a corneal lip of 1.0–1.5 mm.

Clear Corneal Incision

Clear corneal incisions do not require conjunctival dissection. They allow easier access of the phacoemulsification tip and more freedom for manipulations. The incisions are self-sealing and do not require sutures (Table 5.2). During tunneling, the globe may be stabilized by a limbal fixation ring (Mastel Instruments, Rapid City, SD), while a diamond keratome (corneatome) with a 90-degree tip, 45-degree shoulders, and double-beveled edges is entered obliquely just anterior to the limbal vascular arcade. The keratome is advanced approximately 2 mm and its tip is turned posteriorly while it is advanced to perforate Descemet's membrane (Fig. 5.6). The resultant 3-mm incision is sufficient for emulsification and foldable lens implantation.[20] A biplanar incision can be made by changing the angle of penetrance. The internal corneal lip should be at least 1.5 mm to serve as an internal valve. This small incision allows implantation of foldable lenses. The incision is easy to make and eliminates the need for a conjunctival flap and possible resultant bleeding. Manipulations with the phaco tip are facilitated, in contrast to a scleral tunnel incision, which limits lateral tip movement (Table 5.3).

A variant of this incision is the posterior limbal incision, which originates at the posterior limbus within the conjunctiva. The incision extends approximately 1.5–2.0 mm into the clear cornea. The total dimensions of the incision are 3.0 × 3.0 mm. The incision is created with a crescent knife held in an inverted position or with a preset diamond blade while the globe is stabilized. The knife is inserted vertically to a depth of one-third to one-half the scleral thickness. The tunnel is formed with a keratome blade. The instruments currently used for phacoemulsification are described elsewhere.[21]

The incision may enlarge accidentally during surgery.[22] An incision gauge is being designed to prevent this enlargement. Iris prolapse may also occur due to rapid escape of aqueous through the incision.[23] The probability of iris prolapse increases inversely to the fourth power of the radial distance between the iris

---

Table 5.2
Indications for a Clear Corneal Incision

Deep-set eyes
Prominent brow
Filtering bleb
Diffuse scleral thinning
Ocular cicatricial pemphigoid
Anticoagulation/bleeding disorders
Nanophthalmos/high myopia

From Azar DT, Rumelt S. Phacoemulsification. In: Albert DM, Jakobiec FA, eds. *Principles and Practice of Ophthalmology*. 2nd ed. Philadelphia: WB Saunders; 2000:1501, with permission.

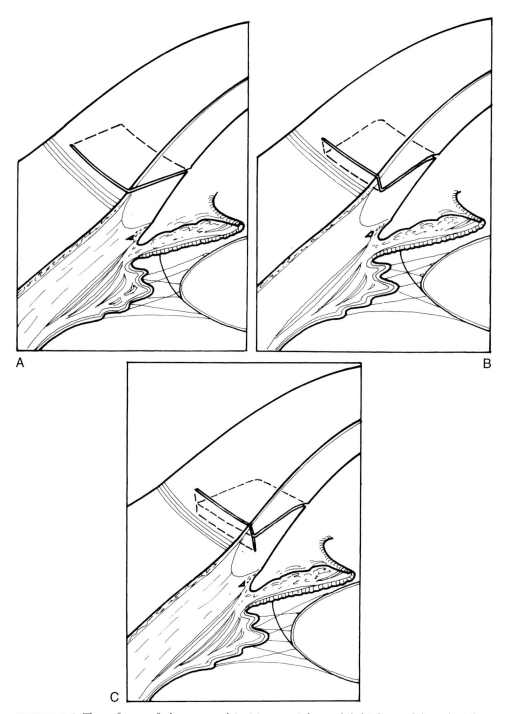

FIGURE 5.6. Three forms of clear corneal incisions: uniplanar *(A)*, biplanar *(B)*, and tripla-nar *(C)*. *(From Azar DT, Rumelt S. Phacoemulsification. In: Albert DM, Jakobiec FA, eds.* Principles and Practice of Ophthalmology. *2nd ed. Philadelphia: WB Saunders; 2000:1504, with permission.)*

and the incision site; thus, the probability is high in posterior internal openings. A paracentesis before pen-etrating the eye when creating the main incision may prevent iris prolapse. However, when prolapse occurs,

the iris may be repositioned and viscoelastic material may be injected. Injury to the iris may also be reduced by coating the tip of the instruments with viscoelastic material and employing low vacuum.

Table 5.3
Advantages and Disadvantages of a Clear Corneal Incision

Advantages
    No sutures
    Easy access with the phacoemulsification tip
    Conjunctival sparing
    No cautery
    Technically easy
Disadvantage
    Descemet's membrane tear

Adapted from Azar DT, Rumelt S. Phacoemulsification. In: Albert DM, Jakobiec FA, eds. *Principles and Practice of Ophthalmology*. 2nd ed. Philadelphia: WB Saunders; 2000:1504, with permission.

Capsulorrhexis

Capsulorrhexis denotes a circular central opening in the anterior capsule (Figs. 5.7 and 5.8). This continuous opening allows the elastic properties of the capsule to be used to express the nucleus from the capsular bag and to place an IOL in the bag without causing radial tears.[24] The radial discontinuity of the capsular opening in other methods ("can-opener" capsulotomy, linear capsulotomy, and capsulopuncture) increases the risk of tears. The tears may extend to the posterior capsule, increasing the likelihood of vitreous loss. The capsule is elastic and may be stretched up to 60% before a radial tear forms.[25] However, in the presence of a radial tear, stretching of the capsule will be transmitted to this focal area of least resistance and cause the tear to extend more radially and posteriorly. In addition, the zonules may be stretched 3.8 mm in middle-age eyes before breaking,[26] with stretchability decreasing by 1.0 mm per decade. These properties allow some degree of manipulation within the bag (e.g., IOL insertion) with greater safety.

Capsulorrhexis prevents rubbing of the iris against the IOL and the formation of posterior synechiae to the IOL (Table 5.4). Small capsular openings make it difficult to remove peripheral cortex and to insert an IOL. Small openings tend to seal and to form fibrous proliferation. With a larger rhexis, more epithelial cells are removed, so the likelihood of anterior proliferation decreases. If the rhexis is larger than the pupil diameter under dim illumination, glare can also be avoided.

Before a capsulorrhexis is performed, the lens stability is evaluated. The surgeon holds the tip of a bent needle or a cystotome against the anterior capsule, and tries to move the lens from side to side (rocking test). The globe is usually stabilized by grasping a paracentesis site or the limbus. The initial tear in the anterior capsule is made near the center to increase the distance of the initial flap from the lens equator.[24] It also allows completion of the rhexis from outside in, eliminating radial discontinuities. A cystotome or a 27- or 30-gauge bent needle at a right angle away from the bevel is introduced into the anterior chamber through a paracentesis or the main incision. The cystotome or needle may be attached to a 3-mL syringe containing a viscoelastic agent. The needle punctures the anterior capsule and sweeps in a curvilinear fashion, passing the center and slashing laterally and circumferentially to create a large capsular flap (Fig. 5.7). The capsular flap is held against the nucleus with the needle tip and is pulled 45 degrees toward the center (45 degrees to the planned course of the rhexis). The needle should always be kept near the edge of the advanced tear (about 1.0 mm from it), especially if radial extension is noted. The needle should be adjusted to this position every 30–45 degrees. If the tear extends to the periphery, the pulling should be changed more toward the center. If a radial tear forms, a flap can be raised with the needle from the tear by making a nick in the flap in the desired position. When there is minimal capsular support to continue the rhexis in the same direction, it may be better to start the rhexis on the other free edge of the capsule in the opposite direction.

Tearing by shearing is produced by folding the flap over the capsule and holding it against the intact capsule while pushing it backward parallel to the planned rhexis (i.e., circumferentially). As the rhexis advances, it may tend to extend further peripherally due to centrifugal forces. Every 1–1.5 hours the position of the needle is changed to be near the advancing edge (approximately 1.0 mm). The extension should not be more than 4 mm from the center, since the zonules may reach this point and capsulorrhexis would

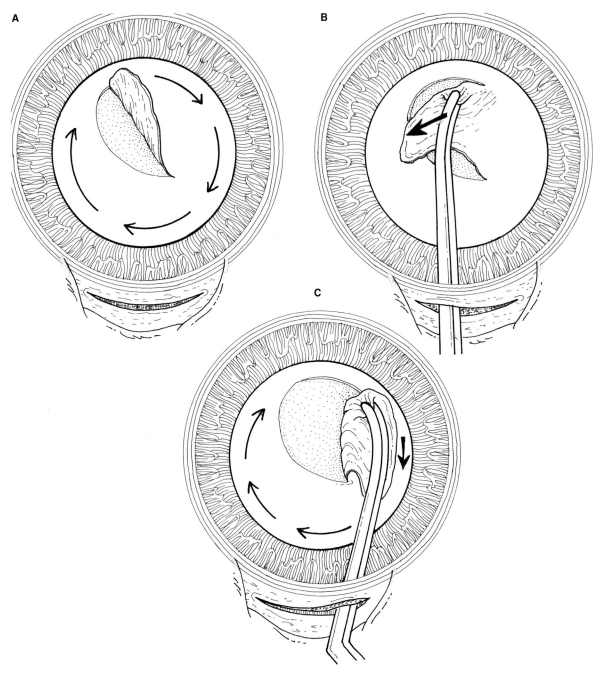

FIGURE 5.7. Stages in capsulorrhexis. *A,* Preparation of anterior capsular flap. *B,* Capsulorrhexis by traction. The forceps pull the flap 45 degrees to the limbus. *C,* Capsulorrhexis by shearing. The flap is flipped and pulled in the direction of the required rhexis (parallel to the limbus). *(From Azar DT, Rumelt S. Phacoemulsification. In: Albert DM, Jakobiec FA, eds.* Principles and Practice of Ophthalmology. *2nd ed. Philadelphia: WB Saunders; 2000:1505, with permission.)*

be impossible. The shearing technique is better controlled than the tearing technique. These maneuvers may also be performed with capsulorrhexis forceps. Shearing the capsule is easier with forceps. The tear direction is monitored and viewed during the capsulorrhexis. Usually a capsulorrhexis of 4.5–5 mm is sufficient to insert an unfoldable implant with a 6.0–7.0 mm optic. The calculated capsulorrhexis diameter when stretched was found to be $2 \times \text{IOL diameter}/\pi$ in order to place nonfoldable lenses in the bag.[27]

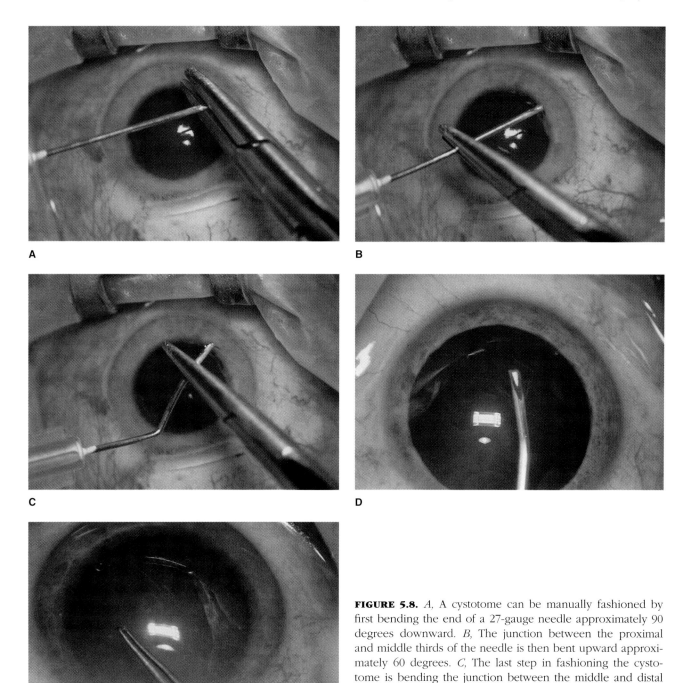

FIGURE 5.8. *A,* A cystotome can be manually fashioned by first bending the end of a 27-gauge needle approximately 90 degrees downward. *B,* The junction between the proximal and middle thirds of the needle is then bent upward approximately 60 degrees. *C,* The last step in fashioning the cystotome is bending the junction between the middle and distal thirds of the needle approximately 15–20 degrees. *D,* The cystotome is used to puncture the anterior lens capsule and begin the capsulorrhexis. *E,* The capsulorrhexis is completed with a Utrata forceps. *(Courtesy of Drs. R. Braunstein and W. J. Stark.)*

In mature or dense subcapsular cataract, the red reflex may be absent and the edge of the capsulorrhexis difficult to visualize. Visualization can be improved by using oblique rather than coaxial illumination. The microscope is focused on the anterior capsule under high magnification. If the margin of the rhexis is still invisi-

ble, injection of 0.05 mL of 10% sodium fluorescein or ICG into the bag will stain the capsule and enhance the view of the rhexis.[28] Hypermature cataract may release soft cortical material into the anterior chamber when the anterior capsule is punctured. Spreading of the material in the anterior chamber may be limited by the

Table 5.4
Advantages of a Capsulorrhexis

Less risk of radial tears and vitreous loss
Possibility of stretching the capsule by 60%
In-the-bag phacoemulsification
In-the-bag IOL implantation

From Azar DT, Rumelt S. Phacoemulsification. In: Albert DM, Jakobiec FA, eds. *Principles and Practice of Ophthalmology.* 2nd ed. Philadelphia: WB Saunders; 2000:1505, with permission.

viscoelastic agent. However, if spreading occurs, the material may be aspirated using the irrigation/aspiration tip prior to continuation of the capsulorrhexis. A posterior capsulorrhexis is the procedure of choice in central posterior capsular tear or posterior polar cataract (posterior capsule plaque) and in certain pediatric patients to avoid late opacification of the capsule.

Hydrodissection and Hydrodelineation

Hydrodissection is the separation of the softer outer nucleus (epinucleus) from the cortex or the whole nucleus from the capsule.[29,30] Hydrodelineation is the separation of the epinucleus from the harder central nucleus (endonucleus) by fluid wave. The successful performance of these maneuvers depends on an intact capsulorrhexis (Table 5.5).

Hydrodissection is performed by injecting BSS under the anterior capsular rim. A 26- or 27-gauge blunt cannula attached to a 2-mL syringe is placed under the capsular rim and advanced toward the equator (Figs. 5.9 and 5.10). Continuous slow irrigation will propel the fluid wave toward the equator and beneath the posterior capsule in the plane of least resistance. Injection of approximately 1 mL into the four quadrants will mobilize the lens within the capsular bag. Injection toward the entry port can be performed through the paracentesis site with a 180-degree Binkhorst cannula.

Hydrodelineation is performed with the same cannula. The cannula's tip, pointing at the equator, is introduced into the nucleus, beneath the soft outer layers and the anterior capsular rim. Fluid injection will separate the epinucleus from the endonucleus. In some cases a circumferential golden ring will appear.

Following complete hydrodissection and hydrodelineation, the nucleus can be rotated within the capsular bag. Rocking the nucleus from side to side with a bent needle helps ascertain its mobility. Hydrodissection and hydrodelineation reduce the nucleus volume for emulsification. The epinucleus protects the capsule from being caught by the phaco tip. However, hydrodelineation leaves cortical material within the bag, and this should be aspirated later. Hydrodissection alone usually leaves no material within the bag and is useful in planned ECCE or in emulsification of soft nuclei. Viscodissection (injection of a viscoelastic agent) is effective for hard nuclei, but more force may be required to inject the agent.[31]

Nucleofracture Techniques

There are numerous ways to remove the endonuclei. All are based on sculpting (central crating or grooving), fracturing into several segments while rotating the nucleus within the bag, and emulsifying each fragment.[32] Surgeons may combine different techniques,

Table 5.5
Advantages of Hydrodissection

Release of cortical-capsular adhesions
Rotation of the lens in the bag
Cushion effect of the fluid (posterior capsule protection)
Nucleus isolation (hydrodelamination)

From Azar DT, Rumelt S. Phacoemulsification. In: Albert DM, Jakobiec FA, eds. *Principles and Practice of Ophthalmology.* 2nd ed. Philadelphia: WB Saunders; 2000:1505, with permission.

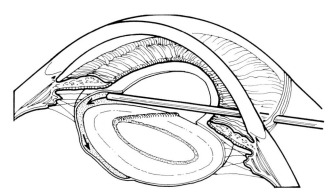

FIGURE 5.9. Hydrodissection and hydrodelineation. A 26-gauge needle is introduced under the anterior capsular rim (hydrodissection) and at the junction of the epinucleus and the nucleus (hydrodelineation), and approximately 1 mL of BSC is slowly injected. *(From Azar DT, Rumelt S. Phaco-emulsification. In: Albert DM, Jakobiec FA, eds.* Principles and Practice of Ophthalmology. *2nd ed. Philadelphia: WB Saunders; 2000:1506, with permission.)*

convert from one to another, and apply their own techniques. It is advisable to start the emulsification at lower power than that anticipated for the specific nucleus in order to avoid capsular tear or sudden anterior chamber collapse and tissue incarceration.

Nucleofracture and emulsification are usually done with high irrigation (high bottle), 50% emulsification power, and moderate aspiration. Emulsification adjacent to the capsule is safer with low vacuum and low power (approximately 10%). The setting may be changed according to the instrument, the nucleofracture technique, and the consistency of the cataract. A safer approach is using a zero vacuum by disconnecting the aspiration line.[33] The irrigated fluid maintains positive pressure in the anterior chamber, and the excess fluid exits via the disconnected aspiration tube. This approach is valuable in cases of zonular dehiscence or iris prolapse. Recently, reverse flow sculpting has been suggested.[34] The irrigation fluid is transferred through the phaco tip while the aspiration is performed through the sleeve. At 70% of maximal linear power, 12–14 mL/min flow, and a vacuum of 80 mm Hg, it is possible to perform deep sculpture up to the capsule without the need for mechanical cracking. The risk of aspirating the capsule or the iris is reduced, since the inflow pushes the capsule away and creates a focal hydrodissection.

Removal of the nucleus is usually performed in the bag (endocapsular; Figs. 5.11 and 5.12) but may be performed in the anterior or posterior chamber following dislocation of the nucleus (extracapsular).[35] When the emulsification is performed in the anterior cham-

ber, the endonucleus is lifted anteriorly and toward the incision from the distal side. An iris hook stabilizes the endonucleus and prevents contact with the cornea. The endonucleus is removed from the equator of the lens rather than from the center. This technique reduces the risk of posterior capsule tears but increases the risk of endothelial cell loss due to the contact between the endothelium and the nucleus or the phaco-emulsification tip.

Divide and Conquer

A large central crater is made through the capsulorrhexis with the phaco tip.[36] The central nucleus is shaved with a 30- to 45-degree phaco tip. The depth of the tip can be estimated by the change in the fundus red reflex.

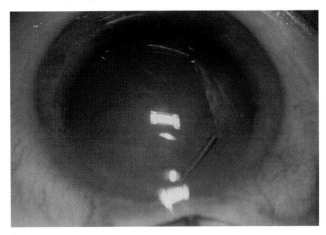

A

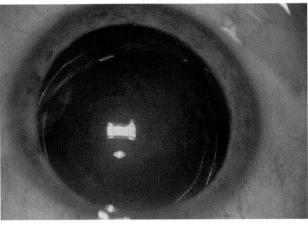

B

FIGURE 5.10. *A,* Hydrodissection is done by injecting balanced salt solution under the tip of the capsulorrhexis into the capsular bag. *B,* After successful hydrodissection, the nucleus and cortex are clearly visible. *(Courtesy of Drs. R. Braunstein and W. J. Stark.)*

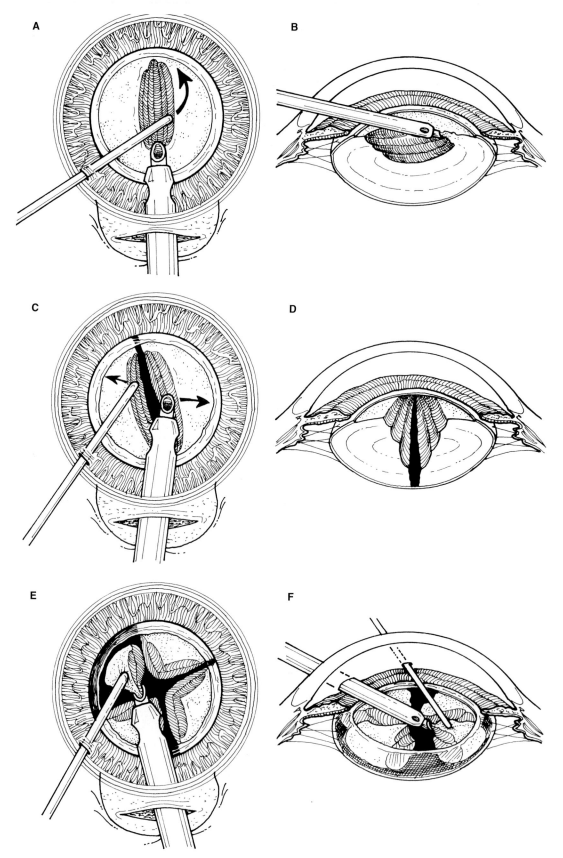

FIGURE 5.11. In situ nucleofracture. Two perpendicular deep grooves are created in the nucleus (*A* to *D*) and each quadrant is phacoemulsified (*E, F*). *(From Azar DT, Rumelt S. Phacoemulsification. In: Albert DM, Jakobiec FA, eds. Principles and Practice of Ophthalmology. 2nd ed. Philadelphia: WB Saunders; 2000:1507, with permission.)*

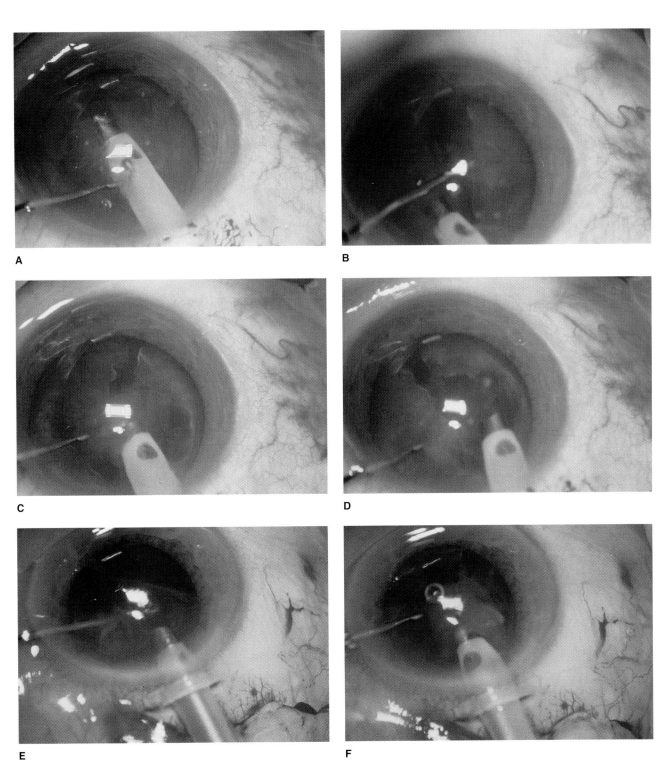

FIGURE 5.12. Nucleofracture technique in situ. *A,* A deep groove is made along the center of the cataract. *B,* The nucleus is cracked by pushing apart the inner sides of the grooved cataract using the phaco tip and the second instrument. *C* and *D,* Additional cracking and debulking are done on each half of the nucleus. *E* and *F,* The remaining nuclear fragments are phacoemulsified and aspirated using the phaco tip. *(Courtesy of Drs. R. Braunstein and W. J. Stark.)*

The surgeon follows the open end of the tip. The sculpted nucleus is fractured bimanually with the phaco tip and a second instrument (cyclodialysis spatula or Sinskey hook). The two instruments anchor the sculpted rim in opposite directions and are slowly pulled apart (Figs. 5.11 and 5.12). The instruments should be positioned close to each other and opposite the entry port. The nucleus is rotated 90 degrees and another crack is created. When this is performed, there is a risk of capsular tear. Individual wedge-shaped sections are brought into the center of the rhexis for emulsification.

In Situ Fracture

Two perpendicular grooves are made with a 30- or 45-degree phaco tip.[37] Each longitudinal groove goes from the entry port to the opposite side through the capsulorrhexis (Fig. 5.13). The nucleus is rotated 90 degrees and a second, slightly deeper groove is sculpted. Then the phaco tip is held against the wall of the groove, a

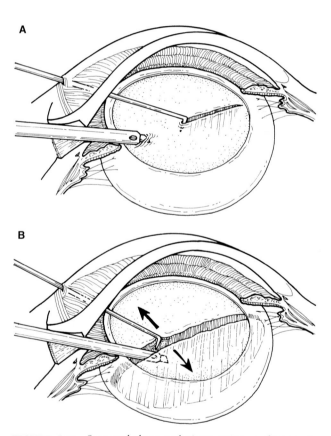

FIGURE 5.13. Stop-and-chop technique using a chopper to break the nucleus. *A,* The chopper engages the distal portion of the nucleus while the phacoemulsification tip stabilizes the proximal portion of the nucleus. *B,* The chopper is pulled toward the phacoemulsification tip, breaking the nucleus. *(From Azar DT, Rumelt S. Phacoemulsification. In: Albert DM, Jakobiec FA, eds.* Principles and Practice of Ophthalmology. *2nd ed. Philadelphia: WB Saunders; 2000:1507, with permission.)*

spatula is held against the other wall, and a crack is formed by moving these instruments in opposite directions. Alternatively, a nuclear cracking forceps with broad, flat tips is used to break the endonucleus. The cross-action handle of the forceps does not cause stretching of the incision, and the forceps control the fracturing better and yield reproducible results. They minimize the risk of capsule tears and do not require deep grooves. Each quadrant is manipulated to the center of the bag and emulsified.

Chip and Flip

Following hydrodelineation, the central endonucleus is sculpted.[38] A cyclodialysis spatula or other hook is used to pull the endonucleus toward the entry port, and the distal part of the endonucleus is emulsified. The endonucleus is rotated and pulled again toward the entry port while this maneuver is repeated. The rest of the endonucleus, which includes the central and posterior portions, is elevated with a second instrument and emulsified. The epinucleus is removed by pulling it with the phaco tip placed opposite the entry port and near the rhexis margin and flipping it with the second instrument.

Crack and Flip

The crack-and-flip technique is a combination of hydrodissection and hydrodelineation, in situ fracture, and chip-and-flip techniques.[39] Two perpendicular grooves are sculpted in the central nucleus and the nucleus is cracked into quadrants. The apex of each quadrant is elevated with the phaco tip and a spatula to engage it in the tip. Segments of hard nuclei may be subdivided with a phacoemulsification tip and a chopper. The small fragments are brought to the phaco tip with a chopper and removed at the level of the capsulorrhexis with low power (10–20%). The epinucleus, which serves as a cushion, is removed by flipping as described previously.

Mini-Lift or No-Lift Multiple Rotations

The mini-lift or no-lift technique is effective for soft lens material.[40,41] Central sculpting is performed. The nuclear rim at the opposite side of the entry port is nipped away from side to side for 4 clock hours with brief bursts of 50% of maximal energy. The nucleus is rotated within the bag and emulsification is repeated. The remaining posterior nuclear disc is elevated with a cyclodialysis spatula and removed by emulsification.

Phaco Chop and Stop-and-Chop Phacoemulsification

The phaco chop technique allows nuclear splitting by engaging the phaco tip in the nucleus at the 12 o'clock rhexis.[42] The phaco tip stabilizes the nucleus while a chopper (a modified lens hook with 1.5-mm 90-degree bent blunt tip) is pulled through the nucleus from the distal end of the rhexis toward the phaco tip (Fig. 5.13). The maneuver can be repeated by rotating the nucleus.

The stop-and-chop technique is similar to the phaco chop technique. A groove is sculpted starting at the middle of the nucleus and ending at the distal edge of the capsulorrhexis or beneath it. Central nuclear sculpting is added in cases of a hard endonucleus. The groove serves as a site for fracture by the phaco tip and the chopper. The instruments are engaged within the walls of the groove and are pulled in opposite directions. The nucleus is rotated and additional sequential breaks as described for the phaco chop technique are made. Each pie-shaped fragment is emulsified before initiating a new break. In this way there is a space in the bag for safer emulsification and removal of the residual fragments.

Victory Groove Phacoemulsification

A V-shaped groove is made in the nucleus.[34] The tip of the V is directed toward the entry port. The nucleus is fractured along its grooves. The pie-shaped wedge is emulsified with the phaco tip in the central portion of the capsulorrhexis. The other two fragments are mobilized into the center and removed. The technique may shorten the operating time.

Cortical Aspiration

With successful hydrodissection, the cortex may be completely separate from the capsule. If a cortical shell is left, it can be teased along the capsulotomy, engaged with the phaco tip, and aspirated (foot pedal in

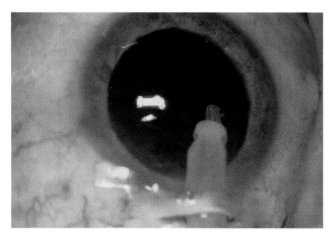

FIGURE 5.14. The cortex is aspirated using the aspiration tip. *(Courtesy of Drs. R. Braunstein and W. J. Stark.)*

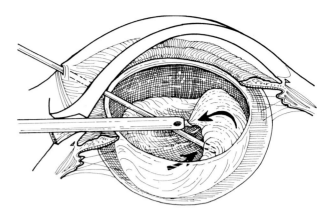

FIGURE 5.15. Removal of the cortex bimanually (cortical bowl) with the phacoemulsification tip and a second instrument. The cortex is engaged with the phacoemulsification tip and flipped with the second instrument. A modification of this technique involves using an aspirating tip as a second instrument to remove subincisional cortex while using the I-A tip for irrigation. *(From Azar DT, Rumelt S. Phacoemulsification. In: Albert DM, Jakobiec FA, eds. Principles and Practice of Ophthalmology. 2nd ed. Philadelphia: WB Saunders; 2000:1508, with permission.)*

position 2) with an aspiration/irrigation tip. The material may be flipped with a second instrument (spatula or cannula) (Figs. 5.14 and 5.15). A 90- or 180-degree curved irrigation/aspiration tip may be used to remove the cortical remnants near the entry port.

Cortex adherent to the posterior capsule is removed by polishing the capsule with a 27-gauge capsular polisher, cannula tip, or the irrigation/apsiration tip.[43] When an irrigation/aspiration tip is used, it is preferable to avoid aspiration and to use the tip as a purely mechanical instrument. Equatorial cortex may be removed following IOL implantation. The IOL distends the bag and keeps the posterior capsule at a distance. The cortex is aspirated with the irrigation/aspiration tip facing the cortex near the edge of the capsulorrhexis.

■ Intraocular Lens Implantation

Viscoelastic material is injected into the anterior chamber, but not directly into the bag, to avoid its entrapment behind the IOL, maintain a deep anterior chamber, and protect the endothelium. If viscoelastics are not used, an anterior chamber maintainer may be used with the bottle in low position. Nonfoldable lenses are made of polymethyl methacrylate (PMMA). The polymer of methylacrylic acid methylester has a refractive index of 1.49 and specific gravity of 1.19 g/mL. The optic size varies from 4.5 to 7.5 mm and the overall diameter (including haptics) from 11.0 to 13.0 mm. Lenses of 11.0–12.0 mm are placed in the bag; 12.5–13.0 mm lenses are placed in the ciliary sulcus. When these lenses are implanted, the incision should be enlarged and the major advantages of the small cataract incision are lost (see Fig. 6.1).

Foldable lenses may be preferred for small incisions. Three types are currently being used: silicone, hydrogel, and acrylic. Silicone has a silicone-oxygen backbone (siloxane) with organic groups attached to the silicone atoms. The side chains determine some of the lens properties (e.g., refractive index).[44] Silicone lenses are available from Allergan, Staar, IOLAB, and Bausch and Lomb Surgical (see Chapter 3).

Hydrogel lenses are usually made of polyhydroxyethyl methacrylate (poly-HEMA). The lenses are rigid in the dehydration state but swell extensively (> 20%) and become soft on contact with water.

Acrylic lenses are cross-linked copolymers of acrylic acids. Acrylic lenses are available from Alcon (Acrysof) (refractive index 1.55)[45] and Ioptex (refractive index 1.47, specific gravity 1.18 g/mL). The high refractive index of these materials allows the production of a thinner optic and reduces the likelihood of iris chafing and posterior synechia formation. The lenses are comparable to PMMA lenses in the rate of posterior capsule opacification (PCO) and damage by Nd:YAG capsulotomy.[46]

The main advantage of foldable lenses is that a large optic can be implanted through a small wound of 2.5–3.5 mm. Decentration of lenses with larger optic would not cause exposure of optic edge and glare.

Foldable lenses are stable and resist hydrolytic and oxidative degradation. The lenses, especially acrylic ones, may cause less inflammatory response and less debris deposition on the lens. Since these lenses also adhere less to the surrounding ocular tissues, they may be easier to explant. They may cause less trauma to the endothelium than the rigid nonfoldable lenses. The main disadvantage of foldable lenses is the unknown long-term in vivo behavior. There is a potential risk of biodegradation and discoloration, especially with hydrogel and silicone lenses.[47–50] These lenses may absorb dye (e.g., fluorescein) and change color. Silicone lenses have a higher tendency to stimulate PCO and increased damage when Nd:YAG capsulotomy is performed.[48] For these reasons, acrylic (Acrysof) and PMMA lenses are preferred over silicone lenses in diabetic and young patients.

Following insertion of the IOL, it is essential to remove the viscoelastic agent in order to avoid postoperative intraocular pressure spikes. BSS injection through the paracentesis and allowing free flow of the vis-

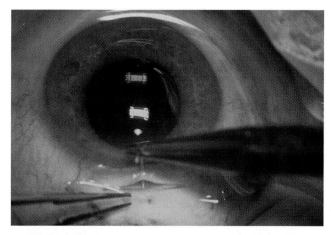

FIGURE 5.16. Scleral tunnel incisions are often closed using single interrupted nylon 10-0 sutures. *(Courtesy of Drs. R. Braunstein and W. J. Stark.)*

coelastic through the main incision may not be sufficient. Irrigation and aspiration of the viscoelastic material may be the only way to minimize residual viscoelastic. Viscoelastic agent trapped between the implant and the posterior capsule may cause a myopic shift. This may be ameliorated by puncture of the posterior capsule beyond the optic margin.

The incisions are usually watertight and self-sealed. The intraocular pressure seals the corneal flanges. The corneal wound and the paracentesis may be hydrated by injecting BSS into the stroma surrounding the opening. A gap in a scleral incision may be closed by horizontal, radial, vertical mattress, or X 10-0 nylon suture (Fig. 5.16). The suture is placed above the scleral tunnel and not at the external wound edge. A horizontal suture is preferred over a radial suture; if radial sutures are used, adequate suture tension should be achieved to minimize astigmatism. The conjunctival incision is closed with cautery prior to subconjunctival injections (Fig. 5.17).

Tight sealing is confirmed during surgery by drying the wound and observing leaking when the intraocular pressure is increased. The seal may also be confirmed with the Seidel test, but this test should not be used with hydrogel or silicone lenses because of the risk of IOL staining. Steroids or nonsteroidal anti-inflammatory agents (diclofenac, flurbiprofen, indomethacin) are used to reduce postoperative inflammation.

■ One-Handed versus Two-Handed Phacoemulsification

Phacoemulsification can be performed using one or two hands. The two-handed technique requires an ad-

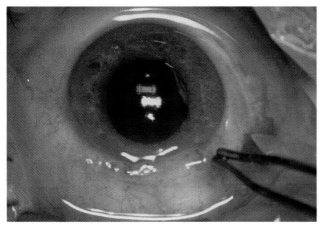

A

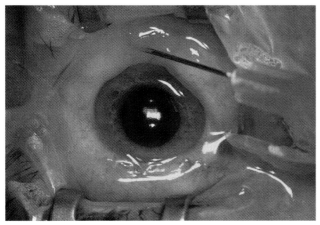

B

FIGURE 5.17. *A,* After the operator confirms that the wound has no leaks, the conjunctiva is cauterized to close it. *B,* A combination of steroid and antibiotic is often injected subconjunctivally in the inferior bulbar conjunctiva. This step may be omitted if topical anesthesia has been used or in the presence a filtering bleb. *(Courtesy of Drs. R. Braunstein and W. J. Stark.)*

ditional opening, usually up to 90 degrees from the main incision. It allows somewhat more control and additional manipulations with a second instrument to break the nucleus, direct nuclear fragments toward the phacoemulsification tip, retract and protect the posterior capsule, and so on. The one-handed technique uses only one intraocular instrument at a time, fewer maneuvers, and fewer entries and exits. The incision is watertight. The one-handed technique may not be suitable for a long operation, hard nuclei, and eyes with poor zonular support. It usually requires more viscoelastic material and more irrigation. The hydrodissection may be performed following central sculpting to avoid nucleus rotation during sculpting.

■ Challenging Situations

Miotic Pupil

A miotic pupil without posterior synechiae or pupillary membrane may be enlarged by stretching.[51] Two instruments, an iris hook and a Lester lens manipulator, are introduced into the anterior chamber. Both may be inserted through the main incision or may be introduced through a paracentesis 1 to 3 clock hours from the incision. One instrument retracts the pupil margin toward the entry port while the other pushes the opposite side of the pupil margin (see Chapter 8). The maneuver is performed slowly for a period of 10–20 seconds, and the stretched position is maintained for 5–10 seconds and repeated perpendicular to the original maneuver. The maneuver causes microsphincterotomies and should be avoided in rubeotic irises. A viscoelastic agent may be injected at the pupil plane to maintain its size.

Alternatively, iris retractors can be positioned in the four quadrants.[52,53] Flexible nylon retractors with adjustable silicone retaining sleeves are easier to manipulate than rigid titanium retractors. The retractors are introduced into the anterior chamber through paracenteses to retract the pupil margin. The paracenteses are made at the anterior limbus with slight posterior declination, so that when the retractors are introduced into the anterior chamber, they will point to the pupil margin. Retraction of the pupil is performed slowly to a diameter of 5.0–5.5 mm. Overstretching should be avoided since it may result in an atonic pupil, chronic inflammation, cystoid macular edema, pigment deposition, or pupillary capture.

An iris ring made of hydrogel (Grieshaber, Schaffhausen, Switzerland) is a compact oval instrument in its dehydrated form. It is inserted through the main incision and placed in the pupillary plane. Upon contact with aqueous humor, the ring expands and captures the pupil margin. Another pupil expander made of silicone is available. It may be inserted following retraction of the proximal pupil margin with an iris-glide retractor.[54] The folded expander is loaded on an insertion spatula so that its folded end extends just beyond the spatula tip. The spatula is placed into the anterior chamber on its side and then rotated 90 degrees. The folded tip of the expander engages the distant margin of the iris and the bulged tabs of the folded expander engage the proximal stretched side of the pupil. The instrument is then withdrawn, allowing the expander to expand (see Chapter 8). An iris spatula is inserted through the paracentesis to hold the expander in place while the iris-glide is removed. Two hooks are placed in the two tabs at the base of the expander to stretch the strab. After insertion of the IOL, the strab is folded inward with an iris hook, lifting the expander and removing it from the eye. Iris retractors or rings are useful in rubeotic irises. They provide a constant pupillary diameter and protect the pupillary margin from the phaco tip.

The pupil may be dilated by various surgical techniques, but this should not be done in the presence of rubeotic irises, chronic uveitis, or coagulopathy. Multiple sphincterotomies may be performed with Vannas scissors. They should not exceed the sphincter muscle width, so as to avoid an atonic pupil. Alternatively, sector iridectomy can be performed and approximated following IOL implantation with a 10-0 nonabsorbable (polypropylene) suture. The suture may be passed through the clear cornea to approximate the free edges of the iridectomy. The suture ends are cut short to prevent contact with the endothelium. The suture restores the normal appearance and function of the sphincter.

Posterior synechiae and a pupillary membrane, which may be evident in eyes with a history of intraocular inflammation (uveitis, rubeosis iridis), are dissected with an iris spatula or bent needle, placed beneath the pupil margin, and swept circumferentially.

Subluxated Lens

Zonular weakness in the absence of clinical evidence of lens subluxation can be confirmed by punching the anterior capsule with a bent needle and rotating the lens from side to side. If the zonules are weak, the lens will move. The movement is directly related to the degree of zonular dehiscence and is greatest opposite the area of dehiscence. This intraoperative test is useful in planning surgery.

A larger capsulorrhexis is performed under a viscoelastic agent in the anterior chamber and over the area of dehiscence. The capsulorrhexis starts in the direction opposite the intact zonules to provide counteraction. The phaco and the irrigation/aspiration tips should be directed toward the weaker side. Therefore, the incision site should be made in the axis of the intact zonules. Viscodissection and viscodelamination are usually effective. If the lens cannot be reached from the intact site, the incision can be made in the weak area. A suture may be passed horizontally along the dehiscent equator to stabilize the lens. Low infusion, low aspiration (25 mL/min), and low vacuum (10 mm Hg) may be employed to remove the endonucleus. The bag may be inflated with viscoelastic material to facilitate IOL insertion. A second instrument such as a spatula may be used to tent the capsule toward the weak area.

An endocapsular ring may be introduced into the capsular bag to prevent it from collapsing and to allow cortex removal and safe IOL implantation.[55] The ring is inserted, then the epinucleus is removed, and the leading haptic of the IOL is inserted into the bag toward the zonular dehiscence. The haptics are oriented in the axis of the zonular dehiscence. The endocapsular ring is left in the bag after IOL implantation.

■ Complications of Phacoemulsification

Various complications have been encountered during cataract surgery. Some are particularly relevant to phacoemulsification (Table 5.6).

A tear in Descemet's membrane may be caused by the phacoemulsification tip or other instrument.[56] It may be prevented by coating the tip with a viscoelastic agent and directing it posteriorly. Small detachments may resolve spontaneously. Large tears may result in corneal edema of the corresponding area of the exposed stroma. They should be repositioned with air or a viscoelastic bubble injected toward the rolled edge. Single 10-0 nylon sutures may be passed through the full corneal thickness to anchor the detached Descemet's membrane. The sutures are removed later. Viscoelastic agent may become trapped under the Descemet's membrane flap. In this case the material usually fails to resorb, and a corneal puncture is required to evacuate it.

Anterior chamber collapse may occur for various reasons.[57] These include insufficient flow (due to phaco sleeve compression, a low bottle, or tube blocking), excessive outflow (a large incision), imbalance between inflow and outflow (high vacuum after occlusion of the phacoemulsification port), and globe compression (by instruments inserted through a long scleral tunnel). Anterior chamber collapse may be prevented by the use of a low vacuum and aspiration rate.

Posterior Capsular Tear

Posterior capsular tears may occur at any stage of the procedure but are more common during cortex removal and nucleofracture. A small radial posterior capsular tear may be covered with viscoelastic material, and then emulsification may proceed. If the tear involves the center of the capsule, a posterior capsulorrhexis may be performed. Lenses with flexible haptics such as a three-piece PMMA lens or a three-piece silicone or acrylic lens are used. When there is some anterior capsular support, a lens of more than 12.5 mm diameter may be placed in the ciliary sulcus. It should have a large optic so that if decentration occurs, the optic margins will not be exposed. When there is no capsular support, an anterior chamber lens is usually preferred over a ciliary sulcus

Table 5.6
Common Complications of Phacoemulsification and Their Management

Complication	Prevention	Management
Descemet's membrane tear	Direct keratome posteriorly	Recognize
	Apply viscoelastic agent	Inject air bubble or viscoelastic agent into anterior chamber
	Use sharp instrument	Suture tear
Posterior capsular tear	Apply viscoelastic agent	Inject viscoelastic agent
	Use smaller capsulorrhexis	Redirect capsulorrhexis
	Use low vacuum	Initiate new capsulorrhexis
	Use second instrument	Use Vannas cutting instrument
		Convert to "can-opener" capsulotomy
Iris prolapse	Create anterior incision	Release speculum and bridle suture
		Direct phaco tip posteriorly
		Use low irrigation
		Perform iridectomy

Adapted from Azar DT, Rumelt S. Phacoemulsification. In: Albert DM, Jakobiec FA, eds. *Principles and Practice of Ophthalmology.* 2nd ed. Philadelphia: WB Saunders; 2000:1512, with permission.

scleral-fixated lens, because it is associated with fewer complications. In some cases, when a radial tear extends beyond the equator, it may be necessary to convert to "can-opener" capsulotomy and perform iris-plane phacoemulsification or ECCE.

Nucleus Dislocation

Nucleus dislocation occurs in 0.3% of procedures.[58] It is more prevalent after ocular trauma and in pseudoexfoliation syndrome, systemic disorders (e.g., Marfan's syndrome), and eyes with hard nuclei that are difficult to remove. Such eyes require optimal akinesia and maximal dilation.

Dislocation of the nucleus into the vitreous cavity results in chronic uveitis in approximately 90% of cases and glaucoma and corneal edema in approximately 50%.[58,59] When lens material is floated in the vitreous, it is usually cortex and can be aspirated, but when it falls onto the retinal surface, it is usually dense nucleus. The surgeon should not be tempted to chase this material because of the increased risk of retinal detachment. The remaining cortex should be cleaned carefully, and an anterior vitrectomy with preservation of the capsule remnants may be performed. An anterior or posterior chamber IOL may be placed unless the hard lens is to be retrieved later through the pupil.

A three-port pars plana vitrectomy is performed for the retained lens particles within 1–3 days, before the development of uveitis and glaucoma. The objective of the vitrectomy is to mobilize the fragments into the middle vitreous cavity and emulsify them. Perfluorocarbone liquid is used to float dropped nucleus. Small fragments are not removed with perfluorocarbone since they may slip over the bubble toward the periphery. The outcome of pars plana vitrectomy is usually good, and visual acuity improves to 20/40 or better in approximately 70% of the patients.[59]

■ Outcome of Phacoemulsification

A visual acuity of 20/40 or better was reported in 92.6% of eyes treated by phacoemulsification performed by third-year residents.[60] Posterior capsular rupture occurred in 9.9% and vitreous loss in 5.5%. The 4-year incidence of retinal detachment following phacoemulsification was 1.17%, compared to 0.9% with ECCE and 1.55% with ICCE.[61] Endophthalmitis was reported in 0.12% of the patients undergoing phacoemulsification or ECCE and in 0.17% of the ICCE patients.[62] The risk increased fourfold when vitreous loss required anterior vitrectomy. No difference in postoperative corneal edema requiring corneal transplantation was reported with different extraction techniques.[63]

■ Current Trends and Alternative Approaches

Several instruments have been designed to reduce the risk of damage to the intraocular tissues, especially the posterior capsule. A handpiece with an ultrasonic cannula was introduced to facilitate hydrodelineation and hydrodissection and to soften hard nuclei (HydroSonics, Alcon Surgical, Fort Worth, TX).[64,65]

A Waterjet device (Pulsatome, Surgijet, Norcross, GA) is an alternative instrument.[66] It is connected to a 2.9-mm tip consisting of two hollow concentric needles. The inner needle supplies a Waterjet; the outer needle aspirates the fluid. The aspiration rate can be adjusted, but the Waterjet is set at 1,000 lb/inch.[2]

Laser fragmentation by Nd:YAG laser (1,064 nm, 250 mJ per pulse, He:Ne aiming beam) is a recent development.[67,68] The instrument (Photon Laser Phacolysis System, Paradigm Medical Industries, Salt Lake City, UT) delivers laser energy through a fiberoptic located in a titanium probe to the nucleus. The shock waves propagate and exit through the tip port, which also aspirates the fragments. This nonvibrating tip allows safer removal of the nucleus and decreases potential damage to the iris or posterior capsule. The diameter of the laser tip is smaller than the phacoemulsification tip and requires a smaller incision (1.6–1.9 mm). The system is air-cooled and the probe is less heated. In the future, other lasers may be used (Er:YAG or Excimer).

Cataract removal using a vortexing approach has also been shown to reduce the time of lens emulsification. This approach, known as catarax surgery, involves making a tiny capsulorrhexis peripheral opening in the anterior lens capsule followed by coupling of the vortexing tip and aspirating the lens contents while maintaining a formed lens bag throughout the procedure. This technique is under investigation by Bausch and Lomb Surgical, but results of clinical studies are not out at the time of this writing.

An alternative for endonucleus removal is manual phacofragmentation instead of phacoemulsification.[69] All stages of phacoemulsification are performed except the use of the phacoemulsifier. Following hydrodissection and hydrodelineation, the endonucleus is brought into the anterior chamber using hooks and is fragmented manually with a bisector. The smaller fragments are removed through the incision.

The nucleus may also be removed by selective hydroexpression (mini-nuc).[70] Following capsulorrhexis, the exposed soft cortex and epinucleus are aspirated with a 4.0-mm cannula up to the level of the hard endonucleus. The endonucleus is released by hydrodelamination and advancement of the 27-gauge cannula under the hard nucleus. The nucleus may be fractured in the anterior chamber and delivered using a plastic glide. The rest of the cortex and the epinucleus are aspirated manually. This method carries the risk of a posterior capsular tear when the cannula is introduced beneath the endonucleus.

■ Future Developments

The ultimate goal of cataract surgery is to replace the cataract with an IOL that can maintain the functions of the normal crystalline lens, including transparency and accommodation. Future procedures may include endocapsular cataract removal through a small capsular puncture by laser or an ultrasonic device[71] to allow retention of the entire capsular bag. Intracapsular injection of antimetabolites such as cyclosporine or 5-fluorouracil may inhibit proliferation of lens epithelial cells. Then a monomer, which can polymerize within the bag without heat release, may be injected. Such a lens substitute should have good elasticity without leakage from the bag following polymerization. A small capsular opening and intracapsular antimetabolites may not be required if a polymerized IOL with high compliance via hinged plate haptics becomes available.

■ References

1. Leaming DL. Practice style and preferences of ASCRS members: 1994 survey. *J Cataract Refract Surg.* 1995; 21:378–385.
2. Allen ED. Understanding phacoemulsification. I. Principles of the machinery. *Eur J Implant Refract Surg.* 1995; 7:247–250.
3. Kelman CD. Phacoemulsification and aspiration. *Am J Ophthalmol.* 1967;64:23–35.
4. Welch CL, Lindstrom RL. Phacoemulsification. In: Lindquist TD, Lindstrom RL, eds. *Ophthalmic Surgery.* St. Louis, Mo: CV Mosby; 1990.
5. Pacifico RL. Ultrasound energy in phacoemulsification: mechanical cutting and cavitation. *J Cataract Refract Surg.* 1994;20:338–341.
6. Study qualifies quality of life after cataract surgery. *Ocular Surg News.* 1996;14(3):32–33.
7. Marr WG, Wood R, Senterfit L, et al. Effect of topical anesthesia on regeneration of corneal epithelium. *Am J Ophthalmol.* 1957;43:606–610.
8. Kershner RM. Topical anesthesia for small incision self-sealing cataract surgery: a prospective evaluation of the first 100 patients. *J Cataract Refract Surg.* 1993; 19:290–292.
9. Anesthesia update. *Ocular Surg News.* 1996;14(5):28–32.
10. Anderson CJ. Subconjunctival anesthesia in cataract surgery. *J Cataract Refract Surg.* 1995;21:103–105.
11. Stevens JD. Curved sub-Tenon cannula for local anesthesia. *Ophthalmic Surg.* 1993;24:121–122.
12. Anderson CJ. Circumferential perilimbal anesthesia. *J Cataract Refract Surg.* 1996;22:1009–1012.

13. Wang HS. Peribulbar anesthesia for ophthalmic procedures. *J Cataract Refract Surg.* 1988;14:441–443.
14. Bloomberg LB. Administration of periocular anesthesia. *J Cataract Refract Surg.* 1986;12:677–679.
15. Hamilton RC. Retrobulbar block revisited and revised. *J Cataract Refract Surg.* 1996;22:1147–1150.
16. Chawla HB, Adams AD. Use of anterior chamber maintainer in anterior segment surgery. *J Cataract Refract Surg.* 1996;22:172–177.
17. Koch PS. Structural analysis of cataract incision construction. *J Cataract Refract Surg.* 1991;17:661–667.
18. Samuelson SW, Koch DD, Kuglen CC. Determination of the maximal incision length for true small-incision surgery. *Ophthalmic Surg.* 1991;22:204–207.
19. Fine IH. Architecture and construction of a self-sealing incision for cataract surgery. *J Cataract Refract Surg.* 1991;17:672–676.
20. Fine IH. Clear corneal incisions. *Int Ophthalmol Clin.* 1994;34:59–72.
21. Guide to hand-held cataract instruments. *Ocular Surg News.* 1996;14(5):44–57.
22. Steinert RF, Deacon J. Enlargement of incision width during phacoemulsification and folded intraocular lens implant surgery. *Ophthalmology.* 1996;103:220–225.
23. Allan BDS. Mechanism of iris prolapse: a qualitative analysis and implications for surgical technique. *J Cataract Refract Surg.* 1995;21:182–186.
24. Gimbel HV, Neuhann T. Development, advantages, and methods of the continuous circular capsulorrhexis technique. *J Cataract Refract Surg.* 1990;16:31–37.
25. Assia EI, Apple DJ, Tsai J, et al. The elastic properties of the lens capsule in capsulorrhexis. *Am J Ophthalmol.* 1991;111:628–632.
26. Assia EI, Apple DJ, Morgan RC, et al. The relationship between the stretching capability of the anterior capsule and zonules. *Invest Ophthalmol Vis Sci.* 1991;32:835–839.
27. Arshinoff A. Mechanics of capsulorrhexis. *J Cataract Refract Surg.* 1992;18:623–628.
28. Hoffer KJ, McFarland JE. Intracameral subcapsular fluorescein staining for improved visualization during capsulorrhexis in mature cataracts [letter]. *J Cataract Refract Surg.* 1993;19:566.
29. Koch DD, Liu JF. Multilamellar hydrodissection in phacoemulsification and extracapsular cataract extraction. *J Cataract Refract Surg.* 1990;16:559–562.
30. Fine IH. Cortical cleaving hydrodissection. *J Cataract Refract Surg.* 1992;18:508–512.
31. Bellucci R, Morselli S, Pucci V, et al. Nucleus viscoexpression compared with other techniques of nucleus removal in extracapsular cataract extraction with capsulorrhexis. *Ophthalmic Surg.* 1994;25:432–437.
32. Cataract techniques allow surgeon better control. *Ophthalmol Times.* 1996;21(30):28–30.
33. Viscoelastic, zero vacuum help cataract surgeons cope with complications. *Ocular Surg News.* 1996;14(3):29.
34. Kelman CD. Reverse-flow victory groove phacoemulsification explained. *Ocular Surg News.* 1996;14(6):30–31.
35. Kelman CD. Phacoemulsification in the anterior chamber. *Ophthalmology.* 1979;86:1980–1982.

36. Gimbel HV. Divide and conquer nucleofracture phacoemulsification: development and variations. *J Cataract Refract Surg.* 1991;17:281–291.
37. Shepherd JR. In situ fracture. *J Cataract Refract Surg.* 1990;16:436–440.
38. Fine IH. The chip and flip phacoemulsification technique. *J Cataract Refract Surg.* 1991;17:966–971.
39. Fine IH, Maloney WF, Dillman DM. Crack and flip phacoemulsification technique. *J Cataract Refract Surg.* 1993;19:797–802.
40. Davidson JA. No lift capsular bag phacoemulsification and dialing technique for no-hole intraocular lens optics. *J Cataract Refract Surg.* 1988;14:346–349.
41. Davidson JA. Bimodal capsular bag phacoemulsification: a serial cutting and suction ultrasonic nuclear dissection technique. *J Cataract Refract Surg.* 1989;15:272–282.
42. Koch PS, Katzen LE. Stop and chop phacoemulsification. *J Cataract Refract Surg.* 1995;20:566–570.
43. Mathey CF, Kohnen TB, Ensikat HJ, et al. Polishing methods for the lens capsule: Histology and scanning electron microscopy. *J Cataract Refract Surg.* 1994;20: 64–69.
44. Boretos JW. *Concise Guide to Biomedical Polymers.* Springfield, IL: Charles C Thomas; 1973.
45. Anderson C, Koch DD, Green G. Alcon AcriSoft acrylic intraocular lens. In: Martin RG, Gills JP, Sanders DR, eds. *Foldable Intraocular Lenses.* Thorofare, NJ: Slack; 1993: 161–177.
46. Oshika T, Suzuki Y, Kizaki H, et al. Two year clinical study of a soft acrylic intraocular lens. *J Cataract Refract Surg.* 1996;22:104–109.
47. Metha KR, Sathe SN, Karyekar SD. The soft intraocular implant. In: Trevor-Roper PD, ed. *The Cornea in Health and Disease. Sixth Congress of the European Society of Ophthalmology.* London, England: Royal Society of Medicine; 1981:859–863.
48. Newmann AC, McCarty DF, Osher RH. Complications associated with Staar silicone implants. *J Cataract Refract Surg.* 1987;13:653–636.
49. Oh KT, Oh KT. Optimal folding axis for acrylic intraocular lenses. *J Cataract Refract Surg.* 1996;22:667–670.
50. Lindstrom RL. Foldable intraocular lenses. In: Steinert RF, ed. *Cataract Surgery: Technique, Complications, and Management.* Philadelphia: WB Saunders; 1995:279–294.
51. Shepherd DM. The pupil stretch technique for miotic pupil in cataract surgery. *Ophthalmic Surg.* 1993;24: 851–852.
52. Nichaminin LD. Enlargement of the pupil for cataract extractions using flexible nylon iris retractors. *J Cataract Refract Surg.* 1993;19:795–796.
53. Masket S. Avoiding complications associated with iris retractor use in small pupil cataract extraction. *Cataract Refract Surg.* 1996;22:168–171.
54. Graether JM. Graether pupil expander for managing the small pupil during surgery. *J Cataract Refract Surg.* 1996;22:530–535.
55. Cionni RJ, Osher RH. Endocapsular ring approach to the subluxated cataractous lens. *J Cataract Refract Surg.* 1995;21:245–249.
56. Walland MJ, Stevens JD, Steele AD, et al. Repair of Des-

cemet's membrane detachment after intraocular surgery. *J Cataract Refract Surg.* 1995;21:250–253.

57. Cionni RJ, Osher RH. Intraoperative complications of phacoemulsification surgery. In: Steinert RF, ed. *Cataract Surgery: Technique, Complications, and Management.* Philadelphia: WB Saunders; 1995:327–340.

58. Lambrow F, Stewart M. Management of dislocated lens fragments during phacoemulsification. *Ophthalmology.* 1992;99:1260–1262.

59. Kim JE, Flynn HW Jr, Smiddy WE, et al. Retained lens fragments after phacoemulsification. *Ophthalmology.* 1994;101:1827–1832.

60. Cruz OA, Wallace GW, Gay CA, et al. Visual results and complications of phacoemulsification with intraocular lens implantation performed by ophthalmology residents. *Ophthalmology.* 1992;99:448–452.

61. Javitt JC, Vitale S, Canner JK, et al. National outcomes of cataract extraction. I. Retinal detachment after inpatient surgery. *Ophthalmology.* 1991;98:895–902.

62. Javitt JC, Vitale S, Canner JK, et al. National outcomes of cataract extraction. II. Endophthalmitis following inpatient surgery. *Arch Ophthalmol.* 1991;109:1085–1089.

63. Canner JK, Javitt JC, McBean AM. National outcomes of cataract extraction. III. Corneal edema and transplant following inpatient surgery. *Arch Ophthalmol.* 1992;110:1137–1142.

64. Brint SF, Blaydes JE, Bloomberg L, et al. Initial experience with the HydroSonics instrument to soften cataracts before phacoemulsification. *J Cataract Refract Surg.* 1992;18:130–135.

65. Anis AY. Hydrosonic intracapsular piecemeal phacoemulsification or "HIPP" technique. *Int Ophthalmol.* 1994; 18:37–42.

66. Cataract waterjet being readied for FDA trials. *Ocular Surg News.* 1996;14(5):35.

67. Laser cataract system vies for domestic, international market. *Ocular Surg News.* 1997;15(1):27.

68. Guide to ophthalmic lasers. *Ocular Surg News.* 1997; 15(1):28–34.

69. Kansas PG, Sax R. Small incision cataract extraction and implantation surgery using a manual phacofragmentation technique. *J Cataract Refract Surg.* 1988;14:328–330.

70. Blumenthal M, Ashkenazi I, Assia E, et al. Small-incision manual extracapsular cataract extraction using selective hydrodissection. *Ophthalmic Surg.* 1992;23:699–701.

71. Hara T, Hara T. Endocapsular phacoemulsification and aspiration (ECPEA): Recent surgical technique and clinical results. *Ophthalmic Surg.* 1989;20:469–475.

Chapter 6

Intraocular Lens Implantation During Cataract Surgery

Stephen U. Stechschulte, Robert T. Ang, and Dimitri T. Azar

Since Harold Ridley's first bold step of intraocular lens (IOL) implantation in 1949, the shape of the lens, the material used for the lens, and surgical techniques have undergone many modifications and improvements.[1] Consequently, the goal of almost all modern cataract surgery is the safe implantation of an IOL that maximizes vision for the lifetime of the patient. In nearly all cases a posterior chamber intraocular lens (PCIOL) is implanted through a small incision after phacoemulsification or through a larger extracapsular wound and placed within the lens capsule.

Several difficulties encountered during surgery and preceding IOL implantation, such as a dense nucleus not responding to phacoemulsification, anterior capsular rents, posterior capsule tears, vitreous prolapse and loss, hyphema, and a dropped nucleus, can influence if or how an IOL is implanted. If the complications are managed properly and if preparations for the IOL implantation are performed properly, certain techniques can be used to ensure IOL implantation with excellent postoperative visual outcomes. The surgeon may use an anterior chamber intraocular lens (ACIOL), place a PCIOL in the bag or sulcus, or suture the superior haptic (a safety suture) or both haptics to the iris or sclera. Alternatively, a surgeon faced with a choroidal hemorrhage or overwhelming vitreal pressure may close the wound and plan for implantation at a later date. How one implants a lens after uncomplicated and complicated surgery and which type of lens one uses in each situation are the subject of this chapter.

■ IOL Implantation After Uncomplicated Phacoemulsification

In the past 15 years cataract surgery has evolved to the point that more than 90% of cases are performed with phacoemulsification and end with the implantation of a foldable PCIOL.[2] The development of phacoemulsification by Charles Kelman made small incisions possible. Small incisions were of little value, however, without small lenses (Fig. 6.1). Consequently, the interest in phacoemulsification waned until smaller, pliable lenses became available.[3]

Silicone elastomers were first used to make foldable lenses and have the longest record of use.[3] They have been implanted in over 1.5 million eyes worldwide. These lenses are very pliable and easy to fold and unfold. First-generation lenses have a tendency to spring open when released from the forceps or injector. These lenses can be used safely if they are unfolded slowly once inside the eye. Reports of capsule rupture secondary to a lens springing open have prompted the use of silicone elastomers that unfold more slowly. Silicone lenses and forceps must be kept dry prior to insertion. These lenses become very slippery and difficult to handle if wet. They have optic diameters between 5.5 and 6.5 mm and, when folded, can be implanted through incisions of 4.0 mm. The optic diameter of some lenses, reduced to 5.5 mm, allows smaller incision lengths but increases the risk for edge glare and halos in patients with large pupils.

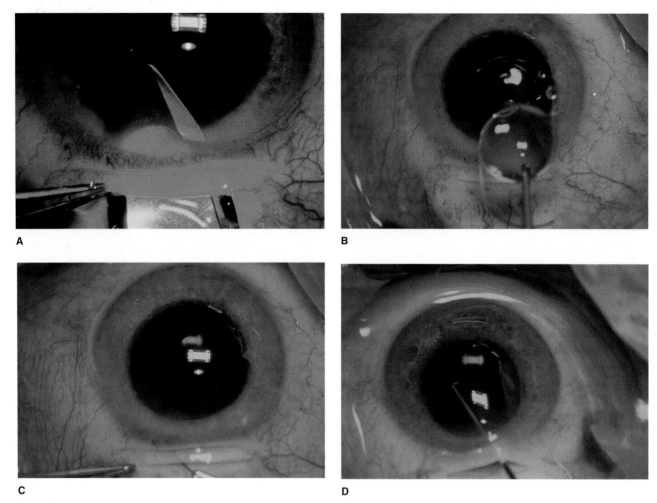

FIGURE 6.1. Three-piece PMMA lens insertion. *A,* The wound is enlarged with a blade just enough to accommodate the nonfoldable PCIOL. *B,* The optic and the leading haptic prior to insertion into the capsular bag. *C,* The trailing haptic is grasped with a forceps and tucked into the capsular bag as well. *D,* Using a Sinskey hook, the operator can dial the PCIOL into place if it is decentered. *(Courtesy of Drs. R. Braunstein and W. J. Stark.)*

Methacrylate-acrylate polymer lenses (acrylic lenses) were developed as an alternative to silicone. Unlike silicone lenses, acrylic lenses can be wetted and open slowly. The surface may be tacky, and the folded lens may adhere to itself. Rarely, this requires the use of a second instrument to help unfold the lens.[4] Before folding an acrylic lens it is best to warm the lens. Even when warmed the lens should be folded slowly. Lenses can crack if folded abruptly and without warming.[5] Because the composition of acrylic lenses is more similar to polymethyl methacrylate (PMMA), acrylic lenses may, like PMMA, be well tolerated over the course of a patient's life. Polyhydroxyethyl methacrylate (poly-HEMA and hydrogel lenses) are the newest type of lenses. They come prerolled and open slowly once inside the eye. HEMA hydrogel lenses, such as the MemoryLens, can be inserted through a 4-mm incision with a long McPherson forceps. These lenses are inserted in the capsule and unfold slowly as they warm over 30 minutes.[6]

Lens injectors first made popular with silicone, single-piece, plate-haptic lenses allow the smallest possible incisions to be used. Plate-haptic lenses may be injected through 3.0-mm incisions (Fig. 6.2), and more recent injectors from Allergan, Alcon, and Bausch and Lomb are advertised to be used with 2.6- and 2.8-mm unenlarged incisions. Kohnen and colleagues showed in cadaveric eyes that corneal tunnel incisions stretch

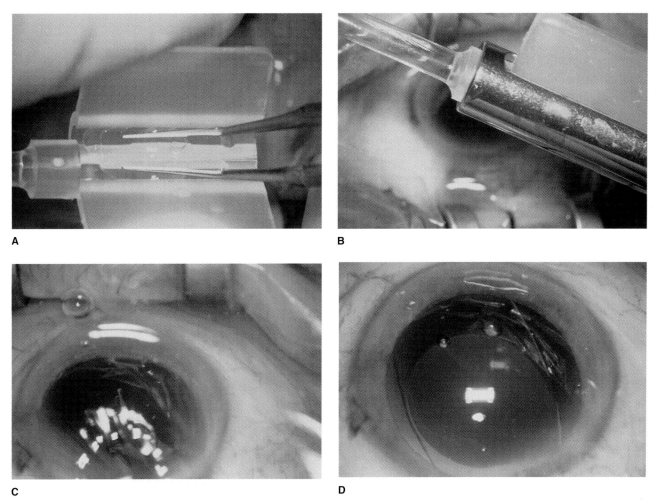

FIGURE 6.2. Plate lens insertion. *A,* The PCIOL is folded inside the injector. *B,* The injector-plunger mechanism is locked and checked. *C,* The PCIOL is slowly injected into the capsular bag. *D,* The PCIOL slowly unfolds inside the capsular bag. *(Courtesy of Drs. R. Braunstein and W. J. Stark.)*

with lens implantation and are enlarged 11% after insertion of foldable IOLs with either forceps or injectors.[7] The smallest incision after insertion of a 20.5-diopter foldable lens was 3.2 mm.

In uncomplicated cases with an intact capsulorrhexis, foldable lenses are commonly inserted with forceps (Fig. 6.3) or through an injector (Fig. 6.2). Folding and inserting forceps are often designed for use with a particular type of lens. The lens is folded with the folder in the operator's nondominant hand. The inserting forceps can then be used in the dominant hand to securely hold the lens. The lens should be inserted so that the leading haptic is on the posterior side of the folded lens and less likely to abrade corneal endothelium. In the eye the lens is guided so that the leading haptic and leading edge of the optic

are under the anterior capsule. The lens is rotated in the eye by pronating the right hand (or supinating the left), and slowly released and unfolded (Fig. 6.3). In general, lenses are folded along the axis parallel to the direction of the haptic optic take-off or along the antiparallel axis. When the lens is folded along the parallel axis, the folder is used to grasp the lens. As the lens begins to fold, the bend in the haptic remains in the plane of the nearer half of the lens. Inserting a lens that has been folded along the parallel axis leaves the trailing haptic out of the wound and requires that the lens be dialed or elbowed into position (Fig. 6.3). Folding the lens along the antiparallel axis allows both haptics to unfold simultaneously in the bag and does not require a dialing or elbowing maneuver.

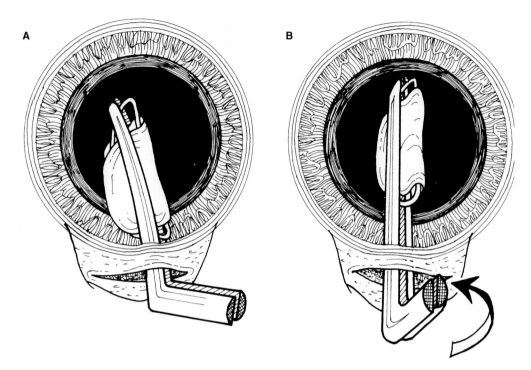

FIGURE 6.3. Foldable IOL with haptics. *A,* The folded PCIOL, with the leading haptic tucked posterior to the optic, is gently inserted into the anterior chamber. *B,* The operator pronates the hand holding the forceps to position the PCIOL before directing it into the capsular bag. *(From Azar DT, Rumelt S. Phacoemulsification. In: Albert DM, Jakobiec FA, eds.* Principles and Practice of Ophthalmology. *2nd ed. Philadelphia: WB Saunders Co; 2000:1509, with permission.)*

In either case, inserting a lens is more difficult without the use of viscoelastics. Viscoelastics make lens insertion safer by ballooning open the capsule and protecting the endothelial surface. Some surgeons advocate the use of different viscoelastics at different times during cataract extraction. A viscoelastic made of smaller molecular weight fragments may more effectively coat and protect the endothelium. Once the lens has been removed, however, the advantage of one type of viscoelastic over another is less distinct. Higher molecular weight viscoelastics are easier to remove after the lens is in place because the material tends to stick together during aspiration. This may be an advantage in preventing postoperative pressure spikes.

If an injector is used, the surgeon must be intimately familiar with its setup and operation before that responsibility can be passed on to the operating room staff. Injectors can jam, crack, fail to release the lens, or shear off a trailing haptic. Unless the surgeon is familiar with the function and disassembly of the injector, a minor problem can become a major complication requiring conversion to extracapsular cataract extraction (ECCE).

The first injector was developed for use with the Starr plate-haptic silicone lens. These injectors worked well, but reports of posterior capsule rupture with rapid injection and late dislocation of lenses into the vitreous after neodymium:yttrium-aluminum-garnet (Nd:YAG) capsulotomy tempered early enthusiasm for plate-haptic lenses and injectors.[8,9] Modifications of the plate-haptic lenses and the availability of newer silicone elastomers have renewed interest in the use of these lenses.

Injectors are designed to direct the lens posteriorly into the inflated capsule, and in the case of the M-Port or Unfolder, the plunger can be withdrawn to reengage the trailing haptic to guide it into the bag. A second instrument placed through a paracentesis port may be used to help direct the lens and trailing haptic into position.

Whether using forceps or loading an injector, the operator must pay attention to the orientation of the lens. In general, posterior chamber lenses are intended to be rotated clockwise. Because PCIOLs are vaulted on average 10 degrees posteriorly, there is a theoretical anterior shift of the lens by 0.7 mm if it is inserted upside-down. A 20-diopter lens displaced anteriorly 1 mm would cause a myopic shift of 1 diopter. The final position of the lens is based on the assumption that the vaulting of the lens is unaffected by capsular contraction and collapse around the lens. In practice the refractive result may be insignificant, given the laxity of the capsule and its tendency to mold around the lens. Halpern and Gallagher examined the results of 457 foldable silicone lens implants, six of which had been inserted upside-down. The range of predicted-achieved correction was + 1.47 to − 1.43 diopters.[10] A more relevant concern may be preventing posterior capsule opacities (PCOs). The incidence of PCOs is significantly higher in cases in which the IOL is not completely in the capsule. Sulcus-fixated or sulcus-capsule-fixated lenses have a much higher rate of PCO.[11] Theoretically, an inverted lens would not have as tight a junction between its posterior surface and the posterior capsule and would thereby allow PCO formation.

Once the lens is safely in the capsule, the irrigation and aspiration port should be used to remove residual viscoelastic. The operator may need to gently depress the IOL in the bag to help viscoelastic behind the lens move forward. Finally, the wound may be sutured or, if watertight, left sutureless.

■ IOL Implantation After ECCE

After successful ECCE, the surgeon has created a 6- to 11-mm wound, removed the lens, and left the posterior capsule intact. In uncomplicated cases the anterior capsulotomy, whether of a "can-opener" or of a continuous curvilinear type, should be visible and without radial tears that would compromise lens centration or propagate posteriorly. In addition, there should be no zonular laxity or areas of dehiscence. In general, wound length is not a consideration after ECCE and a rigid PMMA lens may be used. In the past 7 years some surgeons have advocated small-incision ECCE to reduce the reliance on expensive equipment while maintaining as small a wound as possible.[12–14] Even with small-incision ECCE, the wound must be large enough to accommodate the delivery of the nucleus or nucleus fragments and usually will accommodate a rigid PMMA lens with a 6-mm optic. PMMA lenses have the longest history of use, a low rate of bacterial adherence, may be less irritating in eyes prone to inflammation, are relatively inexpensive, and have high optical quality. Before the lens is placed in the eye the capsule is filled and the corneal endothelium coated with a viscoelastic fluid. The lens is grasped with a long McPherson forceps. Using 0.12-mm forceps in the opposite hand, the operator lifts the front edge of the wound while the lens is inserted. The leading haptic should be directed posteriorly to ensure that the leading haptic and optic edge are under the anterior capsule (see Fig. 6.1B). The trailing haptic should not enter the wound. Before releasing the optic with the McPherson forceps, the operator grasps the trailing haptic at its midpoint with the 0.12-mm forceps to hold the lens in place (see Fig. 6.1C). The end of the trailing haptic, still outside the eye, is grasped with the McPherson forceps with the right hand in a supinated position. By pushing the lens into the eye with the end of the trailing haptic, the operator moves the lens into position, and with pronation of the wrist the haptic can be elbowed into position and released. Before releasing the haptic the operator should ensure that the trailing haptic-optic junction and the elbowed bend in the trailing haptic are beneath the plane of the anterior capsule. If there is doubt, a second instrument such as a Sinskey hook can be used to move the iris and enhance visualization or to inject viscoelastic agent to inflate the capsule more fully. Once the proper position has been ensured the haptic is released under direct visualization and the lens is placed completely in the capsule. This point is emphasized because a lens with one haptic in and one haptic out of the bag is more likely to decenter or provoke inflammation. Ram and colleagues studied 3,493 pseudophakic cadaveric eyes with Miyake-Apple photography and found that only 52% of eyes had lenses completely within the capsular bag. Thirty-four percent had asymmetric sulcus-bag fixation. Asymmetric fixation correlated positively with lens decentration and increased PCO formation.[2]

A properly placed lens should appear centered, with the anterior capsule overlying the haptics. Residual viscoelastic fluid should be irrigated from the eye before the wound is closed with 10-0 nylon sutures.

■ IOL Management After Complicated Phacoemulsification and ECCE

When capsular tears, a dropped nucleus, vitreous loss, or vitreal pressure complicate cataract surgery, the surgeon must carefully manage the problem and then reconsider the type of IOL to be implanted (Fig. 6.4). In phacoemulsification one of the steps most critical to successful surgery is the creation of the capsulotomy. A well-centered and appropriately sized capsulorrhexis allows more consistent in-the-bag placement of the lens and minimizes postoperative lens decentration. A common problem in phacoemulsification is anterior radial tears in the capsule. A tear in the capsule may propagate posteriorly during phacoemulsification, cortex aspiration, or lens implantation. If there is any question regarding the extent of a tear, the surgeon must stop and carefully inspect the tear. A Sinskey hook may be used to retract the iris for clear observation of the peripheral extent of the tear. Often a tear

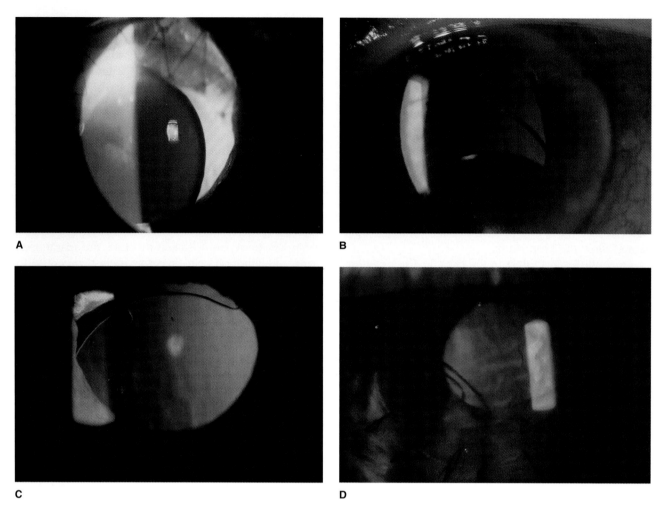

FIGURE 6.4. *A* and *B,* Tears or rents in the anterior or posterior capsule can cause postoperative decentration of the PCIOL laterally *(A)* or inferiorly *(B),* even though the PCIOL was centered intraoperatively. *C,* The optic edge showing through the pupil may cause optical aberrations. *D,* Complete inferior dislocation may simulate aphakia and result in marked reduction of vision.

will stop at the zonular ligament at the midperiphery of the lens. Small tears need not impede intracapsular placement of a lens if placement is done properly. IOL placement should be done with minimal rotational stress on the capsule. Rotating a lens into position may propagate tears beyond the equator and lead to vitreal prolapse. Elbowing the trailing haptic into the bag or using the antiparallel fold to open both haptics in the bag eliminates the need to rotate the lens. The choice of elbowing a haptic or unfolding in antiparallel fashion depends on the location of the tear. Tears that are under the incision or 2 clock hours to either side are best managed by elbowing the haptic into the bag. Anterior capsular rents from 4 to 8 clock hours away from the wound are similarly managed; however, it is more

difficult to control the rotation of the lead haptic, and the risk of tearing the capsule seems greater. Rents 3 or 9 clock hours from the wound should be treated with an antiparallel fold and simultaneous in-the-bag placement of the haptics.

Postoperatively, the lens may decenter because of asymmetric anterior capsule contraction. To prevent this complication the surgeon must balance the anterior capsule rent with three to four additional small tears in the anterior capsular edge with long Gills' scissors. This should be done before removing viscoelastic from the anterior chamber.

Tears in the posterior capsule or anterior rents that propagate posteriorly make IOL selection and placement more difficult because of the high likelihood that the vitreous will prolapse forward. The simpler scenario—the occurrence of posterior rents after the nucleus and the majority of the cortex have been removed—will be addressed first. Isolated posterior rents or holes that are not contiguous with the anterior tears can be managed so that a lens may be placed within the capsule. Rents should be tamponaded with viscoelastic fluid, and a limited anterior vitrectomy can be performed through the tear. A separate infusion cannula in the anterior chamber reduces the likelihood of vitreal hydration. After the vitrectomy, and if the hole is small, a lens can be safely unfolded in the bag. One should anticipate PCO or the need for a capsulotomy if the posterior capsular edge is near the visual axis.

If the posterior rent is large or contiguous with an anterior tear, the lens must be placed in the sulcus. Theoretically a sulcus-placed lens needs only 6 total clock hours of anterior capsule-zonular support—3 hours of support 180 degrees apart. Haptics must be placed precisely and carefully. If there is doubt regarding support, one haptic may be sutured to the iris (a safety suture), both haptics may be sutured to the iris, or both haptics may be sutured to the sclera. What must be emphasized here is the foresight needed to allow these more technically challenging cases to succeed. The surgeon must anticipate which patients may have complicated cataract extraction and plan to have lenses with holes in the optics or eyelets in the haptics available. In patients with a history of trauma, small pupils, dense cataracts, pseudoexfoliation, or zonular dialysis, there is a greater likelihood of capsular tears, vitreal loss, or dropped nuclei.

Unlike isolated posterior capsule tears, where a subsequent pars plana vitrectomy is unlikely, a dropped nucleus will require a second operation. This should affect the choice of lenses because silicone lenses can be more problematic during a vitrectomy. During fluid gas exchange, condensation may form on the back surface of a silicone lens and prevent visualization of the posterior pole. If silicone oil is used the oil can adhere to the back surface of a silicone lens and obscure the view.[15,16] For these reasons, in any complicated cataract surgery, if the likelihood of a secondary pars plans vitrectomy is high, an acrylic or PMMA lens should be implanted.

Vitreal pressure is a problem more often seen in ECCE. The small wounds used in phacoemulsification allow the surgeon to maintain a deep anterior chamber. In ECCE, however, the vitreous can push forward and shallow the anterior chamber, making lens implantation difficult if not impossible. Usually a high molecular weight viscoelastic can be used to fill the chamber and counteract the pressure of the vitreous. If the chamber is still shallow, the wound should be partially closed. This helps to reform the chamber. If need be the wound can be sutured, so that a foldable lens may be inserted.

The surgeon must always be attentive to the possible causes of a shallowing chamber. Choroidal effusions can push the iris forward. Loss of the red reflex may herald choroidal hemorrhage, a potentially catastrophic event. If expulsive, these hemorrhages can result in permanent and complete vision loss. With severe effusions and hemorrhages, the only goal should be to close the wound as rapidly as possible. A lens can always be implanted at a later date under more controlled conditions.

■ Pediatric IOL Implantation

Traditionally, the surgical correction of cataracts in children has stopped short of IOL implantation. Refractive errors are managed with aphakic spectacles or contact lenses. The disadvantages of these techniques are obvious: children and parents may not comply with a unilateral contact lens or tolerate aphakic spectacles for optical or cosmetic reasons. The advantage of being able to change contact lenses as refractions change and the lack of long-term data have stifled the use of IOLs in children. The age at which pediatric cataracts are discovered and removed may be years before the eye is fully mature. This poses an obvious challenge in selecting IOL power and concern if the refraction changes significantly. In 1984 Hiles published results in a large series of IOL implantations in children.[17] The incidence of postoperative complications, including capsular opacification, inflammation, and lens decentration, tempered enthusiasm among pediatric ophthalmologists. In Hiles' study only 23 of the 152 patients who underwent primary IOL implantation had flexible-loop posterior chamber lenses implanted. The results may not be relevant to more modern techniques. Advances in cataract surgery, specifically continuous capsulorrhexis and small wounds, have made intracapsular lens fixation more predictable and presumably have reduced the risks of postoperative complications.

With the longest published follow-up for lens implantation in children approaching 10–15 years, data do not yet exist to lend unqualified support for primary lens implantation in children. However, recent reports are very promising and indicate that at least children with developmental cataracts have excellent visual results after primary lens implantation. Those with traumatic cataracts, despite a slightly higher complication rate, also do well on the basis of visual rehabilitation. For a more extensive discussion, please refer to Chapter 7.

■ References

1. Ridley H. Intra-ocular acrylic lenses. *Trans Ophthalmol Soc UK*. 1951;71:617–621.

2. Ram J, Apple DJ, Peng Q, et al. Update on fixation of rigid and foldable posterior chamber intraocular lenses. Part I. Elimination of fixation-induced decentration to achieve precise optical correction and visual rehabilitation. *Ophthalmology*. 1999;106:883–890.

3. Mazzocco TR. Early clinical experience with elastic lens implants. *Trans Ophthalmol Soc UK*. 1985;104:578–579.

4. Milauskas AT. Current state of acrylic IOLs. *Ophthalmol Pract*. 1994;12:133–136.

5. Carlson KH, Johnson DW. Cracking of acrylic intraocular lenses during capsular bag insertion. *Ophthalmic Surg Lasers*. 1995;26:572–573.

6. Chehade M, Elder MJ. Intraocular lens materials and styles: a review. *Aust NZ J Ophthalmol*. 1997;25:255–263.

7. Kohnen T, Lambert RJ, Koch DD. Incision sizes for foldable intraocular lenses. *Ophthalmology*. 1997;104:1277–1286.

8. Dick B, Schwenn O, Stoffelns B, Pfeiffer N. [Late dislocation of a plate haptic silicone lens into the vitreous body after Nd:YAG capsulotomy: a case report]. *Ophthalmology*. 1998;95:181–185.

9. Tuft SJ, Talks SJ. Delayed dislocation of foldable plate-haptic silicone lenses after Nd:YAG laser anterior capsulotomy. *Am J Ophthalmol*. 1998;126:586–588.

10. Halpern BL, Gallagher SP. Refractive error consequences of reversed-optic AMO SI-40NB intraocular lens. *Ophthalmology*. 1999;106:901–903.

11. Ram J, Apple DJ, Peng Q, et al. Update on fixation of rigid and foldable posterior chamber intraocular lenses. Part II. Choosing the correct haptic fixation and intraocular lens design to help eradicate posterior capsule opacification. *Ophthalmology*. 1999;106:891–900.

12. Bartov E, Isakov I, Rock T. Nucleus fragmentation in a scleral pocket for small incision extracapsular cataract extraction. *J Cataract Refract Surg*. 1998;24:160–165.

13. Bayramlar H, Cekic O, Totan Y. Manual tunnel incision extracapsular cataract extraction using the sandwich technique. *J Cataract Refract Surg*. 1999;25:312–315.

14. Blumenthal M, Ashkenazi I, Assia E, et al. Small-incision manual extracapsular cataract extraction using selective hydrodissection. *Ophthalmic Surg*. 1992; 23:699–701.

15. Hainsworth DP, Chen SN, Cox TA, et al. Condensation on polymethylmethacrylate, acrylic polymer, and silicone intraocular lenses after fluid-air exchange in rabbits [see comments]. *Ophthalmology*. 1996;103:1410–1418.

16. Apple DJ, Federman JL, Krolicki TJ, et al. Irreversible silicone oil adhesion to silicone intraocular lenses: a clinicopathologic analysis. *Ophthalmology*. 1996;103:1555–1561; discussion 1561–1552.

17. Hiles DA. Intraocular lens implantation in children with monocular cataracts: 1974–1983. *Ophthalmology*. 1984;91:1231–1237.

Chapter 7

Intraocular Lenses in Children

Balamurali K. Ambati and Nathalie F. Azar

The management of cataracts in children is complicated by the unique structural characteristic of the
child's eye and by the risk of amblyopia (Fig. 7.1). Visual rehabilitation of pediatric eyes following cataract
removal has been attempted with spectacles (Fig. 7.2),
contact lenses, epikeratophakia, and intraocular lenses
(IOLs).[1] This chapter discusses indications for the use
of IOLs, surgical techniques, materials and sizing, associated refractive issues, and complications, especially
posterior capsular opacification (PCO).

Childhood cataracts are relatively common and account for significant morbidity. Francois reported that
one out of every 250 newborns has some form of congenital cataract (Fig. 7.3), and that 10%–38.8% of cases
of childhood blindness are due to cataracts.[2] Two
other studies found that 13.4%–13.8% of blind children
had congenital cataracts.[3,4] Exhaustive coverage of pediatric cataract surgery (Fig. 7.4) is beyond the scope
of this chapter, and the reader is referred to other published reviews for further information on this topic.[1,5,6]

Using an anterior chamber intraocular lens
(ACIOL), Choyce in 1955 was the first to implant an
IOL in a child.[7] He was followed by Binkhorst, who
used an iridocapsular-fixated IOL in 1959.[8] The use of
IOLs in pediatric cataract surgery has lagged behind
their use in adults because of the changing refractive
status of the developing eye, an increased inflammatory response in children's eyes (which can cause
synechiae, secondary membranes, vitritis, PCO, and occluded or secluded pupils [Fig. 7.5]), and the unknown
effects of a synthetic material in the eye over the lifetime of an individual.[1,5,9] Further, the greater structural
pliability of the sclera in children predisposes such
eyes to scleral collapse on opening of the eye, which
can lead to shallowing of the anterior chamber

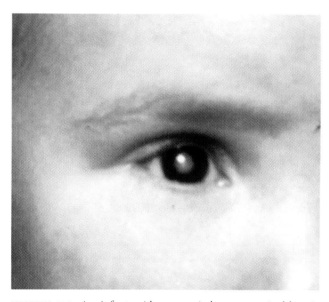

FIGURE 7.1. An infant with congenital cataract. Amblyopia
usually occurs if surgical management is delayed.

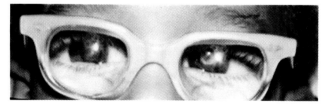

FIGURE 7.2. Visual rehabilitation in a child who has undergone cataract surgery without an IOL for congenital cataracts.
This involves the wearing of aphakic spectacles if the child
cannot tolerate contact lens wear.

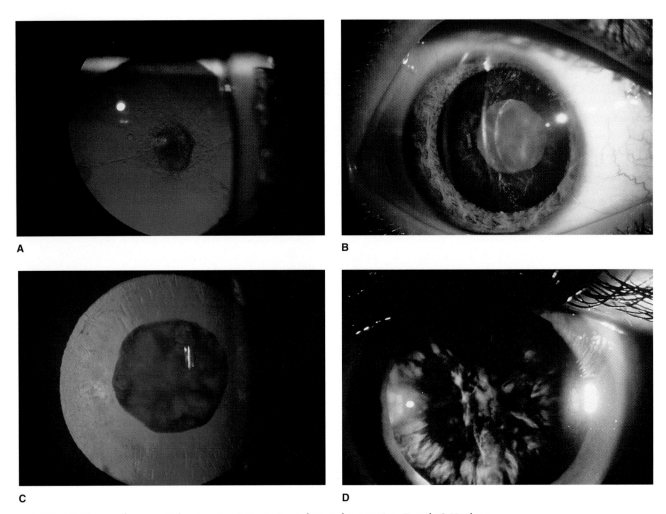

FIGURE 7.3. Types of congenital cataracts. *A,* Posterior subcapsular opacity. *B* and *C,* Nuclear opacity. *D,* Cortical riders.

(damaging the corneal endothelium), vitreous loss, and expulsion of uveal contents.[10]

Initial experience with pediatric IOLs yielded mixed results. Technical advances that have facilitated the implantation of IOLs in children include the development of posterior scleral beveled incisions, continuous curvilinear capsulorrhexis, viscoelastic agents, endocapsular fixation, and Nd:YAG capsulotomy.[1,11]

■ Experience with IOLs in Children: Visual and Refractive Outcomes

Numerous studies have assessed the efficacy and safety of IOLs in children. Awner et al performed cataract extraction, primary posterior capsulotomy (PPC), anterior vitrectomy (AV), and IOL insertion in 12 eyes with congenital cataracts and 9 eyes with traumatic cataracts (Fig. 7.6) (mean patient age was 2 years; mean followup was 12 months).[12] Five of the 12 eyes with congenital cataracts and 6 of the 9 eyes with traumatic cataracts

achieved a final visual acuity of 20/40 or better. Zwaan et al retrospectively reviewed results in 306 eyes, 57% of which had traumatic cataracts and 37% of which had congenital cataracts.[13] A final acuity of 20/40 or better was achieved in 49.3% of the eyes with traumatic cataracts but in only 35.1% of the eyes with congenital cataracts. There was no difference in outcomes between primarily and secondarily implanted IOLs or between capsular bag and sulcus-fixated IOLs. Noncompliance with amblyopia therapy and delay in referral (which worsened amblyopia) accounted for many of the eyes with poorer visual acuity results. PCO occurred in 39% of eyes and fibrin membranes in another 13%. The authors found that the SRK II formula resulted in a refraction within 2 diopters of the targeted goal in 84% of cases (the mean difference was + 0.28 diopter). Dahan and Salmenson performed IOL implantation with PPC and AV in 51 eyes with traumatic cataracts, 20 with developmental cataracts, and 13 with congenital cataracts.[14] They removed one-third of the vitreous anteriorly (dispersing any inflammatory cells

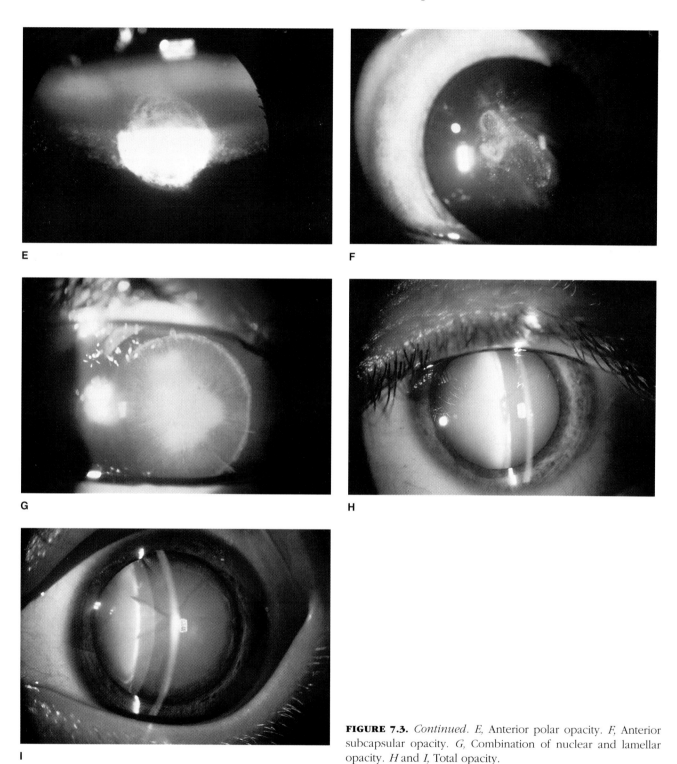

FIGURE 7.3. *Continued. E,* Anterior polar opacity. *F,* Anterior subcapsular opacity. *G,* Combination of nuclear and lamellar opacity. *H* and *I,* Total opacity.

into a larger cavity). To facilitate in-the-bag insertion, they temporarily reduced the diameter of the IOL by compressing the trailing haptic using a 10-0 nylon suture, which was cut once the IOL was inserted to allow the haptic to spring back into the capsular bag fornix. A final visual acuity of 20/40 or better was achieved in 85% of eyes with developmental cataracts, 55% of eyes

with traumatic cataracts, and 7.7% of eyes with congenital cataracts. Similar results have been reported by other groups. Hiles, using ACIOLs, found that among patients who underwent primary IOL implantation, a visual acuity of 20/40 or better was achieved in 65% of eyes with traumatic cataracts and 21% of eyes with congenital cataracts, whereas in eyes treated by secondary

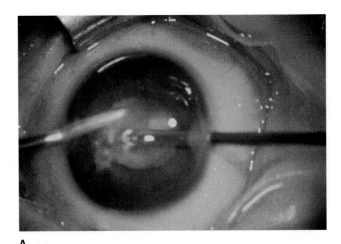

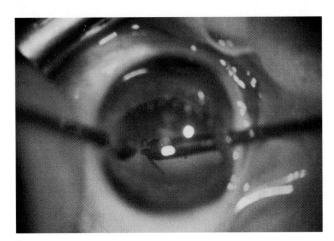

FIGURE 7.4. *A* and *B*, During infantile cataract surgery, an ocutome is used to perform anterior capsulotomy, lens aspiration, posterior capsulotomy, and anterior vitrectomy.

IOL implantation, a visual acuity of 20/40 or better was achieved in 46% of eyes with traumatic cataracts and 10% of eyes with congenital cataracts.[15] Koenig et al performed PCIOL insertion in 8 eyes with traumatic cataracts, 7 of which achieved a visual acuity of 20/40 or better by 10 months. PCO developed in 3 of the 8 eyes and was successfully treated with YAG capsulotomy.[16] The average error of the SRK II formula from the target was + 0.33 diopter. Buckley et al performed IOL implantation with pars plana PPC and pars plana AV in 20 patients (14 with traumatic cataracts, 4 with developmental cataracts, 2 with radiation-induced cataracts), all of whom achieved 20/40 acuity or better.[17] In that study the IOL was placed before PPC and AV were performed, as the IOL is easier to implant in such traumatized eyes while the posterior capsule is still intact; once the IOL was in place, a pars plana approach allowed for a much larger PPC than the standard limbal approach. Hemo and BenEzra presented results in a

series of 20 patients with traumatic cataracts who underwent PPC and AV prior to IOL implantation; in 15 the final acuity was 20/40 or better.[18] Cavallaro et al performed CE/IOL/PPC/AV implantation in 23 eyes (10

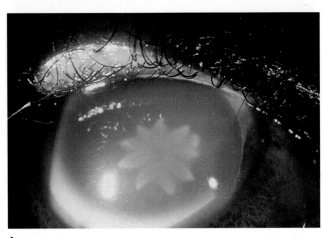

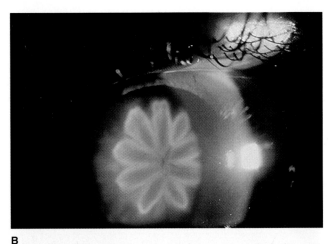

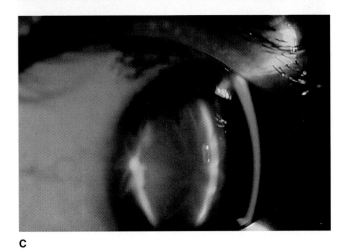

FIGURE 7.5. *A* to *C,* Traumatic cataract. The stellate or rosette-shaped opacity is typically seen in traumatic cataracts.

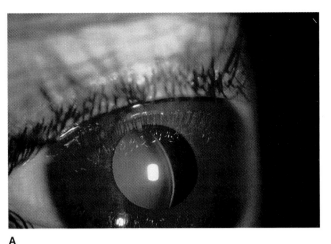
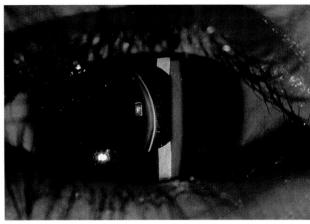

A   **B**

FIGURE 7.6. *A* and *B,* Lens subluxation seen in Marfan's syndrome.

with traumatic cataracts, 11 with developmental cataracts), of which 17 achieved 20/40 acuity or better.[19] This study also found that formulas calculating IOL power were quite inaccurate at short axial lengths. Andreo et al performed a retrospective review of 47 eyes, and found that the average difference between predicted and actual postoperative refractions ranged from 1.2 to 1.4 diopters for all formulas tested (SRK II, SRK-T, Holladay, and Hoffner-Q), comparable to performance in adults.[20] Hiles, studying just traumatic cataracts, found that 62% of patients who had undergone primary IOL implantation and 47% of those who had undergone secondary IOL implantation achieved a visual acuity of 20/40 or better.[21] Basti et al conducted a large, nonrandomized, prospective study of 192 eyes (151 with congenital or developmental cataracts, 41 with traumatic cataracts) that compared the outcome of ECCE/IOL (*n* = 87) versus lensectomy/AV (without IOL placement) (*n* = 23) versus ECCE/PPC/AV/IOL (*n* = 82).[22] There was no significant difference in visual acuity among the three methods studied (in 58 eyes an acuity of 20/40 or better was achieved; acuity was not recordable in 37 eyes). The study did not classify visual outcome with respect to cause of the cataract. Sharma et al performed secondary IOL implantation in 35 patients intolerant of aphakic glasses or contacts; 34 eyes improved, and 15 achieved an acuity of 20/40 or better.[23] Ghosh et al prospectively studied 40 eyes, 20 of which had been treated by ECCE/PCIOL, the other 20 of which had been treated by epilenticular PCIOL placement in the sulcus followed by pars plana lensectomy.[24] Twenty-two eyes had traumatic cataracts and 18 had developmental cataracts; the etiologies were evenly represented in the two groups. Visual acuity of 20/40 or better was achieved in 95% of the eyes that had been treated by epilenticular PCIOL placement and in 65% of

the eyes that did not undergo such treatment, mainly because of the higher rate of PCO in the group. Plager et al implanted PCIOLs in 79 eyes with cataracts (9 with traumatic cataracts, the rest with congenital or developmental cataracts); 79% achieved 20/40 acuity or better after an average follow-up of 2 years, with the rest having limited vision due to amblyopia.[25] DeVaro et al implanted sulcus-fixated secondary IOLs in 11 patients with congenital cataracts and 8 with traumatic cataracts; 3 of the former and 6 of the latter achieved a visual acuity of 20/40 or better.[26] Only 1 patient had a postoperative acuity worse than the preoperative acuity. The mean difference between predicted and actual refraction was − 0.97 diopter. Crouch et al implanted primary IOLs in 24 eyes with developmental cataracts and 10 with traumatic cataracts.[11] After a mean follow-up of 28 months, 21 eyes in the first group and 8 in the second achieved a visual acuity of 20/40 or better. Amblyopia and macular scarring accounted for the poorer vision in the remaining 5 eyes. Sinskey et al implanted IOLs primarily in 11 eyes with developmental cataracts, 8 with traumatic cataracts, and 10 with congenital cataracts.[27] This group also implanted secondary IOLs in 13 aphakic eyes (which had had traumatic cataracts). A visual acuity of 20/40 or better was achieved in 73% of the developmental group, 62.5% of the traumatic primary IOL group, 70% of the traumatic secondary IOL group, and 10% of the congenital group.

When the results of these studies are taken together, the following points may be distilled:

- IOLs are effective in the management of pediatric cataracts.
- Visual outcomes are significantly superior in eyes with developmental cataracts compared to eyes with congenital cataracts.

- Visual outcomes in eyes with traumatic cataracts are comparable to outcomes in eyes with developmental cataracts when no other visually significant posterior segment pathology is present.
- Secondary implantation of IOLs is effective, although not as effective as primary implantation.
- The success of formulas used to predict postoperative refractions in children is comparable to that in adults, except in children with very short axial lengths.
- Management of amblyopia is essential for optimal visual outcome, as it accounts for much of the poorer visual outcomes following IOL implantation.

■ Experience with IOLs in Children: Complications and Their Management

It is generally believed that cataract surgery elicits a far greater inflammatory response in children than in adults.[1,5] The degree of inflammation in children manifests in several ways, but especially as posterior capsular opacification.

Posterior Capsular Opacification

The postoperative development of posterior capsular opacification (PCO) or secondary membranes is the most common complication following pediatric cataract extraction when the posterior capsule is left intact. It is a serious complication, as it can lead to deprivation amblyopia and also impair retinoscopy and, consequently, visual rehabilitation. Hiles and Hered reported an incidence of PCO in 70% in children younger than 6 years.[28] Oliver et al reported an incidence of 44% during the first 3 postoperative months.[29] Gimbel et al found an incidence of 59% over 4 years.[30] Apple et al reported an incidence of nearly 100% over 3 years.[31] Koenig et al, who performed ECCE/PCIOL on 8 eyes, reported 3 cases of PCO, but no other significant complications.[16] Plager et al found that PCO developed within 5 years in all of 69 eyes treated by just CE/PCIOL. The incidence of PCO rose rapidly after 18 months, with PCO present in 50% of eyes within 2 years after surgery.[25] There were only 2 cases of glaucoma, and no posterior segment complications. Several techniques have been developed to prevent or treat PCO, including primary capsulotomy, posterior capsulotomy plus anterior vitrectomy, optic capture, and epilenticular IOL implantation.

Hiles reported a 63% incidence of PCO in eyes treated by CE/IOL/PPC without AV.[15] Zwaan et al reported a 39% incidence of PCO and a 13% incidence

of fibrin membranes in their retrospective review of 306 eyes treated by CE/IOL/PPC.[13] Gupta et al in 1992 reported that 63% of eyes treated by CE/IOL/PPC without AV developed secondary membranes requiring later Nd:YAG laser capsulotomy,[32] presumably because of residual lens epithelium using the anterior vitreous face and posterior surface of the IOL as scaffolding for a fibrotic reaction. This model was proposed to explain why PPC alone is insufficient to preclude the development of PCO.[33,34]

The majority of recent studies have used PPC with AV, which was pioneered by BenEzra in the early 1980s.[35] Mackool and Chatiawala in 1991 described the technique of PPC with AV (which they termed limbal approach retropseudophakic vitrectomy) to remove secondary membranes in 6 cases.[36] Awner et al, who performed CE/IOL/PPC/AV in 21 patients, reported that a pupillary membrane, IOL dislocation, corectopia, and partial pupillary capture of the IOL occurred in 1 patient each; all were surgically corrected.[12] They encountered no PCO, CME, retinal detachments (RD), or other posterior segment complications. Dahan and Salmenson, in a study of CE/IOL/PPC/AV performed on 84 eyes, noted only mild IOL decentration in 2 cases and suture rupture in 3 cases.[14] No cases of PCO, CME, glaucoma, or RD occurred. Cavallaro et al, in a study of CE/IOL/PPC/AV performed on 23 eyes, reported 2 cases of PCO and 1 of IOL decentration.[19] Buckley et al, who performed CE/PCIOL/PPC/AV on 20 eyes, had no cases of PCO; there was 1 case of IOL dislocation and 1 of corectopia.[17]

Two studies have compared different techniques for the management of PCO. Basti et al found that lensectomy with AV in 23 eyes produced no PCO, while the ECCE/PCIOL group of 87 eyes had a 43.7% rate of PCO, and the ECCE/PCIOL/PPC/AV group of 82 eyes had only a 3.7% rate of PCO.[22] Performing AV did not increase the rate of retinal detachment, cystoid macular edema, or vitreous incarceration. BenEzra and Cohen presented results from a large series of both retrospective and prospective studies.[37] In their retrospective analyses of 69 aphakes, 31 eyes in which the posterior chamber was left intact developed PCO, 12 of 16 eyes treated by PPC only developed PCO, and none of 22 eyes treated by PPC with AV developed PCO. In 25 pseudophakes, all 12 eyes with an intact posterior capsule and all 4 eyes treated by PPC only developed PCO, while only 1 of 9 eyes treated by PPC with AV developed PCO. In a prospective series of 28 eyes left with an intact posterior capsule, PCO developed in all children less than 6 years old and in 8 of 10 children more than 6 years old; PCO developed faster in younger children and in pseudophakes. In a prospective analysis of 10 children with bilateral cataracts treated by IOL implantation in both eyes, with PPC and AV performed on one eye and no posterior capsule procedure performed on the fellow eye, PCO developed in all eyes with an intact posterior capsule but in only 1 of 10 eyes that underwent PPC and AV. Eyes with PCO had inferior visual outcomes.

Gimbel and Debroff first described the technique of posterior capsular curvilinear capsulorrhexis (CCC) with optic capture in 1994.[38] In this procedure, the technique of CCC used for an anterior capsulotomy is used to make an opening in the posterior capsule concentric to the IOL with a diameter 1–1.5 mm less than the diameter of the optic. Once the IOL is inserted into the capsular bag, the optic of the IOL is manipulated and pushed first inferiorly and then superiorly through the posterior capsulotomy. This manipulation results in fusion of the anterior and posterior capsule leaflets for 360 degrees, except where they surround the haptic and the haptic-optic junctions. Capsular fusion anterior to the optic theoretically deprives the lens epithelium of the scaffolding needed to produce PCO, without needing to do an anterior vitrectomy. Gimbel presented results in a prospective series of 13 eyes treated by this method in 1996; none of which had developed PCO after a mean follow-up of 19 months.[39] In 1997, Gimbel presented results in another prospective series of 16 eyes treated by this technique with the implantation of heparin-coated IOLs; none of these eyes had developed PCO after a mean follow-up of 3 years.[40] Koch and Kohnen in 1997 published a retrospective review of 20 eyes, in 15 of which posterior CCC (PCCC) was performed, while in 5, the posterior chamber was left intact.[41] Six eyes in the PCCC group also were treated by AV, and in 3 of these 6 optic capture was performed. Five of the 9 eyes not treated by AV underwent optic capture. In this group, only the eyes treated by AV retained clarity of axis. The authors speculated that optic capture may have failed to prevent PCO in this series because the IOL used had an oblique haptic-optic junction, whereas Gimbel's IOL had a 90-degree angle, allowing the optic to protrude below the posterior capsule and enabling the edge of the optic to mechanically block posterior migration of the lens epithelium. Although PCCC is a technically challenging procedure, Koch and Kohnen state that in the young eye it is easier than CCC of the anterior capsule, because the posterior chamber is less rubbery and more resistant to tearing. It should also be noted that PCCC with optic capture improves IOL centration but makes future IOL exchange more difficult.

Tablante et al described the technique of epilenticular PCIOL placement (with sulcus fixation) followed by pars plana lensectomy (PPL).[42] The advantages of this technique are (1) the IOL implantation is independent of the status of the posterior chamber (important in cases in trauma), (2) there is less anterior chamber manipulation and consequently less inflammation, and (3) the lensectomy is minimally affected by scleral collapse and positive vitreous pressure (in young patients, positive vitreous pressure makes anterior chamber maneuvers more difficult). Ghosh et al conducted a prospective randomized trial of epilenticular PCIOL/PPL versus ECCE/PCIOL (20 eyes in each arm) and noted clearly superior results for the former.[24] PCO developed in none of the eyes in the former group, as opposed to 80% of eyes in the latter group.

When PCO does occur, it can be treated with several options. Nd:YAG laser treatment has been shown to be safe and effective in the pediatric population.[43,44] Atkinson and Hiles reported a recurrence rate of 28% after Nd:YAG laser treatment,[44] which is similar to the recurrence rate reported for surgical discission of PCO and secondary IOL implantation.[28] Atkinson and Hiles found that the best results with Nd:YAG capsulotomy occurred when it was performed at the first sign of PCO, as soon as 2–3 weeks postoperatively (sooner than in adults), because early treatment reduced the risk of amblyopia. Retreatment could be done as early as 3 weeks after the first procedure. Mullaney et al reported that intraocular streptokinase was safe and effective in dissolving fibrin membranes.[45]

Other Complications

The development of cystoid macular edema (CME) is of theoretical concern, especially when PPC and/or AV are performed. However, the occurrence of CME has been extremely rare in the studies performed to date. Indeed, the vast majority of studies reviewed here reported no instance of CME in eyes treated by PPC with or without AV.[11–27] Hoyt and Nickel reported that CME developed in 10 of 27 aphakic eyes treated by pars plana lensectomy and AV but in only 1 of 27 aphakic eyes treated by PPC.[46] Morgan and Franklin, in a series of 11 eyes,[47] and Gilbard et al, in a series of 25 eyes,[48] all of which had been treated by PPL and AV, did not report any instance of CME. Poer et al[49] and Pinchoff et al[50] also reported an extremely low incidence of CME in pediatric aphakes, even when AV was performed.

Glaucoma may occur months or even years after cataract surgery.[51–55] Early reports by Binkhorst[8] and by Hiles and Hered,[28] who used principally ACIOLs, noted a relatively high frequency of pupillary block glaucoma. Hiles and Hered recommended that peripheral iridectomy be performed whenever an ACIOL was placed. Vajpayee et al reported results in a series of 16 patients who developed pupillary block glaucoma after

PCIOL implantation.[56] The studies reviewed here all reported no to very few cases of glaucoma; however, the follow-up period in these studies was rather short (usually less than 2 years); hence, no conclusion can be made based on these data.

Early reports indicated an IOL decentration rate of 3%–20%.[57–59] The rate of IOL decentration in the studies reviewed above ranged from 0% to 5%.[11–27] Retinal detachment was extremely rare in the studies discussed above. Success rates for repair are comparable to those in adults.[28,60] Bullous keratopathy, endophthalmitis, and corectopia are also uncommon after pediatric IOL implantation.[1,5]

■ Materials and Sizing

PMMA has the longest history of any material for IOLs; hence, most authors have used one-piece PMMA lenses for children. Sinskey et al reported that polypropylene loop lenses were more flexible and hence easier to insert[27]; however, Apple et al found that polypropylene loops may not be biologically inert in animal models.[61] Silicone and soft acrylic (Acrysof) lenses are coming into favor for use in the adult population because they are flexible. Foldability allows small-incision surgery and thus decreased inflammation, astigmatism, and endothelial damage, as well as faster visual recovery.[62]

Several in vivo and in vitro studies have assessed the effect of various IOL materials on lens epithelial cell (LEC) adherence and the development of PCO, which is thought to be due to proliferation and migration of LECs. In rabbit eyes, Okada et al found that LEC adherence was less to silicone IOLs than to PMMA,[63] correlating with the finding of Cook et al that silicone IOLs developed fewer precipitates on the anterior surface than PMMA IOLs.[64] Versura et al[65] compared four different IOL materials and found that LEC adherence in vitro was highest for PMMA, followed by heparin-coated PMMA, poly-HEMA (polyhydroxyethyl methacrylate), and silicone (least LEC adherence). Majima found that soft acrylic has more LEC adherence than PMMA and silicone, and speculated that higher adherence might decrease LEC migration.[66] Linnola stated the silicone and PMMA are both bioinert, and induce less of an inflammatory reaction than the bioactive Acrysof, which causes more LEC adhesion.[67] He stated that the increased bonding decreased LEC ingrowth and thus PCO. If the edge of the CCC was placed on the optic, it would stay in place; conversely, the adherence of the anterior capsule to Acrysof lenses would make future IOL exchange more difficult. Hollick et al, in a study of 90 adult eyes, reported that Acrysof lenses had fewer LECs on the IOL surface at 3 months and 2 years and more LEC regression than PMMA or silicone IOLs: only 62% of Acrysof lenses exhibited LECs at 2 years, whereas 100% of both PMMA and silicone IOLs and 83% of Acrysof lenses exhibited LEC regression, compared to 15% of PMMA and only 8% of silicone lenses.[68] Nagata et al stated that the sharper optic edges of the Acrysof lens might contribute to the decreased LEC migration and PCO observed with this material.[69] Ursell et al, in a study of 90 adult eyes conducted over 2 years, noted that Acrysof lenses resulted in an 11.8% rate of PCO, compared to 43.7% for PMMA and 33.5% for silicone.[70] To date there is no study comparing rates of PCO in children with different IOL materials.

Motion of the anterior capsule is another consideration in the choice of IOL materials. Joo et al found that CCCs more than 5.5 mm in diameter tended to retract, which could lead to decentration or extrusion of the IOL, while those smaller than 5.0 mm tended to constrict, leading to wrinkling of the posterior capsule and obscuration of the visual axis through phimosis of the anterior capsule.[71] Ursell et al found that anterior capsule movement was less with Acrysof lenses than with PMMA or silicone lenses (capsule motion was slightly more with PMMA than with silicone lenses).[72] Oshika et al reported better clarity of the anterior capsule following placement of Acrysof IOLs.[73] Gonvers et al observed more constriction and fibrosis of the anterior capsule with plate-haptic IOLs than with one-piece PMMA or three-piece silicone or PMMA IOLs, possibly because of contact between the haptics and the anterior capsule.[74]

Thouvenin et al found that treating the surface of PMMA single-piece IOLs with fluorine plasma decreased the secondary cicatricial reaction from 80% to 43%.[75] Fluorine treatment produced a smoother, hydrophobic surface by replacing hydrogen atoms with fluorine atoms on the IOL surface, leading to decreased inflammatory and protein debris on the IOL. Fluorine treatment did not affect the optical or mechanical properties of the IOL. Bechetoille has presented data showing that fluorine-treated IOLs are associated with decreased corneal endothelial damage.[76] Zetterstrom et al found that use of heparin-coated IOLs decreased the inflammatory response in children.[77]

Bluestein et al demonstrated that 90% of human lens growth occurs in the first 2 years of life. In their autopsy study, average capsular bag diameter was 7 mm at birth, 9 mm at age 2, 9.5 mm at age 5, and 10.3 mm at age 16.[78] Dahan in 1987 showed that the use of IOLs with eyelet holes in the haptics and optic reduced the overall diameter of the IOL and facilitated insertion.[79] Assia and Apple showed that the capsular bag in children can tolerate slight oversizing.[80] Based on these data, Wilson et al recommended that capsular IOLs be 10 mm in kids children less than 2 years old and 12–12.5 mm in children more than 2 years old.[81] They recommended IOLs that were of the flexible open-loop, one-piece, PMMA, modified C-loop type. They noted that IOLs placed in the ciliary sulcus in young children would most likely need to be exchanged later on, because the ciliary ring diameter increases steadily throughout childhood, unlike the capsular bag. Wilson et al went on to state that the optimal biomaterial would have enough flexibility for easy insertion into a small eye and yet retain loop memory, as memory allows the loops to re-expand after implantation and keep the original figuration in spite of contractile forces that may occur as the capsule fibroses. Memory also helps reduce tension on zonules, which would be increased if the capsular bag fibrosed and collapsed onto a small IOL while the ciliary ring expanded.

In summary, PMMA continues to be the material of choice for IOLs in children because of its long history of safety. With increasing experience, silicone and Acrysof may come into favor as they offer the potential for foldable IOLs. Acrysof may have the added benefit of decreased PCO and anterior capsule movement due to its increased adhesiveness for LECs; conversely, that would make later IOL exchange more difficult. Coatings with fluorine or heparin may also decrease PCO.

■ Targeting of Refraction

Gordon and Danzis documented that the greatest change in axial length, keratometry, and refractive power occurs in the first 18 months of life.[82] Dahan and Drusedau confirmed that younger children undergo greater myopic shift.[83] Axial length elongation occurs throughout childhood and increases myopia, while thinning of the crystalline lens and corneal flattening, both of which offset myopia, taper off by age 10 years and 3 months, respectively.[84,85] The significant amount of myopic shift in childhood complicates selection of IOL power. Most pediatric ophthalmologists would prefer not to perform future IOL exchange, so they must choose between emmetropia with future myopia or present hyperopia in expectation of a progression toward later emmetropia or mild myopia in adulthood. Some authors have even chosen IOL powers causing myopia to stimulate visual work at near in an attempt to stave off amblyopia, as hyperopia can cause amblyopia.[86] However, the latter seems counterproductive, for significant anisometropia will impede proper visual development. Further, bifocal spectacles and changes in refraction throughout childhood will be needed.

There has been considerable controversy regarding the effect of cataract surgery, IOL implantation, and amblyopia on the refractive growth of the eye. Visual deprivation has been shown to induce axial elongation in animals.[87–89] Lambert et al showed that IOL implantation in neonatal monkeys slowed the growth of axial length over the first year of life relative to the cataractous fellow eye.[90] Sinskey et al presented a case report of a patient with bilateral cataracts in whom the pseudophakic eye grew more slowly than the aphakic eye.[91] In contrast, Enyedi et al, in a prospective series of 83 eyes, found that the myopic shift in refraction and axial lengths of pseudophakic eyes paralleled that of aphakic and normal eyes.[92] They report that the myopic shift was slightly larger than in normal eyes (while the axial length of pseudophakic and normal eyes were not significantly different) and ascribed this difference to the presence of fixed IOL power: in normal ocular development, changes in the lens partly offset the growth of axial length. Flitcroft et al reported that IOL implantation did not significantly affect axial length growth relative to fellow normal eyes.[93] They found that rates of axial elongation and corneal flattening were similar in eyes with congenital and developmental cataracts. Hutchinson et al, in a prospective study of 22 eyes in patients less than 2 years old, found no difference in axial length between pseudophakic and fellow normal eyes over a period of 14 months.[94] McClatchey and Parks, in a mathematical model based on a retrospective series, found that myopic shift was greater in pseudophakic eyes due to a fixed IOL power and not excessive axial length elongation.[95] Von Noorden and Lewis found that patients with unilateral congenital cataracts or unilateral complete blepharoptosis did not consistently have axial elongation in their involved eye.[96] Dahan and Drusedau found that amblyopia increased myopia, whereas Enyedi et al did not.

Dahan and Drusedau recommend that in children less than 2 years old, the IOL power should be chosen to undercorrect the biometry reading for emmetropia by 20%. For children older than 2 years, they recommend undercorrection by 10%. Alternatively, for children younger than 2, they propose that IOL power be based on axial length, as shown in Table 7.1.

Enyedi et al recommend the following:[92]

1. In children up to the age of 7 years, the targeted refraction should be (7 − age in years).
2. In children 8 years old and older, the targeted refraction should be − 1 to − 2 diopters.

Table 7.1
Axial Length versus Recommended IOL Power

Axial Length (mm)	IOL Power (D)
17	28
18	27
19	26
20	24
21	22

IOL power for axial lengths as advocated by Dahan and Drusedau.[83]

Flitcroft et al recommend the following:[93]

1. In children 1–2 months old, the targeted refraction should be +6 diopters.
2. In children 1–4 years old, the targeted refraction should be +3 diopters.
3. In children 5–12 years old, the targeted refraction should be +1 diopters.

In general, the current consensus appears to be aiming for mild hyperopia in expectation of a myopic shift. Of course, IOL selection should be individualized to each patient. For example, if the fellow eye is highly myopic, it might be appropriate to select an IOL aiming for the operate eye to be 1–2 diopters less myopic. In cases of bilateral cataracts, it might be advisable to aim the first eye for emmetropia at adulthood and the second eye for mild myopia at adulthood.

■ Other Surgical Issues

With respect to wound construction and closure, the pediatric eye has less scleral rigidity than the adult eye. Hence, self-sealing sutureless wound construction is less likely to be successful than in adults.[1] Most surgeons use 10-0 nylon for wound closure.[97] However, in children, use of this material may lead to difficulty in removing sutures that cause unacceptable astigmatism or irritation, as suture removal in this population would likely require general anesthesia. Several surgeons use absorbable Vicryl sutures instead.[1]

McDonnell et al recommend a wide anterior capsulotomy to decrease or delay PCO, as PCO begins at the site of apposition of the anterior and posterior capsule leaflets.[98] However, creation of a smaller capsulotomy facilitates lens placement in the bag. The technique of CCC is superior to the traditional "can-opener" capsulotomy. However, capsular tears are much more common with CCC in children than in adults.[1] Wilson et al found that mechanized anterior capsulectomy using a vitrector was easier than CCC and more resistant to tears in children younger than 5 years.[99] Vitrector capsulotomy requires directing the cutting port posteriorly toward the capsule, then applying brief bursts of full suction (250 mm Hg) to engage and cut the capsule.

■ Special Situations

Most surgeons refrain from IOL implantation for microphthalmos because of reports of increased glaucoma[51,100] and the physical dimensions of the eye, which limit the IOL size and also make selection of power more difficult, as power calculation formulas become inaccurate at short axial lengths. IOL implantation is indicated, however, in the management of posterior lenticonus with cataract. In this situation, surgical manipulation of the posterior capsule is difficult and the capsule is more likely to rupture, making IOL placement more difficult.[101] Conditions associated with lens subluxation (Marfan's syndrome, homocystinuria) may be treated with sulcus-fixated IOLs or contact lenses.

■ Comment

Because of distortion of aphakic spectacles, the inconvenience of contact lenses, and postoperative problems associated with epikeratophakia,[1] IOL implantation is becoming increasingly attractive in the management of cataracts in children. The relatively recent IOLAB study[102] reviewed implantation of 1,260 IOLs in pediatric aphakic eyes from 1981 to 1994, and found that they were safe and effective. In 51.8% of patients visual acuity was better than 20/40 at 1 year, and only 15.5% had visual acuity worse than 20/200 at 1 year. As would be expected, older age and secondary cataracts were correlated with better outcomes. Posterior capsule rupture and vitreous loss were the most frequent complications (6.1% and 5.7%, respectively), while CME, glaucoma, corneal edema, and RD rates were all less than 1%. The principal limitation of the study was the high rate of loss to follow-up: 55% of patients were lost to follow-up by 1 year.

If the lack of continuity of care seen in the IOLAB study is typical in the community, the success of IOL use and management of children with congenital cataracts will be vitiated. *Treatment of amblyopia remains essential to optimize visual outcome.* To that end, early intervention is critical in the treatment of cataracts, which is likely one of the main reasons why outcomes in patients with traumatic cataracts undergoing IOL seem consistently superior to outcomes in patients with congenital cataracts.

Implantation of IOLs has become increasingly popular in the pediatric ophthalmology community. In a survey by Wilson et al, 46% of American Association of Pediatric Ophthalmology and Strabismus respondents and 27% of American Society of Cataract and Refractive Surgery respondents stated that they implant IOLs in children.[103] With continued advances in materials, surgical technique, and the treatment of PCO, the use of IOLs in children seems to have a bright future.

■ References

1. Basti S, Greenwald MJ. Principles and paradigms of pediatric cataract management. *Indian J Ophthalmol.* 1995; 43:159–176.
2. Francois J. *Congenital Cataracts.* Springfield, IL: Charles C Thomas; 1963.
3. Merin S, Lapithis AG, Horovitz D, et al. Childhood blindness in Cyprus. *Am J Ophthalmol.* 1972;74:538–542.
4. Fraser GR, Friedman AL. *The Causes of Blindness in Childhood.* Baltimore, MD: Johns Hopkins University Press; 1967.
5. Nelson LB, Wagner RS. Pediatric cataract surgery. *Int Ophthalmol Clin.* 1994;34(2):165–189.
6. Albert DM, Jakobiec FA, eds. *Principles and Practice of Ophthalmology.* Philadelphia: WB Saunders; 1994.
7. Choyce DP. Correction of uni-ocular aphakia by means of anterior chamber acrylic implants. *Trans Ophthalmol Soc UK.* 1958;78:459–470.
8. Binkhorst CD, Gobin MH. Injuries to the eye with lens opacity in young children. *Ophthalmologica.* 1964; 148:169–183.
9. Baker JD, Hiles DA, Morgan KS. Visual rehabilitation of aphakic children. *Surv Ophthalmol.* 1990;34:366–384.
10. Hiles DA, Watson BA. Complications of implant surgery in children. *Am Intraocular Implant Soc J.* 1979;5:24–32.
11. Crouch ER, Pressman SH, Crouch ER. Posterior chamber IOLs: long-term results in pediatric cataract patients. *J Pediatr Ophthalmol Strabismus.* 1995;32:210–218.
12. Awner S, Buckley EG, DeVaro JM, et al. Unilateral pseudophakia in children under 4 years. *J Pediatr Ophthalmol Strabismus.* 1996;33:230–236.
13. Zwaan J, Mullaney PB, Awad A, et al. Pediatric IOL implantation: surgical results and complications in more than 300 patients. *Ophthalmology.* 1998;105:112–119.
14. Dahan E, Salmenson BD. Pseudophakia in children. *J Cataract Refract Surg.* 1990;16:75–82.
15. Hiles DA. IOL implantation in children with monocular cataracts, 1974–1983. *Ophthalmology.* 1984;91:1231–1237.
16. Koenig SB, Ruttum MS, Lewandowski MF, et al. Pseudophakia for traumatic cataracts in children. *Ophthalmology.* 1993;100:1218–1224.
17. Buckley EG, Klombers LA, Seaber JH, et al. Management of the posterior capsule during pediatric IOL implantation. *Am J Ophthalmol.* 1993;115:722–728.
18. Hemo Y, BenEzra D. Traumatic cataracts in young children: correction of aphakia by IOL implanatation. *Ophthalmol Pediatr Gen.* 1987;8:203–207.
19. Cavallaro BE, Madigan WP, O'Hara MA, et al. Posterior chamber IOL use in children. *J Pediatr Ophthalmol Strabismus.* 1998;35:254–263.
20. Andreo LK, Wilson ME, Saunders RA. Predictive value of regression and theoretical IOL formulas in pediatric IOL implantation. *J Pediatr Ophthalmol Strabismus.* 1997; 34:240–243.
21. Hiles DA. Visual rehabilitation of aphakic children: IOLs. *Surv Ophthalmol.* 1990;34:371–379.
22. Basti S, Ravishankar U, Gupta S. Results of a prospective evaluation of three methods of management of pediatric cataracts. *Ophthalmology.* 1996;713–720.
23. Sharma A, Basti S, Gupta S. Secondary capsule-supported IOL implantation in children. *J Cataract Refract Surg.* 1997;23(suppl 1):675–680.
24. Ghosh B, Gupta AK, Taneja S, et al. Epilenticular lens implantation vs extracapsular cataract extraction and lens implantation in children. *J Cataract Refract Surg.* 1997;23:612–617.
25. Plager DA, Lipsky SN, Snyder SK, et al. Capsular management and refractive error in pediatric IOLs. *Ophthalmology.* 1997;104:600–607.
26. DeVaro JM, Buckley EG, Awner S, et al. Secondary posterior chamber IOL implantation in pediatric patients. *Am J Ophthalmol.* 1997;123:24–30.
27. Sinskey RM, Stoppel JO, Amin P. Long-term results of IOL implantation in pediatric patients. *J Cataract Refract Surg.* 1993;19:405–408.
28. Hiles DA, Hered RW. Modern IOL implants in children with new age limitations. *J Cataract Refract Surg.* 1987; 13:493–497.
29. Oliver M, Milstein A, Pollack A. Posterior chamber lens implantation in infants and juveniles. *Eur J Implant Refract Surg.* 1990;2:309–314.
30. Gimbel HV, Ferensowicz M, Raanan M, et al. IOL implantation in children. *J Pediatr Ophthalmol Strabismus.* 1993;30:69–79.
31. Apple DJ, Solomon KD, Jetz MR, et al. Posterior capsular opacification. *Surv Ophthalmol.* 1992;37:73–116.
32. Gupta AK, Grover AK, Gurha N. Traumatic cataract surgery with IOL implantation in children. *J Pediatr Ophthalmol Strabismus.* 1992;29:73–78.
33. Morgan KS, Karcioglu ZA. Secondary cataracts in infants after lensectomies. *J Pediatr Ophthalmol Strabismus.* 1987;24:45–48.
34. Nishi O. Fibrinous membrane formation on the posterior chamber lens during the early postoperative period. *J Cataract Refract Surg.* 1988;14:73–77.
35. BenEzra D, Paez JH. Congenital cataract and IOLs. *Am J Ophthalmol.* 1983;96:311–314.
36. Mackool RJ, Chatiawala H. Pediatric cataract surgery and IOL implantation: a new technique for preventing or excising postoperative secondary membranes. *J Cataract Refract Surg.* 1991;17:62–66.
37. BenEzra D, Cohen E. Posterior capsulectomy in pediatric cataract surgery: the necessity of a choice. *Ophthalmology.* 1997;104:2168–2174.

38. Gimbel HV, DeBroff BM. Posterior capsulorrhexis with optic capture: maintaining a clear visual axis after pediatric cataract surgery. *J Cataract Refract Surg.* 1994; 20:658–664.

39. Gimbel HV. Posterior capsulorrhexis with optic capture in pediatric cataract and IOL surgery. *Ophthalmology.* 1996;103:1871–1875.

40. Gimbel HV. Posterior continuous curvilinear capsulorrhexis and optic capture of the IOL to prevent secondary opacification in pediatric cataract surgery. *J Cataract Refract Surg.* 1997;23:652–656.

41. Koch DD, Kohnen T. Retrospective comparison of techniques to prevent secondary cataract formation after posterior chamber IOL implantation in infants and children. *J Cataract Refract Surg.* 1997;23:657–663.

42. Tablante RT, Lapus JV, Cruz ED, et al. A new technique of congenital cataract surgery with primary posterior chamber IOL implantation. *J Cataract Refract Surg.* 1988;14:149–157.

43. Maltzman BA, Caputo AR, Wagner RS, et al. Neodymium:YAG laser capsulotomy of secondary membranes in the pediatric population. *Am Intraocular Implant Soc J.* 1985;11:572–573.

44. Atkinson CS, Hiles DA. Treatment of secondary posterior capsular membranes with the Nd:YAG laser in a pediatric population. *Am J Ophthalmol.* 1994;118:496–501.

45. Mullaney PB, Wheeler DT, AlNahdi T. Dissolution of pseudophakic fibrinous exudates with intraocular streptokinase. *Eye.* 1996;10:362–366.

46. Hoyt CS, Nickel B. Aphakic cystoid macular edema. *Arch Ophthalmol.* 1982;100:746–749.

47. Morgan KS, Franklin RM. Oral fluorescein angioscopy in aphakic children. *J Pediatr Ophthalmol Strabismus.* 1984;21:33.

48. Gilbard SM, Peyman GA, Goldberg MF. Evaluation for cystoid maculopathy after pars plicata lensectomy-vitrectomy for congenital cataracts. *Ophthalmology.* 1983;90:1201.

49. Poer DV, Helveston EM, Ellis FD. Aphakic cystoid macular edema in children. *Arch Ophthalmol.* 1981;99:249–252.

50. Pinchoff BS, Ellis FD, Helveston EM, et al. Cystoid macular edema in pediatric aphakia. *J Pediatr Ophthalmol Strabismus.* 1988;25:240–243.

51. Parks MM, Johnson DA, Reed GW. Long-term visual results and complications in children with aphakia. *Ophthalmology.* 1993;100:826–840.

52. Chrousos GA, Parks MM, O'Neil JF. Incidence of chronic glaucoma, retinal detachment, and secondary membrane surgery in pediatric aphakic patients. *Ophthalmology.* 1984;91:1238–1241.

53. Simon JW, Mehta N, Simmons ST, et al. Glaucoma after pediatric lensectomy/vitrectomy. *Ophthalmology.* 1991; 98:670–674.

54. Asrani SG, Wilensky JT. Glaucoma after congenital cataract surgery. *Ophthalmology.* 1995;102:863–867.

55. Mills MD, Robb RM. Glaucoma after childhood cataract surgery. *J Pediatr Ophthalmol Strabismus.* 1994;31:355–360.

56. Vajpayee RB, Angra SK, Titiyal JS, et al. Pseudophakic pupillary block glaucoma in children. *Am J Ophthalmol.* 1991;111:715–718.

57. Burke JP, Willsham HE, Young JD. IOL implants for uniocular cataracts. *Br J Ophthalmol.* 1987;73:860.

58. Dutton JJ, Baker JD, Hiles DA, et al. Visual rehabilitation of aphakic children. *Surv Ophthalmol.* 1990;34:365.

59. Kora Y, Inatomi M, Yoshinao F, et al. Long-term study of children with implanted IOLs. *J Cataract Refract Surg.* 1992;18:485.

60. Jungschaffer OH. Retinal detachment after IOL implants. *Arch Ophthalmol.* 1977;95:1203.

61. Apple DJ, Mamalis N, Brady SE, et al. Biocompatibility of implant materials. *Am Intraocular Implant Soc J.* 1984;10:43–66.

62. Steinert RF, Giamporcaro JE, Tasso VA. Clinical assessment of long-term safety and efficacy of a widely implanted silicone IOL material. *Am J Ophthalmol.* 1997; 123:17–23.

63. Okada K, Funahashi M, Iseki K, et al. Comparing the cell populatio on different IOL materials in one eye. *J Cataract Refract Surg.* 1993;19:431–434.

64. Cook CS, Peiffer RL, Mazzocco TR. Clinical and pathologic evaluation of a flexible silicone PCIOL design in a rabbit model. *J Cataract Refract Surg.* 1986;12:130–134.

65. Versura P, Torreggiani A, Cellini M, et al. Adhesion mechanisms of human lens epithelial cells on 4 IOL materials. *J Cataract Refract Surg.* 1999;25:527–533.

66. Majima K. The relationship between morphological changes of lens epithelial cells and IOL optic material. *Jpn J Ophthalmol.* 1998;42:46–50.

67. Linnola RJ. Sandwich theory: bioactivity-based explanation for posterior capsule opacification. *J Cataract Refract Surg.* 1997;23:1539–1542.

68. Hollick EJ, Spalton DJ, Ursell PG, et al. Lens epithelial cell regression on the posterior capsule with different IOL materials. *Br J Ophthalmol.* 1998;82:1182–1188.

69. Nagata T, Wantanabe I. Optic sharp edge or convexity: comparison of effects on posterior capsule opacification. *Jpn J Ophthalmol.* 1996;40:397–403.

70. Ursell PG, Spalton DJ, Pande MV, et al. Relationship between IOL biomaterials and posterior capsule opacification. *J Cataract Refract Surg.* 1998;24:352–360.

71. Joo CK, Shin JA, Kim JH. Capsular opening contraction after continuous curvilinear capsulorrhexis and IOL implantation. *J Cataract Refract Surg.* 1996;22:585–590.

72. Ursell PG, Spalton DJ, Pande MV. Anterior capsule stability in eyes with IOLs made of poly(methylmethacrylate), silicone, and Acrysof. *J Cataract Refract Surg.* 1997;23:1532–1538.

73. Oshika T, Suzuki Y, Kizaki H, et al. Two year clinical study of a soft acrylic IOL. *J Cataract Refract Surg.* 1996; 22:104–109.

74. Gonvers M, Sickenberg, van Melle G. Change in capsulorrhexis size after implantation of 3 types of IOLs. *J Cataract Refract Surg.* 1997;23:231–238.

75. Thouvenin D, Arne JL, Lesueur L. Comparison of fluorine-surface-modified and unmodified lenses for implantation in pediatric aphakia. *J Cataract Refract Surg.* 1996;22:1226–1231.

76. Bechetoille A. Clinical efficiency of fluorinated IOLs in reducing postoperative inflammatory reaction. Presented

at the Symposium on Cataract, IOL, and Refractive Surgery, San Diego, CA, April 1995.

77. Zetterstrom C, Kugelberg U, Oscarson C. Cataract surgery in children with capsulorrhexis of anterior and posterior capsules and heparin-surface-modified IOLs. *J Cataract Refract Surg.* 1994;20:599–601.

78. Bluestein EC, Wilson ME, Wang XH, et al. Dimensions of the pediatric crystalline lens: implications for IOLs in children. *J Pediatr Ophthalmol Strabismus.* 1996;33:18–20.

79. Dahan E. Insertion of IOLs in the capsular bag. *Metab Pediate Syst Ophthalmol.* 1987;10:87–88.

80. Assia EI, Apple DJ. Side-view analysis of the lens: positioning of IOLs. *Arch Ophthalmol.* 1992;110:94–97.

81. Wilson ME, Apple DJ, Bluestein EC, et al. IOLs for pediatric implantation: biomaterials, designs, and sizing. *J Cataract Refract Surg.* 1994;20:584–591.

82. Gordon RA, Donzis PB. Refractive development of the human eye. *Arch Ophthalmol.* 1985;103:785–789.

83. Dahan E, Drusedau M. Choice of lens and dioptric power in pediatric pseudophakia. *J Cataract Refract Surg.* 1997;23:618–623.

84. Mutti DO, Zadnik K, Fusaro RE, et al. Optical and structural development of the crystalline lens in childhood. *Invest Ophthalmol Vis Sci.* 1998;39:120–133.

85. Inagaki Y. The rapid change of corneal curvature in the neonatal period and infancy. *Arch Ophthalmol.* 1986; 104:1026–1027.

86. Huber C. Increasing myopia in children with IOLs. *Eur J Implant Refract Surg.* 1993;5:154–158.

87. Yinon U. Myopia induction in animals following alteration of the visual input during development: a review. *Curr Eye Res.* 1984;3:677–690.

88. Weisel TN, Raviola E. Myopia and eye enlargement after neonatal lid fusion in monkeys. *Nature.* 1977;266:66–68.

89. Von Noorden GK, Crawford ML. Lid closure and refractive error in macaque monkeys. *Nature.* 1978;272:53–54.

90. Lambert SR, Fernandes A, Drew-Botsch C, et al. Pseudophakia retards axial elongation in neonatal monkeys. *Invest Ophthalmol Vis Sci.* 1996;37:451–458.

91. Sinskey RM, Stoppel JO, Amin PA. Ocular axial length changes in a pediatric patient with aphakia and pseudophakia. *J Cataract Refract Surg.* 1993;19:787–788.

92. Enyedi LB, Peterseim MW, Freedman SF, et al. Refractive changes after pediatric IOL implantation. *Am J Ophthalmol.* 1998;126:772–781.

93. Flitcroft DI, Knight-Nanan D, Bowell R, et al. IOLs in children: changes in axial length, corneal curvature, and refraction. *Br J Ophthalmol.* 1999;83:265–269.

94. Hutchinson AK, Wilson ME, Saunders RA. Outcomes and ocular growth rates after IOL implantation in the 1st 2 years of life. *J Cataract Refract Surg.* 1998;14:846–852.

95. McClatchey SK, Parks MM. Theoretic refractive changes after lens implantation in childhood. *Ophthalmology.* 1997;104:1744–1751.

96. Von Noorden GK, Lewis RA. Ocular axial length in unilateral congenital cataracts and blepharoptosis. *Invest Ophthalmol Vis Sci.* 1987;28:750–752.

97. Lavrich JB, Goldberg DS, Nelson LB. Suture use in pediatric cataract surgery. *Ophthalmic Surg.* 1993;24:554–555.

98. McDonnell PJ, Marco MA, Green WR. Posterior capsule opacification in pseudophakic eyes. *Ophthalmology.* 1983;90:1548–1553.

99. Wilson ME, Saunders RA, Roberts EL, et al. Mechanized anterior capsulectomy as an alternative to manual capsulorrhexis in children undergoing IOL implantation. *J Pediatr Ophthalmol Strabismus.* 1996;33:237–240.

100. Egbert JE, Wright MM, Dahlhauser KF et al. A prospective study of ocular hypertension and glaucoma after pediatric cataract surgery. *Ophthalmology.* 1995;102:1098–1101.

101. Cheng KP, Hiles DA, Biglan AW, et al. Management of posterior lenticonus. *J Pediatr Ophthalmol Strabismus.* 1991;28:143–149.

102. Young TL, Bloom JN, Ruttum M, et al. The IOLAB, Inc pediatric IOL study. *J Am Assoc Pediatr Ophthalmic Surg.* 1999;3(5):295–302.

103. Wilson ME, Bluestein EC, Wang XH. Current trends in the use of IOLs in children. *J Cataract Refract Surg.* 1994;20:579–583.

Chapter 8

Intraocular Lens Surgery in Glaucoma

Teresa C. Chen

The management of coexisting cataract and glaucoma is more challenging than the treatment of either problem alone. Cataract and intraocular lens (IOL) surgery is more difficult in the patient with glaucoma. For example, posterior synechiae and miosis from long-term pilocarpine or carbachol treatment complicate cataract extraction. Eyes in patients who have been taking epinephrine compounds can be congested, which may lead to excess bleeding at the time of surgery. Chronic treatment with this and other pharmacologic agents often leads to a breakdown of the blood–aqueous barrier, with increased cells and flare and the development of smudgy macrophage precipitates (resembling keratic precipitates) on the IOL surfaces. These changes are frequently accompanied by a sticky iris, which adheres to the posterior capsule and the IOL in the postoperative period. This may create iris capture of the lens, posterior synechiae, and pupillary block.[1] Pseudoexfoliation, even without glaucoma, not only may make pupillary dilation difficult but also may cause phacodonesis and weakening of the zonules. Both of these factors increase the risk of vitreous loss and lens dislocation intraoperatively. Patients with chronically narrow angles or peripheral anterior synechiae may not tolerate an anterior chamber IOL (ACIOL) as well. Eyes that already have a compromised outflow facility are more likely to have intraocular pressure (IOP) elevation after IOL surgery. Sudden lowering of IOP during surgery in an eye with a high preoperative pressure can also increase the likelihood of a suprachoroidal hemorrhage. Visual rehabilitation is also delayed.

Glaucoma is also more difficult to treat in the patient who has already undergone IOL surgery. Conjunctival scarring from previous operations decreases the success rate of filtering surgery. This scarring can also make dissection more difficult and increase the chance of "buttonholes" in the conjunctiva.[2] If many procedures have already been done, conventional trabeculectomy may not be possible, and either antimetabolites or a tube shunt may have to be used.

This chapter discusses preoperative considerations in a patient who has glaucoma and who needs IOL surgery, guidelines for combined cataract extraction with IOL implantation and trabeculectomy surgery, and the more common complications that occur after combined cataract extraction and trabeculectomy. Emphasis will be placed on postoperative complications that involve elevated IOP.

■ Preoperative Considerations in Patients with Glaucoma and Cataracts

Surgical Options in the Patient with Coexisting Cataract and Glaucoma

There are three basic options for the patient with coexisting glaucoma and cataract: cataract surgery alone, combined cataract and glaucoma surgery, and glaucoma surgery before cataract surgery (two-stage procedure).

Cataract Surgery Alone
Cataract surgery alone may be performed in the glaucoma suspect or in the patient with medically controlled glaucoma and minimal visual field loss. In the latter situation, some surgeons advocate combined cataract and glaucoma surgery if the patient is taking

more than one glaucoma medication. For cataract extraction alone in a glaucoma patient, either small-incision cataract surgery or a clear cornea approach is advantageous in preserving the conjunctiva for future filter surgery.

Combined Cataract and Glaucoma Surgery

With the advent of antimetabolites and small-incision cataract surgery, combined cataract extraction and trabeculectomy surgery has become a better choice for more patients (Fig. 8.1). Combined surgery is a good option in patients with visually significant cataract and glaucoma that is medically well-controlled. It is also an option in patients with marginally significant cataract and poorly controlled glaucoma but who either have a cataract that is expected to progress to visual significance after glaucoma surgery or are unable to tolerate more than one operation.

A combined procedure is also a good option in the patient with advanced glaucoma who would not be able to tolerate a postoperative IOP elevation. Combined procedures may reduce the incidence of postoperative IOP elevation compared to cataract surgery alone,[3,4] and therefore may decrease additional visual field loss in the perioperative period.[3] Moster and colleagues noted that even transient IOP elevation in eyes with advanced chronic glaucoma can result in a loss of at least one line of vision in 25% of eyes.[5]

Combined cataract and glaucoma surgery can be performed either by phacoemulsification and trabeculectomy or by extracapsular cataract extraction (ECCE) and trabeculectomy. Most feel that IOP control is better with the former than with the latter. Some studies question the efficacy of IOP reduction in com-

bined ECCE-trabeculectomy compared to trabeculectomy alone, noting that combined procedures decrease IOP only 3–7.8 mm Hg at 1–2 years postoperatively.[1,6,7] Shields also feels that long-term IOP control is not as predictable as with the two-stage approach.[8] Studies of combined ECCE-trabeculectomy, however, note that in 92%–100% of patients, IOP is less than 21 mm Hg at an average follow-up of 14–16.8 months.[9,10] Other studies report that 42%–72% of patients are off medications postoperatively at an average follow-up of 11–24 months.[1,6,7,9,11,12]

Other investigators feel that at 1-year follow-up, there is no difference in IOP control between patients who underwent combined phacoemulsification-trabeculectomy and those who underwent trabeculectomy alone. This difference in opinion may reflect the possibly greater IOP reduction with phacoemulsification-trabeculectomy than with ECCE-trabeculectomy. Shingleton and colleagues noted an average reduction of 5 mm Hg following phacoemulsification-trabeculectomy and 3 mm Hg following ECCE-trabeculectomy.[13] Wishart et al reported that 79.4% of eyes treated by phacoemulsification-trabeculectomy, compared with 53% of eyes treated by ECCE-trabeculectomy, no longer required glaucoma medications at an average follow-up of 13 months.[12]

In addition to better IOP control, other advantages of phacoemulsification-trabeculectomy over ECCE-trabeculectomy include the smaller incision with phacoemulsification, resulting in reduced inflammation and less suture compression of the angle. Reduced inflammation may contribute to increased bleb formation. With the smaller incision, more conjunctiva is preserved for future operations. Although both techniques appear to result in nearly equal improvement in visual acuity, with 65%–89% of patients gaining 20/40 or better vision,[1,14] recovery of visual acuity is faster after phacoemulsification-trabeculectomy.[13] Even though Hurvitz noted no difference in astigmatism after combined operations incorporating ECCE or phacoemulsification,[15] others have reported less postoperative astigmatism with phacoemulsification.[12] Most studies report about 2 diopters of against-the-rule astigmatism after combined procedures.[1] Wishart also noted a higher rate of postoperative complications after ECCE-trabeculectomy than after phacoemulsification-trabeculectomy.[12] The smaller incision may be safer in patients who are at increased risk for suprachoroidal hemorrhage, and postoperative massage techniques are likely to be safer with a smaller incision.[16]

Other options include one-site surgery (trabeculectomy with cataract extraction through the same incision) versus two-site surgery (trabeculectomy in a superior quadrant with a temporal clear cornea incision for cataract extraction). This is different from the two-stage

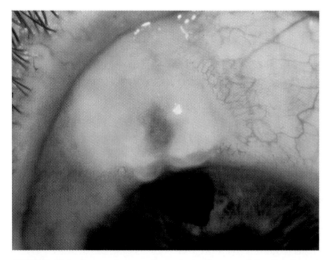

FIGURE 8.1. Appearance of an eye after combined cataract extraction and mitomycin C trabeculectomy.

approach in that both operations are performed at the same sitting. A few reports suggest that similar visual acuity and IOP reduction are achieved with both one-site and two-site surgery.[17] However, the one-site surgery may require more medication to maintain IOP control.[18]

Glaucoma Surgery Before Cataract Surgery (Two-Stage Procedure)

Patients with advanced glaucomatous optic nerve and visual field damage that is uncontrolled with maximal medical therapy may benefit from filtering surgery alone. Even though there may be a visually significant cataract, trabeculectomy surgery alone may result in a lower IOP than would a combined procedure.[15,19,20] Filtering surgery may also cause progression of the cataract. Another disadvantage of this two-stage procedure is that subsequent cataract extraction can cause the filter to fail[1] or may result in a 2–5 mm Hg rise in IOP.[2,21] Subsequent cataract surgery should be done as far away from the bleb as possible. A clear cornea approach should be considered.

Lens-Induced Glaucoma

Certain types of glaucoma are lens-induced and may require only cataract extraction. These include phacolytic glaucoma, lens particle glaucoma, phacoanaphylaxis, phacomorphic glaucoma, and lens dislocation.

Phacolytic Glaucoma

Phacolytic glaucoma results from leakage of high molecular weight lens proteins from a hypermature, or morgagnian, cataract through an intact anterior lens capsule. Macrophages become distended with this lens material and with morgagnian fluid, and subsequently obstruct the intertrabecular spaces.[22] The clinical picture includes corneal edema and an open angle (Fig. 8.2). The anterior chamber may show intense flare and circulating particulate matter. The lens may have white capsular patches or aggregates of macrophages on its anterior surface.[23] Immediate attempts should be made to lower IOP medically. Pilocarpine should be avoided. Patients may also be treated with intensive topical steroids as well as cycloplegics. It is always possible to wait at least 2–3 days before surgical intervention so that the IOP is lowered and the anterior chamber reaction is reduced. The definitive treatment is cataract extraction.[24–26]

Lens Particle Glaucoma

Lens particle glaucoma manifests with an increase in IOP after ECCE, penetrating lens injury, or posterior capsulotomy with a neodymium:yttrium-aluminum-garnet (Nd:YAG) laser. Obstruction to aqueous flow in

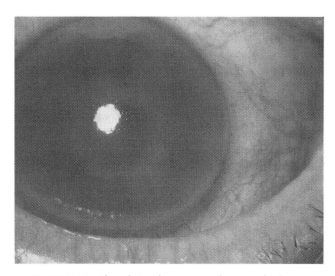

FIGURE 8.2. Phacolytic glaucoma with corneal edema.

these cases is caused by mechanical blockage of the trabecular meshwork by "normal" lens particles. The severity of the glaucoma is usually related to the amount of free cortical material in the aqueous fluid. Considerable free lens material may be seen in the anterior chamber. Therapy is initially medical to lower the IOP. Topical steroids are used, but miotics should be avoided. If glaucoma persists despite attempts at medical management, the remaining cortical material should be removed without delay.[23]

Phacoanaphylaxis

Phacoanaphylactic glaucoma is a severe inflammatory reaction directed against lenticular antigens. It may cause elevation of IOP when the trabecular meshwork is affected by the inflammatory processes or when it becomes obstructed by inflammatory cells. Alternatively, formation of synechiae may result in pupillary block. In some cases hypotony is seen, with hyposecretion by the ciliary body secondary to persistent inflammation. Classically, phacoanaphylaxis manifests 24 hours to 14 days after operative or other trauma to the lens capsule in a patient previously sensitized to lens antigens. However, it has been observed up to 1 year after cataract extraction and up to 59 years after trauma. The intense reaction is clinically demonstrated by lid edema, chemosis, conjunctival injection, corneal edema, heavy anterior chamber reaction, and mutton fat keratic precipitates. Therapy is directed toward lowering the IOP and controlling inflammation; however, surgical removal of the remaining lens material may ultimately be needed. Removal of the posterior capsule may result in resolution of the inflammation, presumably by removing residual cortical material and thereby eliminating the inciting stimulus.[23]

Glaucoma Secondary to Lens Intumescence (Phacomorphic Glaucoma)

A mature or intumescent cataract can precipitate an attack of acute angle-closure glaucoma, also known as phacomorphic glaucoma, in eyes with occludable angles as well as in eyes with wide open angles. Lens swelling can result in angle closure, initially through pupillary block and at later stages through direct displacement of the peripheral iris by the swollen lens against angle structures. In phacomorphic glaucoma, cataract extraction usually normalizes IOP, unless the angle is damaged by peripheral anterior synechiae.[26] The acute attack can be reversed in some cases by laser iridotomy. This may allow the eye to quiet down before cataract surgery. After laser treatment, preoperative mydriasis may be safer. In addition, the surgeon can assess IOP control to determine whether glaucoma and cataract surgery should be performed simultaneously.[27]

Glaucoma Associated with Lens Dislocation

Ectopia lentis occurs when the lens is loosened from some or all of its zonular attachments (Fig. 8.3). The lens either shifts forward, producing pupillary block, or combines its abnormal position with the interposition of vitreous to produce vitreolenticular block.[23] Initially medical treatment is used. If pupillary block is present, other treatments may be used, including corneal depression, laser iridectomy, gonioplasty, laser coreoplasty, and eventually cataract extraction.[23]

Glaucoma Secondary to Retained Lens Fragments

Retained lens fragments may be associated with glaucoma and an IOP greater than 30 mm Hg in 36.8% of

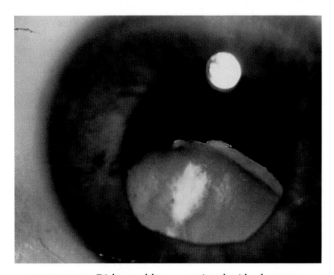

FIGURE 8.3. Dislocated lens associated with glaucoma.

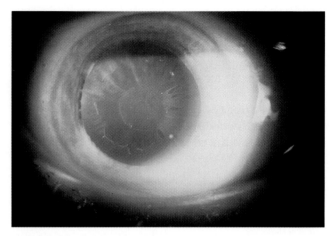

FIGURE 8.4. Pseudoexfoliation material producing a target-like pattern on the anterior lens capsule.

patients before vitrectomy and in 3.2% of patients after vitrectomy. Vitrectomy for removal of retained lens fragments reduces secondary glaucoma. Early vitrectomy generally is recommended, but delayed vitrectomy also has favorable outcomes.[28]

Other Types of Glaucoma

Pseudoexfoliation

There is a significantly higher rate of complications in pseudoexfoliation patients (Fig. 8.4).[29,30] In addition to a higher incidence of glaucoma,[31] these patients have increased intraoperative complications, including zonular weakness, phacodonesis,[32,33] lens dislocation,[32] posterior capsular rupture,[34] vitreous loss,[32] reduced endothelial cell count,[35] and increased fibrinoid reaction with posterior synechiae and IOL cell deposits.[16,36] These patients also may have poor pharmacologic dilation.[34,37–39] Phacoemulsification may be gentler on zonular attachments than ECCE and will facilitate completion of an uncomplicated operation.[13] Supracapsular cataract extraction may also be less traumatic to the zonules than other phacoemulsification techniques. In cases of subluxed lenses, either pars plana lensectomy or intracapsular cryoextraction may be needed.

Glaucoma with Penetrating Keratoplasty

A prolonged increase in IOP occurs in 12%−51% of eyes after penetrating keratoplasty. Open-angle glaucoma after penetrating keratoplasty may be related to a change in the microstructure of the angle after the graft. Progressive angle closure after penetrating keratoplasty is another mechanism. In some, a steroid response may develop. Medical treatment is the first line of care. When this fails, if the angle is open and viable, argon laser trabeculoplasty may be an option. If further

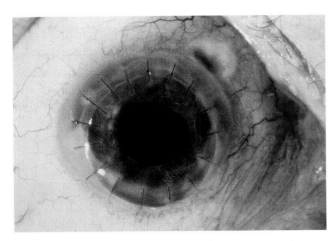

FIGURE 8.5. Appearance of an eye after penetrating keratoplasty and mitomycin C trabeculectomy.

intervention is needed, a drainage seton is an option, as success rates for trabeculectomy are poor in this setting (Fig. 8.5). For eyes with poor visual potential, laser cyclodestruction may be an option.[40]

■ Intraoperative Considerations in Combined Cataract Extraction and Filtering Surgery

Preparation for Surgery

For either cataract extraction or a combined procedure, miotics should be discontinued in order to facilitate pupillary dilation during surgery and minimize postoperative inflammation. If possible, it is also preferable to stop oral aqueous suppressants the evening before surgery. If aqueous production continues to be suppressed postoperatively, the chance of a flat chamber and bleb failure is increased.[41] Phospholine iodide should be discontinued 3 weeks before surgery. Some authors suggest either discontinuing sympathomimetic medications preoperatively or using topical steroids preoperatively to minimize postoperative inflammation.[42] Aspirin or Coumadin products should also be discontinued five to seven days before surgery.

Anesthesia should ideally be topical or retrobulbar. General anesthesia not only increases systemic risks but may also induce postoperative coughing.

Eyes with extremely high preoperative IOPs (>50 mm Hg) may benefit from 1–2 g/kg of intravenous 25% mannitol administered over 45 minutes to avoid sudden decompression of the eye, which may predispose to suprachoroidal hemorrhage.

The α-adrenergic receptor agonist apraclonidine has been shown to be effective in controlling IOP increases

after cataract extraction. Oral carbonic anhydrase inhibitors do not seem especially effective in preventing these IOP increases,[3] although some investigators still consider them helpful.[20]

Intraoperative Considerations

Bridle Suture
A bridle suture is not always needed for a fornix-based conjunctival flap, but it may be useful for a limbus-based flap. A 6-0 silk bridle suture on a tapered needle placed through the perilimbal cornea will minimize manipulation of the conjunctiva.

Fornix-Based versus Limbus-Based Conjunctival Flap
It is always best to limit conjunctival dissection as this will decrease postoperative inflammation. A fornix-based flap is technically easier and quicker to do; however, a limbus-based flap may result in a more formed bleb. A formed bleb ensures separation of the conjunctiva from the sclera, thus decreasing the likelihood that these two surfaces will scar together.[41] A fornix-based flap also does not require repeated handling (it does not need to be draped on and off the cornea).[1] A limbus-based flap may result in fewer bleb leaks,[6,41] which would increase the safety of antimetabolite therapy. Since others have not noted any clear advantage in long-term IOP control in the technically more difficult limbus-based flap,[1,6,43] we recommend the fornix-based flap for combined cataract and glaucoma surgery.

Antimetabolites
Antimetabolites increase the success rates of combined procedures.[44–46] Mitomycin C (MMC) appears to be more effective with respect to IOP control in combined procedures than 5-fluorouracil (5-FU).[8,42] Although 5-FU improves IOP control after filtering surgery alone,[47,48] most of the evidence suggests that postoperative 5-FU injections do not improve IOP control in combined cataract and filtering procedures.[9,19,49–51] Only a few studies indicate that there may be a benefit of 5-FU in combined surgery.[52,53] In general, we recommend MMC over 5-FU for better IOP control in combined procedures.

Either before or after the scleral flap is created, but before the anterior chamber is entered, a pledget or cut Weck-cel saturated with 0.4 mg/mL of MMC is applied subconjunctivally for 2–3.5 minutes.[2,54] Longer application times are reserved for patients at higher risk of filtration failure. Some surgeons prefer to apply the MMC before dissection of the scleral flap, since aqueous concentrations in humans are thought to be higher if the scleral flap is cut first.[55] Care is taken to avoid the cut edges of the conjunctiva. It is extremely important to make sure that the MMC does not get into the eye. Instruments used to handle the MMC should not be used for the rest of the procedure unless they are cleaned thoroughly.

Scleral Flap

A triangular, rectangular, or trapezoidal partial thickness scleral flap may be made with a 3–4 mm base. If a larger diameter optic is placed, the base of the scleral flap may be extended laterally in a linear or curvilinear fashion posterior to the limbus.

Paracentesis

A paracentesis facilitates irrigation and anterior chamber decompression and reformation. An optional maneuver is to decrease IOP in a controlled and gradual fashion via the paracentesis. This may minimize chances of suprachoroidal hemorrhage in eyes with an extremely high preoperative IOP (> 50 mm Hg). When the paracentesis is initially made, a small, controlled amount of fluid is released from the eye to decrease the IOP. After a minute or two, more fluid may be released from the paracentesis site if needed. After the paracentesis is made and viscoelastic agent has been injected into the anterior chamber, the anterior chamber can be entered with a keratome beneath the scleral flap.

Small Pupil

A small pupil is more common in patients with glaucoma than without glaucoma. There are several techniques to enlarge the pupil prior to cataract extraction. The pupil stretch technique is sufficient in most cases. Not only is it simple to perform but it also leaves a cosmetically round pupil. Any posterior synechiae should be first broken with a cyclodialysis spatula. Kuglen or Hirschman iris hooks or Graether collar buttons may be used to stretch the pupil at 12 and 6 o'clock for 20–30 seconds (Fig. 8.6A, *left*). The pupil is then stretched at 3 and 9 o'clock for another 20–30 seconds (Fig. 8.6A *right*). This may be repeated, if necessary, in the oblique meridians.[56] The maneuver creates small sphincter tears located midway between the two instruments.[57] A three-pronged Beehler pupil dilator serves a similar function (Fig. 8.6B).

Other techniques include multiple sphincterotomies.[58] Three radial sphincterotomies at 4:30, 6:00, and 7:30 o'clock are usually sufficient for adequate capsulorrhexis. Occasionally two additional radial sphincterotomies at 3:00 and 9:00 o'clock may be necessary.[59] This may be combined with pupil stretching to enlarge the pupil.[60]

A sector iridectomy can also be done.[61] Although repair of a sector iridectomy is usually not necessary, repair with corioplasty should be considered if the patient strongly desires a round pupil, if an IOL with a small diameter is used, if IOL fixation is other than in the bag, or if the patient has a wide palpebral fissure.[16]

Iris retractors may also be helpful when there are risks with cutting or tearing the iris, such as with rubeosis.[62] Monofilament iris retractors designed by DeJuan are manufactured by Grieshaber (Fig. 8.6C). These retractors have a Silastic sleeve that can be adjusted to yield a triangular or square pupil. Similar iris hooks have been designed by Mackool.[63]

The Graether pupil expander, a device for mechanically dilating the pupil, is a soft silicone ring grooved to engage the iris sphincter and maintain pupil dilation during cataract surgery and IOL implantation (Fig. 8.6D). The pupil expander is preloaded on a disposable insertion tool. Placement of the pupil expander is facilitated by an iris glide retractor that fixates the iris sphincter at the incision prior to insertion of the pupil expander.[64]

These methods, in conjunction with the space-expanding properties of viscoelastic material,[65] may improve visibility during cataract extraction. Iris manipulation should be minimized, as it can contribute significantly to postoperative inflammation.[16,42]

Cataract Extraction and Intraocular Lens Implantation

Most surgeons use a posterior chamber IOL (PCIOL) when possible. Although an anterior chamber lens should be avoided if the angle is compromised, it is not necessarily contraindicated in the presence of glaucoma.[2] Traditionally, ACIOLs have been considered relatively contraindicated in eyes with glaucoma because of an association with IOP increases, peripheral anterior synechiae formation, and corneal endothelial cell loss. Many of the reports of ACIOL complications involved rigid, closed-loop lens designs. The newer semiflexible, open-loop ACIOL design may be a safe alternative for patients in whom intraoperative conditions are not conducive to a sutured lens or if the surgeon is uncomfortable with the procedure. The latter situation is not uncommon, given the infrequent need of putting in a sutured IOL.[16]

When an ACIOL is needed, the lens haptics should be positioned so that they are away from the peripheral iridectomy. Also, when a combined procedure is performed, the filtration portion of the procedure will provide an alternative pathway to control IOP, and the presence of an anterior chamber lens may not hinder postoperative pressure control.[42]

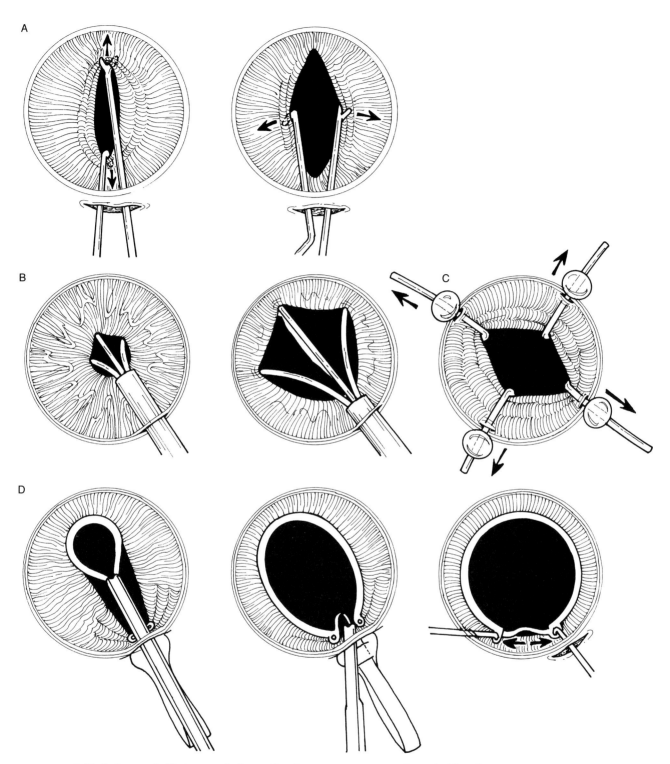

FIGURE 8.6. Techniques of dilating a miotic pupil prior to cataract extraction. *A,* After the posterior synechiae are broken, the pupil is stretched with a Y-hook and a Sinskey hook. *B,* Use of a three-pronged Beehler pupil dilator to achieve the similar result. *C,* Grieshaber iris hooks (retractors) in Silastic sleeves used to create a square pupil. *D,* Use of the preloaded Graether pupil expander assisted by an iris glide retractor (*D, left*) prior to loading, and a Sinskey hook (*D, right*) after iris sphincter engagement. *(From Azar DT, Rumelt S. Phacoemulsification. In: Albert DM, Jakobiec FA, eds. Principles and Practice of Ophthalmology. 2nd ed. Philadelphia: WB Saunders; 2000:1510, with permission.)*

Miotics

Miosis at this point would facilitate the filtration part of the surgery. Intracameral carbachol (Miostat) may also reduce the incidence and severity of postoperative IOP rises. Acetylcholine (Miochol) is short-acting and quickly metabolized by acetylcholinesterase, and provides no long-acting IOP control.[3]

Sclerostomy

By this point, the anterior chamber beneath the scleral flap has already been incised with a keratome. The incision should have been made quite anteriorly through clear cornea. A Kelly Descemet punch is used to complete the trabecular block excision. Because the anterior incision has already been made, the surgeon need only hook the posterior wound margin with the punch and excise the block.[41]

Peripheral Iridectomy

The peripheral iridectomy is then made, ensuring that iris tissue will not block the sclerostomy.

Laser Suture Lysis versus Releasables

The scleral flap may be closed with 10-0 nylon interrupted sutures, which can be lysed later with an argon laser, or with 10-0 nylon releasable sutures. Closure of the scleral flap should allow aqueous to be easily obtainable when pressure is applied to the posterior bed of the flap. This is best demonstrated by filling the anterior chamber with balanced saline solution and observing runoff from the trabeculectomy site.[1]

Conjunctival Closure

Tenonectomy is not routinely done unless a thick Tenon's layer may make laser suture lysis difficult. Conjunctival closure of a fornix-based flap is accomplished with 8-0 Vicryl wing sutures at the medial and lateral extremes of the conjunctival incision. The anterior edge of the conjunctival flap is stretched tight enough to overlap the cornea by a few millimeters.[1] Shingleton and colleagues noted the importance of the very anterior placement of the conjunctival flap upon closure.[13] With this in mind, they did not note any postoperative bleb leaks, despite using the fornix-based conjunctival incision. Conjunctival closure of a limbus-based flap is the same as traditional closure of the usual trabeculectomy.

Postoperative Care

In addition to antibiotic drops, patients who have undergone combined procedures should be treated with topical steroids for 3 months. Although cycloplegic treatment (e.g., with atropine 1%) may be helpful, it is not as critical in pseudophakic patients (in whom anterior chamber shallowing and choroidals are not as common) as it is in phakic or aphakic patients.[41]

In general, if IOP is too high in the first few postoperative days, topical glaucoma treatment or gentle digital pressure may also be tried. The latter may loosen the sutures and open drainage through the scleral flap. If the IOP remains elevated after these more conservative measures, pulling the releasable suture or performing laser suture lysis may be beneficial. If antimetabolites were used, suture releasing or lysis done too early can result in hypotony[55] or may increase the risk of shallow or flat anterior chamber and wound leak.[44] Flap sutures may be cut with an argon laser and Hoskins lens (400–800 mW, 50–100 μm, 0.05–0.1 second).

If early bleb failure is suspected despite laser suture lysis or the pulling of releasable sutures, adjunctive 5-fluorouracil (5-FU) may be tried in 5-mg doses (0.1 mL of 5-FU 50 mg/mL) subconjunctivally 180 degrees away from the bleb. This treatment may be used once or twice a week or more often. 5-FU may even be initiated several months after the initial surgery,[2] and may be used even if mitomycin C was used during the surgery.[55]

■ Postoperative Considerations

Combined trabeculectomy and cataract extraction procedures have a higher complication rate than either procedure alone.[59] This section describes the more common complications that may occur after combined cataract and glaucoma surgery, with special emphasis on complications that involve elevated IOP.

Endophthalmitis/Blebitis

The incidence of endophthalmitis is higher in patients who have undergone combined procedures (1.0%) than in those who have undergone cataract extraction alone (0.15%).[9] The incidence may be even higher in patients who undergo combined procedures that use mitomycin C.[66,67]

Bleb-related endophthalmitis is a virulent form of bleb-related infection in which patients present with rapidly worsening vision, opalescent blebs (white-on-red appearance), intense fibrin and/or hypopyon in the anterior chamber, and florid vitritis. Blebitis is a limited form of bleb-related infection in which patients have intense peribleb conjunctival congestion, opalescent bleb with epithelial defects (a positive Seidel's test in most cases; Fig. 8.7A), with or without anterior chamber reaction, and the absence of vitritis (Fig. 8.7B). Blebitis, which is usually caused by *Staphylococcus epi-*

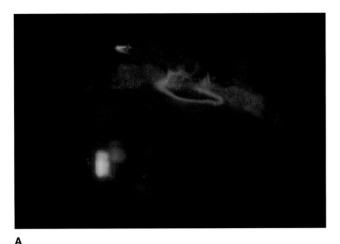

A

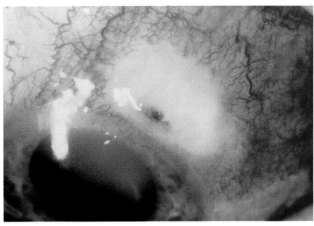

B

FIGURE 8.7. *A,* A positive Seidel test, demonstrating a limbal bleb leak. Pooling of aqueous is highlighted by the fluorescein dye. *B,* Blebitis with injection surrounding the avascular mitomycin C bleb.

dermidis or *S. aureus,* reponds to topical or systemic antibiotics with complete recovery of vision and IOP to preinfection status. Bleb-related endophthalmitis is most commonly caused by *Staphylococcus, Streptococcus,* or *Hemophilus influenzae* and has a poor prognosis despite intensive topical, systemic, and intravitreal antibiotic treatment and vitrectomy.[68,69]

Bleb Leaks

During the first few postoperative days, a small amount of aqueous leakage may occur at the edge of the conjunctival incision (Fig. 8.7A). If the chamber remains formed and the filtration bleb remains elevated, the leak can be observed, since it should stop spontaneously. The patient should limit exertional activities, straining, or bending during this time and protect the eye from rubbing or inadvertent pressure.[1]

Late bleb leaks are more common in eyes that had been treated with mitomycin C.[70] If a late bleb leak is detected or if an early bleb leak persists, aminoglycoside antibiotics to stimulate inflammation may be tried. Aqueous suppressants may slow the flow through the leak and also facilitate healing. A bandage contact lens (20–24 mm) may be helpful. If conservative measures such as autologous blood injection or tissue adhesive fail, the leak may require surgical repair.[71–73]

Hypotony

Hypotony usually occurs when the IOP is less than 5 mm Hg, which can lead to functional and structural changes in the eye. Hypotony may occur in 1.7%–6.0% of combined cataract extraction-trabeculectomy proce-

dures without antimetabolites.[9,74] Although combined surgery with mitomycin C may have higher success rates, it is also associated with a higher incidence of hypotony, 2.2%–9.0%.[51,67,75–79]

Postoperative hypotony has three main causes: a bleb leak, ciliochoroidal detachment, or excess filtration. In the latter, reformation of the anterior chamber and drainage of any choroidal effusions should be performed. Prompt surgical intervention is especially critical, because contact with the IOL produces irreversible corneal endothelial damage.[1] Although a flat chamber with intraocular-corneal touch would seem common with hypotony after combined procedures, the problem, fortunately, is rare.

Hypotony after trabeculectomy alone is more frequent, occurring in 10%–23% of patients so treated.[74] Higher rates of hypotony have been suggested with longer intraoperative use or higher concentrations of mitomycin C, young myopic patients, and early laser suture lysis of the scleral flap. Other studies suggest that these associations do not exist.[67]

Hyphema

Combined procedures are associated with a higher rate of postoperative hyphema (6%–55%)[1,6,14,51,59] than cataract extraction alone (0.87%).[9] In one series of 72 eyes treated by combined cataract extraction-trabeculectomy, Shingleton and colleagues noted no postoperative hyphemas.[13] They attributed this result to anterior dissection of the scleral flap and anterior placement of the sclerotomy. This approach may minimize scleral bleeding from the punch sclerectomy site and posterior bleeding from the peripheral iridectomy site. Postoperative hyphemas usually resolve spontaneously over several days and do not affect the overall success of the trabeculectomy.[1]

Capsulotomy

In some reports combined procedures have been associated with a higher rate of postoperative capsulotomy (12%–19%)[79] than cataract extraction alone (6.55%).[9] Shin and colleagues suggest that mitomycin C application during combined cataract and glaucoma surgery may increase aqueous mitomycin C levels enough to inhibit lens epithelial cell proliferation and result in a decrease in posterior capsular opacification.[80]

Pupillary Capture

Pupillary capture has also been reported to be more common in patients undergoing combined procedures (5.4%–32.4%) than in those undergoing cataract extraction alone (0%–0.57%) (Fig. 8.8).[9,12]

Suprachoroidal Hemorrhage

Suprachoroidal hemorrhage may be more common in eyes with glaucoma. It is also more common in aphakic or highly myopic eyes that have undergone trauma or vitrectomy.[3] If pain and IOP cannot be medically controlled with aqueous suppressants and hyperosmotics, or if the IOP is extremely high, drainage of the suprachoroidal blood may be required. If possible, drainage should be delayed until clot lysis has occurred (3–5 days). Sclerotomies should be placed at or near the center of the choroidal elevation, as determined visually or by ultrasound. If the clot is not fully lysed, a large scleral incision (10–12 mm) may be required to evacuate the clot.[3]

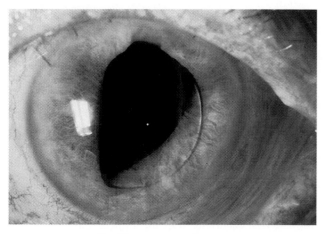

FIGURE 8.8. Pupillary capture after cataract surgery.

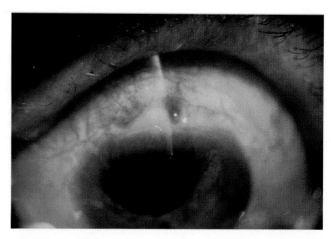

FIGURE 8.9. Slit-lamp beam showing a limbal area of corneal thinning or dellen.

Cystoid Macular Edema

The incidence of cystoid macular edema (CME) in patients who have undergone cataract extraction-trabeculectomy has been reported as 2.7%–9%.[6,77,79] CME in these patients is treated in the same fashion as CME in patients who had cataract extraction alone. If glaucoma medications are being used, it is important to avoid dipivefrin or epinephrine compounds in aphakic patients, who may be susceptible to drug-induced macular edema.

Retinal Detachment

Retinal detachment also occurs more commonly in patients who have undergone combined cataract extraction-trabeculectomy procedures. This is especially true if there were intraoperative complications such as vitreous loss.

Corneal Dellen

Corneal dellen may develop adjacent to elevated blebs (Fig. 8.9). Most dellen resolve with topical lubrication, but bleb revision may be needed in some cases.

■ Postoperative IOP Elevation

Postoperative IOP elevation (≥15 mm Hg) occurs more commonly in patients with glaucoma (23%–40%) than in those without glaucoma (3%).[9,20,51] Studies report increased IOP after cataract extraction in 15%–33% of patients.[1,6,10,12] Some causes included inadequate filtration from tight suturing of the scleral flap, retained viscoelastic agent, or occlusion of the sclerostomy (iris synechiae, fibrin or blood clot, or inadequate creation of fistula intraoperatively). Gonioscopy is vital in distinguishing among the various causes.[1] Causes of postoperative IOP elevations can be classified as either open-angle or angle-closure glaucoma.

Open-Angle Glaucoma

Preexisting Open-Angle Glaucoma

It is generally well accepted that the incidence of postoperative IOP elevation is greater in patients with preexisting glaucoma. When IOP cannot be adequately controlled medically, laser trabeculoplasty may be attempted, but this is less successful in pseudophakic and aphakic patients.[81] If trabeculectomy is eventually needed, success rates are also lower in patients who have previously undergone intraocular surgery.

α-Chymotrypsin-Induced Glaucoma

When intracapsular cataract extraction was more common, α-chymotrypsin-induced glaucoma, also called "enzyme glaucoma," occurred in up to 72% of cases.[20] The onset of IOP rise is usually within 48 hours postoperatively and can last for days or occasionally weeks. Although the effects of α-chymotrypsin on the outflow channels are not thought to be long-lasting, the exact mechanism of enzyme glaucoma is not clearly understood.[20,82,83]

Viscoelastic

Sodium hyaluronate, sodium chondroitin sulfate, and methylcellulose[84] are well-recognized causes of postoperative IOP elevation, especially in eyes with impaired aqueous outflow. Although IOP elevation can still occur, topical β-blockers or oral carbonic anhydrase inhibitors may prevent it. The prophylactic use of acetazolamide should be considered in patients with advanced glaucoma who may not be able to tolerate IOP elevations.[20] It is especially important to make sure that all of the viscoelastic substance is aspirated at the end of the surgery. The IOP elevation usually resolves within 24–72 hours after dissolution of the viscoelastic agent.[3]

Blood or Other Particulate Material

The trabecular meshwork may become temporarily occluded by particulate material such as blood, pigment, inflammatory debris, retained cortical material, or any combination of these. Medical treatment should be relied on until the situation improves. In cases of intractable glaucoma or with impending corneal blood staining, surgical evacuation is indicated.[20]

Idiopathic

IOP may rise following cataract extraction even without any detectable cause. Such idiopathic IOP elevations have been reported in up to 23% of routine cataract extractions, without the use of α-chymotrypsin or viscoelastic substance. Several theories have been proposed, such as trabecular meshwork edema, angle deformation by sutures, and inflammation. Inflammation is thought to cause high IOP by one or more of several mechanisms: breakdown of the blood–aqueous barrier with formation of plasmoid aqueous, presumed compromise of trabecular function caused by postoperative iritis, or the presence of inflammatory cells that block the trabecular spaces.[20]

Corticosteroid-Induced Glaucoma

Topical or systemic corticosteroid use can result in a steroid-induced elevation in IOP. This occurs more frequently in patients with primary open-angle glaucoma, their first-degree relatives, diabetic patients, and patients with high myopia. The IOP elevation may occur within a few weeks of the time corticosteroid treatment is initiated or may be delayed for months to years.[3] After cessation of topical corticosteroid use, the IOP returns to the presteroid level,[85] but the rate at which it falls varies considerably from patient to patient. In rare cases IOP elevation has persisted for months after cessation of corticosteroid use.[86] If medical therapy is unsuccessful in controlling IOP and if the optic nerve is threatened, glaucoma filtering surgery should be performed.[3]

Tenon's Cyst

Tenon's cyst is a fibroelastic growth that typically manifests as elevated IOP 3–4 weeks after surgery. A high, thick-walled, localized bleb with a patent sclerostomy is usually seen.[87] Although Tenon's cysts usually resolve spontaneously in 2–3 months, procedures such as needle or surgical excision may be needed if medical treatment does not control the pressure. If elevated IOP persists, another glaucoma filter procedure with antimetabolites or a tube may be needed.

Pigment Dispersion

Pigment dispersion and increased IOP have been reported with PCIOLs and iris-fixated lenses. Pigment dispersion occurs when the IOL is decentered, tilted, excessively mobile, too small, or reversed in position, creating friction between the lens and the iris pigment epithelium. The pigment particles rubbed off the iris accumulate in the trabecular meshwork. Pressure can increase days to months after cataract surgery but may also improve spontaneously.

Pigment dispersion is different from pigmentary glaucoma. It is distinguished by the temporal relation to surgery, the unilateral state, the geographic loss of pigment, and the absence of Krukenberg's spindle and radial iris transillumination defects. The condition responds to standard medical treatment for glaucoma and to argon laser trabeculoplasty. In some cases, pupillary constriction or dilation may reduce iris chafing. If the pressure is not controlled, the lens should be replaced or stabilized with McCannel sutures.[3]

Ghost Cell Glaucoma

Ghost cell glaucoma is a form of secondary open-angle glaucoma that occurs as a consequence of vitreous hemorrhage. The red blood cells degenerate into ghost blood cells and may pass some weeks later into the anterior chamber through a disruption in the anterior vitreous face,[88] such as after vitrectomy, cataract extraction, or trauma. These rigid, degenerated red blood cells obstruct the trabecular meshwork.[33] Khaki-colored cells floating in the anterior chamber and vitreous cavity may produce a hypopyon-like sediment in the anterior chamber.[20]

If medical treatment is ineffective, removal of the ghost blood cells by anterior chamber irrigation is thought by some to be the procedure of choice.[89] Repeated irrigation may be necessary.[90] Pars plana vitrectomy may be needed in cases of large vitreous hemorrhages to remove the reservoir of ghost blood cells.[91]

Nd:YAG Laser Capsulotomy

Transient IOP elevation, a well-known complication of Nd:YAG posterior capsulotomy, has been reported to occur in 39%–77% of cases.[92–97] Prophylaxis of post-laser-treatment IOP rises is routinely done, because it is difficult to predict who will develop a rise in IOP. No known patient or laser characteristics can reliably predict in which eyes this complication will be seen.[5,92,98–101] Apraclonidine 0.5% or 1.0% is the current standard prophylactic treatment for post-laser-treatment IOP spikes; it may reduce the frequency as well as the magnitude of the IOP rise.[95–97,99,102–108]

Vitreous in the Anterior Chamber

Vitreous in the anterior chamber and its associated inflammation may cause glaucoma through posterior synechiae with pupillary block, peripheral anterior synechiae, sclerostomy site blockage, and other possible mechanisms.

Hyphema

Hyphema after cataract surgery usually occurs from the surgical wound or the iris. The red blood cells released into the anterior chamber become lodged in the trabecular meshwork, raising the IOP.[3]

Lens Particle Glaucoma

Obstruction to aqueous flow may be caused by mechanical blockage of the trabecular meshwork by "normal" lens particles, which may be seen in the anterior chamber.

Uveitis-Glaucoma-Hyphema

The syndrome of uveitis, glaucoma, and hyphema (UGH) has been described in association with anterior chamber lenses and, more rarely, posterior chamber lenses. The syndrome results when the lens is poorly designed, is too mobile, or has coarse finishing characteristics. Affected patients often have a history of a complicated cataract extraction. They often complain of recurrent episodes of blurring (whiteout), presumably due to hyphemas.[3]

Sputtering Hyphema Syndrome (Swan Syndrome)

The sputtering hyphema syndrome, also known as the swan syndrome, results from vascularization of the limbal wound. It manifests with intermittent anterior chamber bleeding and secondary IOP elevation. This syndrome can occur months to years postoperatively. The new vessels in the wound may be seen on gonioscopy.[3,20] Treatment, which should be reserved for patients with disabling recurrences or persistently elevated IOP, includes argon laser goniophotocoagulation, limbal cryopexy, and surgical excision of episcleral vessels.[109]

Angle-Closure Glaucoma

Pupillary block glaucoma presents as a shallowing of the anterior chamber with either no iridectomy or an occluded iridectomy. There is a pressure gradient between the anterior and posterior chambers. This pressure gradient is created by the sequestration of aqueous humor in the posterior chamber because of its inability to pass through the pupil, and results in convexity of the iris. Adhesions may form between the iris, posterior capsule, and IOL and may trap aqueous humor. Pupillary block may also occur in an aphakic eye with an intact anterior hyaloid face. The peripheral iris bows forward to obstruct the trabecular meshwork[23] and causes an iris bombe configuration.[3,110] Treatment includes laser peripheral iridectomy. The most important causes of pupillary block in aphakia and pseudophakia are air bubble (e.g., SF_6 or C_3F_8), vitreous face, posterior lens capsule, an IOL, seclusio pupillae, and silicone oil.[20]

Malignant Glaucoma (Aqueous Misdirection)

Malignant glaucoma currently refers to high IOP with a shallow or flat anterior chamber and a patent iridectomy. It may complicate 2%–4% of eyes after surgery for angle-closure glaucoma.[111] Although this condition classically follows surgery for primary angle-closure glaucoma, it has also been reported after other surgical procedures, such as trabeculectomy, cataract surgery (with or without IOL implantation), laser iridotomy, laser capsulotomy, laser cyclophotocoagulation, seton implantation, scleral buckle, pars plana vitrectomy, and scleral flap laser suture lysis. Malignant glaucoma may even occur spontaneously.[112–116] Shallowing of the central as well as of the peripheral anterior chamber occurs. Although the exact mechanism is unclear, malignant glaucoma is thought to involve posterior misdirection of aqueous into or behind the vitreous. Medical management includes intensive mydriatic-cycloplegic therapy and aqueous suppressants. If medical therapy fails, Nd:YAG capsulotomy and/or hyaloidotomy should be contemplated in aphakic or pseudophakic patients. The anterior hyaloid may eventually require disruption by a vitrectomy.[117–122]

Angle-Closure Glaucoma Without Pupillary Block

Preexisting Chronic Angle-Closure Glaucoma

A gradual, asymptomatic, chronic angle closure and a subsequent rise in IOP result in progressive glaucomatous damage. Peripheral anterior synechiae are almost always present.[123,124] An iridectomy is indicated for most cases of chronic angle closure without visual field loss. However, trabeculectomy might be the best choice in most patients with visual field loss and medically uncontrolled IOP.[123] A combined procedure may be warranted if there is a visually significant cataract, as one study has reported a 60% incidence of IOP rise after cataract extraction alone in eyes with angle-closure glaucoma.[125]

Peripheral Anterior Synechiae

Peripheral anterior synechiae can develop from ACIOLs, a flat chamber, hemorrhage, inflammation, or neovascularization.[3]

Intraocular Lens Haptics (ACIOLs)

The process of secondary angle-closure glaucoma typically begins with broad peripheral synechiae forming at the footplates of the ACIOLs. Recent anterior chamber lens designs with flexible open-loop haptics have reduced the incidence of ACIOL-related erosions and peripheral anterior synechiae.[3]

Prolonged Anterior Chamber Shallowing

When the peripheral anterior chamber is flat or shallow for several days, peripheral anterior synechiae may develop. Aside from reformation of the anterior chamber or surgical intervention in the acute setting, goniosynechialysis may be beneficial in eyes in which the angle closure is of less than 6 months duration.[20]

Inflammation/Hyphema

Complications such as inflammation and hyphema are more common after the combined technique than after cataract extraction alone.[125]

Iris Incarceration in Cataract Incision

If this is left untreated, many cases may develop progressive angle closure, depending on the severity of the iris trauma and the postoperative inflammation.[20]

Neovascular Glaucoma

Most cases of neovascular glaucoma occur after central retinal vein occlusion (CRVO) or secondary to diabetes (Fig. 8.10). The incidence of this glaucoma after CRVO is about 25%–30%, and with diabetes it is about 5% (or 43%–64% of instances of proliferative retinopathy).[126] Carotid occlusive disease is a less common cause. Neovascular glaucoma occurs after 1%–2% of cases of central retinal artery occlusion.[4,126] Neovascularization of the iris consists of a fibrovascular membrane that may grow over the trabecular meshwork. Treatment should be directed to the retina, and panretinal photocoagulation may be beneficial in improving the success rate of trabeculectomy. In many cases tube shunts are needed.

Epithelial Downgrowth

Epithelium gains access to the interior of the eye via a fistula or wound gape. The incidence of this condition

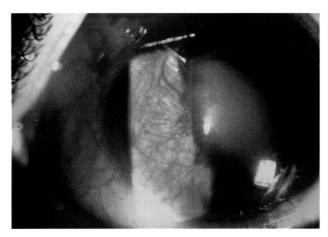

FIGURE 8.10. Neovascular glaucoma. Slit-lamp beam highlights florid neovascularization of the iris.

after cataract surgery is 0%–1.1%[127] and is decreasing with improved wound closure techniques. Glaucoma may occur in 43%[128] to 50%[20] of these patients. As the ingrowth of epithelium spreads over the anterior chamber angle structures, secondary open-angle glaucoma develops. Later, peripheral anterior synechiae may form, and angle closure ensues.[129] Attempts to treat advanced cases of epithelial downgrowth are frequently unrewarding. Several authors, however, have successfully used aqueous shunt devices to treat this glaucoma.[129,130]

Fibrous Downgrowth

Fibrous downgrowth, or the proliferation of variably vascular, fibrocellular tissue inside the eye after surgery or trauma, is similar in several ways to epithelial downgrowth. It is also associated with complicated surgery and can result in glaucoma. Unlike epithelial downgrowth, this process may be self-limiting, and the visual prognosis of medically treated eyes is significantly better than with epithelial downgrowth. The glaucoma in eyes with fibrous downgrowth can be controlled medically in most cases. A drainage seton may be the procedure of choice in cases unresponsive to medical treatment.[127]

Silicone Oil

Intravitreal silicone oil is useful in the management of complex retinal detachments. Risk factors for postoperative elevated IOP include a history of glaucoma[131] and pseudophakia.[132] Although IOP elevation after pars plana vitrectomy and intravitreal silicone oil instillation ranges from 0% to 56%,[133] the frequency of glaucoma after silicone oil treatment can be reduced by an inferior peripheral iridectomy in aphakic and pseudophakic eyes. An inferior iridectomy would allow free passage of aqueous while the lighter oil floats on top.[20] Glaucoma can still develop despite a patent iridectomy.[134] Uncontrolled IOP may benefit from silicone oil removal, glaucoma implants, or cyclodestructive procedures.[135]

■ References

1. Johnson D. Extracapsular cataract extraction, intraocular lens implantation, and trabeculectomy: the combined procedure. *Int Ophthalmol Clin.* 1990;30:209–214.
2. Schuman JS. Surgical management of coexisting cataract and glaucoma. *Ophthalmic Surg Lasers.* 1996;27:45–59.
3. Fang EN, Kass MA. Increased intraocular pressure after cataract surgery. *Semin Ophthalmol.* 1994;9:235–242.
4. Krupin T, Feitl ME, Bishop KI. Postoperative intraocular pressure rise in open-angle glaucoma patients after cataract or combined cataract-filtration surgery. *Ophthalmology.* 1989;96:579–584.
5. Moster MR, Schwartz LW, Spaeth GL, et al. Laser iridectomy: a controlled study comparing argon and neodymium:YAG. *Ophthalmology.* 1986;93:20–24.
6. Simmons ST, Litoff D, Nichols DA, Sherwood MB, Spaeth GL. Extracapsular cataract extraction and posterior chamber intraocular lens implantation combined with trabeculectomy in patients with glaucoma. *Am J Ophthalmol.* 1987;104:465–470.
7. Ohanesian RV, Kim EW. A prospective study of combined extracapsular cataract extraction, posterior chamber lens implantation, and trabeculectomy. *Am Intraocular Implant Soc J.* 1985;2:142–145.
8. Shields MB. Another reevaluation of combined cataract and glaucoma surgery. *Am J Ophthalmol.* 1993;115:806–811.
9. McCartney DL, Memmen JE, Stark WJ, et al. The efficacy and safety of combined trabeculectomy, cataract extraction, and intraocular lens implantation. *Ophthalmology.* 1988;95:754–763.
10. Percival SPB. Glaucoma triple procedure of extracapsular cataract extraction, posterior chamber lens implantation, and trabeculectomy. *Br J Ophthalmol.* 1985;69:99–102.
11. Skorpik C, Paroussis PP, Gnad HD, Menapaoe MR. Trabeculectomy and intraocular lens implantation: a combined procedure. *J Cataract Refract Surg.* 1987;13:39–42.
12. Wishart PK, Austin MW. Combined cataract extraction and trabeculectomy: phacoemulsification compared with extracapsular technique. *Ophthalmic Surg.* 1993;24:814–821.
13. Shingleton BJ, Jacobson LM, Kuperwaser MC. Comparison of combined cataract and glaucoma surgery using planned extracapsular and phacoemulsification techniques. *Ophthalmic Surg Lasers.* 1995;26:414–419.
14. Munden PM, Alward WLM. Combined phacoemulsification, posterior chamber intraocular lens implantation, and trabeculectomy with mitomycin C. *Am J Ophthalmol.* 1995;119:20–29.
15. Hurvitz LM. Combined surgery for cataract and glaucoma. *Curr Opin Ophthalmol.* 1993;4:73–78.
16. Samuelson TW. Management of coincident cataract and glaucoma. *Curr Opin Ophthalmol.* 1993;4:90–96.
17. El Sayyad F, Helal M, El-Maghraby A, Khalil M, El-Hamzawey HH. One-site versus two-site phacotrabeculectomy: a randomized study. *J Cataract Refract Surg.* 1999;25:77–82.
18. Wyse T, Meyer M, Ruderman JM, et al. Combined trabeculectomy and phacoemulsification: a one-site vs a two-site approach. *Am J Ophthalmol.* 1998;125:334–339.
19. Blumenthal M, Glovinsky GY. Surgical consequences in coexisting cataract and glaucoma. *Curr Opin Ophthalmol.* 1995;6:15–18.
20. Tomey KF, Traverso CE. The glaucomas in aphakia and pseudophakia. *Surv Ophthalmol.* 1991;36:79–112.
21. Savage JA, Thomas JV, Belcher CD, Simmons RJ. Extracapsular cataract extraction and posterior chamber intraocular lens implantation in glaucomatous eyes. *Ophthalmology.* 1985;92:1506–1516.

22. Filipe JC, Palmares J, Delgado L, Lopes JM, Borges J, Castro-Correia J. Phacolytic glaucoma and lens-induced uveitis. *Int Ophthalmol*. 1993;17:289–293.

23. Ellant JP, Ostbaum SA. Lens-induced glaucoma. *Doc Ophthalmol*. 1992;81:317–338.

24. Mandal AK. An alternate way to manage patients with morgagnian cataracts and phacolytic glaucoma. *Indian J Ophthalmol*. 1997;45:53–59.

25. Braganza A, Thomas R, George T, Mermoud A. Management of phacolytic glaucoma: experience of 135 cases. *Indian J Ophthalmol*. 1998;46:139–143.

26. Prajna NV, Ramkrishnan R, Krishnadas R, Manoharan N. Lens-induced glaucomas: visual results and risk factors for final visual acuity. *Indian J Ophthalmol*. 1996; 44:149–155.

27. Tomey KF, Al-Rajhi AA. Neodymium:YAG laser iridotomy in the initial management of phacomorphic glaucoma. *Ophthalmology*. 1992;99:660–665.

28. Vilar NF, Flynn HW, Smiddy WE, Murray TG, Davis JL, Rubsamen PE. Removal of retained lens fragments after phacoemulsification reverses secondary glaucoma and restores visual acuity. *Ophthalmology*. 1997;104: 787–792.

29. Drolsum L, Haaskjold E, Sandvig K. Phacoemulsification in eyes with pseudoexfoliation. *J Cataract Refract Surg*. 1998;24:787–792.

30. Scorolli L, Campos E, Bassein L, Meduri R. Pseudoexfoliation syndrome: a cohort study on intraoperative complications in cataract surgery. *Ophthalmologica*. 1998; 212:278–280.

31. Drolsum L, Haaskjold E, Davanger M. Pseudoexfoliation syndrome and extracapsular cataract extraction. *Acta Ophthalmol*. 1993;71:765–770.

32. Schlotzer-Schrehardt U, Naumann GO. A histopathologic study of zonular instability in pseudoexfoliation syndrome. *Am J Ophthalmol*. 1994;118:730–743.

33. Moreno J, Duch S, Larjara J. Pseudoexfoliation syndrome: clinical factors related to capsular rupture in cataract surgery. *Acta Ophthalmol*. 1993;71:181–184.

34. Fine IH, Hoffman RS. Phacoemulsification in the presence of pseudoexfoliation: challenges and options. *J Cataract Refract Surg*. 1997;23:160–165.

35. Naumann GO, Schlotzer-Schrehardt U, Kuchie M. Pseudoexfoliation syndrome for the comprehensive ophthalmologist. *Ophthalmology*. 1998;105:951–968.

36. Drolsum L, Haaskjold E, Davanger M. Results and complications after extracapsular cataract extraction in eyes with pseudoexfoliation syndrome. *Acta Ophthalmol*. 1993;71:771–776.

37. Samuelson TW. Surgical management of coincident cataract and glaucoma. *Curr Opin Ophthalmol*. 1997; 8:39–45.

38. Carpel EF. Pupillary dilation in eyes with pseudoexfoliation syndrome. *Am J Ophthalmol*. 1998;105:692–694.

39. Asano N, Schlotzer-Schrehardt U, Naumann GO. A histopathologic study of iris changes in pseudoexfoliation syndrome. *Ophthalmology*. 1995;102:1279–1290.

40. Doyle JW, Smith MF. Glaucoma after penetrating keratoplasty. *Semin Ophthalmol*. 1994;9:254–257.

41. Samuelson TW, Lindstrom RL. Combined glaucoma filtration surgery and phacoemulsification. *Semin Ophthalmol*. 1992;7:279–285.

42. Samuelson TW. Management of coincident glaucoma and cataract. *Curr Opin Ophthalmol*. 1995;6:14–21.

43. Lemon LC, Shin DH, Kim C, Bendel RE, Hughes BA, Juzych MS. Limbus-based vs fornix-based conjunctival flap in combined glaucoma and cataract surgery with adjunctive mitomycin C. *Am J Ophthalmol*. 1998; 125:340–345.

44. Cohen JS, Greff LJ, Novack GD, Wind BE. A placebo-controlled, double-masked evaluation of mitomycin C in combined glaucoma and cataract procedures. *Ophthalmology*. 1996;103:1934–1942.

45. Carlson DW, Alward WLM, Barad JP, Zimmerman MB, Carney BL. A randomized study of mitomycin augmentation in combined phacoemulsification and trabeculectomy. *Ophthalmology*. 1997;104:719–724.

46. Shin DH, Kim YY, Sheth N, et al. The role of adjunctive mitomycin C in secondary glaucoma triple procedure as compared to primary glaucoma triple procedure. *Ophthalmology*. 1998;105:740–745.

47. Heuer DK, Parrish RK, Gressel MG, Hodapp E, Palmberg PF, Anderson DR. 5-Fluorouracil and glaucoma filtering surgery. II. A pilot study. *Ophthalmology*. 1984;91:384–394.

48. Heuer DK, Parrish RK, Gressel MG, et al. 5-Fluorouracil and glaucoma filtering surgery. III. Intermediate follow-up of a pilot study. *Ophthalmology*. 1986;93:1537–1546.

49. Hennis HL, Stewart WC. The use of 5-fluorouracil in patients following combined trabeculectomy and cataract extraction. *Ophthalmic Surg*. 1991;22:451–454.

50. O'Grady JM, Juzych MS, Shin DH, Lemon LC, Swendris RP. Trabeculectomy, phacoemulsification, and posterior chamber lens implantation with and without 5-fluorouracil. *Am J Ophthalmol*. 1993;116:594–599.

51. Ruderman JM, Fundingsland B, Meyer MA. Combined phacoemulsification and trabeculectomy with mitomycin-C. *J Cataract Refract Surg*. 1996;22:1085–1090.

52. Hurvitz LM. 5-FU-supplemented phacoemulsification, posterior chamber intraocular lens implantation, and trabeculectomy. *Ophthalmic Surg Lasers*. 1993;24:674–680.

53. Cohen JS. Combined cataract implant and filtering surgery with 5-fluorouracil. *Ophthalmic Surg Lasers*. 1990;21:181–186.

54. Mattox C. Glaucoma filtration surgery and antimetabolites. *Ophthalmic Surg Lasers*. 1995;26:473–480.

55. Khaw PT, Migdal CS. Current techniques in wound healing modulation in glaucoma surgery. *Curr Opin Ophthalmol*. 1996;7:24–33.

56. Dinsmore SC. Modified stretch technique for small pupil phacoemulsification with topical anesthesia. *J Cataract Refract Surg*. 1996;22:27–30.

57. Miller KM, Keener GT. Stretch pupilloplasty for small pupil phacoemulsification. *Am J Ophthalmol*. 1994; 117:107–108.

58. Faust KJ. Modified radial iridotomy for small pupil phacoemulsification. *J Cataract Refract Surg*. 1991;17: 866–867.

59. Metz D, Ackerman S, Lish AJ, Kanarek I, Kosowsky K, Ackerman J. Phacotrabeculectomy with posterior chamber lens insertion in early glaucoma. *Ann Ophthalmol.* 1995;27:231–235.

60. Fine IH. Pupilloplasty for small pupil phacoemulsification. *J Cataract Refract Surg.* 1994;20:192–196.

61. Cole MD, Brown R, Ridgeway AEA. Role of sphincterotomy in extracapsular cataract surgery. *Br J Ophthalmol.* 1986;70:692–695.

62. Masket S. Avoiding complications associated with iris retractor use in small pupil cataract extraction. *J Cataract Refract Surg.* 1996;22:168–171.

63. Mackool RJ. Small pupil enlargement during cataract extraction: a new method. *J Cataract Refract Surg.* 1992; 18:523–526.

64. Graether JM. Graether pupil expander for managing the small pupil during surgery. *J Cataract Refract Surg.* 1996;22:530–535.

65. Chen V, Shochot Y, Blumenthal M. Anterior capsulotomy through a small pupil. *Am J Ophthalmol.* 1987; 104:666–667.

66. Shin DH, Ren J, Juzych MS, et al. Primary glaucoma triple procedure in patients with primary open-angle glaucoma: the effect of mitomycin C in patients with and without prognostic factors for filtration failure. *Am J Ophthalmol.* 1998;125:346–352.

67. Nuijts RMMA, Vernimmen RCJ, Webers CA. Mitomycin C primary trabeculectomy in primary glaucoma of white patients. *J Glaucoma.* 1997;6:293–297.

68. Ayyala RS, Bellows AR, Thomas JV, Hutchinson BT. Bleb infections: clinically different courses of "blebitis" and endophthalmitis. *Ophthalmic Surg Lasers.* 1997;28: 452–460.

69. Waheed S, Ritterband DC, Greenfield DS, Liebmann JM, Seedor JA, Ritch R. New patterns of infecting organisms in late bleb-related endophthalmitis: a ten year review. *Eye.* 1998;12:910–915.

70. Greenfield DS, Liebmann JM, Jee J, Ritch R. Late-onset bleb leaks after glaucoma filtration surgery. *Arch Ophthalmol.* 1998;116:443–447.

71. Tomlinson CP, Belcher CD, Smith P, Simmons RJ. Management of leaking filtration blebs. *Ann Ophthalmol.* 1987;19:405–411.

72. O'Connor DJ, Tressler CS, Caprioli J. A surgical method to repair leaking filtering blebs. *Ophthalmic Surg.* 1992; 23:336–338.

73. Kosmin AS, Wishart PK. A full-thickness scleral graft for the surgical management of a late filtration bleb leak. *Ophthalmic Surg Lasers.* 1997;28:461–468.

74. Schubert HD. Postsurgical hypotony: relationship to fistulization, inflammation, chorioretinal lesions, and the vitreous. *Surv Ophthalmol.* 1996;41:97–125.

75. Costa VP, Moster MR, Wilson RP, Schmidt CM, Gandham S, Smith SM. Effects of topical mitomycin C on primary trabeculectomies and combined procedures. *Br J Ophthalmol.* 1993;77:693–697.

76. Zacharia PT, Schuman JS. Combined phacoemulsification and trabeculectomy with mitomycin C. *Ophthalmic Surg Lasers.* 1997;28:739–744.

77. Lederer CM. Combined cataract extraction with intraocular lens implant and mitomycin-augmented trabeculectomy. *Ophthalmology.* 1996;103:1025–1034.

78. Joos KM, Bueche MJ, Palmberg PF, Feuer WJ, Grajewski AL. One-year follow-up results of combined mitomycin C trabeculectomy and extracapsular cataract extraction. *Ophthalmology.* 1995;102:76–83.

79. Yang KJ, Moster MR, Azuara-Blanco A, Wilson RP, Araujo SV, Schmidt CM. Mitomycin-C supplemented trabeculectomy, phacoemulsification, and foldable lens implantation. *J Cataract Refract Surg.* 1997;23:565–569.

80. Shin DH, Kim YY, Ren J, et al. Decrease of capsular opacification with adjunctive mitomycin C in combined glaucoma and cataract surgery. *Ophthalmology.* 1998; 105:1222–1226.

81. Alpar JJ. Glaucoma after intraocular lens implantation: survey and recommendations. *Glaucoma.* 1985;7:241–245.

82. Rauhut D, Rohen JW. Electron microscopic study of the trabecular meshwork in alpha-chymotrypsin glaucoma. *Graefes Arch Klin Exp Ophthalmol.* 1972;184:29–41.

83. Best M, Rabinovitz AZ, Masket S. Experimental alpha-chymotrypsin glaucoma. *Ann Ophthalmol.* 1975;7: 803–810.

84. Morgan RK, Skuta GL. Viscoelastic-related glaucomas. *Semin Ophthalmol.* 1994;9:229–234.

85. Urban RC, Dreyer EB. Corticosteroid-induced glaucoma. *Int Ophthalmol Clin.* 1993;33:135–139.

86. Spaeth GL, Rodrigues MM, Weinreb S. Steroid-induced glaucoma: A. Persistent elevation of intraocular pressure. B. Histopathological aspects. *Trans Am Ophthalmol Soc.* 1977;75:353–381.

87. Campagna JA, Munden PM, Alward WLM. Tenon's cyst formation after trabeculectomy with mitomycin C. *Ophthalmic Surg.* 1995;26:57–60.

88. Campbell DG, Essigmann EM. Hemolytic ghost cell glaucoma. *Ophthalmology.* 1979;97:2141–2146.

89. Campbell DG. Ghost cell glaucoma following trauma. *Ophthalmology.* 1981;88:1151–1158.

90. Montenegro MH, Simmons RJ. Ghost cell glaucoma. *Int Ophthalmol Clin.* 1995;35:111–115.

91. Abu El Asrar AM, Al-Obeidan SA. Pars plana vitrectomy in the management of ghost cell glaucoma. *Int Ophthalmol.* 1995;19:121–124.

92. Flohr MJ, Robin AL, Kelly JS. Early complications following Q-switched neodymium:YAG laser posterior capsulotomy. *Ophthalmology.* 1985;92:360–363.

93. Brown SVL, Thomas JV, Belcher CD III. Effect of pilocarpine in treatment of intraocular pressure elevation following neodymium:YAG posterior capsulotomy. *Ophthalmology.* 1985;92:354–359.

94. Channell MM, Beckman H. Intraocular pressure changes after neodymium:YAG laser posterior capsulotomy. *Arch Ophthalmol.* 1984;102:1024–1026.

95. Cullom RD, Schwartz LW. The effect of apraclonidine on the intraocular pressure of glaucoma patients following neodymium:YAG laser posterior capsulotomy. *Ophthalmic Surg.* 1993;24:623–626.

96. Pollack IP, Brown RH, Crandall AS, et al. Effectiveness of apraclonidine in preventing the rise in intraocular

pressure after neodymium:YAG posterior capsulotomy. *Trans Am Ophthalmol Soc.* 1988;86:461–472.

97. Silverstone DE, Brint SF, Olander KW, et al. Prophylactic use of apraclonidine for intraocular pressure increase after neodymium:YAG capsulotomies. *Am J Ophthalmol.* 1992;113:401–405.

98. Robin AL, Pollack IP. A comparison of neodymium:YAG and argon laser iridotomies. *Ophthalmology.* 1984;91:1011–1016.

99. Robin AL. Medical management of acute postoperative intraocular pressure rises associated with anterior segment ophthalmic laser surgery. *Int Ophthalmol Clin.* 1990;30:2.

100. Glaucoma Laser Trial Research, G., The Glaucoma Laser Trial: I. Acute effects of argon laser trabeculoplasty in intraocular pressure. *Arch Ophthalmol.* 1989;107:1135–1142.

101. Robin AL, Pollack IP, DeFaller JM. Effects of topical ALO 2145 (*p*-aminoclonidine hydrochloride) on the acute intraocular pressure rise after argon laser iridotomy. *Arch Ophthalmol.* 1988;106:308–309.

102. Kitazawa Y, Taniguchi T, Tugiyama K, et al. Use of apraclonidine to reduce acute intraocular pressure rise following Q-switched Nd:YAG laser iridotomy. *Ophthalmic Surg.* 1989;20:49–52.

103. Hong C, Song KY, Park WH, et al. Effect of apraclonidine hydrochloride on acute intraocular pressure rise after argon laser iridotomy. *Korean J Ophthalmol.* 1991;5:37–41.

104. Holweger R, Marefat B. Intraocular pressure change after Nd:YAG capsulotomy. *J Cataract Refract Surg.* 1997;23:115–121.

105. Robin AL. The role of apraclonidine hydrochloride in laser therapy for glaucoma. *Trans Am Ophthalmol Soc.* 1989;87:729–761.

106. Pollack IP, Brown RH, Crandall AS, et al. Prevention of the rise in intraocular pressure following Nd:YAG posterior capsulotomy using topical 1% apraclonidine. *Arch Ophthalmol.* 1988;106:754–757.

107. Rao BS, Badrinath SS. Efficacy and safety of apraclonidine in patients undergoing anterior segment laser surgery. *Br J Ophthalmol.* 1989;73:884–887.

108. Rosenberg LF, Krupin T, Ruderman J, et al. Apraclonidine and anterior segment laser surgery: comparison of 0.5% versus 1.0% apraclonidine for prevention of postoperative intraocular pressure rise. *Ophthalmology.* 1995;102:1312–1318.

109. Jarstad JS, Hardwig PW. Intraocular hemorrhage from wound neovascularization years after anterior segment surgery (Swan syndrome). *Can J Ophthalmol.* 1987;22:271–275.

110. Traverso CE, Tomey KF, Gandolfo E. The glaucomas in pseudophakia. *Curr Opin Ophthalmol.* 1996;7:65–71.

111. Luntz MH, Rosenblatt M. Malignant glaucoma. *Surv Ophthalmol.* 1987;32:73–93.

112. Ruben S, Tsai J, Hitching R. Malignant glaucoma and its management. *Br J Ophthalmol.* 1997;81:163–167.

113. Zacharia PT, Abboud EB. Recalcitrant malignant glaucoma following pars plana vitrectomy, scleral buckle,

and extracapsular cataract extraction with posterior chamber intraocular lens implantation. *Ophthalmic Surg Lasers.* 1998;29:323–327.

114. Liebmann JM, Weinrab R, Ritch R. Angle-closure glaucoma associated with occult annular ciliary body detachment. *Arch Ophthalmol.* 1998;116:731–735.

115. Harbour JW, Lubsamen PE, Palmberg P. Pars plana vitrectomy in the management of phakic and pseudophakic malignant glaucoma. *Arch Ophthalmol.* 1996;114:1073–1078.

116. Saunders PP, Douglas GR, Feldman F, Stern RM. Bilateral malignant glaucoma. *Can J Ophthalmol.* 1992;27:19–21.

117. Little BC, Hitchings RA. Pseudophakic malignant glaucoma: Nd:YAG capsulotomy as a primary treatment. *Eye.* 1993;7:102–104.

118. Brown RH, Lynch MG, Tearse JE, Nunn RD. Neodymium-YAG vitreous surgery for phakic and pseudophakic malignant glaucoma. *Arch Ophthalmol.* 1986;104:1464–1466.

119. Lynch MG, Brown RH, Michels RG, Pollack IP, Stark WJ. Surgical vitrectomy for pseudophakic malignant glaucoma. *Am J Ophthalmol.* 1986;102:149–153.

120. Tsai JC, Barton KA, Miller MH, Khaw PT, Hitchings RA. Surgical results in malignant glaucoma refractory to medical or laser therapy. *Eye.* 1997;11:677–681.

121. Byrnes GA, Leen MM, Wong TP, Benson WE. Vitrectomy for ciliary block (malignant) glaucoma. *Ophthalmology.* 1995;102:1308–1311.

122. Johnson DH. Options in the management of malignant glaucoma. *Arch Ophthalmol.* 1998;116:799–800.

123. Kim YY, Jung HR. Clarifying the nomenclature for primary angle-closure glaucoma. *Surv Ophthalmol.* 1997;42:125–136.

124. Greenidge KC. Angle-closure glaucoma. *Int Ophthalmol Clin.* 1990;30:177–186.

125. Gunning FP, Greve EL. Uncontrolled primary angle closure glaucoma: results of early intercapsular cataract extraction and posterior chamber lens implantation. *Int Ophthalmol.* 1991;15:237–247.

126. Gartner S, Henkind P. Neovascularization of the iris (rubeosis iridis). *Surv Ophthalmol.* 1978;22:291–312.

127. Smith MF, Doyle JW. Glaucoma secondary to epithelial and fibrous downgrowth. *Semin Ophthalmol.* 1994;9:248–253.

128. Weiner MJ, Trentacoste J, Pon DM, Albert DM. Epithelial downgrowth: a 30-year clinicopathological review. *Br J Ophthalmol.* 1989;73:6–11.

129. Peyman GA, Peralta E, Ganiban GJ, Kraut R. Endoresection of the iris and ciliary body in epithelial downgrowth. *J Cataract Refract Surg.* 1998;24:130–133.

130. Costa VP, Katz LJ. Glaucoma associated with epithelial downgrowth controlled with Molteno tube shunts. *Ophthalmic Surg.* 1992;23:797–800.

131. Henderer JD, Budenz DL, Flynn HW, Schiffman JC, Feuer WJ, Murray TG. Elevated intraocular pressure and hypotony following silicone oil retinal tamponade for complex retinal detachment. *Arch Ophthalmol.* 1999;117:189–195.

132. Montanari P, Troiano P, Marangoni P, Pinotti D, Ratiglia R, Miglior M. Glaucoma after vitreo-retinal surgery with

silicone oil injection: epidemiologic aspects. *Int Ophthalmol.* 1997;20:29–31.

133. Honavar SG, Goyal M, Majji AB, Sen PK, Naduvilath T, Dandona L. Glaucoma after pars plana vitrectomy and silicone oil injection for complicated retinal detachments. *Ophthalmology.* 1999;106:169–177.

134. Valone J, McCarthy M. Emulsified anterior chamber silicone oil and glaucoma. *Ophthalmology.* 1994;101: 1908–1912.

135. Nguyen QH, Lloyd MA, Heuar DK, et al. Incidence and management of glaucoma after intravitreal silicone oil injection for complicated retinal detachments. *Ophthalmology.* 1992;99:1520–1526.

Chapter 9

Intraocular Lens Surgery in Uveitis and Scleritis

Panagiota Stavrou and C. Stephen Foster

Cataract, a common complication in patients with uveitis, is a result of the inflammation itself and the use of corticosteroids for its treatment. Chronic low-grade inflammation is thought to have a more pronounced cataractogenic effect than acute attacks of short duration. Similarly, cataract formation in patients with scleritis may be caused by either long-standing anterior uveitis or the use of corticosteroids, and is most common in the necrotizing type of scleritis.

Pathologically, lens abnormalities consisting of localized areas of cellular necrosis surrounded by a zone of hyperplastic lens epithelium occur at the site of posterior synechiae. These focal opacities are difficult to detect clinically, as they lie directly beneath the adherent zone of the synechiae. Inflammation in the posterior chamber leads to changes in the equatorial region of the lens. These changes consist of posterior migration of lenticular epithelium, which undergoes degeneration and hyperplasia, and form the posterior subcapsular type of cataract. Results in experimental animal models also suggest that inflammatory by-products such as phospholipase A, lysosomal enzymes, and oxygen free radicals may lead to lenticular changes. The exact mechanism of posterior subcapsular cataract development in patients receiving corticosteroids is unknown. It has been suggested that electrolyte imbalance following corticosteroid administration may cause abnormal cell metabolism. It is likely that cataract formation in patients with uveitis and scleritis is the result of all of the aforementioned mechanisms.

Indications for Cataract Surgery

The indications for cataract surgery in patients with a history of uveitis or scleritis are visual disability and lens opacities obscuring visualization of the posterior segment. Adequate control of the inflammation for a substantial period of time before surgery is important for satisfactory results. Acute inflammation, usually associated with raised intraocular pressure (IOP) due to acute leakage of lens proteins in cases of hypermature cataract, is an exception in performing surgery on an acutely inflamed eye. Cataract extraction in these patients is therapeutic.

Preoperative Management

The first step in the preoperative management of patients with uveitis or scleritis is to establish a diagnosis of the individual syndrome, in the case of uveitis, and to exclude systemic associated diseases, in the case of scleritis. This is particularly important in preparing the surgical plan and has prognostic value, for after cataract surgery, some uveitis entities are associated with a more favorable visual outcome than others. The diagnostic evaluation includes a comprehensive medical history, an extensive review of systems, clinical assessment, and laboratory investigations. If the initial evaluation is negative, the tests should be repeated every 6–12 months, as nonocular manifestations of systemic diseases such as sarcoidosis may appear months to years after the ocular manifestations.

The visual outcome following cataract extraction in patients with uveitis depends on the success of the surgery itself and the integrity of structures critical for good vision. Hogan et al defined clinically significant inflammation as 1+ cells (5–10 cells per high-power field).[1] Total control of active inflammation (0–2 leukocytes/0.2 mm high slit beam) in the anterior chamber or vitreous body for at least 3 months is considered critical to the success of cataract surgery. Inflammatory activity is assessed by the presence of cells in the anterior chamber and vitreous rather than by the presence of flare, which is due to vascular incompetence of the iris and ciliary body, a consequence of vascular damage from the chronic uveitis. Differentiating between active and old inflammatory cells in the vitreous may be difficult. The clear spaces, or lacunae, within the vitreous should be examined for active cells. If visualization of the fundus is difficult, B-scan ultrasonography and electrodiagnostic testing will be useful.

The patient's treatment is enhanced perioperatively to better modulate surgically stimulated inflammation. Those receiving immunosuppressive therapy continue on the same regimen throughout the perioperative period. Patients who originally required regional or systemic corticosteroids to achieve quiescence but who have had no inflammation for several months or years before surgery are started on oral prednisone (1 mg/kg/d) and an oral nonsteroidal anti-inflammatory drug (NSAID) (diflunisal, 500 mg twice daily) 2 days prior to surgery.[2,3] Intravenous methylprednisolone (1 g) may be considered on the day of surgery for patients with poor compliance with oral treatment.[4] Treatment is also enhanced by the application of topical 1% prednisone sodium phosphate four times daily, 3 days before surgery. Topical 0.25% scopolamine, 1% cyclopentolate hydrochloride, and 10% phenylephrine hydrochloride are applied to the eye to be operated on three times at 30-minute intervals starting 2 hours before surgery.[2–5]

■ Surgical Technique

Cataract surgery in patients with uveitis can be a challenge because of posterior synechiae, small pupils, pupillary membranes, peripheral anterior synechiae, and cyclitic membranes. The method of cataract extraction in patients with uveitis has evolved alongside cataract surgery in general. Phacoemulsification appears to be safer than extracapsular cataract extraction (ECCE), as it is associated with less surgical trauma, resulting in less breakdown of the blood–aqueous barrier and therefore a reduced inflammatory response. Other advantages include a quicker visual recovery and reduced astigmatism. A clear corneal incision may be preferable to a scleral tunnel, particularly in patients with associated scleral thinning from scleritis, and may also eliminate the risk of failure if future drainage surgery is required.

Adequate access to the lens can be achieved by bimanual stretching using a collar-button device to gently pull and push the iris sphincter or using iris retractors (hooks).[5] Alternatively, sphincterotomies or a sector iridotomy (following a peripheral iridectomy) can be performed but may result in a greater postoperative inflammatory response. Intraoperative bleeding may occur, particularly in cases of Fuchs' heterochromic cyclitis (FHC), but can be controlled with the use of viscoelastics to act as a tamponade.

In phacoemulsification, continuous curvilinear capsulorrhexis is the method of choice for anterior capsulotomy. The use of viscoelastics facilitates all the intraocular manipulations. A well-centered capsulorrhexis with a minimum diameter of 6 mm is recommended, as a smaller one may result in phimosis postoperatively.[6] Meticulous aspiration to remove all cortical material is important to avoid postoperative lens-induced inflammation, fibrotic capsule contraction, and posterior capsule opacification (PCO).

Once cataract extraction has been completed, the vitreous is inspected. If significant vitreous debris remains in the visual axis, a pars plana vitrectomy is performed.[5] Combined cataract extraction (pars plana lensectomy or phacoemulsification) and pars plana vitrectomy are recommended in patients with cataract due to juvenile rheumatoid arthritis (JRA)–associated uveitis.[7] This approach ensures complete removal of all cortical material and the lens capsule, which, if left behind, may act as a scaffold in the formation of inflammatory membranes. This complication is relatively common in patients with JRA-associated uveitis and usually eventuates in membrane contraction, ciliary body dysfunction, hypotony, and phthisis.

If the decision has been made to insert an intraocular lens (IOL), an in-the-bag implantation is advised because it ensures good IOL centration and stability. Implantation in the sulcus (theoretically) or in the anterior chamber should be avoided in patients with uveitis to minimize haptic-uveal contact, which may stimulate inflammatory reaction.[5] Furthermore, in patients with FHC, who often have fine abnormal vessels in the drainage angle, an anterior chamber implant could cause bleeding, leading to the uveitis-glaucoma-hyphema syndrome.[8]

There is good evidence that an IOL can be well tolerated by selected patients with specific uveitis syndromes or idiopathic disease. These include FHC, sarcoidosis-associated uveitis, pars planitis, Vogt-Koyanagi-Harada (VKH) syndrome, Adamantiades-Behçet's disease, idiopathic panuveitis, and rheumatoid arthritis. However, the relative and absolute contraindications to IOL implantation are less clear. Overall, IOL implantation should be avoided in cases known to be difficult to control preoperatively and in patients expected to have a long postoperative course and recurrent exacerbations of uveitis.[2-5] There is general agreement that an IOL should be avoided in patients with JRA-associated uveitis. This chronic disease is characterized by the development of posterior synechiae and fibrous membranes. IOLs may act as a scaffold for further fibrous proliferation. Contraction of the fibrous membranes may lead to distortion of the pupil, dislocation of the IOL, and even avulsion of the ciliary body, causing hypotony.

Moorthy et al analyzed the results of cataract surgery with and without IOL in patients with VKH syndrome.[9] They decided whether or not to implant an IOL on the basis of the severity and extent of posterior synechiae found intraoperatively. They recommended that an IOL should not be implanted when extensive posterior synechiae are encountered. Foster has suggested aborting IOL implantation if intraoperative complications arise and the surgeon is not certain that both haptics would be in the bag.[2]

The choice of IOL material is another consideration in patients with uveitis. An all-polymethyl methacrylate (PMMA) lens may avoid the complement-mediated inflammation that may be induced by polypropylene haptics. Although PMMA alone may also stimulate the complement cascade, polypropylene haptics are best avoided. In heparin-surface-modified (HSM) IOLs, heparin is bonded to the PMMA surface to make it hydrophilic, in an attempt to reduce the inflammatory reaction induced by PMMA. The suggested mechanism is that the hydrophilic surface reduces cellular adherence and therefore reduces electrostatic forces, thus preventing the attraction of inflammatory cells and adhesion of fibroblasts to the IOL surface. Despite these theoretical advantages and the favorable results reported in noncontrolled studies,[10] a recent prospective randomized study by Tabbara et al that compared HSM IOLs with PMMA IOLs in 14 patients with uveitis and 11 patients with diabetes found no statistically significant difference between HSM and PMMA IOLs in the number of cellular deposits on the anterior surface of the IOL, the number of adhesions between the iris and IOL, or the number of PCOs.[11] With small-incision phacoemulsification surgery, foldable IOLs are another option. A wide variety of materials are available, including silicone, acrylic, and hydrogel. As yet there are no studies to guide the choice of foldable lenses in uveitic eyes.

■ Postoperative Complications

The most common complications after cataract surgery in patients with uveitis are exacerbation of inflammation, fibrin membrane formation, posterior synechiae formation, a rise in IOP, and inflammatory deposits on the optic of the IOL. Postoperative (or exacerbation of preoperative) cystoid macular edema is also more common in patients with uveitis. Hypotony is a serious complication after cataract surgery in JRA patients. It usually appears in the immediate postoperative period and may be due to occult ciliary body detachment by cyclitic membrane or aqueous hyposecretion secondary to postoperative inflammation.

PCO, another complication after cataract surgery, is due to proliferation, migration, and opacification of lens epithelial cells. Visually significant PCO requires yttrium-aluminum-garnet laser treatment, which carries the risk of IOL damage and dislocation, elevation in IOP, and retinal detachment. Although PCO has been seen in up to 50% of patients with sarcoidosis-associated uveitis, Dana et al reported that the overall incidence of PCO in uveitic eyes, that are properly conditioned for surgery and are treated by modern phacoemulsification/ECCE techniques is similar to the incidence in nonuveitic eyes, after adjusting for age differences between the two groups.[12]

■ Postoperative Treatment

Topical steroids with or without short-acting mydriatics are recommended during the postoperative period and may be required for several months, according to individual response. Systemic steroids are also tapered according to the inflammation (decreased by 5–10 mg/wk) until they are discontinued.[2,5] Foster has included an NSAID (diflunisal) for 2 months after surgery, or longer in the case of macular edema, in which the addition of a topical NSAID may also be beneficial.

■ Visual Outcome

The visual outcome after cataract surgery in patients with uveitis depends on the integrity of structures critical for good vision, such as the macula or optic nerve. Inflammation involving the posterior segment carries a less favorable prognosis than inflammation of the anterior segment. Information from studies reporting on the visual results following cataract surgery in patients with specific uveitis entities are helpful when making the surgical plan and when advising patients on the likely prognosis of their disease.

Akova and Foster reported on 21 eyes that underwent cataract surgery for sarcoidosis-associated uveitis.[13] A posterior chamber IOL was implanted in 19 of the 21 eyes. A visual acuity of 20/40 or better was achieved in 61% of eyes. The causes of poor visual outcome were macular edema, epiretinal membrane, or glaucomatous optic nerve damage. Moorthy et al analyzed the results of cataract surgery in 19 eyes with VKH syndrome.[9] Eleven eyes received an IOL; 13 eyes (68%) achieved a visual acuity of 20/40 or better. Patients who received an IOL had a better visual outcome, but this was thought to be due to milder disease, which allowed IOL implantation, rather than to the presence of the IOL. Complications associated with poor outcome were recurrent inflammation associated with glaucoma, subretinal neovascularization, and long-standing pigmentary disturbances in the macula.

Kaufman and Foster reported the results of cataract extraction in 18 eyes with pars planitis.[14] In 83% of the eyes the final visual acuity was better than 20/40. The causes of poor visual outcome were similar and included macular and optic nerve pathology. Foster and Barrett reported that 75% of eyes that underwent cataract surgery with and without vitrectomy for JRA achieved a stable visual acuity of 20/40 or better.[7] None of their patients had an IOL implanted. Macular pathology, glaucomatous optic nerve damage, chronic hypotony, and amblyopia were responsible for an unfavorable visual result. Ciftci and Ozdemir reported on the results following cataract surgery in patients with Adamantiades-Behçet's disease.[15] Visual acuity worse than 20/200 was seen in 62% of patients and was mainly due to optic atrophy.

O'Neill et al compared IOL versus no IOL implantation after cataract surgery in patients with FHC and found that 93% of pseudophakic eyes and 85% of aphakic eyes achieved a visual acuity better than 20/40.[16] Jones noted that in FHC, preoperative markers of a guarded postoperative prognosis that are associated with increased postoperative inflammation include severe iris atrophy detected on transillumination, severe abnormalities of iris vasculature, and glaucoma.[8] The phenomenon of anterior chamber hemorrhage following paracentesis (Amsler's sign) is common in FCH. Any abrupt change in IOP can provoke subtle hemorrhage in these patients, usually from the vessels in the drainage angle and occasionally from the entire iris surface. This complication can also be provoked by use of the Honan balloon or preoperative mydriasis. As yet there are no studies reporting on the results of cataract surgery in patients with scleritis.

■ Comment

The results following cataract surgery in patients with uveitis and scleritis have improved in recent years as a result of several factors. First, better medical management of inflammation is available during the long period before the need for cataract surgery arises. Various therapies are introduced in stepladder fashion according to the individual patient's response. These therapies include immunomodulatory treatment in patients who are steroid resistant or who develop steroid-induced side effects. With adequate control of inflammation, damage to structures necessary for normal vision (macula, optic nerve, ciliary body, trabecular meshwork) is avoided and cataract development is delayed. Second, better surgical techniques have been developed that are associated with less traumatic intraocular manipulations. These techniques in turn have been facilitated by the development of better microsurgical instruments, viscoelastic materials, and IOL designs and materials. Third, the selection of eyes for IOL implantation has improved.

■ References

1. Hogan MJ, Kimura SJ, Thygeson P. Signs and symptoms of uveitis. I. Anterior uveitis. *Am J Ophthalmol*. 1959;47(5, pt II):155–170.
2. Foster CS. Cataract surgery in patients with uveitis. *Am Acad Ophthalmol Focal Points*. 1994;12:1–6.
3. Foster CS, Fong LP, Singh G. Cataract surgery and intraocular lens implantation in patients with uveitis. *Ophthalmology*. 1989;96:281–288.
4. Okhravi N, Lightman SL, Towler HMA. Assessment of visual outcome after cataract surgery in patients with uveitis. *Ophthalmology*. 1999;106:710–722.
5. Rojas B, Foster CS. Cataract surgery in patients with uveitis. *Curr Opin Ophthalmol*. 1996;7(1):11–16.
6. Davison JA. Capsule contraction syndrome. *J Cataract Refract Surg*. 1993;19:582–589.
7. Foster CS, Barrett F. Cataract development and cataract surgery in patients with juvenile rheumatoid arthritis–associated iridocyclitis. *Ophthalmology*. 1993;100:809–817.
8. Jones NP. Cataract surgery in Fuchs' heterochromic uveitis: past, present, and future. *J Cataract Refract Surg*. 1996;22:261–268.
9. Moorthy RS, Rajeev B, Smith RE, et al. Incidence and management of cataracts in Vogt-Koyanagi-Harada syndrome. *Am J Ophthalmol*. 1994;118:197–204.
10. Stavrou P, Murray PI. Heparin surface modified intraocular lenses in uveitis. *Ocul Immunol Inflamm*. 1994; 2:161–168.
11. Tabbara KF, Al-Kaff AS, Al-Rajhi AA, et al. Heparin surface-modified intraocular lenses in patients with inactive uveitis or diabetes. *Ophthalmology*. 1998;105:843–845.
12. Dana MR, Chatzistefanou K, Schaumberg DA, et al. Posterior capsule opacification after cataract surgery in patients with uveitis. *Ophthalmology*. 1997;104:1387–1394.

13. Akova YA, Foster CS. Cataract surgery in patients with sarcoidosis-associated uveitis. *Ophthalmology*. 1994;101: 473–479.

14. Kaufman AH, Foster CS. Cataract extraction in patients with pars planitis. *Ophthalmology*. 1993;100:1210– 1217.

15. Ciftci OU, Ozdemir O. Cataract extraction in Behçet's disease. *Acta Ophthalmol Scand*. 1996;74:74–76.

16. O'Neill D, Murray PI, Patel BC, Hamilton AMP. Extracapsular cataract surgery with and without intraocular lens implantation in Fuchs heterochromic cyclitis. *Ophthalmology*. 1995;102:1362–1368.

Chapter 10

Intraocular Lenses in the Triple Procedure

Elizabeth A. Davis

■ The Triple Procedure

The cornea is the most commonly transplanted human tissue, and penetrating keratoplasty (PK) is the most successful transplantation procedure performed in the United States.[1] In situations in which a corneal opacity and cataract coexist, PK alone is insufficient for visual rehabilitation. Cataract surgery, either simultaneously or sequentially, must also be performed. Prior to 1960, the standard approach was sequential surgery. However, in 1966 Katzin and Meltzer reported on combined PK and cataract extraction.[2] In 1976, Taylor described intraocular lens (IOL) implantation during this procedure.[3] Initially intracapsular cataract extraction was performed, and thus the first implants were iris-fixated lenses. As the technique of extracapsular cataract extraction (ECCE) evolved, posterior chamber lenses were introduced.[4,5] The success of the triple procedure—combined PK, cataract extraction, and lens implantation or PK and IOL exchange—has been reported by several authors,[6–11] and simultaneous surgery has become more frequent. Clear grafts are achieved in 90% of cases,[8,11] and a best corrected visual acuity of 20/40 or better is achieved in 69%–77% .[9–11]

■ Simultaneous versus Sequential Surgery

Combining keratoplasty with cataract surgery is often preferable to performing these procedures sequentially. Combined surgery allows faster visual rehabilitation. Most patients are able to receive their final optical correction by 8 months after the triple procedure. By contrast, patients who must wait after PK to undergo cataract surgery or secondary IOL implantation for appropriate correction may wait up to 2 years for final correction. Many patients who undergo these operations are elderly and have health problems. By combining the operations in one procedure, the risks and costs of surgery are reduced.

Furthermore, it is known that PK hastens cataract formation. This is likely due to a combination of surgical trauma and inflammation as well as the application of postoperative topical steroid therapy. Martin et al in a multivariate analysis identified age, sex, diagnosis, and the presence of preoperative lens opacities as independent risk factors for cataract extraction after PK.[12] The probability of needing surgery 5 years after PK was 6% for those age 40–49 years, 53% for those 50–59 years, and 100% for those 70 years or older. Women had a significantly higher risk of requiring subsequent cataract surgery. The presence of preexisting lens opacities was associated with an 86% risk of requiring cataract extraction, compared with 15% for those with no preoperative opacity. Additionally, Martin et al found that patients with Fuchs' dystrophy required cataract surgery 36 times more frequently after PK than did patients with keratoconus (73% versus 2%).[12]

Cataract surgery after PK may lead to episodes of graft rejection. Martin et al reported an 18% incidence of rejection after cataract extraction, versus 9% in patients who did not undergo cataract surgery.[12] As well, endothelial cell loss is accelerated by intraocular surgery.[13] Graft survival may thus be compromised by accelerated endothelial loss. Various studies have reported a graft failure rate of 0%–40% after cataract extraction.[14–17]

Some authors have argued that sequential surgery provides a better refractive outcome than simultaneous surgery because the IOL power may be calculated more accurately with known postkeratoplasty keratometry readings.[18] However, several studies have reported acceptable refractive results with the triple procedure. In fact, Pineros et al found no statistically significant difference in visual outcome and refractive status after triple and nonsimultaneous procedures.[19] With experience, the individual surgeon using a particular technique may be able to predict the average posttransplant keratometry readings by reviewing his or her results (see discussion under IOL Power Calculations in the Triple Procedure). This allows for a refractive result within a visually functional range.[20]

■ Penetrating Keratoplasty and Lens Extraction

Although this discussion focuses on IOLs in the triple procedure, a brief summary of the surgical technique of PK and lens extraction is presented.

Pupil Management

For PK with cataract extraction, the pupil should be dilated preoperatively with a mydriatic. If an anterior chamber IOL (ACIOL) is to be removed, the pupil does not have to be altered.

Anesthesia

The triple procedure can be performed with either local or general anesthesia. The choice depends on the indication for surgery, the patient's age, and the patient's ability to cooperate. Local anesthesia may be achieved with a retrobulbar or peribulbar anesthetic and a lid block. A 1:1 mixture of 2% lidocaine without epinephrine and 0.5% bupivacaine with 1 mL of hyaluronidase is commonly used.

Preoperative Intraocular Pressure Control

To minimize the risk of positive posterior pressure with potential vitreous loss and choroidal hemorrhage during open-sky surgery, measures should be taken preoperatively to lower intraocular pressure (IOP). Either a Honan balloon inflated to 30–40 mm Hg or digital pressure applied intermittently for 10–15 minutes should be used. Alternatively, an intravenous hyperosmotic agent can be administered 45 minutes before surgery.

Speculum Placement

After adequate sterile preparation and draping, a wire lid speculum is used to separate the eyelids. Careful inspection should ensure that no pressure is exerted against the globe. In cases of small palpebral fissures, a lateral canthotomy should be performed to obtain adequate exposure.

Scleral Support

When the risk of scleral collapse is high (in young patients or those with myopia or keratoconus), a scleral support ring may be sutured to the eye. Two support rings are commonly used, the Flieringa ring (Fig. 10.1A) and the McNeill-Goldman scleral and blepharostat ring (Fig. 10.1B). These are sutured partial thickness through the sclera with four interrupted 5-0 Dacron sutures.

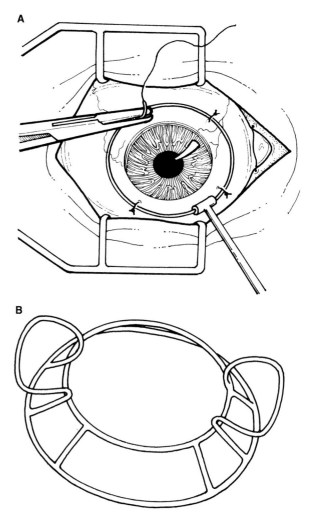

FIGURE 10.1. Scleral support rings to support the globe during penetrating keratoplasty. *A,* A Flieringa ring can be sutured using Vicryl sutures placed through the conjunctiva and episclera. *B,* An alternative to the Flieringa ring is the McNeill-Goldman scleral and blepharostat ring.

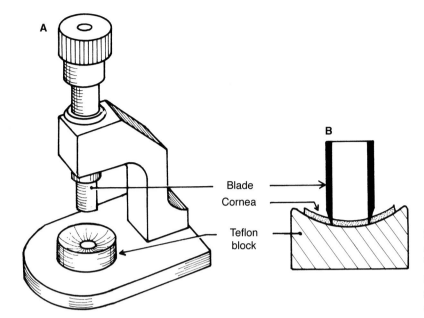

FIGURE 10.2. Donor corneal trephination. *A,* A corneal cutting system includes a trephine and Teflon block. *B,* The donor cornea is positioned endothelial side up on top of the Teflon block and the blade or trephine is applied to the corneal endothelial side.

Suturing and ring placement should be done carefully so as not to distort the cornea, which would cause postoperative astigmatism.

Marking the Corneal Center

The center of the host cornea should be marked with a sterile marking pen. This can be readily done by visually estimating the center and then using calipers to confirm that the position is equidistant from the limbus in four quadrants. A moist corneal shield should then be placed over the eye while attention is turned to the donor cornea on the back table.

Examination of Donor Tissue

The adequacy of the donor tissue should be established prior to surgery. The surgeon should review the tissue bank evaluation and test results and personally inspect the cornea for any opacities, lacerations, or foreign bodies. The storage medium should also be inspected. It should be clear, and if a pH indicator has been added, the color should be pink. Yellow indicates bacterial contamination.

Donor Cornea Trephination

The donor cornea is placed endothelial side up on a Teflon block (Fig. 10.2). The button is punched with a disposable trephine and then placed in a storage medium in a covered container. The scleral rim is sent for microbial culture.

Host Cornea Trephination

Trephination of the host cornea is performed with a manual trephine held perpendicular to the surface (Fig. 10.3). Trephination may be done either full or partial thickness. If partial thickness, the anterior chamber is entered with a sharp blade and the host button is excised with corneal scissors (Fig. 10.4). Some surgeons prefer a vertical incision; others create a posterior beveled ledge. The host button is sent for pathologic examination.

Donor-Host Trephination Disparity

The disparity between donor and host trephination sizes varies among surgeons. Except in cases of keratoconus, most surgeons will cut the graft 0.25–0.50 mm larger than the recipient bed. Depending on the size of the recipient bed (usually 7.0–8.0 mm), this amount of oversizing induces 0–4 diopters of myopia.[21] In cases of keratoconus, some surgeons prefer a 0.25-mm undersized[22] or same size graft.[23,24]

Suturing the Graft

Once the IOL is placed, viscoelastic agent is injected into the anterior chamber to deepen it and to prevent the graft endothelium from touching intraocular structures. The button is then grasped at its edge with toothed forceps, grabbing only epithelium and stroma but not endothelium. The button is placed over the trephined opening. Alternatively, it may be flipped

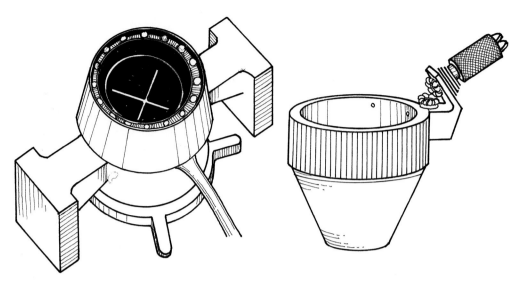

FIGURE 10.3. A suction-type trephination system is used to cut the recipient's corneal button. *Left,* Hessburg trephine. *Right,* Hanna trephine.

over into the recipient bed with a Paton spatula. Four cardinal sutures of 10-0 nylon are then placed at 12, 6, 3, and 9 o'clock. Needle passes should be at 90% depth on both graft and recipient sides. Alignment is critical with these initial stitches. Additional sutures are then placed according to the surgeon's preference and

corneal disease: all interrupted sutures, combined interrupted and running sutures (Fig. 10.5A), or two running sutures (Fig. 10.5B). Much has been written regarding the differences among these techniques and the amount of postoperative corneal astigmatism that results.[25–28] Nevertheless, there is no clear consensus or consistently proven superior technique. To avoid astigmatism and cheesewiring, sutures should not be overly tight. Knots can be buried on either the donor or recipient side but away from the wound. The viscoelastic agent is then aspirated and the anterior chamber is filled with balanced salt solution (BSS) and the wound checked for leaks. If present, these are repaired with sutures. Intraoperative suture adjustment may then be performed to minimize astigmatism. A keratoscope can be used to locate tight sutures. In a prospective randomized study of astigmatism after PK with and without intraoperative suture adjustment, Serdarevic et al found less postoperative astigmatism when suture adjustment was performed during surgery.[29] Whatever suture technique is used, the final postoperative astigmatism is achieved only after all sutures have been removed.

Lens Extraction

If an IOL is present and is to be removed, this is performed as described below (see discussion under Penetrating Keratoplasty and IOL Exchange). If a cataract is present and the lens is to be extracted, this is done next through the corneal opening. If the lens is dislocated, an intracapsular cataract extraction may be done using the cryoprobe. If not, an extracapsular technique is

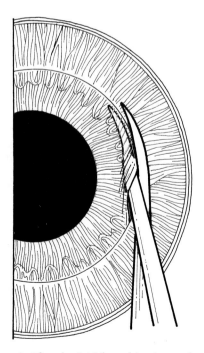

FIGURE 10.4. After the initial trephination and entry into the anterior chamber, the recipient's corneal button is excised using corneal scissors.

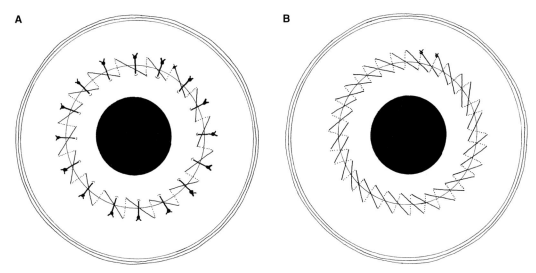

FIGURE 10.5. The corneal button can be sutured with a combination of radial interrupted and continuous sutures (*A*) or two continuous torque-antitorque sutures (*B*).

preferred. In certain instances closed-system phacoemulsification can be performed immediately prior to PK.[30]

First, a capsulotomy is performed either in a "beer-can" fashion with a cystotome or torn as a continuous curvilinear capsulorrhexis (Figs. 10.6A and B). If the nucleus is to be manually expressed with pressure, several radial cuts should be made in the edge of a continuous capsulorrhexis to allow easy lens removal. Pressure is applied with a lens loop or muscle hook at the limbus until one pole of the nucleus presents. The lens may then be speared with a 16-gauge needle, rotated out of the capsule, and lifted out of the eye with a lens loop. Alternatively, if a continuous capsulorrhexis of adequate size is present, the lens may be prolapsed out of the bag with gentle hydrodissection or by using an irrigating lens loop (Fig. 10.6C). Cortical material is then aspirated with either a manual or automated irrigation-aspiration instrument.

IOL Insertion

The choice of IOL and method of fixation vary among surgeons. Insertion techniques are described under IOL Fixation Techniques with Penetrating Keratoplasty.

■ Penetrating Keratoplasty and IOL Exchange

Pseudophakic bullous keratopathy is the most common indication for PK in the United States.[31] The types of IOLs associated with this condition include anterior chamber lenses in 31%–75% of cases, iris-supported lenses in 2%–62% of cases, and posterior chamber lenses in 7%–26% of cases.[21] If bullous keratopathy is unrelated to the IOL itself (e.g., surgical trauma, inflammation, or age-related attrition of endothelial cells), PK should be repeated and the IOL left in place. However, if corneal decompensation is secondary to the particular IOL, the lens should be removed and/or replaced at the time of PK. Lenses classically associated with pseudophakic bullous keratopathy include rigid ACIOLs (e.g., the Choyce lens), closed-loop ACIOLs (e.g., the Azar 91Z, Leiske, Hessburg, and Stableflex lenses), and iris-supported IOLs.

Most IOLs can be safely removed through the PK opening. However, removal may be hampered by the presence of vitreous in the anterior chamber or by encapsulation of the haptics by fibrous tissue. The surgeon must be prepared to perform a Weck-cel or automated anterior vitrectomy to clean up the anterior chamber if necessary. Preoperative gonioscopy should be performed when possible to examine the anterior chamber structures before surgery. This allows the surgeon to determine the condition of the angle, the site of the IOL haptics, and the presence of any encasing fibrous tissue. This knowledge will guide the choice of technique for removing the IOL intraoperatively. Unfortunately, in eyes with corneal opacities, gonioscopy may not be possible. Some have recommended the use of preoperative ultrasound biomicroscopy to assess the anterior chamber angle.[32] This technique may indicate the degree of difficulty likely to be encountered in explanting the IOL.

A

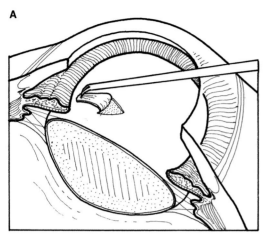

B

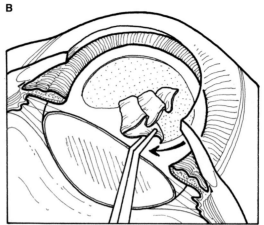

C

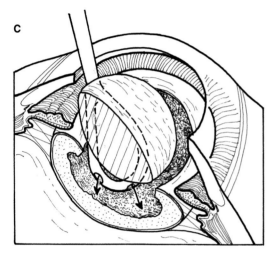

FIGURE 10.6. *A,* A capsulorrhexis is started by puncturing the anterior capsule with a cystotome. *B,* A forceps is used to complete the capsulorrhexis. Pressure is applied with a lens loop at the limbus to present the opposite pole of the nucleus. *C,* Alternatively, an irrigating lens loop can be used to deliver the nucleus. Often the nucleus needs to be speared with a 26-gauge needle.

Rigid ACIOLs like the Choyce lens can usually be removed through the PK opening in one piece by grasping one end of the lens. If this proves difficult, a separate limbal incision may be made to remove the lens and later sutured closed.

Closed-loop ACIOLs can be difficult to remove because of cocooning of the haptics in the angles by fibrous tissue. Vigorous tugging to free the haptics can result in bleeding, iris tears, iridodialysis, and even cyclodialysis. It is safer to cut the haptics at their junction with the optic (Fig. 10.7A). The residual haptic can then be grasped with forceps and rotated out of the cocooning tissue (Fig. 10.7B). If it is physically impossible to remove all of the haptic without traumatizing the angle or uveal tissue, the haptics can be cut as short as possible and left in place. The secondary IOL can be positioned so that it does not impinge on the residual haptic. The Stableflex and Hessburg lenses can be especially difficult to remove because of the presence of four closed-loop haptics that have to be manipulated in the former, and because of the acute angulation of the haptics in the latter.

ACIOLs with positioning holes should also be removed with care because fibrous tissue can grow up through these openings, creating strong adhesions between the iris and the lens. Incomplete lysis of these attachments can result in significant iris damage upon lens removal.

Iris-supported lenses require gentle manipulation as well. Although they have no component extending into the angle, they may be adherent to areas of the iris or vitreous.

Rarely, a PCIOL will have to be removed at the time of PK. The ease of removal depends on the degree of fibrosis of the capsule around the optic and haptics. Using a combination of blunt dissection with a cannula or Sinskey hook and injection of viscoelastic agent to separate the anterior and posterior capsule, the surgeon attempts to free the lens so that it rotates easily. If this is accomplished, the lens is lifted out of the capsule and through the PK opening. If free rotation is not achieved, the optic is removed by cutting the haptics peripherally and leaving them in place. Overly vigorous attempts to remove encapsulated haptics can result in bleeding, ciliary body injury, or even retinal detachment.

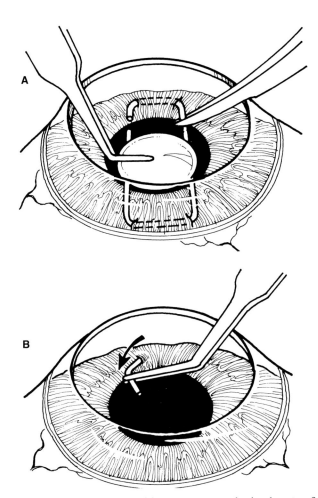

FIGURE 10.7. *A,* A closed-loop ACIOL with the haptics fibrosed over the iris can be removed by cutting the haptics near their junction with the optic. *B,* The residual haptic is removed gently with a forceps.

■ IOL Fixation Techniques with Penetrating Keratoplasty

In the presence of posterior capsular support during the triple procedure, a PCIOL may be inserted. The capsular bag is first inflated with a viscoelastic agent. The optic is then grasped with smooth forceps. After the lens is rinsed with BSS, the leading haptic and optic are inserted through the PK opening into the bag (Fig. 10.8A). The trailing haptic may then be either dialed into position with a Sinskey hook or dunked into position. To dunk the trailing haptic, the surgeon grasps the end of the haptic with a smooth forceps, pushes it over the face of the optic, pronates his or her wrist, and releases the haptic (Fig. 10.8B). The haptic will snap under the anterior capsular leaflet into the capsular fornix. In cases of jeopardized posterior capsule support but adequate anterior capsule support,

the IOL may be placed in the ciliary sulcus. The viscoelastic agent is gently injected between the anterior capsule and the iris to create space. The leading haptic is positioned first under the iris at 6 o'clock, and the trailing haptic is either dunked into position or placed into the sulcus by retracting the superior iris with a hook and positioning the haptic with smooth forceps. The implant is then appropriately rotated and centered (Fig. 10.8C). A miotic is instilled to constrict the pupil.

In the absence of posterior capsular support, the surgeon must select a technique of IOL fixation. Three fixation techniques are commonly used: flexible ACIOL placement, iris suture fixation of a PCIOL, and transscleral suture fixation of a PCIOL. Prior to each technique, an adequate anterior vitrectomy should be performed.

If there is adequate iris support and no angle pathology, an ACIOL may be placed. The pupil is first constricted with a miotic. A viscoelastic agent is then injected into the anterior chamber to separate the peripheral iris from the cornea and open up the angle. The optic of the lens is grasped with a smooth forceps and rinsed with BSS. The leading haptic is inserted through the keratoplasty opening into the inferior angle. This may be done freehand or with the assistance of a lens glide. The surgeon must be wary of trapping the iris between the haptic and the angle. If this occurs, the haptic should be flexed and lifted anteriorly with a hook to release the iris. The haptic is then repositioned in the angle. Next, the trailing haptic is grasped, flexed over the optic, and inserted through the PK opening into the superior angle. During this last manipulation, care should be taken not to induce too much force on the leading haptic as it sits in the angle since it is possible to tear iris structures or create a cyclodialysis.

If there is inadequate iris support or if angle abnormalities preclude ACIOL implantation, a PCIOL may be sutured to the peripheral iris (Fig. 10.9) or in the ciliary sulcus (Fig. 10.10).

The preferred lens for iris suture fixation is a single-piece polymethyl methacrylate (PMMA) PCIOL with two to four positioning holes in the optic. A double-armed 10-0 polypropylene suture is passed through the positioning islets and out through midperipheral iris in mattress fashion (Fig. 10.9). After all sutures have been passed, the lens is positioned posterior to the iris with the haptics in the sulcus. The sutures are then tightened and tied.

To place a transsclerally sutured PCIOL, a single-piece PMMA PCIOL with an islet in each haptic is used. Scleral flaps to cover the exiting sutures are constructed first, usually around the 6 and 12 o'clock meridians. The 3 and 9 o'clock meridians are avoided because of

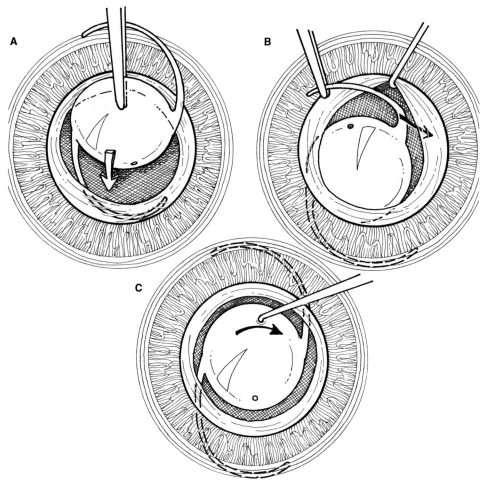

FIGURE 10.8. *A,* The leading haptic is inserted through the open cornea directly into the bag. *B,* An iris hook is used to retract the anterior capsule edge. The trailing haptic is dunked into the bag. *C,* A Sinskey hook is used to dial the PCIOL into place.

the proximity to the long posterior ciliary vessels and nerves. A conjunctival peritomy is fashioned in these areas, and then a scleral flap, either limbus or fornix based, is created. The flap is similar to a trabeculectomy flap, being 50%–75% of the scleral thickness and either triangular or rectangular. A double-armed 9-0 or 10-0 polypropylene suture on a long curved needle (Ethicon CIF-6) is passed through the haptic eyelet.

Each needle is then passed beneath the iris and through the sulcus, exiting in the bed of the scleral flap 1 mm posterior to the limbus. The exiting sutures should be about 2 mm apart. This procedure is repeated for the opposite haptic with a second suture. Then the optic is positioned posterior to the iris with the haptics in the sulcus. Tension is then applied to the sutures until the optic is well centered. The sutures are

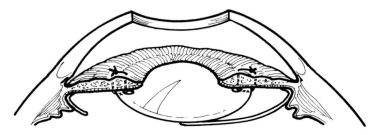

FIGURE 10.9. A PCIOL with positioning holes can be fixated behind the iris by passing sutures through the positioning holes and anchoring them on the iris.

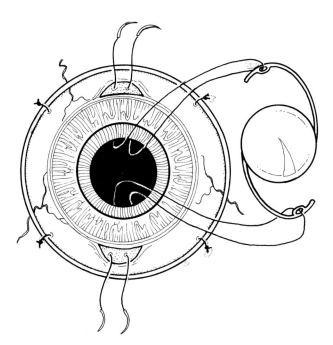

FIGURE 10.10. Prolene 10-0 sutures on curved needles are passed through the hole in each haptic. The needles are then passed through the floor of a previously prepared scleral flap. The Prolene sutures are pulled to position the PCIOL and anchored onto the sclera.

tied, the ends trimmed, and the knots buried. The scleral flaps are secured over the sutures with interrupted 10-0 nylon sutures, and the conjunctiva is replaced at the limbus with interrupted absorbable sutures.

Despite uncomplicated placement of these polypropylene sutures, histopathologic studies have shown that the distal haptics probably lie outside the ciliary sulcus.[33] This may be related to the difficulty of observing the sulcus intraoperatively during suture placement even when limbal indentation is performed. Furthermore, fibrosis of the haptic to the ciliary body does not always occur. Thus the sutures provide the primary support for the lens, preventing dislocation into the vitreous. Nevertheless, several cases of suture removal from transsclerally fixated PCIOLs without lens dislocation have been reported.[34–36]

When an intact posterior capsule is present, almost all surgeons favor implantation of a PCIOL. However, the type of implant to place during PK in the absence of capsular support is much more controversial. ACIOLs are the easiest to insert, but they have been associated with various complications, including corneal endothelial touch, graft failure, iris atrophy, glaucoma, and the uveitis-glaucoma-hyphema syndrome.[37–40] Nevertheless, the newer Kelman-Multiflex-style open-loop anterior chamber lenses are a significant improvement over the previous closed-loop lenses. In long-term studies they

have been shown to be compatible with excellent graft survival and visual acuity.[41] However, these lenses cannot be used without adequate iris support or in the presence of significant angle pathology.

Sutured PCIOLs move the implant away from the corneal endothelium and anterior chamber angle and closer to the nodal point of the eye. They are thus less likely to cause endothelial cell loss, late graft failure, peripheral anterior synechiae, or secondary angle-closure glaucoma.[42] However, suturing a PCIOL is technically much more difficult. Iris-sutured PCIOLs also require adequate iris tissue (Fig. 10.9) and can cause iris chafing, uveitis, and pigment dispersion syndrome.[38,39,41]

Although excellent results have been achieved with transsclerally sutured PCIOLs (Fig. 10.10), complications are not rare. The sutures may erode through the scleral flaps and cause irritation. Additionally, the sutures may loosen or break and cause tilting or dislocation of the optic. A persistent suture extending between intraocular and extraocular environments may provide a tract for bacteria to enter the eye and establish endophthalmitis. Choroidal hemorrhage and detachment can occur from inadvertent injury to the ciliary body. Traction on the peripheral retina or vitreous during suture placement in the sulcus may increase the risk of retinal detachment.[43]

Davis et al performed a retrospective, nonrandomized study of 41 patients who had undergone PK and IOL insertion by either anterior chamber, iris, or transscleral fixation.[44] At a median follow-up of 15 months, the authors found no significant difference among groups in postoperative visual acuity, central corneal thickness, or IOP.

In a prospective randomized study of 176 patients undergoing PK and IOL placement, Schein et al found an increased risk of elevated IOL, cystoid macular edema, IOL dislocation, and graft failure for eyes with scleral fixation versus iris fixation of PCIOLs.[45] The risk of adverse outcomes for eyes receiving a flexible open-loop ACIOL was intermediate but not statistically different from that of the other two groups.

Brunette et al performed a nonrandomized retrospective study comparing the outcomes of PK with anterior or posterior chamber IOL implantation.[46] Although their results did not achieve statistical significance, they found a trend toward better graft survival, visual acuity, and IOP control in the PCIOL group.

■ IOL Power Calculations in the Triple Procedure

With the introduction of the triple procedure in 1976, Taylor stated that "a standard +18.00 diopter lens was used because of the unpredictability of the final refractive error."[3] Although the procedure has evolved considerably since that time, there still is no precise formula to predict preoperatively the IOL power needed to produce postoperative emmetropia.

In standard cataract surgery, IOL power calculation formulas have been developed that achieve postoperative refractive errors within 2 diopters of emmetropia in 71%–100% of cases.[47,48] For these calculations, two variables must be known: axial length and keratometry readings. In any IOL calculation, axial length is the most important factor.[49] Most ultrasonic axial length measurements are accurate within 0.2 mm (0.6 diopter). In cataract surgery, axial length does not change postoperatively. However, after PK, axial length may change, particularly in cases of keratoconus, where the postoperative corneal curvature may be significantly flatter than the preoperative curvature.

The second variable, keratometry readings, can be predicted for routine cataract surgery with high accuracy based on preoperative measurements. In contrast, during a triple procedure, it is not possible to predict the mean postoperative keratometry reading. PK alters the preoperative corneal curvature dramatically, and in eyes with corneal disease it is frequently difficult to obtain accurate preoperative keratometry readings. Some authors have recommended using keratometry readings from either the operative eye, if possible, or the fellow eye to calculate IOL powers.[50] Others have empirically used average keratometry results from their own series of corneal transplants or a corrective factor to their keratometry readings.[49]

Using multiple regression analysis of preoperative and postoperative variables, Crawford et al attempted to derive a predictive formula for the power of the IOL to be implanted during the triple procedure.[11] They were unable to develop a single predictive formula because of the great variation in the postoperative corneal curvature, which could not be predicted from preoperative keratometry values. They found that among surgeons and even among cases treated by the same surgeon, there could be variation in the donor button or recipient bed shape, the pattern of suturing, the depth and tightness of the sutures, and the sizing of the donor-to-host trephination. However, their study suggested that if a single surgeon using a consistent technique subjects his or her variables to multiple regression analysis, there could be an improvement in the IOL power predictability.

Binder examined the refractive results of 43 consecutive triple procedures performed by a single surgeon with the same suturing techniques.[49] Using average postoperative keratometry readings from other transplant procedures and an updated A-constant in the SRK regression formula resulted in a 91% predictability

of a postoperative refractive error within 2 diopters of emmetropia.

Flowers et al performed a study to determine whether second-generation IOL formulas (SRK II, SRK/T, Holladay, Hoffer-Q) were more predictive of appropriate lens powers in the triple procedure.[51] These newer formulas incorporate innovations in IOL design, improvements in A-scan biometry, and the nonlinear relationship between axial length and IOL power. They also allow the use of optimized constants. Their findings suggested that the choice of IOL power formula did not affect IOL power predictions, but personalized constants were critical in improving postoperative refractive estimates.

Several authors have examined the refractive results after the triple procedure when posterior chamber lenses are secured by transscleral fixation. In this situation, predicting the IOL power may be even more challenging because of the variable postoperative location of the transsclerally sutured posterior chamber lens (TS-SPCL). In a study by Djalilian et al, the postoperative refractive results in patients who underwent PK with capsule-fixated PCLs were compared with results in patients who underwent PK with TS-SPCLs.[52] IOL implant power was calculated using the SRK II formula. TS-SPCLs were fixated approximately 0.75 mm posterior to the limbus at the 1:30 and 7:30 o'clock meridians. Theoretically, a TS-SPCL properly fixated in the ciliary sulcus is positioned slightly more anterior than a capsule-fixated PCL, and standard IOL calculations would overestimate the IOL power necessary to achieve emmetropia. Indeed, the authors found slightly more myopia in the TS-SPCL group, but the difference was not statistically significant. In fact, they found the refractive results for each group to be similar.

■ References

1. Council on Scientific Affairs. Report of the Organ Transplant Panel: corneal transplantation. *JAMA.* 1988;259:719–722.
2. Katzin HM, Meltzer JF. Combined surgery for corneal transplantation and cataract extraction. *Am J Ophthalmol.* 1966;62:560.
3. Taylor DM. Keratoplasty and intraocular lenses. *Ophthalmic Surg.* 1976;7:31–42.
4. Kramer SG. Penetrating keratoplasty combined with extracapsular cataract extraction. *Am J Ophthalmol.* 1985;100:129–133.
5. Groden LR. Continuous tear capsulotomy and phacoemulsification cataract extraction combined with penetrating keratoplasty. *Refract Corneal Surg.* 1990;6:459–469.
6. Lee JR, Dohlman CH. Intraocular lens implantation in combination with keratoplasty. *Ann Ophthalmol.* 1977;9:513–518.

7. Alpar JJ. Keratoplasty with primary and secondary lens implantations. *Ophthalmic Surg.* 1979;9:513–518.

8. Buxton JN, Jaffe MS. Combined keratoplasty, cataract extraction with intraocular lens implantation. *Am Intraocular Implant Soc J.* 1978;4(3):110.

9. Hunkeler JD, Hyde LL. The triple procedure: combined penetrating keratoplasty, cataract extraction, and lens implantation. *Am Intraocular Implant Soc J.* 1979;5:222–224.

10. Buxton JN. The triple procedure: corneal graft, intracapsular cataract extraction and intraocular lens. *Contact Intraocular Lens Med J.* 1980;6:409–412.

11. Lindstrom RL, Harris WS, Doughman DJ. Combined penetrating keratoplasty, extracapsular cataract extraction and posterior chamber lens implantation. *Am Intraocular Implant Soc J.* 1981;7:130–132.

12. Martin TP, Reed JW, Legault C, et al. Cataract formation and cataract extraction after penetrating keratoplasty. *Ophthalmology.* 1994;101:113–119.

13. Schiffrin LG, Rich WJ. *The Contact Lens Industry: Structure, Competition and Public Policy.* Health Technology Case Study 31. US Congress, Office of Technology Assessment, 1984.

14. Fine M. Therapeutic keratoplasty and Fuchs' dystrophy. *Am J Ophthalmol.* 1964;57:371–378.

15. Brady SE, Rapuano CJ, Arentsen JJ, et al. Clinical indications for and procedures associated with penetrating keratoplasty, 1983–1988. *Am J Ophthalmol.* 1989;108:118–122.

16. Payant JA, Gordon LW, Van der Zwaag R, et al. Cataract formation following corneal transplantation in eyes with Fuchs' endothelial dystrophy. *Cornea.* 1990;9:286–289.

17. Sharif KW, Casey TA. Penetrating keratoplasty for keratoconus: complications and long-term success. *Br J Ophthalmol.* 1991;75:142–146.

18. Geggel HS. Intraocular lens implantation after penetrating keratoplasty: improved unaided visual acuity, astigmatism, and safety in patients with combined corneal disease and cataract. *Ophthalmology.* 1990;97:1460–1467.

19. Pineros OE, Cohen EJ, Rapuano CJ, et al. Triple vs nonsimultaneous procedures in Fuchs' dystrophy and cataract. *Arch Ophthalmol.* 1996;114:525–528.

20. Davis EA, Azar DT, Jakobs FM, et al. Refractive and keratometric results after the triple procedure: experience with early and late suture removal. *Ophthalmology.* 1998; 105:624–630.

21. Barron BA. Penetrating keratoplasty. In: Kaufman HE, Barron BA, McDonald MB, eds. *The Cornea.* 2nd ed. Boston: Butterworth-Heinemann; 1998:805–845.

22. Girard LJ, Esnaola N, Rao R, et al. Use of grafts smaller than the opening for keratoconic myopia and astigmatism. *J Cataract Refract Surg.* 1992;18:380.

23. Goble RR, Hardman Lea SJ, Falcon MG. The use of the same size host and donor trephine in penetrating keratoplasty for keratoconus. *Eye.* 1994;8:311.

24. Spadea L, Bianco G, Mastrofini MC, et al. Penetrating keratoplasty with donor and recipient corneas of the same diameter. *Ophthalmic Surg Lasers.* 1996;27:425.

25. Assil KK, Zarnegar SR, Schanzlin DJ. Visual outcome after penetrating keratoplasty with double continuous or combined interrupted and continuous suture wound closure. *Am J Ophthalmol.* 1992;114:63.

26. Filatov V, Steinert RF, Talamo JH. Postkeratoplasty astigmatism with single running suture or interrupted sutures. *Am J Ophthalmol.* 1993;115:715.

27. Murta JN, Amaro L, Tavares C, et al. Astigmatism after penetrating keratoplasty: role of suture technique. *Doc Ophthalmol.* 1994;87:331.

28. Filatov V, Alexandrakis G, Talamo JH, et al. Comparison of suture-in and suture-out postkeratoplasty astigmatism with single running suture or combined running and interrupted sutures. *Am J Ophthalmol.* 1996;122:696.

29. Serdarevic ON, Renard GJ, Pouliquen Y. Randomized clinical trial comparing astigmatism and visual rehabilitation after penetrating keratoplasty with and without intraoperative suture adjustment. *Ophthalmology.* 1994;101:990.

30. Malbran ES, Malbran E, Buonsanti J, et al. Closed-system phacoemulsification and posterior chamber implant combined with penetrating keratoplasty. *Ophthalmic Surg.* 1993;24:403.

31. Eye Bank Association of America. *1996 Eye Banking Statistical Report.* Washington, DC: Eye Bank Association of America; 1996.

32. Rutnin SS, Pavlin CJ, Slomovic AR, et al. Preoperative ultrasound biomicroscopy to assess ease of haptic removal before penetrating keratoplasty combined with lens exchange. *J Cataract Refract Surg.* 1997;23:239–243.

33. Lubniewski AJ, Holland EJ, Van Meter WS, et al. Histologic study of eyes with transsclerally sutured posterior chamber intraocular lenses. *Am J Ophthalmol.* 1990;110:237–243.

34. Johnson SM. Results of exchanging anterior chamber lenses with sulcus fixated posterior chamber IOLs without capsular support in penetrating keratoplasty. *Ophthalmic Surg.* 1989;20:465–468.

35. Lindquist TD, Agapitos PJ, Lindstrom RL, et al. Transscleral fixation of posterior chamber intraocular lenses in the absence of capsular support. *Ophthalmic Surg.* 1989; 20:769–775.

36. Davis RM, Best D, Gilbert GE. Comparison of intraocular lens fixation techniques performed during penetrating keratoplasty. *Am J Ophthalmol.* 1991;111:743–749.

37. Insler MS, Kook MS, Kaufman HE. Penetrating keratoplasty for pseudophakic bullous keratopathy associated with semiflexible, closed-loop anterior-chamber lenses. *Am J Ophthalmol.* 1989;107:252–256.

38. Smith PW, Wong SK, Stark WJ, et al. Complications of semi-flexible closed loop anterior chamber lenses. *Arch Ophthalmol.* 1987;105:52–57.

39. Lim ES, Apple DJ, Tsai JC, et al. An analysis of flexible anterior chamber lenses with special reference to the normalized rate of lens explantation. *Ophthalmology.* 1991;98:243–246.

40. Speaker MG, Lugo M, Laibson PR, et al. Penetrating keratoplasty for pseudophakic bullous keratopathy. *Ophthalmology.* 1988;95:1260–1268.

41. Lois N, Cohen EJ, Rapuano CJ, et al. Long-term graft survival in patients with flexible open-loop anterior-chamber intraocular lenses. *Cornea.* 1997;16:387–392.

42. Soong HK, Musch DC, Kowal V, et al. Implantation of posterior chamber intraocular lenses in the absence of lens capsule during penetrating keratoplasty. *Arch Ophthalmol.* 1990;107:660–665.

43. Rajpal RK, Carney MD, Weinberg RS, Guerry RK, Combs JL. Complications of transscleral sutured posterior chamber intraocular lenses. *Ophthalmology*. 1991;98(suppl):144.

44. Davis RM, Best D, Gilbert GE. Comparison of intraocular lens fixation techniques performed during penetrating keratoplasty. *Am J Ophthalmol*. 1991;111:743–749.

45. Schein OD, Kenyon KR, Steinert RF, et al. A randomized trial of intraocular lens fixation techniques with penetrating keratoplasty. *Ophthalmology*. 1993;100:1437–1443.

46. Brunette I, Stulting RD, Rinne JR, et al. Penetrating keratoplasty with anterior or posterior chamber intraocular lens implantation. *Arch Ophthalmol*. 1994;112:1311–1319.

47. Hoffer KJ. Accuracy of ultrasound intraocular lens calculation. *Arch Ophthalmol*. 1981;99:1819–1823.

48. Sanders DR, Retzlaff J, Kraff MC. Comparison of empirically derived and theoretical aphakic refraction formulas. *Arch Ophthalmol*. 1983;101:965–967.

49. Binder PS. Intraocular lens powers used in the triple procedure: effect on visual acuity and refractive error. *Ophthalmology*. 1985;92:1561–1566.

50. Katz HR, Forster RK. Intraocular lens calculation in combined penetrating keratoplasty, cataract extraction and intraocular lens implantation. *Ophthalmology*. 1985;92:1203–1207.

51. Flowers CW, Chang KY, McLeod SD, et al. Changing indications for penetrating keratoplasty, 1989–1993. *Cornea*. 1995;14:583–588.

52. Djalilian AR, George JE, Doughman DJ, et al. Comparison between the refractive results of combined penetrating keratoplasty/transsclerally sutured posterior chamber lens implantation and the triple procedure. *Cornea*. 1997;16:319–321.

Part III

Secondary Intraocular Lenses in Aphakia

Chapter 11

Secondary Anterior Chamber Intraocular Lenses in Aphakia

Bonnie An Henderson and Ivana Kim

Most cataract surgery currently performed in the United States is extracapsular cataract extraction (ECCE) phacoemulsification followed by implantation of a posterior chamber IOL (PCIOL). However, many patients are aphakic secondary to previous intracapsular cataract surgery, torn or unstable posterior capsules from complicated ECCEs, or prior pars plana lensectomies/vitrectomies.

Aphakia can be managed with aphakic spectacles, contact lenses, or surgery (Fig. 11.1). Two categories of IOLs are available for the surgical repair of aphakia with an unstable capsular bag—sutured PCIOLs or ACIOLs. This chapter summarizes the indications for, procedure, and possible complications of implanting secondary ACIOLs in aphakia (Fig. 11.2).

■ Indications and Contraindications

The most common indication for a secondary ACIOL is contact lens intolerance. Because a large percentage of aphakic patients are elderly, it may be difficult for them to manipulate and care for contact lenses. This is especially true for monocular aphakic individuals. Other reasons for contact lens intolerance include problems such as corneal ulceration and corneal vascularization. Indications for secondary ACIOLs also include aphakic spectacle intolerance and aborted primary implantation due to intraoperative complications.[1,2]

ACIOLs are contraindicated in patients with corneal decompensation. Because ACIOLs have been associated with endothelial cell loss and bullous keratopathy,[3–7] a scleral-fixated sutured PCIOL may be a better lens choice in a compromised cornea. Bellucci et al found that in older patients with endothelial cell counts higher than 1.5 cells/mm^2 and no other relevant health or eye problems, insertion of an ACIOL appeared to be a safe alternative to a sutured PCIOL.[8]

For proper ACIOL insertion, the footplate haptics must be tucked into the angle. Therefore, if the angle is abnormal because of peripheral anterior synechiae or previous iris trauma or surgery, an ACIOL may be contraindicated. ACIOLs should be avoided in patients with glaucoma and compromised drainage.[9]

Another possible contraindication to ACIOL implantation may be the presence of vitreous in the anterior chamber.[10] In patients with a ruptured anterior hyaloid face, Kraff et al found a 16% chance of vitreous loss at the secondary procedure.[4] Wong et al reported that 28% of eyes in which the vitreous was manipulated during implantation of a secondary IOL experienced retinal complications.[10] However, in Wong's series the ACIOLs implanted were closed-loop lenses. These older-style ACIOLs were subsequently shown to be associated with a higher incidence of retinal problems.[11] The role of preoperative vitreous in the anterior chamber remains controversial.

■ Preoperative Preparation

A complete ocular examination is essential prior to secondary lens implantation. The findings will help the surgeon assess potential risks and determine the appropriate operative technique.

The cornea, specifically the endothelium, must be assessed. Many authors advocate the use of specular microscopy before surgery. Lass et al noted no significant difference in the amount of cell loss after 1 year between open-loop ACIOL and sutured PCIOL.[12]

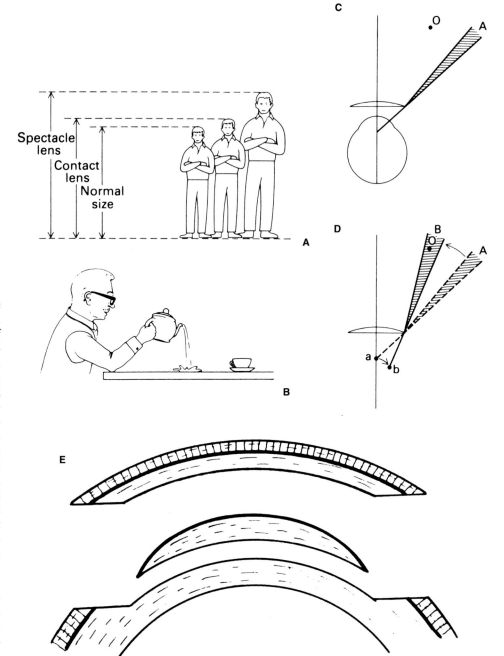

FIGURE 11.1. Alternative methods of correcting aphakia. *A,* Relative magnification of spectacle correction and contact lens correction of aphakia. *B,* With aphakic spectacles, magnification is accompanied by wrong estimation of distances. *C* and *D,* Jack-in-the-box phenomenon. This is explained by the ring scotoma (*B*) as the viewer moves the gaze from point A to object O. *E,* In keratophakia, a segment of the cornea is removed and sewn over a donor button that has been ground to the desired power. (A *to* D, *from Elkington AR, Frank HJ.* Clinical Optics. *Boston: Blackwell; 1984, with permission.* E, *from Kaufman HF.* The correction of aphakia. *Am J Ophthalmol. 1980;89:1–10, with permission from Elsevier Science.)*

Although these studies evaluated the results in patients undergoing PK and IOL implantation and not simple secondary IOL placement, the factors that cause endothelial cell loss after surgery should theoretically remain comparable.

To our knowledge, no studies have compared the percentage of endothelial cell loss in secondary ACIOL placement of the open-loop flexible lenses and cell loss in placement of sutured PCIOLs. In a study reported by Bellucci et al, one patient who underwent secondary ACIOL implantation of a flexible open-loop lens developed corneal decompensation after 15 months, compared with no patient in the sutured PCIOL group.[8] However, the change in endothelial cell counts before and after surgery were not given, so that the two groups cannot be compared. Similarly, Lyle and Jin stated that the presence of preoperative corneal disorders may increase the risk of a poor visual outcome, but no statistically significant quantitative data were given.[7]

Intraocular pressure (IOP) and cup-to-disc ratio measurements should be performed to rule out possible glaucoma. Gonioscopy is also helpful in determining the status of the angle. If peripheral anterior synechiae (PAS) are present, the location of the wound can be al-

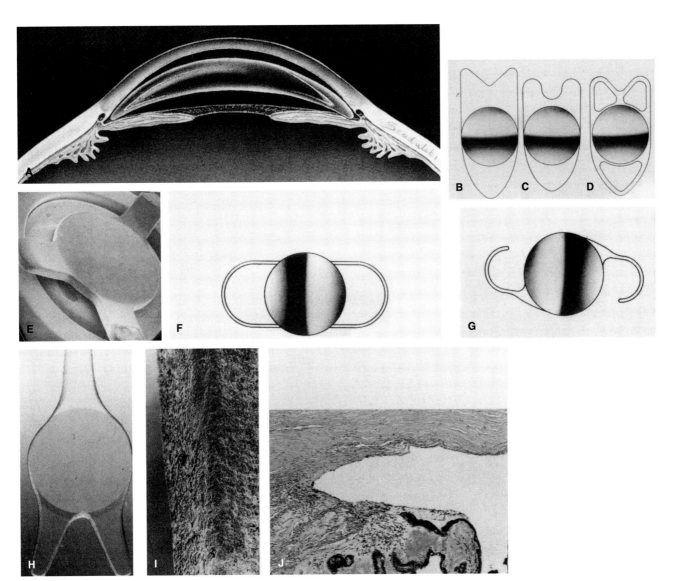

FIGURE 11.2. Early anterior chamber lenses. *A,* Baron ACIOL. *B,* Strampelli rigid ACIOL. *C,* Choyce Mark I ACIOL. *D,* Boberg-Ans three-point ACIOL. *E,* Ridley tripod ACIOL. *F,* Dannheim closed-loop ACIOL. *G,* Barraquer J-loop ACIOL. *H,* Rigid tripod IOL. *I,* Electron microscopy of the IOL edge in H. *J,* Light microscopy showing indentation of the angle recess caused by the Choyce Mark I ACIOL. *(Modified from Apple DJ, Mamalis N, Olson RJ, Kincaid MC. Evolution, Designs, Complications, and Pathology. Baltimore: Williams & Wilkins; 1989, with permission.)*

tered to plan for optimal placement of the footplate haptics. Iris evaluation is necessary to avoid placing the ACIOL haptic in the site of a prior iridectomy.

Because the presence of vitreous in the anterior chamber may be related to the visual outcome of the surgery, a careful evaluation of the anterior chamber and anterior hyaloid face will allow the surgeon to prepare for a vitrectomy. Since the development of postoperative cystoid macular edema (CME) and retinal detachment has been linked to anterior vitreous adhesions and incarcerations, it is important to perform a complete anterior vitrectomy.[13]

The appropriate strength of the proposed ACIOL is determined by the A constant of the lens, the keratometry readings, and the axial length. Because prior cataract surgery, especially intracapsular surgery, can alter the corneal curvature, the keratometry measurements must be recent. Care must be taken to use the appropriate A constant for each particular ACIOL (see Chapter 4).

The axial length of the globe is measured by A-scan ultrasonography. Ultrasound waves are emitted by a transducer to form sound beams. As the waves propagate and strike eye tissues (interfaces), reflections or echoes are recorded.[14] As the sound beam continues through the eye, the energy emitted from the transducer gradually attenuates.

A-scan biometry can be performed by two different methods. In the more common method, applanation, the transducer probe is placed directly on the patient's cornea. The probe can be manually placed by a hand-held or stand-held technique. In the hand-held technique, the patient is seated and the transducer probe is centered on the cornea perpendicularly. In the stand-held technique, the probe is held by a spring-loaded holder and a headrest is used. This technique is preferable to the hand-held technique because the chance of compressing the cornea is less.[15] An accurate axial measurement is crucial for correct lens power; a 0.3-mm error in length can result in a 1-diopter error in IOL power.[16]

Axial length can also be measured by the immersion method. The patient is positioned supine and a scleral cup is placed over the eye. The cup, which is open at both ends, is placed under the upper and lower lids and then filled with saline. The transducer probe is suspended above the eye in the saline but not in direct contact with the cornea. The advantage of the immersion technique is elimination of excessive compression on the cornea.

The A-scan instrument must be calibrated every day. The sound velocity must also be altered for the type of lens in the measured eye (see Chapter 4).[14]

■ Surgical Procedure

Prior to the procedure, the surgeon must plan the steps and determine the necessary equipment for the secondary implantation. After adequate anesthesia is achieved, exposure of the globe is optimized. If the exposure is not sufficient, consideration can be given to placing a bridle suture through the superior rectus muscle. An important step in achieving a successful implantation is sizing the IOL. The horizontal limbal "white-to-white" diameter is measured with calipers. The length of the IOL should be 1 mm greater than this distance.

If the patient has a large amount of astigmatism, the wound can be placed at the axis of the steep meridian. However, many surgeons believe that a temporal incision is optimal to avoid sites of prior peripheral iridectomies and any PAS.[18] A conjunctival peritomy is performed for the 6–6.5 mm scleral groove in the chosen axis. The groove is made 1–2 mm posterior to the limbus. The tunnel is carried into peripheral cornea. The anterior chamber is entered with a keratome.

A careful vitrectomy is performed (Fig. 11.3A). Acetylcholine chloride (Miochol) is injected to con-

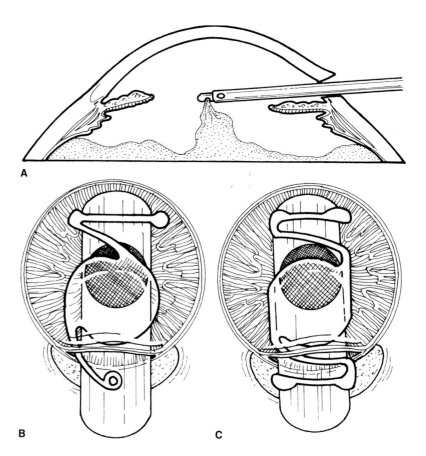

FIGURE 11.3. Anterior chamber lens insertion. *A,* A mechanical vitrectomy may be necessary to clear vitreous that is anterior to the iris plane. *B* and *C,* A plastic glide can be used to facilitate insertion of Kelman flexible three-point fixated (*B*) and four-point fixated (*C*) IOLs. The glide may also be helpful in holding back loose vitreous. *(From Azar DT, Clamen Glazer L, Flikier P. Secondary intraocular lens implantation. In: Albert DM, Jakobiec FA, eds.* Principles and Practice of Ophthalmology. *Vol 2. Philadelphia: WB Saunders; 2000: 1524, with permission.)*

A

B

C

strict the pupil. A viscoelastic solution is placed to maintain the anterior chamber. The wound is widened to its full length. A plastic sheets guide is slipped on top of the iris to facilitate lens placement. The ACIOL is then placed over the sheets guide (Figs. 11.3B and C). The leading/inferior footplate is tucked into the angle. The sheets guide is removed. The trailing footplate is then held firmly and tucked under the scleral edge of the incision as the sclera is retracted with forceps. Both haptic footplates should be secured at the level of the ciliary body band. The optic can be gently pressed to check the stability of the placement. Iris tuck should be avoided. A peripheral iridectomy is performed if needed. The viscoelastic solution is removed. The wound is closed with interrupted 10-0 nylon sutures.

■ Complications

Iris Tuck

At the time of lens implantation, peripheral iris tissue may become entrapped between the haptics or footplates of the IOL and the angle anteriorly or the ciliary body posteriorly, resulting in iris tuck. If the IOL is angled too posteriorly as it is advanced across the anterior chamber, it will push iris ahead of it, creating an anterior tuck. Posterior tuck can occur if the superior (or temporal) feet are pushed posteriorly with too much force or if the ACIOL is too long. In addition to proper sizing of the IOL, ensuring that the iris is horizontal, not concave, prior to IOL insertion can help prevent iris tuck.

Pupil ovaling in the long axis of the ACIOL is pathognomic of iris tuck. The ovaling may initially be extremely subtle but often will increase postoperatively. If a round pupil is not observed during surgery, the IOL should be partially withdrawn and reinserted. With the flexible open-loop ACIOLs, lifting the IOL with a spatula and pressing the involved haptic with a microhook frequently corrects the tuck.

Some cases of iris tuck are well-tolerated by the patient; others result in pain, persistent inflammation, and CME. In these situations, inflammation may persist despite IOL removal, and the pupil remains ovoid as a result of adhesions in the tucked area. Therefore, prevention, involving meticulous technique and vigilant inspection at the time of surgery for any indication of iris tuck, should be the mainstay of management for this condition.[19,20]

Cystoid Macular Edema

The incidence of CME following secondary IOL implantation varies from 1.2% to 7.7%. In a study of 348 cases of secondary lens implantation, Lyle and Jin reported that CME was the major complication, occurring in 6% of eyes.[7] They noted higher rates of CME in eyes with vitreous prolapse, previous ICCE, and anterior vitrectomy at the time of secondary implantation. Other reports have also noted an association between complicated surgery and CME.[11,21] Additionally, Shammas and Milkie reported a reduced incidence of CME when secondary lens implantation was performed 1 year or more after cataract surgery.[22] In Lyle and Jin's series, there was no significant difference in the incidence of CME between ACIOL implantations and PCIOL implantations (68% with scleral suture fixation). However, Wong et al found a higher incidence of CME in ACIOL than in PCIOL cases.[10]

Corneal Endothelial Decompensation

Corneal endothelial decompensation leading to corneal edema has long been associated with rigid closed-loop ACIOLs and iris-fixated lenses, with the reported prevalence as high as 15% in some series.[23] Endothelial damage has been attributed to chronic inflammation secondary to various factors such as sharp edges from poor manufacturing and mechanical erosion of fine loops into uveal tissue. In addition, intermittent touching of the cornea because of improper vaulting of lenses and toxicity from sterilizing methods and incomplete removal of polishing compounds were thought to play a role.

In a study of 4,104 explanted anterior chamber lenses, Auffarth et al found that corneal pathology was the most frequent complication associated with explantation (65.1% of cases) and that closed-loop ACIOLs were responsible for almost 80% of cases of corneal pathology.[24] Their analysis of implantation to explantation ratios, normalized explantation rates, actual versus expected complications, and duration of implantation reveals that the modern, flexible, open-loop ACIOLs are much safer than the older-style lenses. The explantation rate is approximately five times lower for open-loop ACIOLs than for closed-loop styles. Most complications with open-loop ACIOLs occurred in the first postoperative year, suggesting that these complications are mostly related to surgical problems. Kraff et al measured endothelial cell counts in cases of secondary anterior chamber lens implantation and found 9.4% cell loss with rigid and semirigid lenses 3 months postoperatively and 3.2% cell loss with the newer flexible lenses.[25]

More recent studies of secondary implantation with open-loop ACIOLs report rates of corneal edema as low as 1.2%.[26] However, these results are based on relatively short-term follow-up. Sawada et al from Japan reported complications of *primary* implantation of Simcoe and

Kelman ACIOLs at a mean follow-up of 9 years 7 months.[27] Bullous keratopathy occurred in 14% of all eyes (nine with Simcoe lenses implanted, three with Kelman lens), and only one of the eyes sustained intraoperative complications. The mean endothelial cell density in all eyes was $1,722 \pm 704$ cells/mm^2. The authors attributed the corneal endothelial cell damage to contact between the lens haptic and the angle and suggested that the broader area of contact between the haptic of the Simcoe lens and the angle accounted for the higher prevalence of corneal edema in eyes with that lens. Although the lack of nonsteroidal anti-inflammatory agents and viscoelastics in Japan during the period of this study may have influenced the complication rates, these results still demonstrate the potential for corneal decompensation even with the newer ACIOL designs.

Iritis and Hyphema

Ellingson first described the uveitis-glaucoma-hyphema (UGH) syndrome in 1977.[28] He found that rigid, Choyce-type anterior chamber lenses with warped, poorly polished footplates were associated with these findings. A high incidence of UGH syndrome was seen with closed-loop lenses (Fig. 11.4). The latter is a semi-flexible closed-loop IOL that was withdrawn from the market in 1983.[29] Newer, flexible lens designs and improved manufacturing have essentially eliminated this complication. Recent studies of secondary ACIOL implantation with open-loop flexible models show rates of iritis and hyphema of 0.9% to 1%.[7,11]

Glaucoma

Early studies involving rigid anterior chamber lenses found rates of angle fibrosis of up to 60% and, in one study, a PAS formation rate of 48%.[30] With such angle

pathology, glaucoma would be an expected complication of anterior chamber lens implantation (Fig. 11.5). Downing and Parrish noted a yearly increase in the number of patients with elevated IOP in a series of 200 eyes implanted with Choyce-Tennant rigid anterior chamber lenses.[31] By the seventh postoperative year, 7% of the patients required treatment for glaucoma. Sawada et al found an 11.6% rate of late-onset glaucoma in 86 eyes with Simcoe and Kelman lenses at a mean follow-up of 9 years 7 months. The 1983 FDA report on IOLs showed the rates of secondary glaucoma at 1 year to be 1.2% for anterior chamber lenses and 0.5% for posterior chamber lenses. The incidence of glaucoma in cases of secondary anterior chamber implantation with flexible lenses is 1.7%–5.6% in recent series.[7,11]

Shammas and Milkie studied the visual results of secondary ACIOL implantation in 17 eyes with preexisting glaucoma.[22] In eyes with a cup-to-disc ratio of 0.6 or lower and IOP controlled with a single medication, they did not find a reduction in visual acuity or a significant change in cup-to-disc ratio or visual field. In four patients with advanced cupping and visual field loss who had undergone previous filtration surgery, the visual acuity remained the same in three eyes but decreased by two lines in one eye in which there was a postoperative IOP increase. This small series suggests that implantation of an ACIOL may be safe in selected patients with preexisting glaucoma. However, given the trend toward increasing IOL, it may be prudent to avoid anterior chamber lens implantation in such cases, if possible.

Irregular Pupil

Pupil deformation can be a late complication of anterior chamber lens implantation. Although not a serious complication, certain cases may result in diplopia and

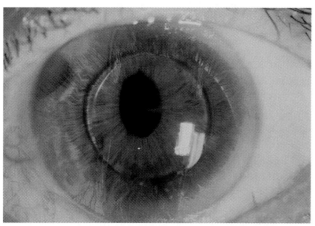
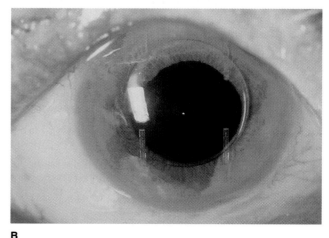

A **B**

FIGURE 11.4. UGH syndrome following Leiske lens insertion, with ovalization of the pupil more evident before (*A*) than after (*B*) pupil dilation. (*Courtesy of Dr. S. Yoo.*)

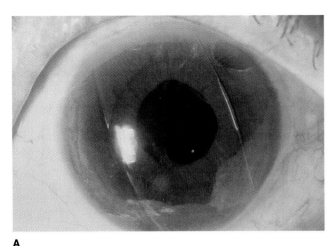
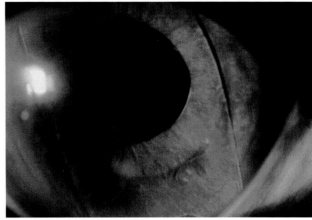

A   **B**

FIGURE 11.5. *A,* Glaucoma development after Choyce lens implantation. *B,* Higher magnification showing relationship between the IOL and the iris plane. *(Courtesy of Dr. S. Yoo.)*

glare. Sawada et al found a 31.9% incidence of pupil deformation at 18 months postoperatively with the Simcoe lens and 16.7% incidence with the four-point fixation Kelman lens.[27] After a mean follow-up of 9 years 7 months, the rates were 55% and 58% respectively. However, Sawada et al studied the results of primary implantation performed at a time when sodium hyaluronate was unavailable in Japan. A recent report by Bayramlar et al noted a 23% incidence of pupil deformation after secondary ACIOL implantation with the Ophtec AC260T lens.[32] The incidence of pupil deformation after implantation in the same series was 31%. The follow-up time was 12–31 months.

■ Conclusions

The high rate of complications seen with the older style ACIOLs in the 1980s resulted in curtailment of the use of anterior chamber lenses and a search for methods of securing posterior chamber lenses in the absence of scleral support. However, in light of more recent studies demonstrating significantly lower complication rates with the flexible open-loop ACIOLs, anterior chamber implantation warrants reconsideration as a valuable option in appropriate clinical situations.[33–41] Bellucci et al compared the results of secondary implantation of anterior chamber versus scleral-fixated posterior chamber IOLs in a small series.[8] They found that although the rate of vision-threatening complications was approximately 6% for both groups, the cases involving scleral-fixated PCIOLs had more intraoperative and postoperative complications and required longer surgery. Similarly, Lass et al found no significant difference in graft clarity, visual outcome,

IOP control, and endothelial survival between eyes treated with Kelman-style ACIOLs and eyes treated with iris-sutured PCIOLs 1 year after PK.[12] Although longer-term prospective studies are necessary, it appears that there will continue to be a role for anterior chamber lens implantation.

In aphakic cases requiring secondary IOL implantation in the absence of posterior capsular support, the surgeon may need to set an age limit below which ACIOL implantation should be replaced by sutured PCIOL. This limit should depend on the surgeon's familiarity, experience, and success with sutured PCIOLs. For younger aphakic patients the potential intraoperative complications with sutured PCIOLs are outweighed by the long-term complications of ACIOLs, which may make the former option of a PCIOL preferable (see Chapter 14). For older aphakic patients or for patients with limited life expectancy, the long-term complications of ACIOL will be outweighted by the ease, simplicity, and lower complication rate of ACIOL implantation, thus favoring this option. Frequent evaluations by individual surgeons of the possible short- and long-term surgical outcomes of ACIOL implantation versus other surgical options remain the cornerstone for the decision-making process in the treatment of aphakia in the absence of lens support.

■ References

1. Kraff MC, Sanders DR, Lieberman HL, et al. Secondary intraocular lens implantation. *Ophthalmology.* 1983;90: 324–326.
2. Sanders DR, Kraff MC. Computerization of intraocular lens data. *Am Intraocular Implant Soc J.* 1980;6:156–159.

3. Ridley H. Intraocular acrylic lenses: 10 years' development. *Br J Ophthalmol.* 1960;44:705–712.

4. Apple DJ, Hansen SO, Richards SC, et al. Anterior chamber lenses. Part II. A laboratory study. *J Cataract Refract Surg.* 1987;13:175–189.

5. Apple DJ, Brems RN, Park RB, et al. Anterior chamber lenses. Part I. Complications and pathology and a review of designs. *J Cataract Refract Surg.* 1987;13:157–174.

6. Hahn TW, Kim MS, Kim JH. Secondary intraocular lens implantation in aphakia. *J Cataract Refract Surg.* 1992;18: 174–179.

7. Lyle WA, Jin J. Secondary intraocular lens implantation: anterior chamber vs posterior chamber lenses. *Ophthalmic Surg.* 1993;24:375–381.

8. Bellucci R, Pucci V, Morselli S, et al. Secondary implantation of angle-supported anterior chamber and scleral-fixated posterior chamber intraocular lenses. *J Cataract Refract Surg.* 1996;22:247–252.

9. Leatherbarrow B, Trevett A, Tullo AB. Secondary lens implantation: incidence, indications, and complications. *Eye.* 1988;2:370–375.

10. Wong SK, Koch DD, Emery JM. Secondary intraocular lens implantation. *J Cataract Refract Surg.* 1987;13:17–20.

11. Biro Z. Results and complications of secondary intraocular lens implantation. *J Cataract Refract Surg.* 1993;19: 64–67.

12. Lass JH, DeSantis DM, Reinhart WJ, et al. Clinical and morphometric results of penetrating keratoplasty with one-piece anterior-chamber or suture-fixated posterior-chamber lenses in the absence of lens capsule. *Arch Ophthalmol.* 1990;108:1427–1431.

13. Spaide RF, Yannuzzi LA. Post-cataract surgery cystoid macular edema. *Clin Signs Ophthalmol.* 1992;13:2–15.

14. Shammas HJ. *Intraocular Lens Power Calculations.* Glendale, CA: News Circle Publishing House; 1996.

15. Steinert RF, Fine IH, Gimbel HV, et al, eds. *Cataract Surgery: Technique, Complications, and Management.* Philadelphia: WB Saunders; 1995:25.

16. Sanders DR, Kraff MC. Improvement of intraocular lens power calculation using empirical data. *Am Intraocular Implant Soc J.* 1980;6:263–267.

17. Sanders DR, Retzlaff J, Kraff MC. Comparison of empirically derived and theoretical aphakic refraction formulas. *Arch Ophthalmol.* 1983;101:965–967.

18. Jaffe NS. *Atlas of Ophthalmic Surgery.* 2nd ed. Baltimore: Mosby-Wolfe; 1996.

19. Clayman HM. *The Surgeon's Guide to Intraocular Lens Implantation.* Thorofare, NJ: Slack; 1985:65–83.

20. Clayman HM, Jaffe NS, Galin MA. *Intraocular Lens Implantation: Techniques and Complications.* St. Louis, MO: CV Mosby; 1983:52–81.

21. David R, Yagev R, Shneck M, et al. The fate of eyes with anterior chamber intra-ocular lenses. *Eur J Ophthalmol.* 1993;3:42–46.

22. Shammas HJF, Milkie CF. Secondary implantation of anterior chamber lenses. *Am Intraocular Implant Soc J.* 1983; 9:313–316.

23. Sugar A. An analysis of corneal endothelial and graft survival in pseudophakic bullous keratopathy. *Trans Am Ophthalmol Soc.* 1990;87:762–801.

24. Auffarth GU, Wesendahl TA, Brown SJ, et al. Are there acceptable anterior chamber intraocular lenses for clinical use in the 1990s? *Ophthalmology.* 1994;101:1913–1922.

25. Kraff MC, Lieberman HL, Sanders DR. Secondary intraocular lens implantation: rigid/semi-rigid versus flexible lenses. *J Cataract Refract Surg.* 1987;13:21–26.

26. Ellerton CR, Rattigan SM, Chapman FM, et al. Secondary implantation of open-loop, flexible, anterior chamber intraocular lenses. *J Cataract Refract Surg.* 1996;22:951–954.

27. Sawada T, Kimura W, Kimura T, et al. Long-term follow-up of primary anterior chamber intraocular lens implantation. *J Cataract Refract Surg.* 1998;24:1515–1520.

28. Ellingson FT. The uveitis-glaucoma-hyphema syndrome associated with the Mark VIII anterior chamber lens implant. *Am Intraocular Implant Soc J.* 1978;4:50–53.

29. Hagan JC. A comparative study of the 91-Z and other anterior chamber intraocular lenses. *Am Intraocular Implant Soc J.* 1984;10:324–328.

30. Moses L. Complications of rigid anterior chamber implants. *Ophthalmology.* 1984;91:819–825.

31. Downing JE, Parrish CM. Long-term results with Choyce-Tennant anterior chamber intraocular lens implants. *J Cataract Refract Surg.* 1986;12:493–498.

32. Bayramlar H, Hepsen IF, Cekic O, et al. Comparison of the results of primary and secondary implantation of flexible open-loop anterior chamber intraocular lens. *Eye.* 1998;12:826–828.

33. Arkin MS, Steinert RF. Secondary intraocular lenses. In: Steinert RF, Fine IH, Gimbel HV, et al, eds. *Cataract Surgery: Technique, Complications, and Management.* Philadelphia: WB Saunders; 1995:302–313.

34. Beehler CC. A review of 100 cases of flexible anterior chamber lens implantation. *Am Intraocular Implant Soc J.* 1984;10:188–190.

35. Lim ES, Apple DJ, Tsai JC, et al. An analysis of flexible anterior chamber lenses with special reference to the normalized rate of lens explantation. *Ophthalmology.* 1991;98:243–246.

36. Mamalis N, Crandall AS, Pulsipher MW, et al. Intraocular lens explantation and exchange. *J Cataract Refract Surg.* 1991;17:811–818.

37. Sinskey RM, Amin P, Stoppel JO. Indications for and results of a large series of intraocular lens exchanges. *J Cataract Refract Surg.* 1993;19:68–71.

38. Smith PW, Wong SK, Stark WJ, et al. Complications of semiflexible, closed-loop anterior chamber intraocular lenses. *Arch Ophthalmol.* 1987;105:52–57.

39. Smith SG, Lindstrom RL. *Intraocular Lens Complications and Their Management.* Thorofare, NJ: Slack; 1988.

40. Stark WJ, Worthen DM, Holladay JT, et al. The FDA report on intraocular lenses. *Ophthalmology.* 1983;90:311–317.

41. Weene LE. Flexible open-loop anterior chamber intraocular lens implants. *Ophthalmology.* 1993;100:1636–1639.

Chapter 12

Secondary Posterior Chamber Intraocular Lenses: Bag- and Sulcus-Fixation

Samir A. Melki and Dimitri T. Azar

Extracapsular cataract extraction (ECCE) without intraocular lens (IOL) implantation is rarely a result of unavailability of IOLs at the time of surgery, especially in developed countries.[1] More commonly it reflects an intraoperative decision to leave the patient aphakic because of unforeseen events. An unanticipated rise in posterior vitreous pressure, intraoperatively, intraocular bleeding, suspected suprachoroidal hemorrhage, and uncontrollable patient movement are among the reasons why a surgeon may defer IOL implantation. Other contraindications to IOL implantation include a history of recently active uveitis.[2]

Secondary implantation of IOLs may therefore occur early (days to weeks) or late (months to years) after cataract extraction. When the initial surgery is performed in an extracapsular fashion (manually or by phacoemulsification), the surgeon should take advantage of any remaining capsular support to aim for implantation in the posterior chamber. The sooner the eye is rehabilitated for safe IOL implantation, the greater are the chances for placement within the capsular bag. Although modern anterior chamber IOLs (ACIOLs) have significantly reduced the incidence of associated complications, a posterior chamber IOL (PCIOL) is still more desirable if the implantation risks do not outweigh the benefits. A patient with a history of uveitis may be better served with a sulcus placement because of easier explantation.

■ Surgical Planning

A thorough preoperative evaluation is mandatory when implantation of secondary IOLs is planned. A review of the patient's surgical history and a meticulous slit-lamp examination can help avoid intraoperative complications and guide the surgeon in deciding on the best location for the secondary IOL. The data collected should provide the necessary information about the status of the capsular bag (Fig. 12.1).

The time elapsed since cataract extraction is probably the factor most predictive of irreversible intracapsular adhesions with bag collapse. Other factors that can lead to intracapsular adhesions or iridocapsular synechiae are listed in Table 12.1. Figure 12.2 illustrates anterior capsular phimosis in the presence of a PCIOL. This condition may signal incomplete removal of lens material and may be seen in the absence of an IOL in the bag. Frequently, cortical remnants settling in the anterior chamber may suggest possible intraoperative surgical problems during the primary procedure (Fig. 12.3). If the posterior capsule is intact or if a small tear is present, in-the-bag placement should be contemplated at the earliest opportunity to preserve optimal chances for success. A history of trauma or pseudoexfoliation may alert the surgeon to possible zonular compromise.[3] The history or presence of intraocular inflammation could signal a greater likelihood of intracapsular adhesions or peripheral anterior synechiae (PAS). The presence of a posterior capsular tear should steer the surgeon to plan a possible anterior vitrectomy at the onset of the procedure. Knowledge of prior intraoperative events can also help in deciding on the size and model of IOL to use. If the surgeon implanting the secondary IOL was not present during the initial procedure, every effort should be made to obtain the operative note. When that information is not available, it is wisest to plan the surgery anticipating a reoccurrence of intraoperative surgical complications.

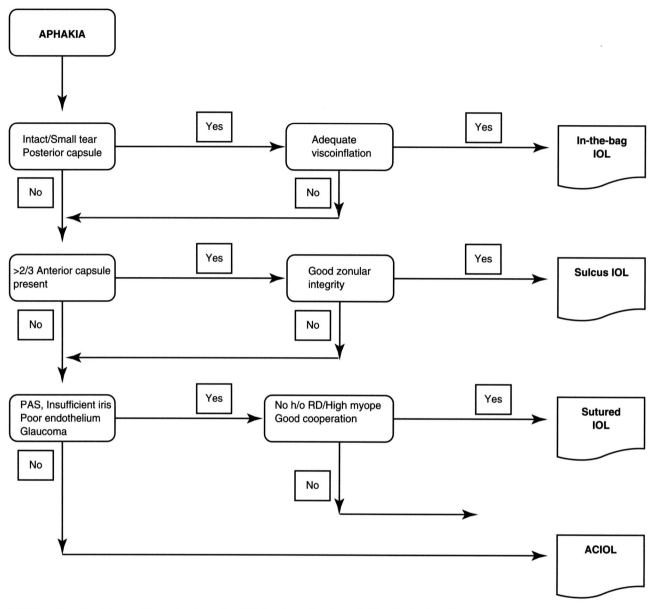

FIGURE 12.1. Decision-making algorithm for IOL implantation in aphakia. In-the-bag insertion should be attempted only after the surgeon has ensured adequate posterior capsular support and adequate viscoinflation. Good zonular integrity is necessary for sulcus IOL insertion. Otherwise, an ACIOL or a sutured PCIOL may be implanted.

A clear indication of significantly compromised capsular support should prepare the surgeon for the possibility of an ACIOL versus an iris- or sulcus-fixated lens. For this reason, a careful gonioscopic examination of the anterior chamber to detect any PAS is essential. Poor or asymmetric pupillary dilation is an indication of posterior iridocapsular synechiae. Evaluation of the corneal endothelium will provide more data to help in deciding between anterior and posterior chamber IOL placement. The presence of glau-

coma is usually a contraindication to ACIOL implantation (see Fig. 12.1).

■ Surgical Technique

If secondary IOL implantation is performed late (>12 weeks) after the original cataract surgery, incision at a new surgical site (i.e., temporal) might be preferable to avoid wound bleeding and possible PAS formation.

Table 12.1
Factors Suggesting Synechiae or Intracapsular Adhesions

Predisposing historical factors
    Uveitis
    Prolonged postoperative intraocular inflammation
    Long-standing aphakia
Clues on clinical examination
    Irregular or peaked pupil
    Small or shrunken anterior capsular opening (phimosis) (see Fig. 12.2)
    Lens or cortical remnants (see Fig. 12.3)

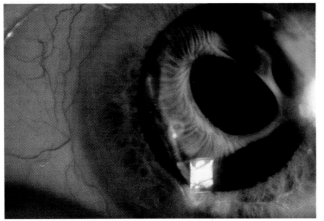
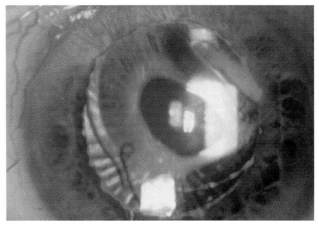

A   **B**

FIGURE 12.2. Anterior lens capsular contraction following cataract surgery (*A*) resulted in IOL decentration, which is evident on retroillumination (*B*).

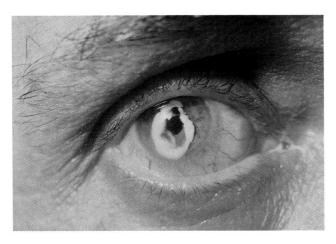

FIGURE 12.3. Sommering ring cortical remnants floating and settling in anterior chamber.

Once the anterior chamber is entered, a blunt cannula can be gently introduced under the anterior capsular edge at multiple locations, followed by injection of viscoelastic material. Any adhesions between the iris and the anterior capsule can be gently broken, aiming to free 360 degrees of the capsular-pupillary space. Attention is then directed to the space between the anterior and the posterior capsule. Viscoelastic material is slowly injected under the anterior capsule, with the aim of viscodissecting any capsular fibrosis. If viscoinflation of the bag is not successful, additional manipulation is not indicated, and implantation in the sulcus should be the next choice.

The presence of any vitreous or lens and cortical remnants should be dealt with prior to IOL implantation, preferably by automated vitrectomy under low infusion to prevent hydration of the vitreous body. Some advocate a pars plana approach for better removal of subincisional vitreous. Once the anterior and posterior chambers are free of vitreous, cortical cleanup can be achieved by switching the vitrectomy port to an aspiration mode. If this setting is not available, regular irrigation/aspiration is performed. The benefit of aggressive cortical removal should always be weighed against the risk of causing additional capsular damage.

If in-the-bag placement is ruled out because of inadequate support, a careful examination of the anterior capsule will guide the subsequent surgical steps. Using a collar-button or similar instrument, the operator gently displaces the iris to expose the anterior capsule (Figs. 12.4 and 12.5). An intact third of the anterior capsule is usually considered adequate for safe sulcus placement. Assessment of zonular integrity is more difficult. Loose or absent zonules at the 6 o'clock position can, for example, lead to the well-known "sunset syndrome." A history of pseudoexfoliation, traumatic cataract formation, or significant intraoperative manipulation should alert the surgeon to the possibility of zonular compromise. In such a situation, consideration should be given to scleral or iris fixation to prevent postoperative lens displacement. Viscoelastic material is then injected to fill the anterior chamber, with the operator making sure to insert the cannula last in the sulcus space to expand it in preparation for lens implantation. The IOL is then inserted through the wound with a Kelman-McPherson forceps, directing the haptic elbow between the iris and capsule inferiorly. The trailing haptic is then inserted as described previously (see Chapters 5 and 6). IOL rotation should be avoided if at all possible to prevent future damage to the capsule or migration of the haptic toward the pars plana or through a present peripheral iridectomy. Consideration should be given to a surgical iridectomy if unusual postoperative inflammation is expected. This will avert the possibility of pupillary block glaucoma from iridocapsular adhesions.

A sulcus-placed IOL should be checked for adequate centration and stability. To do so, the operator applies gentle pressure at the limbus with the plastic end of a microsponge applicator. An inward movement followed by sudden release mimics postoperative eye movement. A significant displacement of the IOL should prompt the surgeon to consider a larger IOL or suturing to the iris or sclera.[4]

Placing IOLs in the ciliary sulcus carries the risk of several complications. Intraoperatively, injury to the ciliary body might lead to heavy bleeding. This can

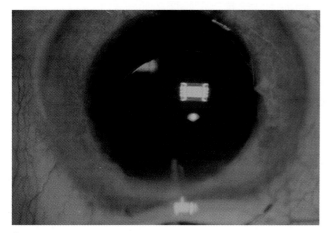
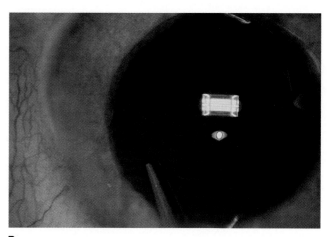

A   **B**

FIGURE 12.4. In-the-bag IOL insertion. The inferior haptic is secured in the bag (*A*) prior to pronation of the superior haptic into the bag (*B*).

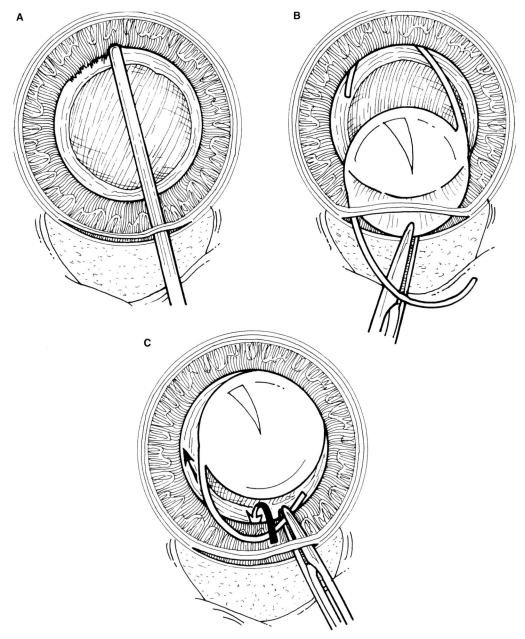

FIGURE 12.5. Posterior chamber IOL insertion in the ciliary sulcus. *A,* Adhesions between the iris and the anterior lens capsule are gently severed. *B,* The distal haptic is inserted into the sulcus, avoiding the adhesions between the anterior and posterior capsule. *C,* The proximal haptic is inserted into the posterior chamber. *(From Azar DT, Clamen Glazer L, Flikier P. Secondary intraocular lens implantation. In: Albert DM, Jakobiec FA, eds. Principles and Practice of Ophthalmology. Vol 2. Philadelphia: WB Saunders; 2000:1527, with permission.)*

also occur postoperatively, with progressive erosion and possible perforation of the ciliary body. Other complications include decentration, pupillary block glaucoma from posterior synechiae formation, and pupillary capture of the optic. Iris chafing, if significant, can also result in abundant pigment release and pigmentary glaucoma.

■ IOL Choice

The different types of ACIOLs and PCIOLs are discussed in Chapter 3. Stable positioning of sulcus IOLs is more dependent on the optic and haptic-haptic dimensions than is positioning of ACIOLs and PCIOLs. A minimal optic size of 6.0 mm and a haptic-haptic diameter of 13 mm are usually preferred. This will diminish the likelihood of postoperative decentration. Single-piece, all-polymethyl methacrylate (PMMA) lenses are ideal, as the greater plastic memory of PMMA loops better resists external forces and hence decentration. A sulcus IOL is placed more anteriorly than accounted for by the A constant (unless specified otherwise by the manufacturer); 1–1.5 diopters should be subtracted from the calculated IOL power to prevent a myopic shift.[5]

■ References

1. Pe'er J, Wood M. Intraocular lens implantation in developing countries. *J Cataract Refract Surg.* 1990;16:621–623.

2. Foster CS, Stavrou P, Zafirakis P, et al. Intraocular lens removal in patients with uveitis. *Am J Ophthalmol.* 1999;128:31–37.

3. Naumann GO, Schlotzer-Schrehardt U, Kuchle M. Pseudoexfoliation syndrome for the comprehensive ophthalmologist: intraocular and systemic manifestations. *Ophthalmology.* 1998;105:951–968.

4. Uthoff D, Teichmann KD. Secondary implantation of scleral-fixated intraocular lenses. *J Cataract Refract Surg.* 1998;24:945–950.

5. Safar AN, Melki SA, Adi M. Avoiding myopic shift by cutting power of the IOL 1–1.5 D when implanted in the ciliary sulcus [abstract]. Presented at a meeting of the American Society of Cataract and Refractive Surgery, San Diego, 1998.

Chapter 13

McCannel Sutures and Secondary Iris-Fixated Intraocular Lenses

M. Farooq Ashraf and Walter J. Stark

Intraocular lens (IOL) implantation has revolutionized the visual rehabilitation of patients undergoing cataract surgery. IOLs are rarely decentered in the presence of an intact capsule, intact zonules, and continuous curvilinear capsulorrhexis with placement of the IOL within the capsular bag. The surgeon must be familiar with the McCannel suture technique, which is extremely valuable in the management of IOL decentration. Furthermore, he or she must anticipate potential capsular instability preoperatively, be prepared to modify the cataract procedure intraoperatively, and manage IOL complications secondary to capsular pathology postoperatively. Options for IOL placement with capsular instability include implantation of an anterior chamber IOL (ACIOL) or a scleral- or iris-fixated posterior chamber IOL (PCIOL). This chapter discusses iris fixation of PCIOLs in cases of aphakia and inadequate capsular support, as well as the use of the McCannel suture technique to manage IOL decentration.

Indications for and Contraindications to Iris-Fixated PCIOLs and McCannel Sutures

The indications for iris fixation of an IOL include:

- Aphakes: monocular, cannot wear contact lens, require good peripheral vision
- No capsular support
- Poor capsular support that would result in IOL instability
- Poor zonular support that would result in IOL instability

The contraindications include:

- Active uveitis
- Iridonesis
- Pigment dispersion
- Lack of adequate iris tissue

Biometry

Measuring the axial length is one of the most important functions of ophthalmic ultrasound, and the most common use for such measurements is for IOL calculations. A variety of echographic equipment is available for measuring axial length (see Chapter 4). In general, an A-scan that has a screen display is recommended so that the echogram can be visualized as the scan is being performed. The examination of aphakic and pseudophakic eyes is slightly different from that of phakic eyes. The speed of sound through the average phakic eye is 1,550 meters per second (m/s).[1] As discussed in Chapter 4, this value changes for aphakic and pseudophakic eyes with different types of IOL materials and with silicone oil. In the aphakic eye, a sound velocity of 1,532 m/s is used.[1] In pseudophakic eyes with a polymethyl methacrylate (PMMA) implant, 0.4 mm is added to the axial length using the aphakic velocity of 1,532 m/s; with an acrylic lens, 0.2 mm is added, and with a silicone lens, 0.8 mm is subtracted.[1] With iris fixation of PCIOLs, a slight modification of the lens implant power must be made. Most regression formulas assume that the lens will be implanted in the capsular bag. However, fixation of the PCIOL to the iris moves the lens forward, or anterior to the capsular bag position. To account for this, the lens power must be decreased accordingly. We usually decrease the lens power by 0.25–0.50 diopter. If a different type or size of lens is used in place of the planned PCIOL, the new A constant must be taken into consideration.

■ Surgical Considerations

A zonular dialysis itself does not prevent IOL placement in the posterior chamber. If zonular integrity is compromised by 4–5 clock hours, the surgeon may still consider IOL placement in the capsular bag. Once the lens is placed in position, little manipulation or rotation should be done, to prevent prolapse in the vitreous. For small zonular dialysis, the haptics may be placed in the ciliary sulcus in areas away from the dialysis site. If there is a large zonular dehiscence or questionable capsular support, there should be little hesitation in fixating the IOL to the sclera or iris. More often the McCannel suture is utilized when IOL decentration is noted following cataract surgery. The techniques described in the following section will familiarize the surgeon with the use of the McCannel technique both in primary and secondary situations.

■ Surgical Techniques

McCannel Sutures

McCannel sutures may be used in cases of partial capsular support of only one haptic or in cases of no capsular stability for both haptics in primary surgery. McCannel sutures could also be used in cases preexisting malpositioned PCIOLs. We use McCannel sutures in aphakia if there are capsular or zonular ruptures, and in pseudophakia if there are deformed haptics, or unstable IOLs.

For planned procedures in aphakia, a retrobular block is followed by routine preparation and draping of the patient. Paracentesis incisions are made at the 3 and 9 o'clock positions using a Ziegler blade. The anterior chamber is filled with viscoelastic agent. Any vitreous in the anterior chamber must be removed before the lens is inserted. This is preferably done with a vitrectomy unit. The lens is inserted into the eye and can be rotated with two Sinskey hooks (Fig. 13.1). After the IOL is rotated into the anterior chamber, the optic of the lens is kept in the pupillary axis or elevated to induce pupillary capture (Fig. 13.2). A miotic agent such as acetylcholine is then injected intracamerally. As the iris constricts, the optic will remain centered and the pupil will become peaked along the axis of the haptic-optic junction. The course of the haptics will be out-

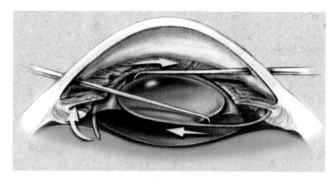

FIGURE 13.1. The PCIOL can be rotated with Sinskey hooks to keep it in the pupillary axis, release any adhesions, and position the haptic in the sulcus, particularly if one haptic is in the sulcus and the other is in the capsular bag.

lined against the posterior surface of the iris, making suture placement straightforward.

A single-armed 10-1 polypropylene (Prolene) suture on a CIF or CTC needle (Ethicon, Somerville, NJ) is placed through the peripheral cornea, through the iris, and underneath the haptic, to exit through the iris and peripheral cornea (Fig. 13.3). The needle is cut off, and both suture ends are retrieved through a paracentesis tract with a Sinskey or Lester hook (Fig. 13.4). The suture ends are tied securely at the paracentesis site, the knot is trimmed, and the iris is pushed back to its normal position (Fig. 13.5). After the haptics have been stabilized with one or two sutures, the optic is repositioned behind the iris (Fig. 13.6). Sutures tied too tightly or with an excessively large bite of iris may cause peaking of the pupil or bunching of the iris. Any

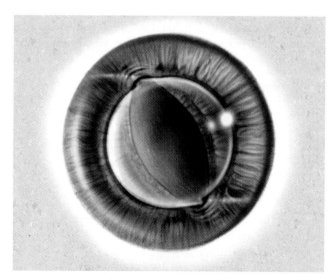

FIGURE 13.2. Pupillary capture is induced and the iris is constricted to outline the course of the haptics against the posterior surface of the iris.

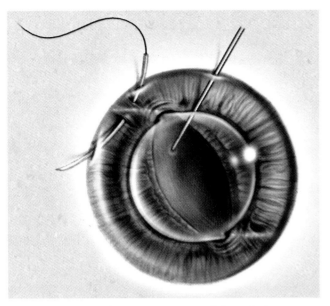

FIGURE 13.3. A Prolene suture is passed through the cornea, through the iris, underneath the haptic, and out through the iris and peripheral cornea.

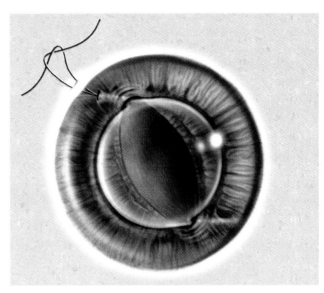

FIGURE 13.5. The suture ends are tied securely and the knot is trimmed.

viscoelastic material or vitreous remaining in the anterior chamber is then removed.

For preexisting malpositioned PCIOLs, a similar procedure is performed as described previously. However, we tend to use Sinskey hooks inserted at each paracentesis site to lyse any capsular lesions. A McCannel suture may be placed in one or both haptics, depending on the stability of the lens during the primary procedure.

The third option for iris fixation of PCIOLs is during penetrating keratoplasty (PK). The technique is similar. After the corneal cap has been removed and vitrectomy performed if necessary, a one-piece PCIOL with a 7-mm-diameter optic is placed into the posterior chamber with the optic elevated above the pupillary axis. This will cause the haptics to impinge on the iris, and a 10-0 Prolene suture is passed through the mid-

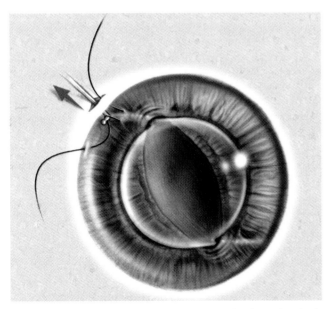

FIGURE 13.4. A paracentesis incision is made through which the sutures ends are retrieved with a Sinskey or Lester hook.

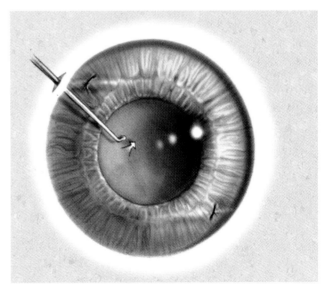

FIGURE 13.6. The iris is pushed back to its normal position. The optic is repositioned behind the iris.

peripheral iris, under the haptic, and out of the iris. The suture ends are tied securely onto the iris.

A one-piece PCIOL with two positioning holes in the optic may be used. Fixation is achieved using a double-armed 10-0 Prolene suture on a BV 100–4 (Ethicon) needle. The sutures are placed through the midperipheral iris, usually at the 3 and 9 o'clock positions. Each suture also passes through the positioning hole of the lens. The suture is then tied between the iris and lens.

Iris Claw Lens

An alternative technique for iris fixation of an IOL is implanting an iris-fixated lobster-claw lens, which does not require suture fixation. A paracentesis incision is made at the 3 and 9 o'clock positions and acetylcholine is injected into the anterior chamber. After a conjunctival peritomy, a partial-scleral-thickness groove 5–6 mm long is made 1–2 mm posterior to the limbus. The groove is then tunneled anteriorly to just beyond the limbus. The anterior chamber is entered and the lens is inserted and positioned. The lens is fixated by grasping the midperipheral iris such that it impinges on the haptic claws at the 3 and 9 o'clock positions. A peripheral iridectomy is performed, followed by scleral wound closure with 10-0 nylon sutures. The surgical technique is very similar to that used for phakic Artisan lenses (see Chapter 21). However the use of forceps through the horizontal paracenteses is favored in aphakic patients (instead of using the inclavation hooks).

■ Iris-Fixated Lenses

As discussed in Chapter 1, iris-fixated lenses have been used since the early days of lens implantation. In the 1950s these lenses were of two general kinds, based on the method of fixation: iris clip lenses, in which the lens was fixated onto the pupillary border of the iris, usually by four clips, and iridocapsular lenses, in which the haptic was ultimately fixated by adhesions between the lens capsule and the iris. The theoretical advantages of these prepupillary lenses were minimal interference with the pupil, avoidance of pupillary block, and easy access to the pupil in case of capsular opacification.

Prior to modern lens production, these lenses were sterilized and stored in sodium hydroxide. In the early years of lens implantation, lens power was empirically based on the average power of the lens in every age group. The surgical procedure involved general anesthesia, and operating magnification was obtained using 2× loupes. In children and young adults with a clear cortex, needling was performed to ripen the cataract. This made aspiration and removal easier. In older patients, cataract removal and lens implantation were done in a single procedure. Lens implantation was abandoned if vitreous was present in the anterior chamber or if the iris did not constrict sufficiently. Before viscoelastic agents became available, air was used to deepen the anterior chamber. There was a time when an intracapsular technique was preferred over extracapsular cataract extraction (ECCE), owing to the formation of capsular opacification associated with the latter. It was commonly believed that capsular opacities would resorb spontaneously with the aid of warm compresses and pupillary dilation. When they did not, needling was performed.

The Food and Drug Administration's regulation of IOLs began in February 1978, and by August 1979, the most frequently implanted IOLs were iris-fixated lenses (46%), followed by ACIOLs (30%), iridocapsular lenses (18%), and PCIOLs (6%).[2] Since that time posterior chamber lenses have accounted for the majority of IOL implants in the United States.

Surgical Outcomes and Reported Clinical Results

Pupil-supported IOLs were popular 20–30 years ago. These early lenses were plagued by problems such as interference with the papillary sphincter, irritation of the iris, cystoid macular edema (CME), and lens dislocation. The newer-generation iris-fixated lenses, extensively modified in design, afford improved microsurgical instrumentation and are associated with a significant decrease in early complications.

Several retrospective studies have compared the three lens implantation techniques with no capsular support. Menezo and colleagues evaluated the visual outcomes and complications of iris-fixated (worst claw lens) and scleral-fixated IOLs in primary (ECCE or ICCE without capsular support) and secondary (aphakia) implantation.[3] The retrospective study included 101 patients. Visual acuity in the primary implantation groups was similar in both lens types. However, in the secondary implantation group, the percentage of patients with a postoperative visual acuity of 20/40 or better was significantly higher in the group with iris-fixated IOLs than in the group with scleral-fixated IOLs (87.5% versus 54.6%). Corneal complications, including transient corneal edema and bullous keratopathy, were observed more frequently in the group with sutured sulcus-fixated lenses. The incidence of lens malposition was slightly higher in the scleral-fixated lens group. The overall conclusion was that the incidence of postoperative complications common to both IOL types in primary or secondary implantation did not differ significantly. The authors concluded that since the Worst claw lens is fixated to the midperipheral portion of the iris, it does not interfere with the normal physiology of the iris or the angle structures. Because implantation of this lens requires a shorter operating time than scleral fixation techniques and because removal or replacement of the lens, if needed, is easy, use of the Worst claw lens is associated with a low incidence of intraoperative and postoperative complications.

Speaker et al reviewed the results of PK for 102 cases of pseudophakic bullous keratopathy with respect to the IOL, coexisting abnormalities, and management of the IOL at surgery.[4] The lenses implanted included 43 ACIOLs, 50 iris-supported lenses, and 9 PCIOLs. The graft failure rate after 2 years of follow-up was 60% for ACIOLs, 9% for iris-supported lenses, and 0% in the PCIOLs. The authors reported good results with retention of iris-supported lenses after 12–24 months of follow-up; after 36 months one graft failure occurred (out of ten eyes). Visual acuity was worst for retained rigid ACIOLs at PK. The authors recommended that closed-loop ACIOLs and unstable lenses of any type be removed or exchanged and that well-fixated PCIOLs and iris clip IOLs be retained at the time of PK.

Schein et al randomized 176 consecutive patients with pseudophakic corneal edema who underwent PK with IOL exchange.[5] The secondary IOLs were either a flexible open-loop ACIOL or a PCIOL fixated to the sclera or the iris. Randomization produced comparable groups at baseline. A complications index was constructed based on the major outcomes of glaucoma escalation, CME, IOL dislocation, and graft failure. The likelihood of adverse outcome was greatest for scleral fixation for all principal outcomes except graft failure, which was least likely to be associated with scleral-fixated lenses. IOL dislocation and CME occurred least frequently in the iris fixation group. Iris fixation was associated with significantly less CME than anterior chamber implantation and scleral fixation ($P = 0.02$ for both). The risk of complications was significantly lower for the iris fixation group than for the scleral fixation group of PCIOLs. The authors concluded that transscleral fixation of PCIOLs at PK for pseudophakic corneal edema is associated with a greater risk of adverse outcome than is iris fixation.

In a retrospective study, Price and Whitson suture-fixated 233 IOLs to the iris during PK.[6] Seventy-two procedures were performed on aphakic eyes, and the rest entailed secondary IOL implantation. After a follow-up of 12–68 months, 59.5% of patients achieved a visual acuity of 20/40 or better and 74% achieved a visual acuity of 20/80 or better. Seven patients had graft failures, two had dislocated IOLs, and there were ten

cases of endophthalmitis. The authors felt that suture fixating a PCIOL to the iris offered multiple advantages over ACIOL placement and was technically easier than scleral fixation of a PCIOL during PK.

In a similar study, Lass et al retrospectively analyzed clinical and endothelial function after PK for pseudophakic bullous keratopathy with the insertion of either an open-loop ACIOL or iris fixation of a PCIOL.[7] They reviewed the records of 49 patients with respect to graft clarity, visual outcome, intraocular pressure (IOP), and endothelial survival 1 year after PK. They found no statistically significant difference in the parameters between the two procedures.

Davis et al reported similar results after comparing ACIOL, scleral-fixated PCIOL, and iris-fixated PCIOL placement following PK for pseudophakic bullous keratopathy.[8] With a median follow-up of 15 months, there was no significant difference in visual acuity, central corneal thickness, or IOP among the three lens fixation procedures.

Pseudophakodenesis is a feature of iris clip IOL implants that can occur with even minor eye movements. Using high-speed cinematography, Jacobs et al studied degree of movement of the Fyodorov iris clip lens implant after ICCE.[9] This implant is similar to the Binkhorst iris-fixated lens implant. The maximum tilt with eye movement of the lens implant was 20 degrees in one patient. The authors concluded that if the anterior chamber is greater than 3.0 mm, it would be impossible for the lens to come into contact with the corneal endothelium. There was a very negligible change in the forward movement of the lens with change in posture, measured in the prone and supine positions. Miller and colleagues in a similar study that also used high-speed cinematography noted significant phacodonesis upon eye movement.[10] They studied various iris-supported IOLs in patients who had previously undergone ICCE. The maximum tilt of the IOL implant was 24 degrees. They noted that violent motions of the eye could be significant enough to stretch and compress the iris such that the IOL could potentially contact the endothelial surface of the endothelium, especially in an eye with a shallow anterior chamber. They concluded that newer lens designs and extracapsular surgery would significantly reduce this effect.

Complications

The potential complications of iris-fixated lenses may be similar to those of scleral-fixated lenses, but the actual incidence may be lower. These complications include elevated IOP, IOL malposition/subluxation, CME, uveitis, retinal detachment, corneal complications, pupillary distortion, vitreous hemorrhage, hyphema, diplopia, pseudophakodonesis, and endophthalmitis. Theoretically, iris-sutured lenses may cause more inflammation as a result of irritation of uveal tissue because of suspension of the relatively heavy IOL from the iris. Pathology specimens from iris-sutured PC lenses exhibit mild to moderate local inflammation, but this has not been shown to be clinically significant.[11] Soong et al reported a corneal graft rejection rate of 3.8% in patients with iris-fixated PCIOLs, which is not significantly different from the rate reported with other IOL fixation techniques.[12]

■ Conclusions

Suturing a PCIOL with the McCannel technique is a viable alternative in aphakia. When performed systematically, the McCannel technique for suturing PCIOLs is extremely helpful, not only with aphakia and for treating IOL decentration, but also to prevent this complication in eyes with inadequate posterior capsular support. This technique and the use of aphakic iris-claw lenses may lead to complications including uveitis, hyphema, and pupillary distortions. However, the majority of patients seem to do well, especially if these techniques are avoided in patients with active uveitis, iridodonesis, pigment distortion, and lack of adequate iris tissue.

■ References

1. Burne SF. *A-Scan Axial Eye Length Measurements: A Handbook for IOL Calculations.* Mars Hill, NC: Grove Park; 1995:11–12.

2. Worthen DM, Boucher JA, Buxton JN, et al. Interim FDA report on intraocular lenses. *Ophthalmology.* 1980;87:267–271.

3. Menezo JL, Martinez MC, Cisneros AL. Iris-fixated Worst claw versus sulcus-fixated posterior chamber lenses in the absence of capsular support. *J Cataract Refract Surg.* 1996;22:1476–1484.

4. Speaker MG, Lugo M, Laibson PR, et al. Penetrating keratoplasty for pseudophakic bullous keratopathy: management of the intraocular lens. *Ophthalmology.* 1988;95:1260–1268.

5. Schein OD, Kenyon KR, Steinert RF, et al. A randomized trial of intraocular lens fixation techniques with penetrating keratoplasty. *Ophthalmology.* 1993;100:1437–1443.

6. Price FW Jr, Whitson WE. Visual results of suture-fixated posterior chamber lenses during penetrating keratoplasty. *Ophthalmology.* 1989;96:1234–1240.

7. Lass JH, DeSantis DM, Reinhart WJ, et al. Clinical and morphometric results of penetrating keratoplasty with one-piece anterior-chamber or suture-fixated posterior-chamber lenses in the absence of lens capsule. *Arch Ophthalmol.* 1990;108:1427–1431.

8. Davis RM, Best D, Gilbert GE. Comparison of intraocular lens fixation techniques performed during penetrating keratoplasty. *Am J Ophthalmol.* 1991;111:743–749.

9. Jacobs PM, Cheng H, Price NC. Pseudophakodonesis and corneal endothelial contact: direct observations by high-speed cinematography. *Br J Ophthalmol.* 1983;67:650–654.

10. Miller D, Doane MG. High-speed photographic evaluation of intraocular lens movements. *Am J Ophthalmol.* 1984;97:752–759.

11. Cameron JD, Apple DJ, Sumsion MA, et al. Pathology of iris support intraocular lenses. *Implant.* 1987;5:15–24.

12. Soong HK, Musch DC, Kowal V, et al. Implantation of posterior chamber intraocular lenses in the absence of lens capsule during penetrating keratoplasty. *Arch Ophthalmol.* 1989;107:660–665.

Chapter 14

Sulcus Suture-Fixated Posterior Chamber Intraocular Lenses*

Liane Clamen Glazer and Dimitri T. Azar

Secondary intraocular lens (IOL) implantation refers to IOL insertion at a time remote from the initial cataract extraction (or, less commonly, from the trauma that led to loss of the lens). There are several issues to consider when deciding on the type of IOL to be used for a secondary implant. First, a secondary IOL implant following an intracapsular cataract extraction (ICCE) must either be placed in the anterior chamber, sutured to the iris, or sutured in the posterior chamber because of the lack of posterior capsular support following an ICCE. Following an extracapsular cataract extraction (ECCE) that has left an intact capsule, the surgeon can, theoretically, implant a posterior chamber IOL (PCIOL). However, even in the rare instances in which the posterior capsule is open, without fused walls, it is always necessary to have ciliary sulcus placement of secondary PCIOLs, because secondarily inserted lenses typically fail to fixate to the capsule (probably because of the lack of an inflammatory response). Thus, sutured PCIOLs are becoming more popular, and may be placed in an eye that has been treated by either ICCE or ECCE. This chapter describes a variety of techniques for ciliary sulcus fixation of IOLs.

■ Internal Landmarks for Scleral-Sutured IOL Implantation

The anterior chamber of the eye is formed by the cornea and a small portion of the sclera anteriorly and by the iris, a segment of the ciliary body, and a variable area of the anterior surface of the lens posteriorly. The anterior chamber angle is at the periphery of the anterior chamber; it is formed by the trabecular tissue (the ligamentum pectinatum iridis), the spaces of Fontana, and the canal of Schlemm. Sodium hyaluronate 1% or air can be injected into the anterior chamber to prevent its collapse during IOL insertion.[1] After an ACIOL insertion, an IOL that rests in the anterior chamber angle can cause complications such as iris inflammation, pigment dispersion, or—as occurred with steeper, early editions of ACIOLs—corneal endothelial cell loss (see Chapter 11).

The posterior chamber is bounded by the ciliary processes and the clefts between them, the lens (resting in its capsular bag) and the lens suspensory ligament, and the pigment epithelium of the iris. The ciliary sulcus, where a sutured PCIOL rests, is the area between the iris and the zonules of the lens.

The surgeon who implants a ciliary sulcus–fixated IOL will need to know the exact location of the ciliary sulcus in relation to the corneoscleral limbus (see Chapter 2). The posterior surgical limbus is defined as the location where the white of the sclera meets the blue-gray zone of the corneoscleral limbus. In a study of 21 cadaver eyes, Duffey et al determined that the average scleral exit site of a suture passed from the inside of the eye perpendicularly through the ciliary sulcus was 0.94 mm posterior to the surgical limbus in the vertical axis (6 and 12 o'clock), 0.87 mm in the oblique meridians (1 and 7 o'clock), and 0.50 mm in the horizontal axis (3 and 9 o'clock) (Fig. 14.1).[2] If true ciliary sulcus fixation is achieved, one can avoid contact with the major arterial circle of the iris (located in the ciliary body) as well as with the entire ciliary body, thereby decreasing the risk of acute hemorrhage in the operative and immediate postoperative period.

*Modified from: Azar DT, Clamen L, Flikier P. Secondary intraocular lens implantation. In: Albert DM, Jakobiec FA, eds. *Principles and Practice of Ophthalmology*. 2nd ed. Philadelphia: WB Saunders;2000, with permission.

171

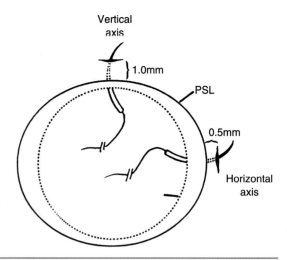

FIGURE 14.1. Surgical entrance for ciliary sulcus fixation. *(From Duffey RJ, Holland EJ, Agapitos PJ, Lindstrom RL. Anatomic study of transsclerally sutured intraocular lens implantation.* Am J Ophthalmol. *1989;108: 300–309, with permission from Elsevier Science.)*

Table 14.1
A Comparison of Techniques for Scleral-Sutured Posterior Chamber Intraocular Lenses

Technique	Advantages	Disadvantages
Classic ab externo technique for ciliary sulcus fixation[7]	Technical ease Good alternative when ACIOL cannot be implanted Avoids risk of passing needles out of the eye Surgeon's view not obscured	Requires large incision (slower visual rehabilitation) Sutures can erode into subconjunctival space (inadequate scleral flap) One-point scleral fixation (less stable)
Classic ab interno technique with ciliary sulcus fixation[4]	Technical ease Avoidance of iris fixation More precise placement of scleral fixation sutures (decreasing risk of IOL decentration)	Increased risk of hitting anterior ciliary arteries at 3 o'clock and 9 o'clock Increased risk of hemhorrage, damage to ciliary body, retinal complications (ab interno approach) One-point scleral fixation
Small-incision ab externo technique with ciliary sulcus fixation[8]	Smaller incision: earlier recovery of visual function, corneal shape preservation Same benefit as classic ab externo approach	One-point scleral fixation
Knotless ab externo technique with ciliary sulcus fixation[9]	Safer ab externo approach Looping suture around haptics is easier than tying square knots Suture loop may create more secure fixation than knots	Technically difficult to insert needle in reverse position One-point scleral fixation
Ab interno technique with two-point ciliary sulcus fixation[10]	More stable two-point fixation Can be used with IOLs without eyelets	Technically challenging because of many loops of suture Ab interno approach is more dangerous
Ab interno technique with pars plana fixation[3]	Avascularity of pars plana Less risk of hemorrhagic complications and retinal detachment Can avoid contact between IOL, iris, and pars plicata (decreasing risk of pigment dispersion)	Ab interno approach is more dangerous One-point scleral fixation without iris support

Another relevant surgical landmark is the pars plana—the smooth, flat posterior surface of the ciliary body. This region is relatively avascular and is located anterior to the retina. (The scalloped posterior margin of the pars plana fits into the edge of the ora serrata, which is the very beginning of the retina.) The pars plana is therefore a safe point at which to traverse the sclera and choroid to enter the vitreous. For instance, in Teichmann's technique of sutured PCIOL implantation (described below), the operator is advised to enter the globe via the pars plana by inserting the needle parallel to the iris plane, 3–5 mm behind the limbus.[3]

■ Indications for Scleral-Sutured IOLs

The posterior chamber is the normal anatomic position of the human lens. Thus, placement of the IOL in the posterior rather than the anterior chamber reduces the risk of bullous keratopathy, damage to anterior chamber angle structures, damage to corneal endothelium, pupillary block glaucoma, and pseudophakodonesis (see Chapters 11 and 13). In addition, positioning the lens closer to the rotational center of the eye, just anterior to the vitreous face, helps reduce the centrifugal forces on the lens and stabilize the ocular contents, thereby decreasing the probability of complications such as iritis, cystoid macular edema (CME), and retinal detachment. Another advantage of positioning the lens closer to the nodal point and center of rotation of the eye is the superior optical properties accrued by the lens in this position.[4] In an eye without an intact posterior capsule, however, a PCIOL can be inserted only if it is sutured to either the sclera or the iris.

The indications for placement of a PCIOL fixated to the sclera include the following:

- An eye that has undergone ECCE and now has either a fibrosed anteroposterior capsule with extensive posterior synechiae or zonular or posterior capsule tears
- An eye with inadequate capsular or zonular support
- An aphakic eye in a patient who is contact lens intolerant
- An eye that has undergone ICCE
- For a secondary IOL implanted in combination with penetrating keratoplasty
- In patients less than 70 years old, to avoid the risk of corneal decompensation and other late-onset ACIOL complications (see Chapter 11)

Suture-fixated IOLs were first introduced by Parry in the 1950s.[5] PCIOLs designed for suturing to the sclera have eyelets on both haptics as well as large-diameter optics (6.5–7.0 mm) to decrease the risk of decentration. Although suture-fixated lenses are technically difficult to insert, they often yield good results when implanted as secondary IOLs. There are many methods for scleral fixation of PCIOLs. A few of the most promising techniques are described in the next section and compared in Table 14.1. Future advances in this area, such as endoscope-assisted suture fixation of PCIOLs, described by Jürgens et al,[6] could help ease the technical difficulty of implanting these lenses.

■ Surgical Techniques

Preferred Technique: Classic Ab Externo Technique with Ciliary Sulcus Fixation

In 1991, Lewis published a brilliant, technically facile technique for ab externo sulcus fixation of the PCIOL (Fig. 14.2).[7] By definition, the ab externo technique avoids passing a needle from the inside of the eye to the outside through the sclera. The surgeon's view is never obscured, because all manipulation occurs in the iris plane. Thus, the risk of hemorrhage, retinal detachment, and lens malposition is reduced because the potential inaccuracies of suture placement inherent to the ab interno technique are avoided. One disadvantage of the Lewis method is that the one-point fixation of the suture to the sclera creates a less stable fixation than a two-point fixation would (Fig. 14.3).

The basic surgical technique for ab externo sulcus fixation of a posterior chamber secondary lens is as follows:

1. A conjunctival peritomy is created superiorly from the 4 o'clock to the 10 o'clock position. Then, at the 4 and 10 o'clock positions, a partial-thickness limbal-based triangular scleral flap 3 mm high and 2 mm wide is made.
2. Next, a 7-mm corneal scleral wound is made and a complete anterior vitrectomy is performed. The anterior chamber and retropupillary space are filled with viscoelastic agent.
3. A straight needle carrying a 10-0 polypropylene suture is placed through the 10 o'clock scleral bed parallel to the iris and 0.8–1.0 mm posterior to the posterior surgical limbus. The needle tip is directed through the sulcus and behind the iris until it is visualized behind the pupil.
4. In a similar manner, a 28-gauge needle on a standard insulin syringe is inserted through the 4 o'clock scleral bed. The tip of the syringe should be seen through the pupil.
5. The straight needle is inserted into the barrel of the 28-gauge needle and the syringe is withdrawn from the eye. (The syringe will be carrying with it the straight needle and suture.) A taut segment of 10-0

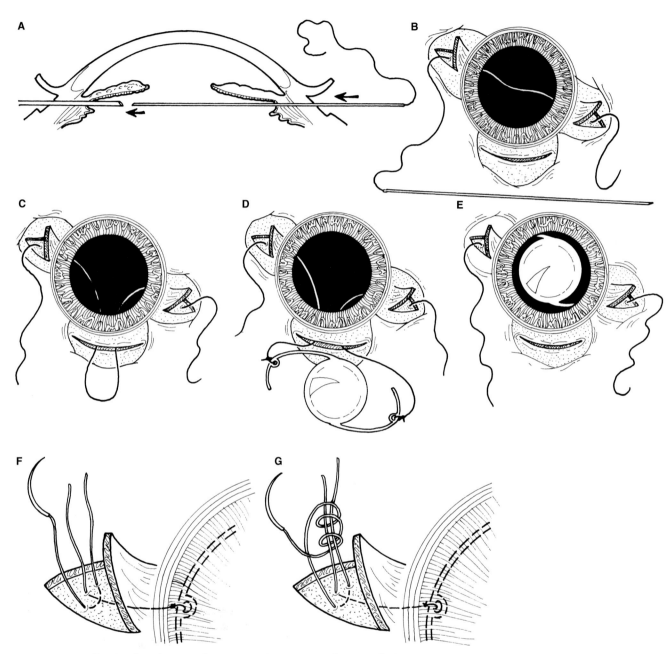

FIGURE 14.2. Classic ab externo technique. *A,* Cross-sectional view of ab externo needle placement. The straight needle is inserted into the barrel of a 28-gauge needle on an insulin syringe. *B,* As the syringe is withdrawn from the eye, it will carry with it the 10-0 propylene suture such that the suture straddles the eye. *C,* A loop of suture is delivered through the corneal scleral incision. *D,* The loop is cut and the free ends are tied to the haptics of the lens. *E,* The lens is inserted into the ciliary sulcus. *F,* The lens is dialed into position as slack is removed from the sutures. *G,* A second suture is used to take a short scleral bite anterior to the exit of the first suture. The short ends of both sutures are tied in a square knot. *(Adapted from Lewis JS. Ab externo sulcus fixation. Ophthalmic Surg. 1991;22: 692–695, with permission.)*

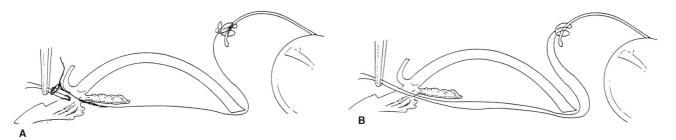

FIGURE 14.3. One-point versus two-point fixation of sutured PCIOLs. One-point fixation to the sclera (*A*) provides less support than two-point fixation (*B*). (*From Azar DT, Clamen L, Flikier P. Secondary intraocular lens implantation. In Albert DM, Jakobiec FA, eds.* Principles and Practice of Ophthalmology. *2nd ed. Philadelphia: WB Saunders; 2000:1530, with permission.*)

polypropylene will remain in the eye, extending from sulcus to sulcus. The operator withdraws a loop of this suture with a hook through the corneal scleral wound.

6. The loop of suture is cut and one end is securely tied to the superior haptic, the other end to the inferior haptic. The lens is slid into the sulcus and rotated into position while slack is removed from the attached sutures.

7. With a second 10-0 polypropylene suture on a half-circle needle, the operator takes a short bite in the 4 o'clock scleral bed just anterior to the first suture's exit. The short end of this suture is sutured to the IOL-fixated suture; this is considered a single "hybrid" suture. The long end of the second polypropylene suture is tied to the hybrid suture in a square knot with four throws.

8. The same steps are followed in the 10 o'clock scleral bed.

9. The scleral flaps are closed and the conjunctiva is reapproximated.

Alternative Technique No. 1: Classic Ab Interno Technique with Ciliary Sulcus Fixation

In 1990, Smiddy and colleagues described a technique for implanting scleral-fixated PCIOLs that is technically straightforward and produces good visual results with a low rate of complications (Fig. 14.4).[4] This technique allows more precise placement of the scleral fixation sutures, thereby decreasing the risk of IOL decentration. The main disadvantage of this method is the risk of hemorrhage associated with going from inside the eye outward through the sclera at the 3 o'clock and 9 o'clock positions. Also, the decreased stability of the one-point fixation of the sutures to the sclera allows occasional lens decentration.

The basic steps for ab interno scleral fixation of a PCIOL are given following.

1. The eye is prepared preoperatively by maximally dilating the pupil and applying a Honan pressure cuff to diminish vitreous volume. A 4-0 silk bridle suture is placed at the insertion of the superior rectus muscle to stabilize the eye.

2. A modified J-loop PCIOL with a 7.0-mm optic is selected. If a polymethyl methacrylate (PMMA) haptic with a knob is not available, a thermal cautery is placed within a few millimeters of the tip of each haptic to blunt the tip by forming a knob. A 6-inch double-armed 10-0 polypropylene suture is bisected with a standard needle and the two free ends of the suture are tied to the apex of each haptic with several square knots. The IOL with attached sutures is placed outside the operative field.

3. Next, the operator fashions an 8.0-mm-long fornix-based conjunctival flap with separate radial incisions at the 3 o'clock and 9 o'clock meridians. Wet field cautery is used to obtain hemostasis before a 7.5-mm biplanar stepped groove is made at the superior surgical limbus.

4. After entering the anterior chamber with a sharp paracentesis knife, the surgeon may have to perform a moderately extensive anterior vitrectomy with a mechanical vitrector. Viscoelastic medium is then injected into the anterior chamber to coat the corneal endothelium and displace any residual vitreous posteriorly.

5. The 7.5-mm limbal incision is gently completed with the corneoscleral scissors.

6. The prepared IOL is brought back into the surgical field and placed just superior to the incision. Using a standard nonlocking needle holder, the operator grasps the needle attached to the IOL. This needle is then passed through the surgical incision, through the pupil, behind the iris, and out through the sclera 1.0 mm posterior to the corneoscleral limbus in the 3 o'clock meridian. Forceps with the tops open are used to provide counterpressure

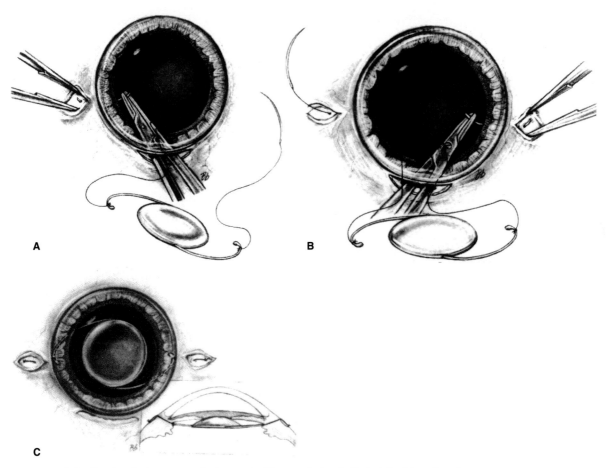

FIGURE 14.4. Classic ab interno technique. *A,* After a shelved, limbal incision has been made, the needle is passed transclerally 1 mm posterior to the limbus in the 3 o'clock meridian. The operator applies gentle counterpressure with the forceps externally while passing the suture through the sclera. *B,* The second needle and the polypropylene suture are passed transsclerally in a similar manner at the 9 o'clock meridian. *C,* A properly positioned scleral-fixated lens with haptics oriented in the 3 o'clock and 9 o'clock meridians. The operator makes a midthickness scleral pass with the needle and ties the suture to itself. *(From Smiddy WE, Sawusch MR, O'Brien TP, Scott DR, Huang SS. Implantation of scleral-fixated posterior chamber intraocular lenses.* J Cataract Refract Surg. *1990;16:691–696, with permission.)*

while the needle is being passed through the sclera (Fig. 14.4A). The other IOL-attached needle is passed through the sclera at the 9 o'clock meridian in backhand fashion (Fig. 14.4B).

7. With the lens forceps, the operator introduces the IOL into the eye while the assistant adjusts the tension of the polypropylene sutures externally. To ensure proper final orientation of the lens, the implant's orientation is adjusted so that the 9 o'clock haptic is introduced first. Grasping the tip of the superior haptic with an angled McPherson forceps, the operator rotates the haptic over the optic while depressing the optic posteriorly with the forceps tip. Once the elbow of the haptic is below the iris, it is directed toward the ciliary sulcus by the oper-

ator's pronating the hand holding the angled forceps.

8. The IOL must be secured by one-point scleral fixation, since only one suture comes off each haptic. Each needle is passed through the half-thickness sclera 1 mm posterior to the exit site, leaving a loop in the suture so that the suture can be tied to itself. The suture ends are left approximately 2 mm long so that they will lie flat under the conjunctiva, which is sewn over the knot using 8-0 chromic suture. The superior groove and conjunctival flap are closed in the usual fashion. In its final position, the implant rests in the posterior chamber with the haptics oriented in the 3 o'clock and 9 o'clock meridians (Fig. 14.4C).

Alternative Technique No. 2: Small-Incision Ab Externo Technique with Ciliary Sulcus Fixation

Regillo and Tidwell published a modified version of the Lewis technique for suturing a PCIOL (Fig. 14.5).[8] Their method utilizes a foldable silicone lens to allow for a smaller incision. A smaller incision decreases the risk of intraocular fluid loss and hypotony, thereby improving globe stability during lens insertion and suturing. With a smaller incision, patients often achieve earlier recovery of visual function and better preservation of corneal shape. By obviating limbal-incision suturing, the small-incision method requires less time in the operating room and reduces astigmatism.

The Regillo-Tidwell procedure includes the following steps:

1. A standard three-port pars plana vitrectomy is completed. The two superior sclerotomies are closed, with the inferotemporal infusion left in position but turned off.
2. Two triangular partial-thickness scleral flaps are created at the limbus in the 3 o'clock and 9 o'clock meridians in preparation for passing the transscleral fixation suture.
3. A 4-mm keratome is used to create a small, self-sealing, clear corneal incision near the temporal aspect of the limbus.
4. With the needle holder, the operator grasps a single double-armed 10-0 polypropylene suture with a straight needle on one end. The straight needle is passed through the bed of the temporal scleral flap and retrieved within the barrel of a 28-gauge needle placed through the opposite scleral bed, as described by Lewis (Fig. 14.5A). A Sinskey hook is used to externalize a loop of suture through the clear corneal incision. The ends of the loop are cut, and each free end is sutured to one haptic of a foldable silicone IOL (Fig. 14.5B).
5. The lens is folded along the 12 and 6 o'clock axis with positive action forceps. The folded lens is inserted through the 4-mm corneal incision with the leading haptic on the posterior aspect of the lens implant and opened up just behind the level of the iris plane (Fig. 14.5C). Folding and inserting the lens in this fashion keeps the leading haptic in the proper orientation throughout the maneuver. The trailing haptic rotates 180 degrees during unfolding and is not advanced through the corneal wound until after the lens itself has unfolded in the eye. In this way, rotation of this haptic into its ultimate orientation at 9 o'clock takes place safely outside the anterior chamber. This haptic is then inserted completely through the corneal wound and allowed to fall under the iris temporally. A gentle pull on the two sutures will bring both haptics into the desired 3 o'clock and 9 o'clock positions of the ciliary sulcus.
6. The sutures are permanently tied down into the bed of the scleral flap in the following manner. First the operator creates a loop, using the needles already present on the two ends to make a small, partial-thickness scleral pass adjacent to the exiting suture. The end with the needle is tied to the loop in its own suture material (Fig. 14.5D). Finally, the suture ends are trimmed, and the scleral flap is draped over the knot. The corneal incision is usually watertight and may not require any sutures.

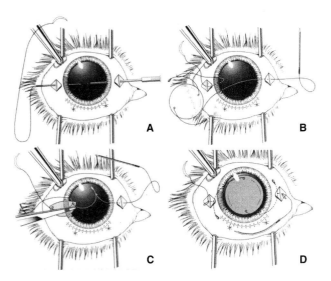

FIGURE 14.5. Small-incision ab externo technique. *A,* The straight needle end of a 10-0 polypropylene suture is inserted through the bed of the scleral flap temporally. The straight needle is retrieved within the barrel of a 28-gauge needle. *B,* The single, transscleral suture is externalized through the temporal corneal incision and the loop is cut. The two free ends are tied to the haptics of the silicone lens. *C,* The folded silicone lens is inserted through the 4-mm corneal incision. *D,* The lens is secured in the ciliary sulcus with the haptics in the 3 o'clock and 9 o'clock positions. *(From Regillo CD, Tidwell J. A small-incision technique for suturing a posterior chamber intraocular lens.* Ophthalmic Surg Lasers. *1996;27:473–475, with permission.)*

Alternative Technique No. 3: Knotless Ab Externo Technique with Ciliary Sulcus Fixation

In 1995, Eryildirim published a technique for inserting a sutured PCIOL by an ab externo approach (Fig. 14.6).[9] Eryildirim's manner of looping the suture around the haptics is easier than tying square knots around the haptics and may create a more secure fixation than knots would. The difficulty of the second step, in which the surgeon inserts the needle in reverse position, from the inside out, might be alleviated by a trick the author describes. Although Eryildirim's method leaves the surgeon with two lines of suture at each scleral clock hour at the end of the operation, these sutures cannot be used to do a more stable two-point fixation because the two strands exit through the same port.

The basic steps of Eryildirim's procedure follow:

1. Scleral flaps 3 × 3 × 3 mm are created at the 2 o'clock and 8 o'clock positions, 1 mm from the posterior limbus.
2. The straight needle is inserted into the globe 1 mm from the limbus to make a port. The needle is then drawn back and inserted again in the reverse position (Fig. 14.6C).
3. Using a lens dialer the operator captures the suture and pulls it through the corneal incision, thereby creating a loop in the suture.

4. The procedure is repeated on the other port.
5. The suture is passed into the eyelet of a monoblock PMMA lens with eyelets on its haptics. Then the suture loop is pulled through the eyelet such that the loop can go over the IOL and straddle the haptic (Fig. 14.6H). Tightening the suture locks it in place.
6. The second suture loop is passed into the second eyelet. This time, the loop is passed over the haptic (rather than over the entire IOL) to lock the suture over the eyelet (Figs. 14.6K to O).
7. The IOL is implanted in the posterior chamber and the sutures are tightened.
8. Using a needle holder, the operator curves the straight needles and passes them through the sclera beneath the flaps. The sutures are tied together, creating a one-point fixation.
9. The sutures are cut long so that the ends do not erode the scleral flaps and conjuctiva. The scleral flaps are not closed. The conjunctiva should be closed by cautery.

Eryildirim describes some tricks that may be helpful during two difficult steps of this procedure. First, it is often hard to find the entrance port while inserting the needle in reverse position. Before inserting the needle into the eye to make a port, the surgeon can mark the entrance point with a pre-inked marking pad. Touch

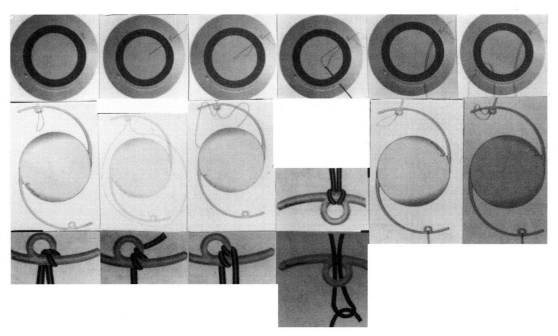

FIGURE 14.6. Knotless ab externo technique. *(From Eryildirim A. Knotless scleral fixation for implanting a posterior chamber intraocular lens. Ophthalmic Surg. 1995;26:82–84, with permission.)*

the needle with the ink pad, and when the needle passes through the sclera, ink will remain on the surface of the sclera, leaving a blue circle with a hole in the center. Second, it is often difficult to pass the two-fold polypropylene suture through the eyelet of the haptic (Fig. 14.6G). To solve this problem, the surgeon can pass an 8-0 silk suture through the eyelet and then use that as a guide for the 10-0 suture (Fig. 14.6P).

Alternative Technique No. 4: Ab Interno Technique with Two-Point Ciliary Sulcus Fixation

This technique may result in very stable fixation of the IOL: the fixation to the sclera is a stable two-point fixation since two sutures exit the sclera at two different spots (Fig. 14.7).[10] This method can be used with IOLs that do not have eyelets, but it is best suited for IOLs

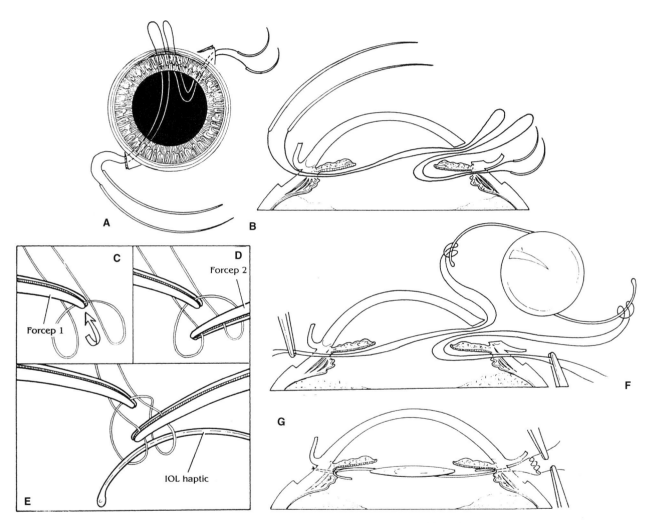

FIGURE 14.7. Ab interno technique with two-point fixation. *A* and *B,* Two limbal-based, partial-thickness scleral flaps are dissected, 180 degrees apart. A double-armed suture is passed on a long needle through the incision and the pupil, under the iris, through the ciliary sulcus, and out through the sclera 1–1.5 mm posterior to the limbus. The other needle of the double-armed suture is passed in a similar manner, exiting 1 mm lateral to the first exit site. These steps are shown from the surgeon's perspective (*A*) and from a side view (*B*). *C* to *E,* A girth hitch is used to affix the haptics to the double-armed suture. *F,* The haptics are positioned in the ciliary sulcus by gently drawing up on the suture ends with tying forceps. *G,* Once the lens has been centered, the superior and inferior loops are tied with a 3-1-1 surgeon's knot. *(From Mead MD, Sieck EA, Steinert RF. Optical rehabilitation of aphakia. In Albert DM, Jakobiec FA, eds.* Principles and Practice of Ophthalmology: Clinical Practice. *Vol 1. Philadelphia: WB Saunders; 1994:641–656, with permission.)*

with two eyelets on each haptic. The procedure is technically challenging because of the loops of suture involved.

The steps are as follows:

1. The eye is prepared in the usual fashion, including the removal of vitreous from the anterior chamber, iris plane, and anterior vitreous cavity.
2. Two limbal-based, partial-thickness scleral flaps are dissected, 180 degrees apart (Fig. 14.7A).
3. A double-armed 10-0 polypropylene suture on a long needle (e.g., Ethicon CIF 4 or CTC-6) is grasped with a needle holder. The suture is passed through the surgical entrance wound and pupil, under the iris, through the ciliary sulcus, and out through the sclera 1–1.5 mm posterior to the limbus under the scleral flap (Fig. 14.7B).
4. The other needle of the double-armed suture is passed on a similar path, but exits the eye about 1 mm lateral to the first exit site.
5. Steps 3 and 4 are repeated for the superior fixation suture. This suture uses a strong, short needle such as the Ethicon TG 160-8. The needles are rotated backward through the pupil and behind the iris such that they exit through the superior ciliary sulcus.
6. A girth hitch is used to fixate the superior and inferior IOL haptics to their respective double-armed sutures (Figs. 14.7C to E).
7. The haptics are placed into position in the ciliary sulcus by passing the inferior and then the superior haptics behind the pupil while gently drawing the sutures through the sclera (Fig. 14.7F).
8. Once the IOL has been centered, the superior and inferior loops are tied using a 3-1-1 surgeon's knot. The suture ends are trimmed short (Fig. 14.7G).

9. After the corneoscleral limbal wound has been closed in the usual fashion, the scleral flaps are closed at their corners with an 8-0 or 9-0 Vicryl suture on a spatula needle. Finally, the conjunctiva is sutured over the scleral flap.

Alternative Technique No. 5: Ab Interno Technique with Pars Plana Fixation

The pars plana fixation technique, originally described by Girard in 1981, never became as popular as the ciliary sulcus fixation technique. However, significant improvements in lens design and materials as well as changes in surgical technique could make pars plana fixation an alternative surgical approach.[3] The pars plana is relatively avascular and lies anterior to the retina; thus, one can avoid hemorrhagic complications and retinal detachments by making incisions through the sclera and choroid into the vitreous at the level of the pars plana. Other advantages of a pars plana fixation include the chance to avoid contact of the IOL, iris, and pars plicata. Pigment dispersion could also be avoided, since the only area in direct contact with the haptic of the IOL should be the nonpigmented inner layer of the pars plana.

A few modifications in the shape and size of the standard PCIOL would be required for pars plana fixation (Fig. 14.8):

1. The diameter of the lens must be increased to about 17 mm and the diameter of the biconvex optic to 7 mm.
2. The haptics must be angled backward at 10 or 20 degrees, according to the surgeon's preferred loca-

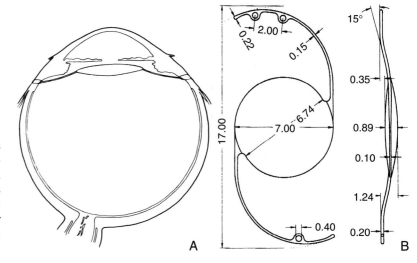

FIGURE 14.8. Ab interno technique with pars plana fixation. *A,* Diagram of the cross-section of a globe with the pars plana PCIOL in place. *B,* Morcher's prototype of the pars plana IOL. *(From Teichmann KD. Pars plana fixation of posterior chamber intraocular lenses. Ophthalmic Surg. 1994;25: 549–553, with permission.)*

tion of the optic in relation to the iris. (The surgeon should aim to avoid iris touch, and to leave a space of at least 1 mm between lens and iris. If the lens is in this position, the A constant should be in the same range as for in-the-bag placement.)

3. PMMA is the material of choice for a pars plana–fixated IOL. This polymer will provide sufficient stability against torque and tilt.

4. Preferably, the IOL would have an eyelet on each haptic to facilitate suture fixation and permit burying the knots. Alternative methods of burying the knots include covering them with scleral flaps or a scleral groove. For more stable fixation, it is best to use three-point fixation, with one of the haptics carrying two eyelets (Fig. 14.8B).

The basic steps of Teichmann's pars plana fixation technique[3] follow:

1. A suture is tied around each of the three eyelets of the lens. Then the IOL is inserted in the preferred fashion, typically through a superior limbal incision. It is best to orient the IOL vertically or obliquely from superonasally to inferotemporally.

2. The pars plana fixation will proceed from inside the eye out. During pars plana fixation, the long ciliary arteries, positioned at 3 o'clock and 9 o'clock, may be injured. Therefore, sutures cannot be placed in the horizontal plane. The ora serrata is located 5–6 mm posterior to the limbus, and the vascular pars plicata of the ciliary body ends a little less than 3 mm from the limbus. Therefore, to enter the pars plana safely, the operator should enter the sclera 3–5 mm behind the limbus, keeping the needle path parallel to the iris plane.

3. For increased IOL stability, either two-point fixation of the sutures or double transscleral pars plana fixation should be used. The two strands of each suture could be placed radially, such that they are on the same longitudinal meridian but 3.0 and 3.5 mm from the posterior surgical limbus. Alternatively, they could be placed limbus-parallel: both at the same distance from the limbus but 2 mm apart. In either case, it is important to place these double sutures exactly opposite each other relative to the center of the cornea in order to avoid lens tilt.

4. Teichmann notes that for greater stability, one can secure the two sutures attached to the haptic with two eyelets inferotemporally, about 3.0 or 3.5 mm from the posterior limbus, measured on the scleral surface. The operator then secures the haptic with the single eyelet and one suture by creating iris-parallel stitches inserted 3.0 and 3.5 mm from the limbus on the scleral surface, superonasally.

■ Scleral-Sutured Pediatric IOLs

Worldwide, approximately 200,000 children are blind from cataracts.[11] Thus, the issue of IOLs in children is clearly significant. Most surgeons agree that when cataracts are removed from children less than 2 years old, the lenses should not be replaced with IOLs. Rapid ocular growth during the first 2 years of life makes it very difficult to select the appropriate IOL power. However, there is still considerable debate over the appropriate age for IOL implantation and the best type to use. In many cases the cataract is removed and the child is left aphakic, dependent on a contact lens or spectacles.

Children who are aphakic may require secondary IOLs in a variety of cases, including children with congenital monocular cataracts who have had the cataracts removed and subsequently have become resistant to using contact lenses, eyes that have experienced a trauma preventing primary placement of IOLs, and children with bilateral aphakia who develop intolerance to contact lenses or spectacles.[12]

Two commonly used IOL implantation techniques in children are in-the-bag PCIOLs and sulcus-fixated IOLs. A study reviewing the results of IOL placement in children ages 2–16 years found no significant differences in visual outcome and complications (at 13 months' average follow-up) between capsular bag and sulcus-fixated IOLs.[13] It could be argued, however, that rather than implant in-the-bag PCIOLs in children, it is better to perform posterior capsulectomies and vitrectomies followed by ciliary implantation of sulcus–fixated IOLs. Determining the size of the capsular bag is often difficult for in-the-bag implantation in children, and opacification of the posterior capsule (PCO) often occurs rapidly in younger patients.[14] One review of 146 eyes found that 8.5 years after pediatric IOL implants, PCO had occurred in 81.5% of eyes.[15] Nd:YAG laser capsulotomies, which have their own set of complications, are limited to older, more cooperative patients. On the other hand, it can be argued that, PCIOL in-the-bag implantation is best for children because only capsular fixation will sequester the implant from vascularized tissues.[16] Of course, with secondary IOL implantation, it is often impossible to achieve fixation of the IOL to the posterior capsule because of the lack of inflammatory response. Longer-term follow-up should help establish the best type of secondary IOL implants for children.

■ Complications of Scleral-Sutured PCIOLs

There is a risk of unusual but serious complications with scleral-sutured IOLs, including retinal detachment, hemorrhagic choroidal detachment, persistent CME, and late lens dislocation.[17] Sundmacher and colleagues found a 12% rate of severe complications with scleral-sutured PCIOLs.[18] A retrospective review of 32 patients with scleral-fixated PCIOLs found postoperative complications in 11 patients; however, 30 patients maintained their visual acuity long term.[19]

Cystoid Macular Edema

Cystoid macular edema, with its associated decrease in visual acuity, is a frustrating but common complication after scleral-sutured PCIOL implantation. Some 9%–36% of patients with scleral-sutured lenses and penetrating keratoplasty may sustain this complication.[17,18]

Glaucoma

Glaucoma is another potential complication of scleral-sutured PCIOLs. Glaucoma after an implant occurs even more frequently when the implant operation is performed at the same time as penetrating keratoplasty. Holland and colleagues suspected that scleral-sutured lenses were associated with glaucoma. They found new-onset ocular hypertension in 30.3% of patients after a penetrating keratoplasty with a scleral-sutured PCIOL.[20]

Lens Decentration

Lens tilt or decentration is found in 5%–10% of patients after scleral-sutured PCIOL implantation.[18] Proper polypropylene suture placement and tension are important in avoiding this complication.

Retinal Detachment

There seems to be an increased risk of retinal detachment with sutured PCIOLs. Soong et al reported a 2.3% risk of retinal detachment after corneal transplant combined with iris sutured PCIOL implantation.[21] The location of the haptics posterior to the ciliary body adjacent to the pars plana, rather than in the ciliary sulcus, may increase the risk of retinal detachment.[22,23]

Uveitis

One must consider carefully the risks versus benefits of fixating an IOL in diabetics and in patients with a history of recurrent anterior uveitis.

Choroidal Detachment

Transscleral sutures are thought to increase the risk of choroidal detachment. Heidemann and Dunn found that 3.6% of scleral-sutured PCIOLs were associated with this complication, although these were nonexpulsive.[17]

■ Capsular Tension Rings

In 1991, Hara and colleagues developed an "equator ring" which could maintain the circular contour of the capsular bag after cataract extraction.[24] This ring, also known as capsular tension ring, has been used in patients with zonular dialysis to successfully maintain the circular contour of the capsular bag and prevent IOL decentration. Now, when a surgeon is presented with an eye with broken or loose zonules, there are more options than implanting a sutured PCIOL or an ACIOL.

Currently two types of capsular tension rings are available: the open PMMA rings, manufactured by Morcher and Ophtec (Groningen, Holland), and the closed silicone rings. Although the Ophtec ring is injected into the capsular bag with an inserter and the Morcher ring is implanted into the bag with a forceps, these rings are similar in design, and both come in two sizes (12.5 mm compressible to 10.0 mm and 14.5 mm compressible to 12.0 mm). The surgeon selects the ring size based on the size of the corneal white-to-white diameter.

Several clinical studies with small sample sizes have demonstrated the efficacy of the capsular tension ring. Gimbel et al presented 14 cataract surgery cases with loose or broken zonules that were managed with PMMA capsular tension rings.[25] At 2–11 months after surgery, no observable decentration of the IOL had occurred in any of these cases. The study concluded that the capsular tension ring may provide five potential benefits for cataract surgery patients with zonular dialysis: (1) the ring stabilizes the capsule and enhances safety and efficacy during phacoemulsification and PCIOL implantation, (2) it maintains the circular contour of the capsular bag, (3) it reduces IOL decentration by providing additional support to the bag and by decreasing the incidence of postoperative bag shrinkage, (4) it may help to avoid vitreous herniation, and (5) it may inhibit lens epithelial cell proliferation on the posterior capsule by compression, which could reduce the incidence of secondary cataract.[25] A similar study was performed by Cionni and Osher in four patients who had extensive traumatic zonular dialysis. Using PMMA capsular tension rings, phacoemulsification and PCIOL in-the-bag implantation was successfully performed. At 4–10 months after surgery, all four patients had well-centered IOLs that afforded excellent vision with no complications.[26]

A recent in vitro study utilizing pig and cadaver eye models supported previous clinical data. This study demonstrated that PCIOLs implanted alone were significantly decentered when the capsular bag zonular support was cut in one quadrant of the meridian. However, no IOL decentration was observed when the tension ring and the IOL were implanted together. When PCIOLs alone were implanted into isolated capsular bags, they became oval, whereas the circular shape of the bags was preserved when both the IOL and the tension ring were placed in the bag.[27]

Although no published studies have compared PMMA and silicone rings, studies in animals have shown that the silicone capsular tension ring maintains the circular contour of the capsular bag in rabbits.[28] If more studies provide similar results, both PMMA and silicone capsular tension rings may become more frequently used in the management of zonular dialysis in cataract surgery.

■ Conclusions

Secondary IOL implantations have been reported to account for 6% of all IOL implantations.[29] In the future, the frequency of secondary IOL implantations will likely decrease, as most IOL implantations will be done at the time of cataract removal. However, there will still be a need for secondary IOL implantations: in cases with severe complications during cataract surgery, in eyes requiring IOL exchange, in children who have had a congenital cataract removed before the age of 1 year, or after an ocular trauma when IOL implantation is postponed. With a good technique, such as one of the five surgical methods described in this chapter, ciliary sulcus fixation is a very good approach for secondary IOL implantation.

■ References

1. Kanski JJ, Packard RBS. *Cataract and Lens Implant Surgery: A Systematic Manual.* New York: Churchill Livingstone; 1985.
2. Duffey RJ, Holland EJ, Agapitos PJ, et al. Anatomic study of transsclerally sutured intraocular lens implantation. *Am J Ophthalmol.* 1989;108:300–309.
3. Teichmann KD. Pars plana fixation of posterior chamber intraocular lenses. *Ophthalmic Surg.* 1994;25:549–553.
4. Smiddy WE, Sawusch MR, O'Brien TP, et al. Implantation of scleral-fixated posterior chamber intraocular lenses. *J Cataract Refract Surg.* 1990;16:691–696.
5. Apple DJ, Price FW, Gwin T, et al. Sutured retropupillary posterior chamber intraocular lenses for exchange or secondary implantation: the 12th Annual Binkhorst Lecture, 1988. *Ophthalmology.* 1989;96:1241–1247.
6. Jürgens I, Lillo J, Buil JA, et al. Endoscope-assisted transscleral suture fixation of intraocular lenses. *J Cataract Refract Surg.* 1996;22:879–881.
7. Lewis JS. Ab externo sulcus fixation. *Ophthalmic Surg.* 1991;22:692–695.
8. Regillo CD, Tidwell J. A small-incision technique for suturing a posterior chamber intraocular lens. *Ophthalmic Surg Lasers.* 1996;27:473–475.
9. Eryildirim A. Knotless scleral fixation for implanting a posterior chamber intraocular lens. *Ophthalmic Surg.* 1995;26:82–84.
10. Mead MD, Sieck EA, Steinert RF. Optical rehabilitation of aphakia. In: Albert DM, Jakobiec FA, eds. *Principles and Practice of Ophthalmology: Clinical Practice.* Vol 1. Philadelphia: WB Saunders; 1994:641–656.
11. Foster A, Gilbert C, Rahi J. Epidemiology of cataract in childhood: a global perspective. *J Cataract Refract Surg.* 1997;23:601–604.
12. Biglan AW, Cheng KP, Davis JS, et al. Results following secondary intraocular lens implantation in children. *Trans Am Ophthalmol Soc.* 1996;94:353–379.
13. Zwaan J, Mullaney PB, Awad A, et al. Pediatric intraocular lens implantation: surgical results and complications in more than 300 patients. *Ophthalmology.* 1998;105:112–119.
14. Simons BD, Siatkowski RM, Schiffman JC, et al. Surgical technique, visual outcome, and complications of pediatric intraocular lens implantation. *J Pediatr Ophthalmol Strabismus.* 1999;36:118–124.
15. Malukiewicz-Wisniewska G, Kaluzny J, Lesiewska-Junk H, et al. Intraocular lens implantation in children and youth. *J Pediatr Ophthalmol Strabismus.* 1999;36:129–133.
16. Wilson ME. Intraocular lens implantation: has it become the standard of care for children? [editorial]. *Ophthalmology.* 1996;103:1719–1720.
17. Heidemann DG, Dunn SP. Transsclerally sutured intraocular lenses in penetrating keratoplasty. *Am J Ophthalmol.* 1992;113:619–625.
18. Sundmacher R, Althaus C, Wester R, et al. Two years' experience with transscleral fixation of posterior chamber lenses. *Dev Ophthalmol.* 1991;22:89–93.
19. McCluskey P, Harrisberg B. Long-term results using scleral-fixated posterior chamber intraocular lenses. *J Cataract Refract Surg.* 1994;20:34–39.
20. Holland EJ, Daya SM, Evangelista A, et al. Penetrating keratoplasty and transscleral fixation of posterior chamber lens. *Am J Ophthalmol.* 1992;114:182–187.
21. Soong HK, Musch DC, Kowal V, et al. Implantation of posterior chamber intraocular lenses in the absence of lens capsule during penetrating keratoplasty. *Arch Ophthalmol.* 1989;107:660–665.
22. Price FW Jr, Whitson WE, Collins K, et al. Explantation of posterior chamber lenses. *J Cataract Refract Surg.* 1992;18:475–479.

23. Lubniewski AJ, Holland EJ, Van Meter WS, et al: Histologic study of eyes with transsclerally sutured posterior chamber intraocular lenses. *Am J Ophthalmol.* 1990;110: 237–243.

24. Hara T, Hara T, Yamada Y. "Equator ring" for maintenance of the completely circular contour of the capsular bag equator after cataract removal. *Ophthalmic Surg.* 1991; 22:358–359.

25. Gimbel HV, Sun R, Heston JP. Management of zonular dialysis in phacoemulsification and IOL implantation using the capsular tension ring. *Ophthalmic Surg Lasers.* 1997;28:273–281.

26. Cionni RJ, Osher RH. Endocapsular ring approach to the subluxed cataractous lens. *J Cataract Refract Surg.* 1995; 21:245–249.

27. Sun R, Gimbel HV. In vitro evaluation of the efficacy of the capsular tension ring for managing zonular dialysis in cataract surgery. *Ophthalmic Surg Lasers.* 1998;29:502–505.

28. Hara T, Hara T, Sakanishi K, Yamada Y. Efficacy of equator rings in an experimental rabbit study. *Arch Ophthalmol.* 1995;113:1060–1065.

29. Kraff MC, Sanders DR, Lieberman HL, et al. Secondary intraocular lens implantation. *Ophthalmology.* 1983;90: 324–326.

Part IV

Intraocular Lens Complications

Chapter 15

Anterior Segment Complications of Intraocular Lens Surgery

Robert T. Ang and Dimitri T. Azar

Several complications involving the anterior segment may follow cataract extraction with anterior or posterior intraocular lens (IOL) implantation. These complications may arise from poor lens design, variable surgical techniques and predisposing ocular disorders. Recent improvements in IOL design and in surgical techniques, however, have reduced the incidence of these complications.

While it is difficult to determine the incidence of every complication, a good indicator is the relative incidence of anterior segment complications requiring IOL explantation or exchange.[1-7] In a study by Mamalis et al of 102 patients who underwent IOL explantation or exchange prior to 1991, 68 (66.7%) had anterior chamber IOLs (ACIOLs), 18 (17.6%) had iris-fixated lenses, and 16 (15.7%) had posterior chamber IOLs (PCIOLs).[1]

The most common style of ACIOL removed was the Leiske lens (35.3%), followed by the Dubroff lens. The most common indications were pseudophakic bullous keratopathy (PBK), uveitis-glaucoma-hyphema (UGH) syndrome, and IOL dislocation. The most commonly removed iris-fixated IOLs were the Binkhorst two-loop (38.9%), Platina (22.2%), Binkhorst four-loop (16.7%), and Medallion (16.7%) lenses. The most common indication was PBK. The most commonly removed PCIOL was the modified J-loop (68.6%). The most common indications for PCIOL removal were lens dislocation and PBK.

The average interval from implantation to IOL removal for iris-fixated lens was 72.5 months, for the ACIOL, 41.7 months, and for the PCIOL, 16.7 months.[1] PCIOLs were removed much earlier probably because of the great proportion of lenses removed for malpositioning, which occurs much sooner than problems secondary to chronic inflammation, PBK, UGH, and cystoid macular edema (CME).[1] This chapter discusses the etiology and pathogenesis of IOL malpositioning, anterior chamber inflammation, glaucoma, PBK, and capsular opacification.

■ IOL Malpositioning

IOL malpositioning may account for the majority of cases where the PCIOL is removed. The common types of malposition include IOL decentrations ("sunset syndrome," "sunrise syndrome," horizontal decentration, and "windshield-wiper syndrome") and pupillary capture.[2]

IOL Decentration

In two postmortem studies published between 1985 and 1986, the frequency of optic decentration was between 47% and 57%.[3,4] Decentration was associated with asymmetric haptic placement. In the classic study by Apple et al of 75 autopsy eyes, the most common combination of loop placements was one loop in the bag and one loop in the sulcus (occurring in 47% of eyes). In 32% both loops were in the bag, in 17% both loops were in the sulcus, and in 4% one or both loops were on the pars plana.[3] A study by Champion et al similarly showed 54% of PCIOLs having one loop in the bag and the other in the sulcus.[4]

Despite recent improvements in surgical techniques for cataract, asymmetric IOL placements persist.[1-6] Most commonly the inferior haptic is inserted into the capsular bag while the superior haptic is placed in the ciliary sulcus, predisposing a superior movement of the optic if inferior capsular contraction occurs. In addition, lack

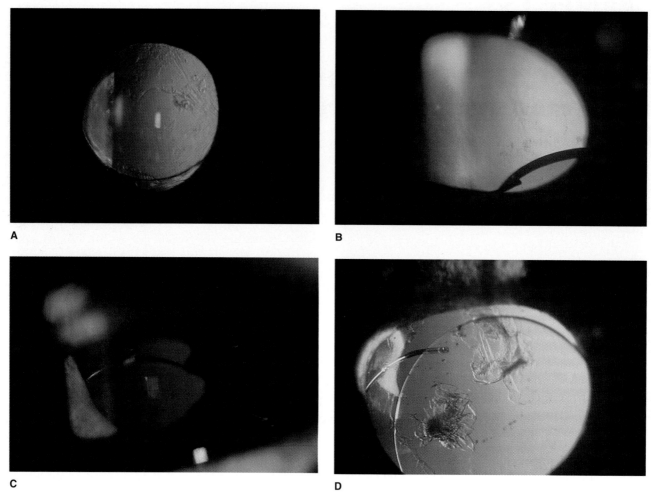

FIGURE 15.1. *A*, When the PCIOL is displaced upward, it is termed "sunrise syndrome." *B* and *C*, In the "sunset syndrome," the PCIOL is displaced downward and the optic is clearly visible. *D*, The "east-west syndrome" occurs when the PCIOL is decentered along the horizontal meridian. Cortical remnants are visible in this figure.

of superior zonular integrity allows the PCIOL to migrate, giving rise to the "sunrise syndrome" (Fig. 15.1A). Less frequently, the PCIOL may subluxate inferiorly, causing the "sunset syndrome" (Figs. 15.1B and C). Zonular dehiscence in the horizontal meridian can give rise to the "east-west syndrome," (Fig. 15.1D). Poorly sized IOLs may cause a pendular motion in the posterior chamber (pseudophakodonesis), creating the "windshield-wiper syndrome." With ACIOLs, iris tuck may occur when an ACIOL haptic entraps peripheral iris tissue as it is being slid over the iris into the anterior chamber angle (Figs. 15.2A and B).[5] Iris tuck is less likely to occur with PCIOLs. In a study by Hakin et al, 60% of 110 eyes had gonioscopic evidence of implant loops indenting the iris from behind, causing anterior iris tuck. Possible causes included sulcus-implanted haptics or haptic loops that were in the bag but excessively angulated anteriad.[6]

With the advent of ACIOL improvements allowing better fixation of ACIOLs in the anterior chamber angle, decentration became less common (unless the IOL was missized). With PCIOLs, Obstbaum reported that using one-piece polymethyl methacrylate (PMMA) IOLs with larger optics and angulated haptics reduced the incidence of decentration.[7] In terms of IOL material, Hayashi et al found no statistically significant differences in extent of decentration and tilt between PMMA, silicone, and acrylic lenses over a 12-month observation period.[8]

ACIOLs can rotate (Figs. 15.2C and D), and chafe the anterior iris, causing anterior chamber inflammation, or may erode their footplates into the angle, causing recurrent hyphema and uveitis, resulting in UGH. PBK may also result from contact with the corneal endothelium. Implantation of the PCIOL into the ciliary sulcus may cause pigmentary glaucoma, recurrent hy-

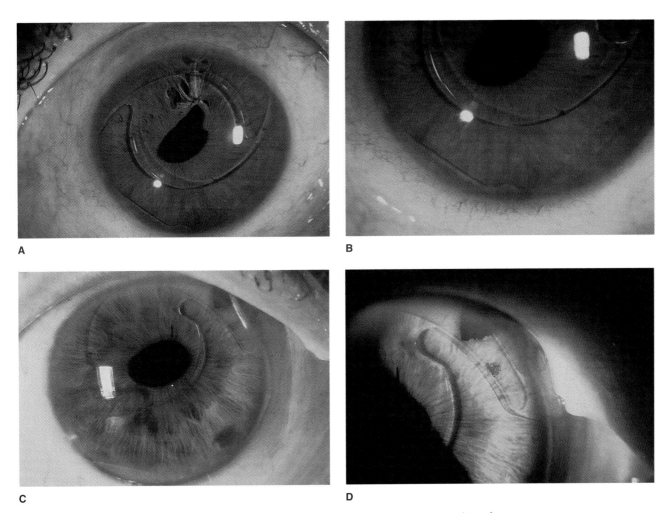

FIGURE 15.2. *A* and *B,* An ACIOL can trap peripheral iris tissue, causing iris tuck. *C* and *D,* If the ACIOL rotates, the haptic end can enter the peripheral iridectomy.

phema, and UGH syndrome.[2] The treatment of IOL decentration is discussed in Chapter 13, 14, and 18.

Pupillary Capture

Pupillary capture results from the entrapment of the entire optic or a portion of the optic in the pupillary aperture while the rest of the lens is positioned behind the iris (Fig. 15.3).[9–16] The reported incidence of pupillary capture is 1%–14%. It is reported to be lower with angled than with uniplanar-haptic rigid IOLs (1% versus 3%).[9,10] The incidence is 0%–1.5% when the IOL is placed in the bag, compared to 1.5%–14% when the IOL is placed in the sulcus.[9–12] Bartholomew recently reported a 3.9% incidence with rigid PCIOLs but no cases of capture with foldable lenses.[13] However, several cases of pupillary capture have been reported with silicone and acrylic IOLs.[14–16] Pupillary capture usually occurs 30–60 days after surgery, although it can occur as early as 5 days postoperatively.[17] Bartholomew, on the other hand, noted a mean time of 14 weeks between surgery and pupillary capture.[13] An increased incidence of pupillary capture was associated with several conditions. It developed significantly more often ($P < 0.001$) in eyes treated by combined glaucoma and cataract extraction surgery versus eyes treated by ECCE; in eyes treated by "can-opener" capsulotomy versus eyes treated by capsulorrhexis; in eyes with angle-closure glaucoma versus no glaucoma; in eyes treated by manual extraction versus phacoemulsification; with sulcus versus in-the-bag implantation; with large-optic (7.0 mm) versus, small-optic (5.0–6.0 mm) IOLs; and with a one-piece versus a two-piece IOL.[13]

The causes of pupillary capture are wound leakage, a shallow anterior chamber, pupil dilation, a sulcus fixation, capsule contraction, persistent iritis, and posterior synechiae.[1,2,9–17] Two cases of pupillary capture after in-the-bag fixation of a three-piece silicone

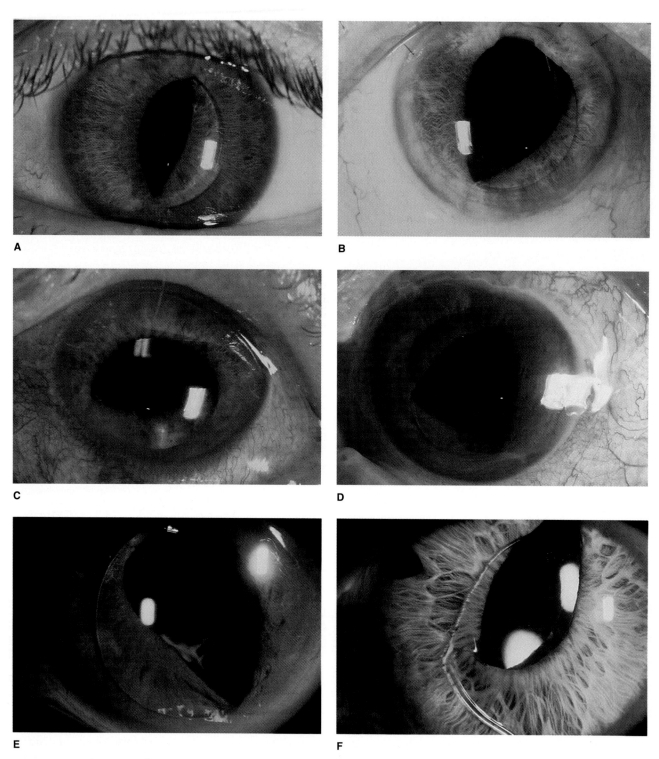

FIGURE 15.3. *A* to *F,* Pupillary capture occurs when part or all of the IOL is entrapped by the pupillary aperture. The "cat's-eye" pupil is typical of pupillary capture *(A).*

IOL through a continuous curvilinear capsulorrhexis (CCC) have been reported. Marcus et al noted that wound leakage and choroidal detachment seemed to have induced the pupillary capture, which was fol-

lowed by pupillary block.[14] Bucci and Lindstrom attributed the cause of their case of pupillary capture to incomplete anterior rotation of the flexible haptics.[15] Nagamoto et al reported pupillary capture of an

AcrySof (soft polyacrylic) lens implanted through a round 6-mm CCC, and suggested two possible mechanisms for pupillary capture.[16] The first possibility was that contraction of the capsular bag forced the optic anteriorly, causing pupillary capture, iridocapsular synechiae, and subsequent pupillary block. The second possibility was that the iridocapsular synechiae caused the pupillary capture. An IOL with a larger overall length and harder haptics, such as the AcrySof lens, can transmit the mechanical force of the capsular contraction more efficiently than smaller IOLs with more flexible haptics. This can lead to anterior vaulting, dislocation of the IOL, and pupillary capture.[16]

Partial pupillary capture produces elongation of the pupil, causing the "cat's-eye" pupil. This is often more than just a cosmetic problem, since contact between the edge of the IOL optic and the iris can result in chronic uveitis and IOL deposits, posterior capsule thickening and opacification, lens tilt, CME, and pupillary block glaucoma.[13] Pupillary capture has become rare because of capsular bag implantation and the popular use of haptics angled 10–15 degrees anteriorly, which maintains the optic farther from the iris plane and pupil. Nonsurgical methods of reversing the capture may be attempted by dilation Trendelenburg positioning, and reconstriction of the pupil. External pressure over the haptics may be helpful before the development of synechiae. Iritis should be treated. The neodymium:yttrium-aluminum-garnet (Nd:YAG) laser is used to create an iridectomy if relative pupillary block is suspected. The surgical technique of IOL tapping is described in Chapter 18.

■ Anterior Chamber Inflammation

Anterior chamber inflammation results from breakdown of the blood–aqueous barrier. Its manifestations include: a cellular response on the anterior surface of the IOL (Fig 15.4), and on the posterior capsule. The incidence of persistent iritis in patients who have undergone extracapsular cataract extraction (ECCE) and PCIOL implantation ranges between 0.3% and 3.3%.[18] (See Chapter 9.)

Poorly positioned anterior chamber and iris-supported IOLs can cause chronic iris chafing, leading to breakdown of the blood–aqueous barrier. Using gonioscopy, Numa et al observed that the haptics of ACIOLs placed either on the peripheral iris or between the scleral spur and the iris root, in contact with the ciliary band, led to chronic irritation that caused subclinical inflammation and disruption of the blood–aqueous barrier.[19] One such example is the Dubroff-style (Intermedics Pharmacia, Monrovia, CA) ACIOL, a flexible,

open, thin-loop lens, which was found to erode into the peripheral angle.[20] Iris-fixated or iris-supported IOLs can cause similar inflammation because of anterior chafing from pseudophakodonesis.[21] The iris erosions caused by PCIOLs are usually radial and midperipheral, and appear about 1 year after implantation (Fig. 15.5A). In a study of pseudophakic iris chafing, Mastropasqua et al found that 184 (20%) of 920 eyes developed this condition.[22] Friction between the posterior iris surface and the loops located in the ciliary sulcus causes the release of pigment into the anterior chamber. This can lead to pigment dispersion syndrome or pigmentary glaucoma. Amino and Yamakawa reinforced Mastropasqua's findings and reported that anterior chamber flare measurements, even more than 2 years after surgery, were higher in eyes with sulcus-to-sulcus IOL fixation than in eyes with in-the-bag fixation.[23] These findings are consistent with the concept that the main reason for anterior chamber inflammation after cataract surgery is contact between the IOL optic and the iris.

Two different methods have been reported for the evaluation of anterior chamber inflammation associated with IOL materials.[24–27] One method uses the inflammatory cytologic response, which consists of a small-cell response initially and a giant-cell response later. Shah and Spalton postulated that giant cells are probably formed by the fusion of small cells on the IOL surface or by migration of macrophages from adjacent uveal tissue.[24] Hollick et al found a statistically significant association between IOL material and small- and giant-cell grades.[25] Silicone IOLs had significantly more small cells than PMMA or acrylic lenses. AcrySof lenses had no giant cells. Silicone IOLs appeared to have giant cells on their surface for a longer time than PMMA lenses. However, the investigators concluded that all three types of foldable IOLs produced a mild degree of nonspecific foreign body response that resolved over the study period without significant sequelae. (See Chapter 9).

The other methods used by Miyake et al involved laser flare and cell measurements to assess inflammation. Three months after IOL implantation, laser flare and cell findings were significantly higher for PMMA IOLs than for heparin-surface-modified (HSM) IOLs ($P < 0.01$), and silicone IOLs had significantly higher findings than acrylic and memory lenses ($P < 0.01$), but laser flare and cell findings did not differ significantly between acrylic and memory lenses.[26] This study confirmed that HSM IOLs resulted in less severe postoperative inflammation. Miyake et al also observed that the memory lens, composed of hydrogel and PMMA, was the most biocompatible among the foldable lenses, followed by acrylic and silicone lenses.[26]

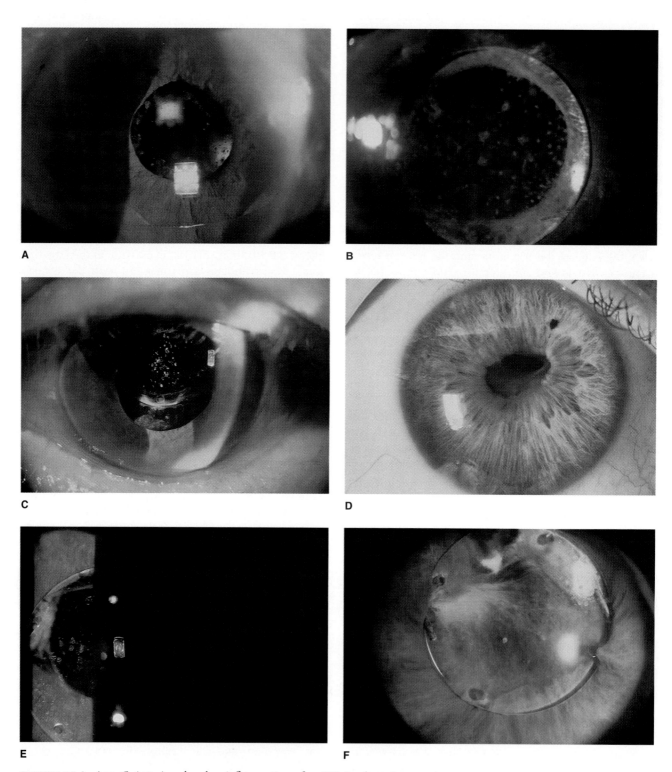

FIGURE 15.4. *A* to *C*, Anterior chamber inflammation after IOL implantation can be seen as pigment deposits on the IOLs *(A,B)*, which may be difficult to differentiate from YAG laser burns *(C)*. *D*, Synechia formation can occur between the iris and IOL and lead to lens pupillary capture *(E)*, or fibrous membrane *(F)*.

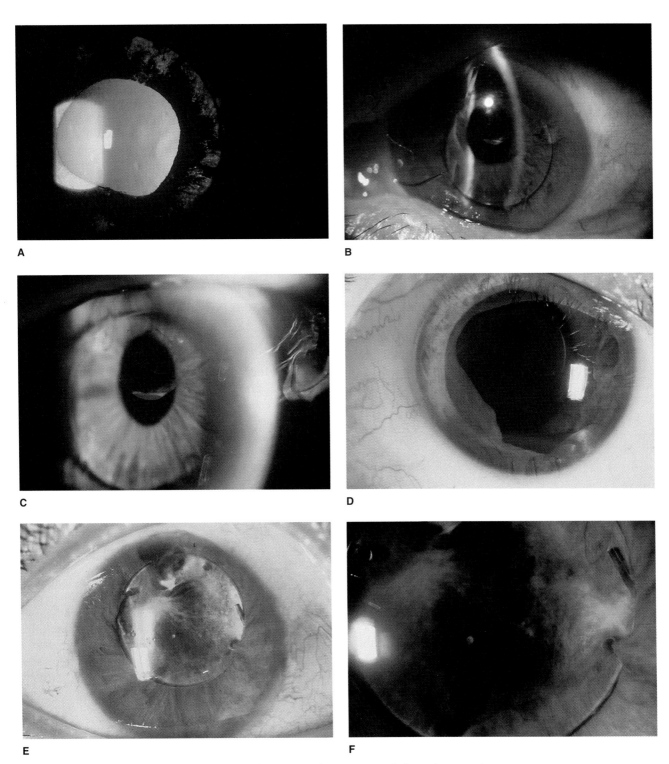

FIGURE 15.5. *A,* Transillumination defects and pigment release can result from the posterior iris rubbing against the IOL implanted in the sulcus. *B* to *D,* Blood in the anterior chamber can be due to mechanical trauma causing injury to the iris and angle structures. *E,* Complete occlusion by a pupillary membrane can cause pupillary block glaucoma. *F,* Higher magnification shows residual iridocapsular adhesions after optic capture.

A different conclusion was reached by Schauerberger et al, who found no significant differences in the course of postoperative inflammation between the Pharmacia 920 silicone lens, the Alcon AcrySof, the Bausch and Lomb Hydroview, and the MemoryLens.[27] They concluded that because of the high biocompatibility of current foldable IOLs, the differences may have been only subclinical.

Anterior chamber inflammation may also be related to the haptic material. Polypropylene undergoes superficial surface alteration after long-term contact with uveal tissue, as revealed by electron microscopy.[28,29] Drews has demonstrated that cracking and flaking may occur.[29] Contact with the posterior iris can lead to liberation of iris pigment and alteration of the blood–aqueous barrier. Injury to and microlacerations of blood vessels in the iris may occur (Figs. 15.5B to D). Microhyphema has been noted in 5% and 3% of anterior chamber and iris-fixated lenses, respectively, after cataract extraction.[30] One of the sequelae of hyphema is red blood cells clogging the trabecular meshwork, resulting in the UGH syndrome.

Occasionally, postoperative IOL-related sterile hypopyon occurs a few days after surgery, mimicking microbial endophthalmitis.[31] This entity, also called toxic lens syndrome, is a sterile intraocular inflammation presumably secondary to residual polishing compounds on the lens surface, to defective IOL haptics or optics, and to excessive anterior segment manipulation.[31]

■ Glaucoma

Uveitis-Glaucoma-Hyphema Syndrome

The triad of uveitis, glaucoma, and hyphema was first described by Ellingson in 1977.[32–34] It can occur with any type of IOL but is mainly ascribed to poorly manufactured ACIOLs, although it can also follow PCIOL implantations. UGH, or Ellingson's syndrome, is a rare complication of IOL implantation that results from mechanical trauma inflicted on the angle or iris by the haptics or optic of an IOL.[32] In 1980, Worthen et al reported the incidence of secondary glaucoma resulting from uveitis after lens implantation to be 6.3% with an ACIOL, 3.9% with an iris-fixated lens, and 3.5% with a PCIOL.[30] The incidence has since sharply declined as a result of refinements in IOL design, better manufacturing techniques, better quality control, and improved surgical techniques. The latest incidence reported by Berger et al in 1995 was a low 0.259%.[32]

The presumed mechanism of UGH is mechanical irritation of the iris from unpolished, roughened haptics. The condition was initially described with ACIOLs such as the Choyce Mark VII ACIOL, but it was later reported also for flexible ACIOLs and PCIOLs.[34] With PCIOLs, sulcus fixation of one or both haptics causes similar trauma to the posterior iris and surrounding tissues and vessels. The unstable sulcus fixation was confirmed by rocking of the IOL and extrusion of the haptic, leading to hyphema.[33] The development of glaucoma can be caused by two mechanisms: a pigmentary dispersion syndrome (Fig. 15.5A), resulting in dense pigment deposition in the trabecular meshwork, and a secondary hemolytic glaucoma (Figs. 15.5B to D), in which macrophages containing red blood cell debris accumulate in the trabecular meshwork and obstruct the aqueous outflow.[34] (See Chapter 8.)

For mild cases of UGH, treatment with topical steroids, systemic carbonic anhydrase inhibitors, and laser trabeculoplasty is advised. If vision is decreased or if there is excessive uveal touch, persistent uveitis, or retinal injury, rotation of the IOL to reposition the loops in a symmetric in-the-bag position can be done, or the IOL can be explanted.[34]

Pupillary Block Glaucoma

Pupillary block occurs when the IOL blocks the flow of aqueous through the pupil. It was initially reported to be more common with anterior chamber and iris-fixated lenses,[35–37] but it has been reported with PCIOLs as well.[38–40] In pupillary block secondary to ACIOLs and iris-fixated lens, the optic of the lens can act as a flap valve to occlude the pupil.[35] With PCIOLs, disruption of the zonules during lens nucleus delivery or irrigation and aspiration can result in forward movement of the vitreous and consequently of the IOL.[39,40] Pseudophakic pupillary block can also occur after the formation of adhesions between the pupillary margin after excessive postoperative inflammation[40] (Figs. 15.5E and F). The risk of this complication is higher in diabetic patients, probably because of abnormal permeability of the blood–aqueous barrier.[41] Contraction of the capsular bag can force the optic anteriorly, causing sequentially pupillary capture, iridocapsular synechiae, and pupillary block.[16]

Pseudophakic pupillary block is not a benign event, as it may lead to synechiae formation and angle-closure glaucoma (Figs. 15.5E and F). While Samples et al advocate routine peripheral iridectomy,[38] we believe this is not indicated, insofar as the prevalence is quite low with newer IOL designs and modern surgical techniques (see Chapter 8).

Malignant Glaucoma

Malignant glaucoma is a process in which anterior aqueous flow is obstructed and aqueous is misdirected posteriorly. Duy and Wollensak reported two cases of pseudophakic malignant glaucoma and theorized that surgical trauma caused the vitreous base to separate from the pars plana, permitting aqueous to flow into the vitreous, displacing the IOL and iris forward.[42] Reed et al reported a similar case and attributed the initiating factor to be direct apposition of the ciliary processes to the optic of the IOL in a small eye.[43] They hypothesized that a 7-mm optic crowds the anterior segment of small eyes. The periphery of the IOL lying adjacent to the ciliary processes creates a relative block of aqueous flow to the anterior chamber, forcing it to be misdirected into the vitreous cavity. The expanded volume of the vitreous cavity causes a forward movement of the hyaloid, ciliary processes, posterior capsule, IOL, and iris (see Chapter 8). Reed et al suggest that a cardinal feature predisposing an eye to iatrogenic malignant glaucoma is a short axial length, which includes nanophthalmic eyes.[43]

■ Pseudophakic Bullous Keratopathy

The initial experience and subsequent reports regarding intracapsular cataract extraction (ICCE), ECCE, ACIOLs, and iris-fixated IOLs have documented progressive endothelial cell loss.[44–56] Taylor and colleagues reported that less than 1% of patients with ECCE and PCIOL developed clinically significant PBK.[46] In a review of 1,100 corneal transplants, DeLuise found that 0.8% of all penetrating keratoplasties for PBK were associated with PCIOLs.[47]

The corneal endothelium consists of a monolayer of nonregenerative cells responsible for maintaining corneal clarity. Ohara et al showed that endothelial cell density decreases from 3,410 to 2,777 per mm^2 from the second to the ninth decade of life.[50] From that, it was surmised that the loss in endothelial cell density with aging ranges from 8.36 to 17.4 cells/mm^2 per year. In comparison, the cell loss with ACIOLs was 112 cells/mm^2 per year, while with PCIOLs it was 31.6 cells/mm^2 per year. If the endothelial cell density decrease of 112 cells/mm^2 per year continues at a steady rate, all patients would develop PBK within 20 years.[19]

It has been suggested that quantitative measurements of cellular structure (polymegathism and pleomorphism) are more sensitive indications of endothelial damage and function than changes in cell density. Matsuda et al found marked polymegathism and pleomorphism in the endothelium of ACIOL-implanted eyes postoperatively, suggesting that ACIOLs may retard the endothelial remodeling that normally occurs in eyes that received PCIOLs with intracapsular fixation. They postulated that polymegathism and pleomor-

phism were indicative of low functional reserve of the monolayer and may be an early sign of continuing cell loss.[52]

Endothelial cell loss related to IOL may be caused by direct mechanical trauma (intermittent touch syndrome) due to excessive vaulting of an ACIOL, lens mobility (pseudophakodonesis) of an undersized or poorly fixated IOL (tilting, rocking, or rotating), or IOL malposition (Figs. 15.6A to D).[2] Even peripheral corneal-IOL contact has the potential to cause central endothelial dysfunction by stimulating cell migration from the central cornea to the periphery (Figs. 15.6E and F).[53] IOLs with designs (e.g., semiflexible closed-loop design) associated with corneal decompensation include the Leiske Style 10 (Surgical Corp, Goleta, CA), the Optical Radiation Corporation model 11 Stableflex (Azusa, CA), the Intermedics Hessberg model 024 (Intraocular Inc, Pasadena, CA), and the Pannu ACIOL (Allergan Medical Optics, Irvine, CA).[2]

Erosion of an IOL into uveal tissue may also lead to damage of the corneal endothelium.[2] Inflammation is often the mechanism for late corneal decompensation associated with closed-loop ACIOL designs that erode into the peripheral iris, anterior chamber angle, and ciliary body.[2] Because the inflammation is often very mild, careful examination is required to reveal subtle anterior chamber reaction and fine inflammatory precipitates on the IOL surface.[2,55] (See Chapters 13 and 18).

It is believed that at least 600 cells/mm^2 are needed to provide adequate corneal deturgescence.[47] Coli et al reported findings in a series of 102 eyes with anterior chamber or iris-plane IOLs and signs of progressive endothelial damage and concluded that corneal decompensation may be prevented if the IOLs are removed before a critical degree of endothelial cell loss or dysfunction occurs.[56] However, most observers believe that once PBK has occurred over a wide area, even removal may not prevent the occurrence of total corneal decompensation. The definitive treatment for PBK is penetrating keratoplasty (see Chapter 10).

■ Anterior Capsular Opacification

Anterior capsular opacification (ACO) is also called anterior capsule fibrosis or anterior subcapsular opacification (Fig. 15.7). Compared with posterior capsular opacification (PCO), ACO usually occurs much earlier, sometimes as early as 1 month after cataract surgery.[57] Hara et al found that postoperative ACO is composed of fibroblast-like cells, presumably transformed from lens epithelial cells and collagen. They based this assumption on a previous study by Font and Brownstein, which found that LECs can metamorphose into fibroblast-like

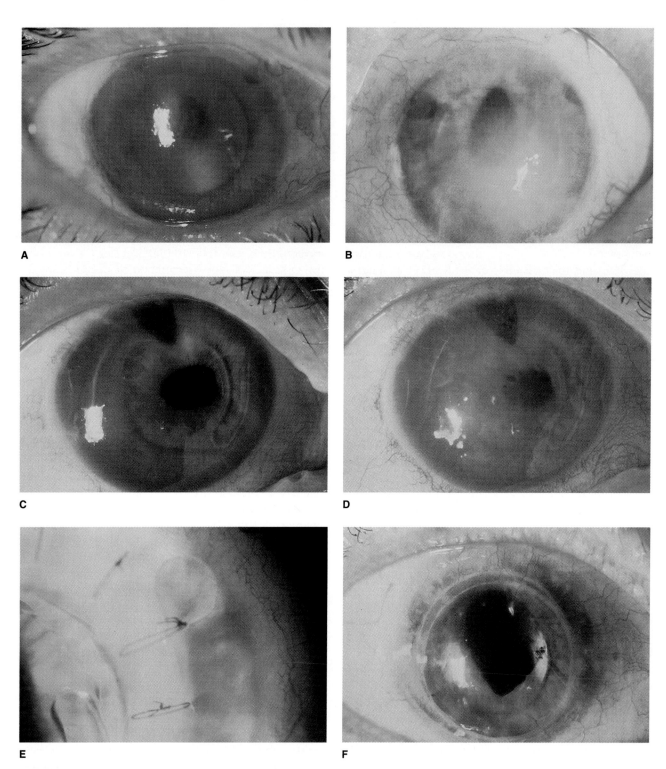

FIGURE 15.6. *A* to *D*, Constant or intermittent touch of an ACIOL on the cornea can progressively lead to pseudophakic bullous keratopathy. *E* and *F*, The haptic end can touch the peripheral corneal endothelium and lead to graft failure.

cells and produce type 4 collagen.[58] Ishibashi et al reinforced these findings by doing an ultrastructural analysis which showed that the cellular components of ACO had characteristics of LECs; the extracellular matrix con-

sisted of collagen fibrils, basal-lamina-like material, and microfibrils.[59]

The formation of ACO can be affected by innate characteristics of the IOL, such as lens material and lens

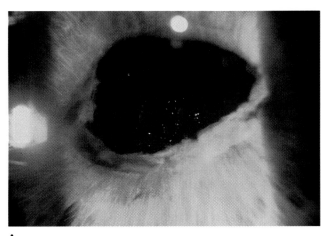
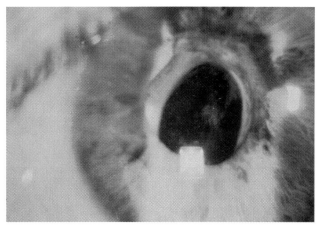

A   B

FIGURE 15.7. *A* and *B,* The rim of the anterior capsule is clearly visible due to opacification.

design. With regard to lens material, Miyake et al found that the biocompatibility of a lens surface is related to its hydrophilicity, that is, its contact angle of water and oil.[60] The more hydrophilic lenses had less postoperative inflammation and slower ACO formation. Among the rigid IOLs that were tested, HSM IOLs had significantly less inflammation and slower ACO formation than PMMA IOLs after 3 months postoperatively. Among the foldable IOLs, the memory lenses (hydrogel and PMMA) had significantly less inflammation and opacification, followed by the acrylic lenses; the silicone lenses had significantly more inflammation and greater opacification after 3 months postoperatively.[60] With regard to lens design, Werner et al demonstrated that among four silicone IOL groups examined, the group with plate-haptic silicone design had a significantly higher rate of ACO than the three-piece (loop-haptic) designs. This difference is probably due to the relatively larger area of contact of the plate-haptic silicone material with the anterior capsule, exposing a larger surface area for stimulating cell proliferation and fibrosis.[61]

Although the formation of ACO may be clinically noticeable, ACO usually has very little deleterious effect on vision. Among its sequelae are fibrous contraction of the capsule causing IOL decentration, capsular phimosis, and obstruction causing difficulty in examining the retinal periphery. Only if the visual axis is obstructed will active intervention be needed.[61]

■ Posterior Capsular Opacification

Posterior capsular opacification (PCO) is the most common complication of cataract surgery and IOL implantation. Clinical findings include fibrous membrane and Elschnig pearl formation. Clinically, the Elschnig pearls

develop several months to several years after surgery and are caused by LEC migration at the equatorial zone. In contrast, fibrous opacity develops 2–6 months postoperatively and is caused by fibrous metaplasia of LECs beneath the anterior capsule. Elschnig-type PCO was found to be more common in PMMA IOL-implanted eyes and the fibrous type was found to be more common in silicone IOL-implanted eyes (Figs. 15.8A and B).[62]

The reported incidence of PCO ranges from 10% to 50% on follow-up ranging from 6 to 80 months postoperatively.[63] The incidence range is wide because different authors have used different definitions of PCO. Sundelin and Sjostrand defined clinically significant PCO as (1) a reduction in visual acuity by two lines compared with best corrected visual acuity early in the postoperative period; (2) PCO seen against red reflex by ophthalmoscopy; (3) PCO visible within the central area of the pupil seen on slit-lamp examination; and (4) patient reports of glare, reduced vision, or both. If the patient had another vision-reducing eye disease, all criteria had to be fulfilled except the first one. With this definition, Sundelin and Sjostrand found an incidence of 43% sight-limiting PCO at a mean follow-up of 60 months.[64] The 5-year PCO incidence in their study is comparable to that in other long-term follow-up studies with a high incidence. It shows that PCO is a major complication of ECCE, and that almost half of patients will need to undergo postoperative neodymium:yttrium-aluminium-garnet (Nd:YAG) laser capsulotomy before the end of the fourth postoperative year.

However, a standardized method for assessing, measuring, and monitoring PCO is still needed. Different authors have used a variety of methods for quantifying PCO. Hayashi et al analyzed images obtained using Scheimpflug videophotography.[65] Clark et al used a semiquantitative and subjective system to assess PCO,[66]

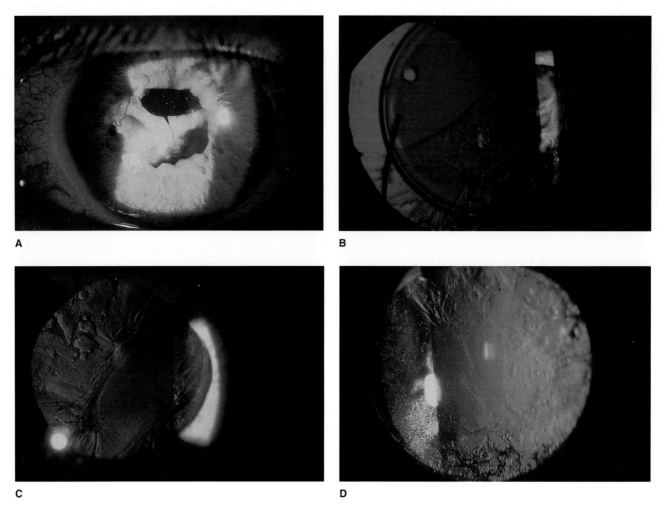

FIGURE 15.8. *A* to *D,* Migration of lens epithelial cells onto the center of the posterior capsule leads to posterior capsule opacity.

while Tan et al used both glare testing and contrast sensitivity.[67,68] In the absence of universal, standardized methods and equipment for assessing PCO, between-study comparisons of incidences and surgical indications will be difficult.

PCO results from the proliferation and migration of LECs onto the central region of the posterior capsule. Several studies comparing the incidence of PCO among various PCIOLs have provided evidence that IOL material and IOL design affect the development of PCO.

Using bovine collagen sheets and rabbit lens capsules, Oshika et al demonstrated that the adhesive force to the lens capsule differs significantly among lens materials. The collagen sheet adhered most strongly to the acrylic IOL, followed by the PMMA IOL, while the silicone IOL showed no adhesion.[69] A more adhesive material such as foldable acrylic may retard the source of PCO from extending to the visual axis on the posterior capsule, possibly by acting as a mechani-

cal barrier or by minimizing capsule wrinkling and limiting the space between the IOL and capsule. Histologic observation suggested that PMMA and acrylic foldable IOLs inhibited LECs and lens fibers at the optic edge from proliferating and migrating toward the center of the posterior capsule. This inhibitory effect was more prominent with acrylic foldable IOLs, with fewer LECs found on both the posterior capsule and the posterior surface of the IOL. In eyes with silicone IOLs, abundant proliferated tissue, including LECs, was seen on the posterior capsule, while almost no LECs were found on the posterior surface of the silicone IOL.[69] Versura et al reinforced Oshika's findings and tested the adhesion of human LECs to PMMA, HSM PMMA, hydrogel, and silicone IOLs. They observed that adhesion was greatest with PMMA IOLs and least with silicone IOLs. HSM PMMA and hydrogel IOLs exhibited intermediate properties.[70]

Of the PMMA, silicone, and acrylate lenses, it is thought that PCO is greatest in patients implanted with

Table 15.1
Incidence of PCO with Different IOL Materials

Material	PCO Incidence (%) at Measurement Interval	
	90 Days	**2 Years**
PMMA	96	100
Silicone	93	100
Polyacrylic	46	62

Data from Hollick EJ, Spalton DJ, Ursell PG, Pande MV. Lens epithelial cell regression on the posterior capsule with different intraocular lens materials. *Br J Ophthalmol.* 1998;82: 1182–1188.

the PMMA lens and least with the acrylate lenses. At 3-year follow-up, the average percentage PCO for implanted PMMA lenses was 56%, for silicone lenses it was 40%, and for polyacrylic lenses it was 10%.[71] The higher refractive index of polyacrylic (1.55) compared with silicone (1.41–1.46) and PMMA (1.49) allows polyacrylic IOLs to have much thinner optics, suggesting that bulk cannot explain the reduced LEC migration.[71]

Polyacrylic IOLs have a more defined and squarer optic edge than the other two implants. A study by Nagata and Watanabe found a significant decrease in PCO with sharp optic edges.[72] It has been proposed that the sharp edge acts as a mechanical barrier to LEC migration onto the posterior capsule (the barrier effect). This could explain the decreased number of cells on the posterior capsule with polyacrylic lenses but does not explain the phenomenon of LEC regression.[71–75] Nishi and Nishi showed that a PMMA IOL with sharp rectangular edges created a similarly sharp bend and complex frill in the posterior capsule at which LEC migration was inhibited. This effect was equivalent to that of the polyacrylic IOL of similar design. This study suggests that the preventive effect of the polyacrylic IOL on PCO may be design dependent.[73] Posterior convexity of the IOL optic is also thought to reduce LEC migration by mechanically producing apposition of the posterior lens surface to the capsule: the "no space, no cells" theory. Peng et al suggested three possible reasons why increased adhesion between the IOL and the capsule could lead to less PCO:[74] (1) There is less space for cells to grow into ("no space, no cells"). (2) Tight adhesion may sequester the IOL and LECs away from growth factors and nutrients in the aqueous or vitreous, such as transforming growth factor-β (TGF-β), which promotes LEC proliferation. (3) As the capsule and IOL become adherent, physical compression may "squeeze out" cells, causing atrophy of LECs already in the capsular space.[71] But the best barrier effect by far appeared to be created by the squared-off, truncated, relatively thick optic edge, which confined the cells peripheral to the optic within the region of Soemmering's ring. The squared-edge optic seems to provide the maximum impediment to growth and migration of cells behind the IOL optic.[74]

Hollick et al demonstated in vivo that LECs can progress, regress, or remain stable under the IOL over a 2-year period.[75] They attributed these occurrences to the type of IOL used (Tables 15.1 and 15.2). At 90 days postoperatively LECs were present in the posterior capsule in 96% of patients in the PMMA group, 93% in the silicone group, and 46% in the polyacrylic group. At 2 years postoperatively all patients with PMMA and silicone IOLs had LECs on the posterior capsule, while only 62% in the acrylic group did so. These rates are higher than those reported in other series. Of the eyes with LECs at day 90, in the PMMA group, 81% showed progression between day 90 and 2 years, 4% remained stable, and 15% showed regression. In the silicone group, 84% progressed, 8% stayed stable, and 8% regressed. In the acrylic group, none showed LEC progression, 17% remained stable, and 83% demonstrated marked LEC regression. The increased incidence in

Table 15.2
Fate of PCO from Day 90 to 2 Years, by Lens Material

Material	Progressed (%)	Remained Stable (%)	Regressed (%)
PMMA	81	4	15
Silicone	84	8	8
Polyacrylic	0	17	83

Data from Hollick EJ, Spalton DJ, Ursell PG, Pande MV. Lens epithelial cell regression on the posterior capsule with different intraocular lens materials. *Br J Ophthalmol.* 1998;82:1182–1188.

PCO at 2 years in the polyacrylic group resulted not from LEC progression but from delayed LEC migration onto the posterior capsule in 16% of patients who had no LECs at 90 days. This study showed that a statistically significant relation exists between lens type and whether LECs in the posterior capsule progress, regress, or remain stable, with more progression seen with PMMA and silicone lens and more regression seen with polyacrylic lenses. The explanation for regression is probably the tight adhesive relation between the polyacrylic IOL and the capsular bag, exerting compression on the LECs that are present and causing them to regress and atrophy. Alternatively, tight adhesion might restrict access to nutrients and growth factors by the migrant LECs, leading to regression. This study suggested that the adhesion takes some weeks to establish, during which time some LECs may already have migrated.[75]

PCO may be successfully treated by Nd:YAG laser capsulotomy (see Chapter 18). Patients with PMMA lenses had the greatest need for Nd:YAG surgery and patients with acrylate lenses had the least need.[63] Kim et al found that silicone lenses induce PCO and the need for Nd:YAG laser treatment about twice as fast as do PMMA lenses.[62] The mean interval from cataract surgery to Nd:YAG laser capsulotomy in their study was 31.82 months for patients with PMMA lenses and 15.03 months for patients with silicone lenses.[62] Nd:YAG capsulotomy, however, has the disadvantages of inconvenience and cost to the patient and several medical complications, such as damage to the IOL, intraocular pressure elevation, CME, retinal detachment, IOL subluxation, and localized endophthalmitis exacerbation.

Given the high incidence of PCO, surgeons have tried to develop ways to inhibit its development. A popular surgical technique to eliminate LECs at the time of surgery is to polish the lens capsule with a blunt rough cannula. Nishi designed a capsule-bending ring made of PMMA that had a sharp edge to create a sharp, discontinuous capsule bend in the fornix.[76] The idea was to induce contact inhibition of the migrating LECs after cataract surgery. Another attempt to enhance the barrier effect was Hoffer's design of a 360-degree ridge.[74] Clark et al demonstrated the effectiveness of a new immunotoxin (IMT) to inhibit PCO following cataract surgery.[66] The IMT is specific to human LECs and has been shown to be cytotoxic to these cells in vitro.

■ References

1. Mamalis N, Crandall AS, Pulsipher MW, et al. Intraocular lens explantation and exchange. *J Cataract Refract Surg.* 1991;17:811–818.

2. Carlson AN, Stewart WC, Tso PC. Intraocular lens complications requiring removal or exchange. *Surv Ophthalmol.* 1998;42:417–440.

3. Apple DJ, Park SB, Merkley KH, et al. Posterior chamber intraocular lenses in a series of 75 autopsy eyes. Part 1. Loop location. *J Cataract Refract Surg.* 1986;12:358–362.

4. Champion R, McDonnell PJ, Green WR. Intraocular lenses: histopathologic characteristics of a large series of autopsy eyes. *Surv Ophthalmol.* 1985;30:1–32.

5. Apple DJ, Mamalis N, Loftfield K, et al. Complications of intraocular lenses: a historical and histopathological review. *Surv Ophthalmol.* 1984;29:1–54.

6. Hakin K, Batterbury M, Hawksworth N, et al. Anterior tucking of the iris caused by posterior chamber lenses with polypropylene loops. *J Cataract Refract Surg.* 1989; 15:640–643.

7. Obstbaum SA. Posterior chamber intraocular lens dislocations and malpositions. *Aust NZ J Ophthalmol.* 1989;17: 265–270.

8. Hayashi K, Harada M, Hayashi H. Decentration and tilt of polymethyl methacrylate, silicone, and acrylic soft intraocular lenses. *Ophthalmology.* 1997;104:793–798.

9. Lindstrom RL, Herman WK. Pupil capture: prevention and management. *Am Intraocular Implant Soc J.* 1983; 9:201–204.

10. Kratz RP, Mazzocco TR, Davidson B, Colvard DM. The Shearing intraocular lens: a report of 1,000 cases. *Am Intraocular Implant Soc J.* 1981;7:55–57.

11. Brazitikos PD, Roth A. Iris modifications following extracapsular cataract extraction with posterior chamber lens implantation. *J Cataract Refract Surg.* 1991;17:269–280.

12. Pallin SL, Walman GB. Posterior chamber intraocular lens implant centration: in or out of "the bag." *Am Intraocular Implant Soc J.* 1982;8:254–257.

13. Bartholomew RS. Incidence, causes, and neodymium: YAG laser treatment of pupillary capture. *J Cataract Refract Surg.* 1997;23:1404–1408.

14. Marcus DM, Azar DT, Boerner C, Hunter DG. Pupillary capture of a flexible silicone posterior chamber intraocular lens [letter]. *Arch Ophthalmol.* 1992;110:609.

15. Bucci FA, Lindstrom RL. Total pupillary capture with a foldable silicone intraocular lens. *Ophthalmic Surg.* 1991; 22:414–415.

16. Nagamoto S, Kohzuka T, Nagamoto T. Pupillary block after pupillary capture of an AcrySof intraocular lens. *J Cataract Refract Surg.* 1998; 24:1271–1274.

17. Lavin M, Jagger J. Pathogenesis of pupillary capture after posterior chamber intraocular lens implantation. *Br J Ophthalmol.* 1986;70:886–889.

18. Stark WJ, Leske MC, Worth DM, et al. Trends in cataract surgery and intraocular lenses in the United States. *Am J Ophthalmol.* 1983;96:304–310.

19. Numa A, Nakamura J, Takashima M, Kani K. Long-term corneal endothelial changes after intraocular lens implantation: anterior vs posterior chamber lenses. *Jpn J Ophthalmol.* 1993;37:78–87.

20. Lee DA, Price FW Jr, Whitson WE. Intraocular complications associated with the Dubroff anterior chamber lens. *J Cataract Refract Surg.* 1994;20:421–425.

21. Bahn CF, Sugar A. Endothelial physiology and intraocular lens implantation. *Am Intraocul Implant Soc J*. 1981;7:351–363.

22. Mastropasqua L, Lobefalo L, Gallenga PE. Iris chafing in pseudophakia. *Doc Ophthalmol*. 1994;87:139–144.

23. Amino K, Yamakawa R. Long-term results of out-of-the-bag intraocualr lens implantation. *J Cataract Refract Surg*. 2000;26:266–270.

24. Shah SM, Spalton DJ. Natural history of cellular deposits on the anterior intraocular lens surface. *J Cataract Refract Surg*. 1995;21:466–471.

25. Hollick EJ, Spalton DJ, Ursell PG, Pande MV. Biocompatibility of poly(methyl methacrylate), silicone, and AcrySof intraocular lenses: randomized comparison of the cellular reaction on the anterior lens surface. *J Cataract Refract Surg*. 1998;24:361–366.

26. Miyake K, Ota I, Miyake S, Maekubo K. Correlation between intraocular lens hydrophilicity and anterior capsule opacification and aqueous flare. *J Cataract Refract Surg*. 1996;22:764–769.

27 Schauerberger J, Kruger A, Abela C, et al. Course of postoperative inflammation after implantation of 4 types of foldable intraocular lenses. *J Cataract Refract Surg*. 1999;25:1116–1120.

28. Apple DJ, Mamalis N, Brady SE, et al. Biocompatibility of implant materials: a review and scanning electron microscopy study. *Am Intraocular Implant Soc J*. 1984;10:53–66.

29. Drews RC. Polypropylene in the human eye. *Am Intraocular Implant Soc J*. 1983;9:137–142.

30. Worthen DM, Boucher JA, Buxton JN, et al. Interim FDA report on intraocular lenses. *Ophthalmology*. 1980;87:267–271.

31. Meltzer D. Sterile hypopyon following intraocular lens surgery. *Arch Ophthalmol*. 1980;98:100–104.

32. Berger RR, Kenyeres AM, Vlok AN. Incomplete posterior UGH syndrome: different iatrogenic entity? *Int Ophthalmol*. 1995;19:317–320.

33. Aonuma H, Matsushita H, Nakajima K, et al. Uveitis-glaucoma-hyphema syndrome after posterior chamber intraocular lens implantation. *Jpn J Ophthalmol*. 1997;41:98–100.

34. Van Liefferinge T, Van Oye R, Kestelyn P. Uveitis-glaucoma-hyphema syndrome: a late complication of posterior chamber lenses. *Bull Soc Belge Ophtalmol*. 1994;252:61–66.

35. Van Buskirk EM. Pupillary block after intraocular lens implantation. *Am J Ophthalmol*. 1983;95:55–59.

36. Schrader CE, Belcher CD, Thomas JV, et al. Pupillary and iridovitreal block in pseudophakic eyes. *Ophthalmology*. 1984;91:831-837.

37. Werner D, Kaback M. Pseudophakic papillary block glaucoma. *Br J Ophthalmol*. 1977;61:329–333.

38. Samples JR, Bellows AR, Rosenquist RC, et al. Pupillary block with posterior chamber intraocular lenses. *Arch Ophthalmol*. 1987;105:335–337.

39. Willis DA, Stewart RH, Kimbrough RL. Pupillary block associated with posterior chamber lenses. *Ophthalmic Surg*. 1985;16:108–109.

40. Naveh N, Rosner M, Blumenthal M. Pseudophakic pupillary block glaucoma with posterior-chamber intraocular lens. *Glaucoma*. 1985;7:262–265.

41. Weinreb RN, Wasserstrom JP, Forman JS, Ritch R. Pseudophakic pupillary block with angle closure glaucoma in diabetic patients. *Am J Ophthalmol*. 1986;102: 325–328.

42. Duy TP, Wollensak J. Ciliary block (malignant) glaucoma following posterior chamber lens implantation. *Ophthalmic Surg*. 1987;18:741–744.

43. Reed JE, Thomas JV, Lytle RA, Simmons RJ. Malignant glaucoma induced by intraocular lens. *Ophthalmic Surg*. 1990;21:177–180.

44. Bourne WM, Kaufman HE. Endothelial damage associated with intraocular lenses. *Am J Ophthalmol*. 1976;81:482–485.

45. Waring GO III, Welch SN, Cavanaugh HD, et al. Results of penetrating keratoplasty in 123 eyes with pseudophakic or aphakic corneal edema. *Ophthalmology*. 1983;90:25.

46. Taylor DM, Atlas BF, Romanchuk KG, et al. Pseudophakic bullous keratopathy. *Ophthalmology*. 1983;90:19–24.

47. DeLuise VP. Complications of intraocular lenses. *Int Ophthalmol Clin*. 1987;27:195–204.

48. Liesegang TJ, Bourne WM, Ilstrup DM. Short- and long-term endothelial cell loss associated with cataract extraction and intraocular lens implantation. *Am J Ophthalmol*. 1984;97:32–39.

49. Rao GN, Stevens RE, Harris JK, et al. Long-term changes in corneal endothelium following intraocular lens implantation. *Ophthalmology*. 1981;88:386–397.

50. Ohara K, Tsuru T, Inoda S. Morphometric parameters of the corneal endothelial cells. *Nihon Ganka Gakkai Zasshi*. 1987;91:1073–1078.

51. Hoffer KJ. Corneal decompensation after corneal endothelial cell count. *Am J Ophthalmol*. 1979;87:252–253.

52. Matsuda M, Miyake K, Inaba M. Long-term corneal endothelial changes after intraocular lens implantation. *Am J Ophthalmol*. 1988;105:248–252.

53. Hoffer KJ. Anterior chamber lens exchange. *J Cataract Refract Surg*. 1992;19:536–537.

54. Apple DJ, Mamalis N, Olson RJ, Kincaid MC. *Intraocular Lenses: Evolution, Designs, Complications, and Pathology*. Baltimore: Williams & Wilkins; 1989. p255–270.

55. Maynor RC Jr. Lens-induced complications with anterior chamber lens implants: a comparison with iris supported and posterior chamber lenses. *Am Intraocular Implant Soc J*. 1983;9:450–452.

56. Coli Af, Price FW Jr, Whitson WE. IOL exchange for anterior chamber lens-induced corneal endothelial damage. *Ophthalmology*. 1993;100:384–393.

57. Hara T, Azuma N, Chiba K, et al. Anterior capsule opacification after endocapsular cataract surgery. *Ophthalmic Surg*. 1992;23:94–98.

58. Font RL, Brownstein S. A light and electron microscopic study of anterior subcapsular cataracts. *Am J Ophthalmol*. 1974;78:972–984.

59. Ishibashi T, Araki H, Sugai S, et al. Anterior capsular opacification in monkey eyes with posterior chamber intraocular lenses. *Arch Ophthalmol*. 1993;111:1685–1690.

60. Miyake K, Ota I, Miyake S, Maekubo K. Correlation between intraocular lens hydrophilicity and anterior capsule opacification and aqueous flare. *J Cataract Refract Surg.* 1996;22(suppl 1):764–769.

61. Werner D, Pandey SK, Escobar-Gomez M, et al. Anterior capsule opacification: a histopathological study comparing different IOL styles. *Ophthalmology.* 2000;107:463–471.

62. Kim MJ, Lee HY, Joo CK. Posterior capsule opacification in eyes with a silicone or poly (methyl methacrylate) intraocular lens. *J Cataract Refract Surg.* 1999;25:251–255.

63. Clark D. Posterior capsule opacification. *Curr Opin Ophthalmol.* 2000;11:56–64.

64. Sundelin K, Sjostrand J. Posterior capsular opacification 5 years after extracapsular cataract extraction. *J Cataract Refract Surg.* 1999;25:246–250.

65. Hayashi K, Hayashi H, Nakao F, Hayashi F. Reproducibility of posterior capsule opacification measurement using Scheimpflug videophotography. *J Cataract Refract Surg.* 1998;24:1632–1635.

66. Clark DS, Emery JM, Munsell MF. Inhibition of posterior capsule opacification with an immunotoxin specific for lens epithelial cells: 24 month clinical results. *J Cataract Refract Surg.* 1998;24:1614–1620.

67. Tan JC, Spalton DJ, Arden GB. Comparison of methods to assess visual impairment from glare and light scattering with posterior capsule opacification. *J Cataract Refract Surg.* 1998;24:1626–1631.

68. Tan JC, Spalton DJ, Arden GB. The effect of neodymium:YAG capsulotomy on contrast sensitivity and the evaluation of methods for its assessment. *Ophthalmology.* 1999;106:703–709.

69. Oshika T, Nagata T, Ishii Y. Adhesion of lens capsule to intraocular lenses of polymethylmethacrylate, silicone, and acrylic foldable materials: an experimental study. *Br J Ophthalmol.* 1998;82:549–553.

70. Versura P, Torreggiani A, Cellini M, Caramazza R. Adhesion mechanisms of human lens epithelial cells on 4 intraocular lens materials. *J Cataract Refract Surg.* 1999;25: 527–533.

71. Holick EJ, Spalton DJ, Ursell PG, et al. The effect of polymethacrylate, silicone, and polyacrylic intraocular lenses on posterior capsule opacification 3 years after cataract surgery. *Ophthalmology.* 1999;106:49–54.

72. Nagata T, Watanabe I. Optic sharp edge or convexity: comparison of effects on posterior capsule opacification. *Jpn J Ophthalmol.* 1996;40:397–403.

73. Nishi O, Nishi K. Preventing posterior capsule opacification by creating a discontinuous sharp bend in the capsule. *J Cataract Refract Surg.* 1999;25:521–526.

74. Peng Q, Visessook N, Apple DJ, et al. Surgical prevention of posterior capsule opacification. Part 3. Intraocular lens optic barrier effect as a second line of defense. *J Cataract Refract Surg.* 2000;26:198–213.

75. Hollick EJ, Spalton DJ, Ursell PG, Pande MV. Lens epithelial cell regression on the posterior capsule with different intraocular lens materials. *Br J Ophthalmol.* 1998;82: 1182–1188.

76. Nishi O. Posterior capsule opacification. Part 1. Experimental investigations. *J Cataract Refract Surg.* 1999;25:106–117.

Chapter 16

Posterior Segment Complications of Intraocular Lens Surgery

Jayakrishna Ambati

While modern cataract surgery has become a finely tuned and nearly flawless procedure, it is not entirely uneventful. Even "uncomplicated" cataract surgery can be complicated by the development of visually disabling conditions such as cystoid macular edema (CME). Posterior segment complications can range from the mere disconcerting to the frankly devastating. The shift from intracapsular cataract extraction to small-incision phacoemulsification has transformed the landscape of intraoperative and postoperative complications. As an example, although the incidence of retinal detachment (RD) has declined, the loss of lens fragments has become more common. This chapter presents the most commonly encountered retinal and choroidal sequelae of cataract and intraocular lens (IOL) surgery.

■ Crystalline Lens Dislocation

The widespread use of phacoemulsification has been accompanied by a concomitant rise in the incidence of dislocated crystalline lens fragments into the vitreous cavity.[1] This complication occurs at a rate of approximately 1 to 15 per 1,000 cases.[2,3] Predisposing factors include deep-set eyes, a hard nucleus, small pupils, and traumatic cataract. Patients with pseudoexfoliation or Marfan's syndrome who suffer from zonular weakness are at particular risk for lens luxation. The surgeon can reduce the chance of lens dislocation by vigilantly observing the status of the posterior capsule, utilizing the lowest possible vacuum and power settings and infusion pressures. Directing forces away from known areas of zonular weakness during capsulorrhexis is essential.

Nuclear fragments of the lens may dislocate posteriorly into the vitreous cavity during delivery or phacoemulsification, usually in the setting of a posterior capsular tear or zonular dialysis. Retention of an unencapsulated nucleus can cause significant inflammation and phacolytic glaucoma, in contrast to dislocated lenses with intact capsules, which can be innocuous.[1]

If dislocation occurs intraoperatively and the nucleus remains on the anterior hyaloid face, it is prudent to attempt extraction, either with a loop or with a cryoprobe. This maneuver may be facilitated by using viscoelastic material to float the nucleus anteriorly. Aggressive maneuvers to retrieve a lens that has already migrated posteriorly are rarely successful and can be complicated by accidental retinectomy, giant retinal tears, RD, a macular hole, vitreous hemorrhage, and CME. These complications can sometimes lead to a situation in which recovery of visual acuity is abysmal, particularly if a giant retinal tear is created.[4]

If vitreoretinal consultation is available at hand, immediate posterior vitrectomy and removal of the nucleus is recommended. If such assistance is not immediately available, then removal of residual cortex and anterior vitrectomy with a low infusion rate is warranted. Although placement of an IOL is not contraindicated, it also can be deferred to the time of vitrectomy. After wound closure the patient should be treated with topical antibiotics and corticosteroids and referred promptly for posterior segment surgery.

Recommendations about the timing of vitrectomy are controversial. Although some studies suggest a higher incidence of complications with delayed vitrectomy,[1] other reports claim that the timing of vitrectomy is not significantly associated with postoperative sequelae.[5-7] Although small fragments of nucleus (less than one-quarter of the whole) may safely be observed, both the patient and the eye will benefit from prompt removal of larger fragments.

After posterior vitrectomy the nucleus generally settles on the retinal surface, from which it can be lifted, fragmented, and aspirated. The vitreous cutter can be employed to remove soft cortex, while harder cortical material and nuclear fragments should be engaged with the phacofragmentor. Perfluorocarbon liquid can be used to float the fragment off the retinal surface. Large fragments may require limbal extraction, but this approach may increase the risk of RD because of vitreous traction on the retinal periphery. Eyes managed by pars plana vitrectomy usually achieve satisfactory visual outcomes. Recent series report that approximately 70% of eyes so treated achieve a visual acuity of 20/40 or better.[5,6,8] However, removal of the lens is not absolute prophylaxis against chronic uveitis, CME, epiretinal membrane, glaucoma, RD, and corneal decompensation. As expected, the presence of these pathologies is associated with a poor visual outcome.

■ IOL Dislocation

Dislocation of an IOL into the vitreous is quite rare, ranging from 0.2% to 1.8% of cases.[9,10] Most often it is due to capsule shrinkage and late posterior capsular tears. Pseudoexfoliation is a risk factor for IOL dislocation as well. Posterior chamber IOLs (PCIOLs) have been reported to dislocate into the vitreous cavity after neodymium:yttrium-aluminum-garnet (Nd:YAG) laser capsulotomy as a result of the tangential stresses exerted by the IOL on the compromised posterior capsule. The placement of a plate silicone lens when anterior capsular integrity has been compromised is highly undesirable, as it can lead to IOL migration. Management alternatives include observation and aphakic correction with a contact lens, extraction and replacement with an anterior chamber IOL (ACIOL), or replacement of the IOL in the posterior chamber. Surgical intervention is warranted in the event of contact lens intolerance or the development of complications (CME, chronic uveitis, vitreous hemorrhage, epiretinal membrane, and RD) due to the retained IOL.

Pars plana vitrectomy is generally superior to limbal approaches. If the IOL is damaged or has long, flexible haptics preventing stable optic positioning, then IOL exchange is desirable. Silicone IOLs are more difficult to reposition than polymethyl methacrylate (PMMA) lenses because of structural instability. Ciliary sulcus fixation without sutures is prudent only if there is at least 180 degrees of peripheral capsular support. Scleral suture fixation is required in the event of less capsular support. Iris suture fixation is yet another option. IOLs with small optic zones or interhaptic distances are less stable when suspended by scleral sutures, and can also present undesired optic edge effects. ACIOL placement may be associated with a slightly increased risk of bullous keratopathy, but this is less of an issue with modern haptic designs. The use of perfluorocarbon liquids greatly facilitates extraction and repositioning of the IOL. Special instrumentation may be required to remove silicone IOLs.[11–13] Large IOLs may require bisection for removal. Although intraocular scissors can aid in this task, a disposable instrument such as a myringotomy blade can also serve this purpose (see Chapter 17, Figs. 17.5 to 17.8).

■ Complications of Nd:YAG Laser Capsulotomy

The decision to perform laser posterior capsulotomy should not be made cavalierly. Far from being innocuous, this procedure is associated with a fourfold increase in the risk of developing RD.[14] This is probably due to loss of hyaluronic acid from the vitreous humor and subsequent destabilization of the vitreous matrix, leading to perturbations in the vitreoretinal interface.[15,16] A history of RD in the fellow eye, myopia, youth, and male sex are augmenting risk factors for RD after laser capsulotomy.[14,17,18]

Other complications such as vitritis, macular hole formation,[19] CME,[20–23] and endophthalmitis[22] have rarely been reported. It has been suggested that the risk of CME is minimized by increasing the duration between cataract surgery and laser capsulotomy, although this is not a universal finding. In diabetic patients, there is an increased risk of neovascular glaucoma,[24] probably because of the disruption of a diffusion barrier (the posterior capsule) to angiogenic growth factors. The use of acrylic or modern silicone IOL designs has been reported to reduce the incidence of posterior capsule opacification (PCO), and consequently the need for Nd:YAG laser capsulotomy.[25–27] Intraoperative polishing of the posterior capsule may also reduce the incidence of PCO.

■ Cystoid Macular Edema

Cystoid macular edema is the most common complication of uneventful cataract surgery. The exact incidence of CME following cataract extraction is unknown. Estimates range widely because of variability in defining the entity on angiographic or clinical bases and differences in follow-up duration. Whereas angiographic evidence of CME is quite prevalent (10%–20% in ECCE), clinically symptomatic CME is less common (1%–3% in ECCE).[28,29]

CME may be asymptomatic or may manifest with decreased vision, central scotoma, or metamorphopsia.[30] Fundus examination reveals granularity to the fovea with possible loss of the sharp foveal reflex. Yellow white spots or frank cystoid spaces may be seen as well. Chronic CME leads to atrophic or pigmentary disturbances in the retinal pigment epithelium. Fluorescein angiography reveals early pinpoint punctate retinal hyperfluorescence. Late frames demonstrate filling of the intraretinal cystoid spaces, leading to the classic pattern of pettaloid hyperfluorescence. Associated optic nerve head leakage is frequent. Although fluorescein angiography is invaluable in assessing the presence of CME, the degree of leakage does not correlate with visual acuity.[31]

Although CME can occur in the absence of obvious surgical complications, it is more likely to occur in the setting of posterior capsular rupture of frank vitreous loss.[32] For this reason, the use of low-vacuum, low-aspiration phacoemulsifucation can be invaluable in reducing the likelihood of posterior capsular tears because paroxysmal shallowing or collapse of the chamber is minimized. The obscurity of the pathogenesis of CME has spawned myriad explanations for its occurrence: vitreous traction, vascular instability, disruption of the blood–ocular barrier, ocular hypotony, endophthalmodonesis, and inflammation mediated by prostaglandin synthesis. The last of these is generally accepted as perhaps the most important factor in the development of CME.[31]

The usual time course of appearance of CME is 1–3 months after surgery.[30,33] It is rare, but not unknown, for CME to occur months or years later.[34] Although most cases resolve spontaneously, about 1% persist on a chronic basis (>6 months in duration).[33,35] Such a chronic course accompanied by poor visual outcome is often heralded by the presence of optic disc leakage. These eyes require treatment for 2–3 months before visual improvement can occur.[36,37]

Topical cyclooxygenase inhibitors (NSAIDs) used preoperatively and postoperatively reduce the incidence of angiographic CME but have not conclusively been shown to improve visual acuity. A significant exception is ketorolac, which when used preoperatively and postoperatively significantly decreased angiographic CME in a double-masked, randomized, placebo-controlled study.[29] Two double-masked, placebo-controlled studies have reported significant beneficial visual effects of ketorolac tromethamine in treating chronic clinical CME.[36,37] No nonsteroidal anti-inflammatory drug (NSAID) has been shown to be superior to others in its class. It is important to note that patients with diabetes mellitus or hypertension also benefit from NSAID use.[31] Because of the high incidence of spontaneous resolution of CME, it may be advisable to defer treatment for 6 months after surgery. The treatment of CME by NSAIDs within the first 6 months has not been shown to improve visual outcome compared to treatment with placebo.[31] However, the presence of marked retinal thickening and decreased vision within the first 2–3 months may warrant earlier treatment.

Although corticosteroids have not been shown to reduce CME in a prospective randomized fashion, there is general clinical agreement on their use, and they appear to have a synergism with NSAIDs in suppressing prostaglandin production. While sub-Tenon's capsule steroid injections appear to benefit some patients, it should be noted that this mode of administration results in significant systemic absorption as well.[38] Acetazolamide may have a role in CME as well, especially when the retinal pigment epithelium's pumping ability has been compromised. Acetazolamide's adverse effects are intolerable by a substantial proportion of patients. In addition, CME tends to recur on discontinuation of the drug.[39]

Pars plana vitrectomy can be highly beneficial in selected patients. The Vitrectomy Aphakic Cystoid Macular Edema Study recommended that intervention be delayed until visual acuity has stabilized for 2–3 months, and that surgery be undertaken before visual acuity drops below 20/80, and within 2 years of surgery.[40] Vitrectomy in pseudophakic chronic CME has been promising in cases refractory to medical therapy and with evidence of vitreous adherence to anterior segment structures.[41] The Nd:YAG laser also has been used to cut vitreous strands adherent to the wound, with promising results.[42]

Unlike diabetic macular edema, which responds to laser photocoagulation, postcataract CME does not benefit from laser photocoagulation, probably due to the diffuse leakage from the retinal vasculature.[31]

■ Vitreomacular Traction Syndrome

Vitreomacular traction syndrome (VMTS) occurs as a result of persistent traction on the foveal region by an attached posterior hyaloid and can lead to visual loss by macular distortion, avulsion of retinal vessels, retina hole formation, or frank traction detachment of the macula. The diagnosis can be particularly challenging to establish because the vitreous attachment may be subtle. Diligent biomicroscopy will reveal a thickened posterior hyaloid face that remains attached, and a foveal depression that is obscured or appears cystic. Fluorescein angiography typically reveals diffuse late leakage in the macula but without optic nerve staining, in contrast to CME. Ultrasonography may aid in the diagnosis by demonstrating that the posterior hyaloid face is detached in the periphery but attached at the posterior pole. Optical coherence tomography may be helpful not only in appreciating vitreomacular traction but also in surgery.[43] It is not clear whether VMTS in pseudophakic patients is preexistent or a result of changes in the vitreous induced by cataract surgery.

The natural history of this condition is poor, with most eyes undergoing deterioration in visual acuity, usually due to the development of cystoid changes in the macula that persist.[44] Spontaneous vitreomacular separation is unusual. Pars plana vitrectomy with detachment of the posterior hyaloid can successfully restore vision. Anatomic success is accompanied by visual improvement in VMTS in more than 60% of eyes without macular detachment.[45,46] In cases of traction macular detachment, however, a macular attachment rate of almost 80% is undermined by minimal visual recovery.[47]

■ Retinal Detachment

Retinal detachment is an uncommon but potentially devastating complication of cataract surgery. The incidence of RD after ECCE is far less than after ICCE.[14,48,49] Most large studies report an incidence of approximately 1%.[48,50,51] Although most RDs occur within 6 months after surgery,[52] pseudophakia confers a persistent increased risk: even 6 years after cataract extraction, pseudophakic patients have a 7.5-fold excess risk compared to matched controls.[50]

The principal preexisting risk factors for postoperative RD are high myopia, lattice degeneration of the retina, a history of RD in the fellow eye, a family history of RD, vitreoretinal hereditary degenerations, and subluxated lenses.[18,53–55] High myopia (axial length > 26 mm) confers an 8-fold excess risk, whereas lattice degeneration is associated with a 10-fold excess risk.[18]

Loss of vitreous or crystalline lens fragments and suprachoroidal hemorrhage are intraoperative factors that predispose to RD. Intraoperative disruption of the posterior capsule is associated with a 13-fold increase in risk for RD.[18] Nd:YAG laser capsulotomy is associated with a fourfold increase in risk.[14,18] The underlying mechanism in both cases is probably related to loss of hyaluronic acid from the vitreous humor, which destabilizes the vitreoretinal interface.[15,16] Endophthalmitis and IOL dislocation are postoperative risks for the development of RD. Postoperative trauma results in a fourfold increase in relative risk.[18]

The prophylactic treatment of asymptomatic peripheral retinal lesions (e.g., lattice degeneration) with cryopexy or laser photocoagulation is controversial. A large fraction of RDs occur in areas thought to be normal, and most areas of retinal pathology do not evolve into RDs.[56–58] Prophylaxis itself is not innocuous, as it can cause macular edema, macular pucker, posterior RD, lens opacities, and corneal lesions.[59] However, there is general agreement that suspicious retinal lesions (e.g. symptomatic retinal tears or atrophic holes, asymptomatic horseshoe or flap tears with fluid, and tears with more than 1 disc diameter of fluid) merit retinopexy.[60] The most important intraoperative contribution to reducing the risk of RD is gentle phacoemulsification with preservation of the posterior capsule. There appears to be no difference in RD incidence between ECCE by phacoemulsification versus manual expression.[18,49,61,62]

The diagnosis of pseudophakic RD is rendered difficult by the location of retinal breaks in these cases. They are quite anterior, often near the vitreous base. Patient self-monitoring of symptoms is essential to early diagnosis. Scleral buckling alone often is sufficient to reattach the retina. The reattachment rate is quite high, with rates upward of 90% reported in modern series.[55] In cases of posterior retinal breaks, significant vitreous traction, or proliferative vitreoretinopathy, vitrectomy is necessary. Pneumatic retinopexy is not particularly successful in aphakic or pseudophakic eyes.[63–65]

■ Choroidal Detachment

Choroidal effusions generally develop intraoperatively and can be recognized by the anterior displacement of the iris and vitreous as well as by a change in the red reflex. This development should be managed by wound closure and elevation of the intraocular pressure to tamponade the fluid. It should be noted that choroidal effusions can lead to suprachoroidal hemorrhage by causing traction. Choroidal hemorrhage is an ominous complication that should be addressed by rapid wound closure and drainage of blood via sclerostomies posterior to the ora serrata, sometimes in multiple quadrants. An expulsive hemorrhage, the abattoir of the cataract surgeon, is heralded by darkening of the red reflex, gaping of the wound, prolapse of the iris, and possible expulsion of intraocular contents. Risk factors for this catastrophe include systemic or ocular hypertension, diabetes mellitus, blood dyscrasias, anticoagulation therapy, old age, arteriosclerosis, myopia, glaucoma, ocular inflammation, and an intraoperative pulse above 90 beats per minute. Although this complication is rare (0.2%),[66] quick management by wound closure, often with digital pressure, is necessary to salvage any hope of useful vision.

Postoperative choroidal serous detachment can develop 24–48 hours after surgery, increase in size for 2–3 days, and then spontaneously subside in approximately 2 weeks. It is associated with ocular hypotony, sometimes caused by poor wound closure or inflammatory ciliary body shutdown. Although serous choroidal detachments are generally innocuous and resolve spontaneously, "kissing" choroidals may require drainage of the suprachoroidal space, as may significant anterior chamber shallowing accompanied by intractable secondary angle-closure glaucoma or corneal decompensation. Some authors have reported success with systemic corticosteroids.

■ Photic Retinopathy

Actinic retinal damage produced by exposure to light from the operating microscope has been reported in patients undergoing cataract extraction both with and without implantation of an IOL. Angiographic studies have reported a 3%–7.4% incidence of photic retinopathy in eyes undergoing cataract surgery, with the frequency directly related to the duration of surgery.[67,68] These lesions are characteristically, well-circumscribed, intensely hyperfluorescent areas with central pigment mottling. Interestingly, most of these lesions are parafoveal and often spare the foveal avascular zone. Late development of choroidal folds can complicate the picture.[69] Rarely, choroidal neovascularization can develop secondary to photic retinopathy. Although exposure to light for 7.5 minutes has been shown to produce retinal lesions in monkeys,[70] cataract surgery of 60 minutes or longer has been associated with the development of photic maculopathy in humans.[68,71,72]

Histologic examination reveals damage to the inner and outer photoreceptor segments, swelling of the retinal pigment epithelium, and disruption of the retinal pigment epithelial tight junctions.[70] Thus, the phototoxicity is due not to photocoagulation but to cellular damage secondary to light interaction with cellular components, leading to the formation of toxic oxygen radicals.

The major modifiable intraoperative factors in the development of photic maculopathy are the duration of light exposure, the tilt of the microscope, and the intensity of illumination. Therefore, intraoperative exposure to light should be minimized by operating under the least possible light intensity, altering the angle of incident light into a nonaxial ray, and using a corneal protector when intraocular visualization is not needed (e.g., during suturing). Merely moving the microscope light to the peripheral cornea is not sufficient, for the prismatic effect of the eye results in the direction of peripheral rays of light into the center. Ultraviolet filters in the operating microscope are protective.[73]

■ Clear Lens Extraction

Clear lens extraction (CLE) to correct myopia is controversial because of the potentially deadly posterior segment complications such as RD and endophthalmitis.[74,75] The incidence of postoperative RD after CLE has decreased over time, perhaps because of smaller incisions and improved surgical techniques. Still, the risk of RD is higher in these patients than in nonmyopic patients undergoing phacoemulsification. The incidence of RD has ranged from 0% to 7.3%.[57,76–78] There is no significant difference in incidence or RD with or without intraoperative posterior capsule rupture. However, RD occurs twice as frequently in patients who underwent posterior capsulotomy than in those who did not undergo any postoperative procedure performed on the posterior capsule.

A wide anterior capsulorrhexis would facilitate future retinal examinations. Placement of an IOL with a large optic may be beneficial in limiting anterior movement of the vitreous, especially after Nd:YAG laser capsulotomy. This would have a salutary effect in reducing the risk of retinal tears. The utility of prophylactic laser photocoagulation or cryotherapy for asymptomatic peripheral retinal lesions is suspect. Many studies have failed to demonstrate any reduction in retinal detachment rates as a result of these preoperative maneuvers. Nevertheless, there are limited data suggesting some beneficial effects of prophylactic treatment of asymptomatic retinal lesions in highly myopic patients prior to cataract surgery. Therefore, some authors have advocated cerclage prophylaxis, and have claimed a low rate of postoperative RD in highly myopic eyes.[79]

It should be noted that the frequent need for Nd:YAG laser posterior capsulotomy following CLE[76,80] raises the specter of RD and CME. Therefore, the patient should be clearly informed not only of the potentially devastating complications accompanying CLE but also of surgical alternatives, such as refractive surgery, which is associated with fewer posterior segment complications. Postoperatively, periodic examinations of the retinal periphery and treatment of degenerative lesions should be performed on a regular basis.

■ Phakic IOLs

Placement of an IOL in a phakic eye has emerged as an alternative to refractive surgery or CLE in patients with high refractive errors. Although no posterior segment complications have been consistently reported as a result this procedure,[81] well-controlled, long-term studies on the posterior segment complications of this procedure are lacking. CME secondary to uveal inflammation is a possible consequence both because of iris touch and because of the creation of a peripheral iridotomy. The possible secondary development of a cataract carries with it the concomitant complications outlined previously.[82]

References

1. Blodi BA, Flynn HW Jr, Blode CF, et al. Retained nuclei after cataract surgery. *Ophthalmology.* 1992;99:41–44.

2. Leaming DV. Practice styles and preferences of ASCRS members: 1994 survey. *J Cataract Refract Surg.* 1995;21:378–385.

3. Pande M, Dabbs TR. Incidence of lens matter dislocation during phacoemulsification. *J Cataract Refract Surg.* 1996;22:737–742.

4. Aaberg TM Jr, Rubsamen PE, Flynn HW Jr, et al. Giant retinal tear as a complication of attempted removal of intravitreal lens fragments during cataract surgery. *Am J Ophthalmol.* 1997;124:222–226.

5. Kim JE, Flynn HW Jr, Smiddy WE, et al. Retained lens fragments after phacoemulsification. *Ophthalmology.* 1994;101:1827–1832.

6. Borne MJ. Tasman W, Regillo C, et al. Outcomes of vitrectomy for retained lens fragments. *Ophthalmology.* 1996;103:971–976.

7. Gilliland GD, Hutton WL, Fuller DG. Retained intravitreal lens fragments after cataract surgery. *Ophthalmology.* 1992;99:1263–1269.

8. Kapusta MA, Chen JC, Lam WC. Outcomes of dropped nucleus during phacoemulsification. *Ophthalmology.* 1996;103:1184–1187.

9. Stark WJ, Maumenee AE, Dangel ME, et al. Intraocular lenses: experience at the Wilmer Institute. *Ophthalmology.* 1982;89:104–108.

10. Smiddy WE, Ibanez GV, Alfonso E, Flynn HW Jr. Surgical management of dislocated intraocular lenses. *J Cataract Refract Surg.* 1995;21:64–69.

11. Carlson AN, Apple DJ, Garrett SN, et al. Dislocation of silicone plate design IOLs following Nd:YAG laser capsulotomy. *Ophthalmology.* 1995;102(suppl):126.

12. Gonzalez GA, Irvine AR. Posterior dislocation of plate haptic silicone lenses. *Arch Ophthalmol.* 1996;114:775–776.

13. Schneiderman TE, Johnson MW, Smiddy WE, et al. Surgical management of posteriorly dislocated silicone plate haptic intraocular lenses. *Am J Ophthalmol.* 1997;123:629–635.

14. Javitt JC, Tielsch JM, Canner JK, et al. National outcomes of cataract extraction: increased risk of retinal complications associated with Nd:YAG laser capsulotomy. *Ophthalmology.* 1992;99:1487–1498.

15. Österlin S. On the molecular biology of the vitreous in the aphakic eye. *Acta Ophthalmol.* 1977;55:353–361.

16. Österlin S. Macromolecular composition of the vitreous in the aphakic owl monkey eye. *Exp Eye Res.* 1978;26: 77–84.

17. Koch DD, Liu JF, Gill EP, Parke DW II. Axial myopia increases the risk of retinal complications after neodymium-YAG laser posterior capsulotomy. *Arch Ophthalmol.* 1989;107:986–990.

18. Tielsch JM, Legro MW, Cassard SD, et al. Risk factors for retinal detachment after cataract surgery: a population-based case-control study. *Ophthalmology.* 1996;103:1537–1545.

19. Blacharski PA, Newsome DA. Bilateral macular holes after Nd:YAG laser posterior capsulotomy. *Am J Ophthalmol.* 1988;105:417–418.

20. Bukelman A, Abrahami S, Oliver M, Pollack A. Cystoid macular edema after neodymium:YAG laser posterior capsulotomy: a prospective study. *Eye.* 1992;6:35–38.

21. Steinert RF, Puliafito CA, Kumar SR, et al. Cystoid macular edema, retinal detachment, and glaucoma after Nd:YAG laser posterior capsulotomy. *Am J Ophthalmol.* 1991;112:373–380.

22. Stark WJ, Worthen D, Holladay JT, et al. Neodymium:YAG lasers: an FDA report. *Ophthalmology.* 1985;92:209–212.

23. Lewis H, Singer TR, Hanscom TA, et al. A prospective study of cystoid macular edema after neodymium:YAG laser posterior capsulotomy. *Ophthalmology.* 1987;94:478–482.

24. Weinreb RN, Wasserstrom JP, Parker W. Neovascular glaucoma following neodymium-YAG laser posterior capsulotomy. *Arch Ophthalmol.* 1986;104:730–731.

25. Ram J, Apple DJ, Pena Q, et al. Update on fixation of rigid and foldable posterior chamber intraocular lenses. Part II. Choosing the correct haptic fixation and intraocular lens design to help eradicate posterior capsule opacification. *Ophthalmology.* 1999;106:891–900.

26. Hollick EJ, Spalton DJ, Ursell PG, Pande MV. Lens epithelial cell regression on the posterior capsule with different intraocular lens materials. *Br J Ophthalmol.* 1998;82:1182–1188.

27. Hayashi H, Hayashi K, Nakao F, Hayashi F. Quantitative comparison of posterior capsule opacification after polymethylmethacrylate, silicone, and soft acrylic intraocular lens implantation. *Arch Ophthalmol.* 1998;116:1579–1582.

28. Kraff MC, Sanders DR, Jampol LM, et al. Prophylaxis of pseudophakic cystoid macular edema with topical indomethacin. *Ophthalmology.* 1982;89:885–890.

29. Flach AJ, Stegman RC, Graham J, Kruger LP. Prophylaxis of aphakic cystoid macular edema without corticosteroids: a paired comparison, placebo controlled double-masked study. *Ophthalmology.* 1990;97:1253–1258.

30. Irvine SR. A newly defined vitreous syndrome following cataract surgery. *Am J Ophthalmol.* 1953;36:599–619.

31. Flach AJ. The incidence, pathogenesis and treatment of cystoid macular edema following cataract surgery. *Trans Am Ophthalmol Soc.* 1998;96:557–634.

32. Miami Study Group. Cystoid macular edema in aphakic and pseudophakic eyes. *Am J Ophthalmol.* 1979;88:45–48.

33. Gass JD, Norton EW. Cystoid macular edema and papilledema following cataract extraction. *Arch Ophthalmol.* 1966;76:646–661.

34. Mao LK, Holland PM. "Very late onset" cystoid macular edema. *Ophthalmic Surg.* 1988;19:633–635.

35. Jampol LM. Cystoid macular edema following cataract surgery. *Arch Ophthalmol.* 1988;106:894–895.

36. Flach AJ, Dolan BJ, Irvine AR. Effectiveness of ketorolac tromethamine 0.5% ophthalmic solution for chronic aphakic and pseudophakic cystoid macular edema. *Am J Ophthalmol.* 1987;103:479–486.

37. Flach AJ, Jampol LM, Weinberg D, et al. Improvement in visual acuity in chronic aphakic and pseudophakic cystoid macular edema after treatment with topical 0.5% ketorolac tromethamine. *Am J Ophthalmol.* 1991;112:514–519.

38. Weijtens O, van der Sluijs FA, Schoemaker RC, et al. Peribulbar corticosteroid injection: vitreal and serum concentrations after dexamethasone disodium phosphate injection. *Am J Ophthalmol.* 1997;123:358–363.

39. Tripathi RC, Fekrat S, Tripathi BJ, Ernest JT. A direct correlation of the resolution of pseudophakic cystoid macular edema with acetazolamide therapy. *Ann Ophthalmol.* 1991;23:127–129.

40. Fung WE. The national, prospective, randomized vitrectomy study for chronic aphakic cystoid macular edema: progress report and comparison between the control and nonrandomized groups. *Surv Ophthalmol.* 1984;28:569–576.

41. Harbour JW, Smiddy WE, Rubsamen PE, et al. Pars plana vitrectomy for chronic pseudophakic cystoid macular edema. *Am J Ophthalmol.* 1995;120:302–307.

42. Katzen LE, Fleischman JA, Trokel S. YAG laser treatment of cystoid macular edema. *Am J Ophthalmol.* 1983;95:589–592.

43. Munuera JM, Garcia-Layana A, Maldonado MJ, et al. Optical coherence tomography in successful surgery of vitreomacular traction syndrome. *Arch Ophthalmol.* 1998;116:1388–1389.

44. Hickichi T, Yoshida A, Trempe CL. Course of vitreomacular traction syndrome. *Am J Ophthalmol.* 1995;119:55–61.

45. Smiddy WE, Michels RG, Glaser BM, deBustros S. Vitrectomy for macular traction caused by incomplete vitreous separation. *Arch Ophthalmol.* 1988;106:624–628.

46. McDonald HR, Johnson RN, Schatz H. Surgical results in the vitreomacular traction syndrome. *Ophthalmology.* 1994;101:1397–1403.

47. Melberg NS, Williams DF, Balles MW, et al. Vitrectomy for vitreomacular traction syndrome with macular detachment. *Retina.* 1995;15:192–197.

48. Javitt JC, Vitale S, Canner JK, et al. National outcomes of cataract extraction. I. Retinal detachment after inpatient surgery. *Ophthalmology.* 1991;98:895–902.

49. Ninn-Pedersen K, Bauer B. Cataract patients in a defined Swedish population, 1986–1990. V. Postoperative retinal detachments. *Arch Ophthalmol.* 1996:114:382–386.

50. Norregaard JC, Thoning H, Andersen TF, et al. Risk of retinal detachment following cataract extraction: results from the International Cataract Surgery Outcomes Study. *Br J Ophthalmol.* 1996;80:689–693.

51. Nissen KR, Fuchs J, Goldschmidt E, et al. Retinal detachment after cataract extraction in myopic eyes. *J Cataract Refract Surg.* 1998;24:772–776.

52. Smith PW, Stark WJ, Maumenee AE, et al. Retinal detachment after extracapsular cataract extraction with posterior chamber intraocular lens. *Ophthalmology.* 1987;94:495–504.

53. Lindstrom RL, Lindquist TD, Huldin J, Rubenstein JB. Retinal detachment in axial myopia following extracapsular cataract surgery. In: Caldwell DR, ed. *Cataracts. Trans New Orleans Acad Ophthalmol.* 1988:253–268.

54. Alldredge CD, Elkins B, Alldredge OC Jr., et al. Retinal detachment following phacoemulsification in highly myopic cataract patients. *J Cataract Refract Surg.* 1998;24:777–780.

55. Yoshida A, Ogasawara H, Jalkh AE, et al. Retinal detachment after cataract surgery. *Ophthalmology.* 1992;90: 460–465.

56. Delaney WV Jr, Oates RP. Retinal detachment in the second eye. *Arch Ophthalmol.* 1978;96:629–634.

57. Barraquer C, Cavelier C, Mejia LF. Incidence of retinal detachment following clear-lens extraction in myopic patients: retrospective analysis. *Arch Ophthalmol.* 1994;112: 336–339.

58. Kanski JJ, Daniel R. Prophylaxis of retinal detachment. *Am J Ophthalmol.* 1975;79:197–205.

59. Zweng HC, Little HL, Hammond AH. Complications of argon laser photocoagulation. *Trans Am Acad Ophthalmol Otolaryngol.* 1974;78:OP194–OP204.

60. American Academy of Ophthalmology. *Preferred Practice Pattern: Retinal Detachment.* San Francisco: American Academy of Ophthalmology; 1990.

61. Ranta P, Kevela T. Retinal detachment in pseudophakic eyes with and without Nd:YAG laser posterior capsulotomy. *Ophthalmology.* 1998;105:2127–2133.

62. Powe NR, Schein OD, Gieser SC, et al. Synthesis of the literature on visual acuity and complications following cataract extraction with intraocular lens implantation. *Arch Ophthalmol.* 1994;112:239–252.

63. Grizzard WS, Hilton GF, Hammer ME, et al. Pneumatic retinopexy failures: cause, prevention, timing, and management. *Ophthalmology.* 1995;102:929–936.

64. Chen JC, Robertson JE, Coonan P, et al. Results and complications of pneumatic retinopexy. *Ophthalmology* 1988; 95:601–608.

65. McAllister IL, Meyers SM, Zegarra H, et al. Comparison of pneumatic retinopexy with alternative surgical techniques. *Ophthalmology.* 1988;95:877–883.

66. Taylor DM. Expulsive hemorrhage. *Am J Ophthalmol.* 1974;78:961–966.

67. Gomolin JE, Koenekoop RK. Presumed photic retinopathy after cataract surgery: an angiographic study. *Can J Ophthalmol.* 1993;28:221–224.

68. Khwarg SG, Linstone FA, Daniels SA, et al. Incidence, risk factors, and morphology in operating microscope light retinopathy. *Am J Ophthalmol.* 1987;103:255–263.

69. Johnson RN, Schatz H, McDonald HR. Photic maculopathy: Early angiographic and ophthalmoscopic findings and late development of choroidal folds. *Arch Ophthalmol.* 1987;105:1633–1634.

70. Irvine AR, Wood I, Morris BW. Retinal damage from the

illumination of the operating microscope: an experimental study in pseudophakic monkeys. *Trans Am Ophthalmol Soc.* 1984;84:239–260.

71. McDonald HR, Irvine AR. Light-induced maculopathy from the operating microscope in extracapsular cataract extraction and intraocular lens implantation. *Ophthalmology.* 1983;90:945–951.

72. Robertson DM, Feldman RB. Photic retinopathy from the operating room microscope. *Am J Ophthalmol.* 1986;101:561–569.

73. McIntyre DJ. The eclipse filter. *Ophthalmology.* 1985;92:361–365.

74. Javitt JC. Clear-lens extraction for high myopia: is this an idea whose time has come? *Arch Ophthalmol.* 1994;112:321–323.

75. Goldberg MF. Clear-lens extraction for axial myopia: an appraisal. *Ophthalmology.* 1987;94:571–582.

76. Colin J, Robinet A. Clear lensectomy and implantation of low-power posterior chamber intraocular lens for the correction of high myopia: a four-year follow-up. *Ophthalmology.* 1997;104:73–77.

77. Verzella F. Microsurgery of the lens in myopia for optical purposes. *Cataract.* 1984;1:8–12.

78. Lyle WA, Jin GJ. Phacoemulsification with intraocular lens implantation in high myopia. *J Cataract Refract Surg.* 1996;22:238–241.

79. Centurion V. Retinal detachment following clear lens extraction. Reported in Werblin TP. Barraquer Lecture 1998. Why should refractive surgeons be looking beyond the cornea? *J Refract Surg.* 1999;15:357–376.

80. Lyle WA, Jin GJC. Clear lens extraction to correct hyperopia. *J Cataract Refract Surg.* 1997;23:1051–1056.

81. Sanders DR, Martin RG, Brown DC, et al. Posterior chamber phakic IOL for hyperopia. *J Refract Surg.* 1999;15:309–315.

82. Trindade F, Pereira F. Cataract formation after posterior chamber phakic intraocular lens implantation. *J Cataract Refract Surg.* 1998;24:1661–1663.

Chapter 17

Intraocular Lens Explantation

Jeffrianne S. Young and Mary Gilbert Lawrence

Cataract extraction is routinely accompanied by intraocular lens (IOL) implantation. Although IOL implantation generally is a highly successful procedure, a small percentage of patients develop severe inflammation, endophthalmitis, and other complications secondary to IOL placement that require removal or repositioning of the IOL. This chapter focuses on the indications, techniques, and outcomes of IOL removal.

■ Indications for IOL Removal

Indications for surgical intervention of IOL-associated complications have changed over the past two decades as IOL design and implantation techniques have evolved. In nine recently published case series of IOLs requiring repositioning, removal, or exchange, 52% were anterior chamber intraocular lenses (ACIOLs), 30% were posterior chamber intraocular lenses (PCIOLs), and 18% were iris-fixated lenses (Table 17.1). The figure for ACIOLs is probably lower today because the flexible, three-point and four-point fixation, one-piece polymethyl methacrylate (PMMA) open-loop ACIOLs now available have significantly lower complication rates.[1-4] Suture and metal claw iris-fixated lenses have fallen into disuse owing to continued problems with inflammation, cystoid macular edema (CME), and corneal damage.[4-7] PCIOLs have become increasingly popular. Foldable PCIOLs made of acrylic, hydrogel, and silicone allow much smaller incisions. Complication rates have decreased with the use of sutureless PCIOLs in the presence of adequate capsulo-zonular support.[4]

Recently, phakic IOLs have gained popularity for the reversible correction of high myopia (although new permanent laser techniques, such as photorefractive keratectomy and laser in situ keratomileusis are increasingly popular; see Chapter 19).[8] The complications associated with phakic IOLs include inappropriate power, dislocation, inflammation, cataract formation, endothelial cell damage, corneal edema, and retinal detachment (RD), as well as such extremely rare complications as endophthalmitis and choroidal hemorrhage.[8-10] (See Chapters 20–22 for further discussion of the complications of phakic IOLs.) In a review of nine published studies, the most common complications of anterior chamber, posterior chamber, and iris-fixated lenses that required removal or exchange included dislocation, pseudophakic bullous keratopathy (PBK), optical symptoms, inflammation, corneal decompensation, glaucoma, and CME.

Depending on the extent of IOL dislocation, secondary complications may occur. A "subluxated IOL" is when an IOL becomes extremely decentered such that only a small fraction of the pupillary opening is adequately covered. Subluxated IOLs may cause optic symptoms such as diplopia and glare.[11] In more severe cases, subluxated IOLs may cause corneal decompensation and PBK from direct IOL-endothelial touch.[12,13] A luxated IOL is completely dislocated into the posterior segment of the eye. Dislocated IOLs may also lead to pupillary capture, uveitis, hyphema, chronic CME, corneal edema, retinal traction, and subsequent RD.[14-19]

IOL-related inflammation may also require surgical intervention. Endophthalmitis may follow either an acute course or a delayed, low-grade chronic course.[20,21] The most common cause of chronic endophthalmitis is *Propionibacterium acnes*, although coagulase-negative *Staphylococcus epidermis, Streptococcus, Actinomyces, Achromobacter, Corynebacterium,* and *Nocardia* have also been implicated.[17,20,22-24] Since the pathogens are

211

Table 17.1
Recent Studies of Indications for IOL Repositioning, Removal, and/or Exchange

Study, Year	No. of Eyes with IOL Removal	Type of Intraocular Lens		
		ACL	PCL	IFL
Sawada et al, 1998[15]	14	14	—	—
Osher et al, 1995[11]	68	24	33	11
Smiddy et al, 1995[16]	78	18	59	1
Busin et al, 1995[17]	52	16	31	5
Sinskey et al, 1993[2]	79	48	15	16
Doren et al, 1992[18]	101	54	8	39
Mamalis et al, 1991[3]	102	68	16	18
Noecker et al, 1989[12]	33	25	2	6
Busin et al, 1987	27	22	—	5
Total[d]	554	289	164	101
Percent of total	100%	52%	30%	18%

sequestered and colonize both on the IOL and inside the capsular bag, the condition is often refractory to antibiotic therapy.

In addition, chronic sterile inflammation may result from faulty lens design or inappropriate lens sizing. For example, an ACIOL that is too short may rotate in propeller-like fashion in the anterior chamber, causing inflammation and corneal endothelial cell loss. Peripheral anterior synechiae (PAS) may develop around the haptics, serving as a bridge for the migration of endothelial cells and subsequent corneal decompensation.[11,15,25]

Rare indications for IOL removal include ocular trauma,[26] expulsive choroidal hemorrhage, cyclodialysis cleft,[27] and severe neodymium:yttrium-aluminum-garnet (Nd:YAG) laser-induced IOL damage.[28]

■ Nonsurgical Approaches to IOL Complications

Conservative medical management may be adequate in the absence of immediate surgical indications for IOL removal, such as inflammation and mechanical retinal damage. For instance, in a mild case of anterior chamber inflammation (trace cell and flare) without associated symptoms or reduced visual acuity, topical steroids may be appropriate.[11] Patients with chronic CME may be treated with a combination therapeutic trial of a nonsteroidal anti-inflammatory agent and topical steroids.[11,19] Elderly patients with low endothelial cell counts and peripheral cornea edema may fare better with topical sodium chloride than with surgical intervention.[29]

In some cases, surgical intervention may not involve IOL removal or exchange. For instance, IOL-associated glaucoma may be treated adequately by pars plana vitrectomy, provided that a pathway for aqueous flow to the anterior chamber is established.[30] Rare complications such as hypotonus cyclodialysis cleft formation secondary to IOL implantation may require argon laser photocoagulation if proven refractory to pharmacologic therapy.[27] Patients with endophthalmitis should undergo immediate vitrectomy only if vision is severely impaired (light perception only). Patients with less severe visual loss may be adequately treated with tap biopsy and injection of appropriately fortified antibiotics.[20,31]

Condition(s) Requiring Removal

Dislocated	PBK	Optical Symptoms[a]	Endophthalmitis	Corneal Decompensation[b]	UGH	Glaucoma	CME	Uveitis	Other[c]
—	9	—	—	—	—	2	—	2	1
20	—	25	—	9	6	8	5	15	5
78	—	68	15	8	—	7	10	—	16
15	15	2	17	—	—	—	—	—	3
33	10	10	—	12	8	1	2	—	3
7	69	—	6	—	9	3	—	—	7
16	41	2	1	8	16	5	4	—	9
4	17	—	—	4	1	—	2	5	—
4	—	—	14	2	—	8	2	—	9
Total[d] 177	161	107	53	43	40	34	25	22	53
32%	29%	19%	10%	8%	7%	6%	5%	4%	10%

ACIOL, anterior chamber intraocular lens; PCIOL, posterior chamber intraocular lens; IFL, iris-fixated intraocular lens; PBK, pseudophakic bullous keratopathy; UGH, uveitis-glaucoma-hyphema syndrome; CME, chronic macular edema.

[a] Optical symptoms include incorrect lens power, decreased visual acuity despite best-corrected vision, glare, monocular diplopia, and unwanted optical images.

[b] Corneal decompensation includes corneal edema, corneal ulcers, corneal perforation, and failed corneal transplants.

[c] Other include the following: Sawada—deformation of pupil (1); Osher—iris tuck (5); Smiddy—hyphema (6), vitreous hemorrhage (4), pupillary capture (2), cataract wound dehiscence (2), choroidal folds (1), epiretinal membrane (1); Busin (1995)—traumatic expulsion (3); Sinskey—traumatic subluxation (2), pupillary capture (1); Doren—retinal detachment (7); Mamalis—pupillary capture (2), iris laceration (1), miscellaneous (6); Busin (1987)—hyphema (2), senile macular degeneration (3), retinal detachment (1), hemiretinal vein occlusion (1), surgical wound leak (2).

[d] Indications add up to more than 100% because some studies (Osher, Busin [1987]) reported patients with multiple indications for IOL removal.

■ Surgical Techniques for IOL Removal

Preoperative Evaluation

A thorough ocular examination is mandatory prior to IOL removal. Bilateral best corrected visual acuity is determined and slit-lamp microscopy is performed. Keratometry, ultrasonography, pachymetry, and, in some cases, specular microscopy with endothelial cell count may be performed to assess the health of the cornea. Surgical trauma should be avoided in regions of endothelial cell loss. A low cell count (<700 cells/mm^3) alone is not an adequate criterion for deciding whether or not to perform concomitant penetrating pseudophakic keratoplasty (PK) with IOL removal. However, in the setting of corneal edema and a low cell count, concomitant PK may be indicated. In the absence of microcystic corneal edema, eyes with corneal pachymetry measurements greater than 600 μm may also require concomitant PK.[25]

Gonioscopy may be performed to determine the location of IOL haptics, PAS, and possible subluxated haptics through peripheral iridectomies. The presence and location of vitreous in the anterior chamber will determine the extent of vitrectomy required during the procedure. Dilation of the pupil is necessary to determine the amount of peripheral capsular support, followed by complete dilated fundus ophthalmoscopy. If there is evidence of CME, fluorescein angiography may be necessary. Review of the operative report, lens type, and power may be helpful in making a preliminary decision to reposition, remove, or exchange the IOL.

The timing of surgery is also important. An improperly implanted IOL is ideally repaired during initial implantation, if possible. Severe complications such as severe endophthalmitis or RD may require immediate surgical intervention. In less severe cases, the timing of surgery may depend on the presence and amount of inflammation and fibrosis. Early intervention may in fact be preferable, since fibrotic material has had minimal time to develop.

Removal of ACIOLs

Open-loop ACIOL removal is performed essentially by reversal of IOL implantation. In the absence of

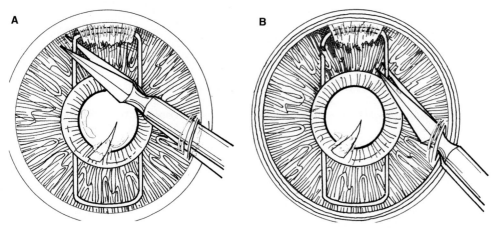

FIGURE 17.1. *A* and *B*, A technique for removal of a closed-loop ACIOL with PAS or fibrotic coccoon covering footplates of the haptic. The inferior haptic is severed with a haptic cutter inserted through the paracentesis wound. The ACIOL can then be explanted and the remaining haptic part pulled out of the coccoon.

synechiae, it may be possible to remove the IOL without severing the haptics from the optic. Viscoelastic material is injected into the anterior chamber. The haptics are removed by carefully rotating the lens and backthreading the haptics out of the anterior chamber. A spatula may be inserted into the wound to serve as a ramp to prevent snagging of the iris or wound edges.[11,19,25] If synechiae are present, a closed-loop ACIOL removal technique may be necessary.

Closed-loop ACIOL removal is more complex, because the filamentous haptics may have become enveloped by fibrotic material. Significant bleeding and iridodialysis may result from direct pulling on the haptics. For this reason, the haptics must instead be threaded out via fibrotic tunnels until they are free within the anterior chamber. This may be accomplished by carefully cutting each haptic so that the U-shaped loop is transformed into an L-shape, with one side of the haptic loop cut close to the optic and the other side cut as close to the angle as possible (Fig. 17.1). Filling the anterior chamber with viscoelastic material may minimize damage to intraocular structures during piecemeal removal of the IOL. A spatula may be used as a ramp under the optic. After the optic is removed, the remaining haptics are carefully threaded out of the fibrotic cocoon into the anterior chamber for removal. It may be necessary to leave behind remaining portions of the haptics rather than risk unnecessary damage to the iris and ciliary sulcus. The haptics should be cut as close to the angle as possible. If the vitreous face is broken, a vitrectomy may be necessary. (See discussion under Removal of PCIOLs—Anterior Approach for the management of vitreous in limbus approach procedures.)

When a haptic is subluxed into a peripheral iridectomy or the incision wound, repositioning may be adequate. In some cases an iris tuck may be corrected by flexing, lifting, and repositioning the haptic.[11]

Removal of Iris-Fixated IOLs

Dislocated and malpositioned iris-fixated IOLs may be removed or exchanged for ACIOLs or PCIOLs. Rarely, iris-fixated IOLs may be surgically repositioned in cases in which an extensive explantation procedure is too risky.

The technique for removal of an iris-fixated lens depends on whether the lens has dislocated into the anterior or the posterior vitreous. Successful removal often requires synechiae separation with or without anterior vitrectomy. If the lens has dislocated into the anterior vitreous, two stab incisions are made anteriorly. A C-shaped hook may be used to capture a visible haptic. The lens is subsequently guided back through the pupil into the anterior chamber. A second hook is placed under the lens to keep the lens from dropping back into the vitreous. After the lens has been safely manipulated into the anterior chamber, an intracameral miotic may be given to constrict the pupil. A spatula may be used to guide the lens past the scleral lip. All vitreous adhesions should be removed. If the lens has dislocated into the posterior vitreous, the technique used is identical to that for removing a PCIOL dislocated into the posterior vitreous, described in a later section.

If the repositioning of an iris-fixated lens is necessary, two limbal incisions are made just anterior to the corneoscleral junction to avoid hemorrhage. Viscoelastic material should be avoided if possible, because it is difficult to remove without disturbing the vitreous. Two microhooks may be inserted through the incisions for haptic manipulation. One hook is used to retract and depress the iris while the other is used to elevate and decenter the optic. The haptics are repositioned and topical miotics are given to ensure IOL fixation.[11,19,25]

Removal of PCIOLs

Anterior Approach

As with iris-fixated lenses, the surgical approach for removing a PCIOL depends on whether it has dislocated into the anterior or the posterior vitreous. Preoperative assessment of the presence and amount of vitreous in the anterior chamber is also important, since it may influence the surgical approach used. If only a small amount of vitreous is present in the anterior chamber, a limbal approach may be adequate, whereas a large amount of vitreous may require a pars plana or combined approach. Regardless, all accessible vitreous should be removed to minimize postoperative inflammatory and tractional complications.[16] This section describes limbus techniques for dislocated PCIOLs. The technique for anterior maneuvering or removal of the PCIOL from the anterior vitreous is discussed in the next section.

Removal of a PCIOL depends on whether the lens is located in the ciliary sulcus or in the capsular bag. In either case, it is important to identify both the configuration and the precise location of each haptic within the sulcus. Enlarged haptic tips or eyelets may be difficult to manipulate through a tunnel of fibrosis. If the lens is in the sulcus, injection of viscoelastic material may ease manipulation of the haptics. Continued resistance indicates that the haptics must be severed for piecemeal removal of the IOL. If haptic removal proves too difficult and risks permanent damage to the sulcus or capsular bag, the haptics may be trimmed as close as possible to the ciliary sulcus and left in place. If the lens is within the capsular bag, the lens may be rotated to free the haptics, then dialed into the anterior chamber for removal. Resistance to rotation requires severing the optic from the haptics. If a severed haptic is adherent within the leaflets of the capsule, the bag may be opened by injection of viscoelastic material. Again, haptics too difficult to remove may be cut and left behind. Closed-loop PCIOLs also require piecemeal IOL removal, but excessive fibrosis may require that the closely cut haptics be left behind.[19,25]

Repositioning a dislocated PCIOL may be possible in some cases. If the dislocation is due to asymmetric haptic placement (one haptic in the capsular bag, one

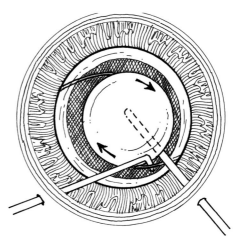

FIGURE 17.2. Repositioning or removal of a PCIOL using the Sinskey hook and spatula.

in the sulcus) but the capsule remains intact, it may be possible to rotate the lens with a one- or two-hook technique so that each haptic assumes a new, secure position within the sulcus (Fig. 17.2). Then gentle manipulation of the optic toward each haptic (Osher's "bounce test") ensures that the lens will spontaneously recenter (Fig. 17.3).[11] Even in the presence of significant fibrosis, endocapsular fixation of a dislocated PCIOL that remains encapsulated may be possible. A 30-gauge cannula may be inserted to bluntly develop a plane between the fused anterior and posterior capsule leaflets. Viscoelastic material may be injected to reopen the capsular bag and provide access for the surgeon to rotate the IOL into place.[11]

Management of the vitreous is crucial for all limbal approach procedures. If the anterior chamber fills with vitreous, vitrectomy may be necessary. If there is only minimal vitreous prolapse, a more limited dry technique may be performed. This involves filling the anterior chamber with viscoelastic material and inserting the vitrectomy handpiece without irrigation (Fig. 17.4). Proper management of the vitreous is also necessary at the end of the procedure. Removal of the viscoelastic material from the anterior chamber risks additional vitreous prolapse. Osher et al suggest a preventive technique whereby a 30-gauge cannula on a 3-mL air syringe is inserted through a second incision, with air injected as the I/A tip is removed. The air maintains a deep chamber so that balanced salt solutions may be safely exchanged in small aliquots.[11]

Posterior Approach

A variety of pars plana techniques are available for removal, retrieval, and repositioning of a subluxated PCIOL. The precise location of the optic and haptics

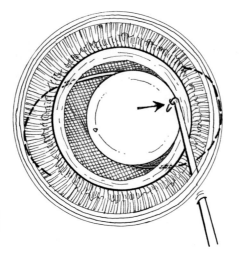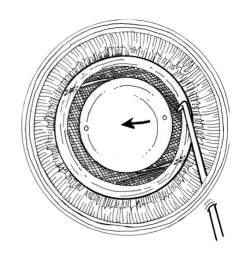

FIGURE 17.3. Osher's "bounce test" to ensure that the lens will spontaneously recenter.

should be determined, as well as the design, size, stability, and condition of the PCIOL. If capsulozonular support is adequate, repositioning by capsular support is often ideal.[16] In the absence of adequate capsular support, iris or scleral suture fixation may be used. Some lenses are not amenable to repositioning. For instance, foldable silicone lenses are less stable than all-PMMA lenses, and lenses with a smaller optic and smaller interhaptic distances are less stable for scleral sutures.[11] Preexisting damage to the haptic or coexisting ocular conditions may also prevent successful repositioning. In some cases a subluxated PCIOL may prove too difficult to retrieve without permanently damaging the retina.

Regardless of whether dislocation or removal is planned, incisions must be made to retrieve the dislo-

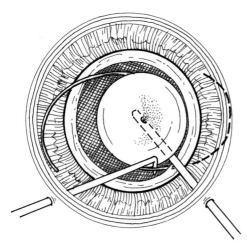

FIGURE 17.4. A Sinskey hook is used to dial the haptic into the anterior chamber (anterior to the iris), and a vitrectomy handpiece is used through a side port incision to relieve vitreous traction as the IOL is manipulated and removed.

cated PCIOL. The locations of the sclerotomies vary, depending on the purpose of the incision. Posterior sclerotomies are preferred by many because they reduce the risk of iris root damage and intraoperative bleeding. However, repositioning through posterior incisions results in IOL fixation more posteriorly to the iris diaphragm. Typically, an incision is made 3 mm posterior to the surgical limbus for intraoperative manipulation and 1.0–1.5 mm posterior to the limbus for scleral suture fixation of PCIOLs. Separate sclerotomies are made 3 mm posterior to the limbus for vitrectomy to avoid damage to fixation sutures, iris root, and ciliary body.[11]

Initial retrieval of a subluxated PCIOL from the posterior vitreous is often the most difficult step. Numerous methods have been described that involve grasping one of the dangling haptics. If the lens is only minimally subluxated or if the peripheral region of the haptic is hidden from view, the cut end of a one-armed suture may be wrapped around the midportion of the haptic and guided back through the sclerotomy. Other techniques for looping the first IOL include introducing a suture loop by threading it down the internal shaft of a needle, creating optic positioning holes for the suture, using three- and four-point fixation, and sewing the suture to the internal lip of the sclerotomy.[32–34] However, techniques involving externalization of the haptic may risk damage to peripheral retinal structures while the haptic is dragged through the vitreous base.

If the lens is completely dislocated into the posterior segment, it may be possible to float the IOL up to the anterior vitreous for further maneuvering by injecting temporary liquid perfluorocarbon (perflubron) (Fig. 17.5).[35–37] If the PCIOL is not too heavy, the dislocated lens will float up into the anterior vitreous immediately posterior to the iris, and loop sutures may be placed around the haptics (Fig. 17.6). First one haptic is

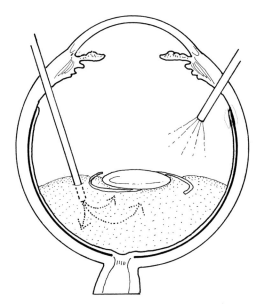

FIGURE 17.5. Technique for removal of luxated PCIOL from vitreous cavity via flotation with perfluorocarbon liquid injection. The IOL may then be maneuvered anteriorly for removal through an enlarged pars plana incision or maneuvered into the anterior chamber for removal through a limbal incision.

successfully looped and guided into the ciliary sulcus, then the second haptic is secured. The lens may be properly centered in the sulcus by maneuvering the sutures.[11]

Regardless of the retrieval method used, proper suture fixation placement is critical for successful repositioning (except when capsular support is utilized); this should be kept in mind during the planning of IOL removal. The ciliary sulcus is located approximately 0.8 mm posterior to the surgical limbus. Excessive torsion on the PCIOL may be avoided by proper suture placement.[16] The surgeon must also decide whether or not to create a scleral flap. Osher et al have described two suturing techniques (Fig. 17.7).[11] Some authors have suggested temporary externalization of the haptic through the sclerotomy for suture knot fixation.[38] Endophthalmitis has been reported following scleral suture fixation in cases without scleral flaps, presumably because the pathogens entered the eye along the suture tract.[16]

If explantation of the PCIOL is necessary, the lens is first guided into the anterior chamber (and removed as previously described). Older designs of PCIOLs required substantial enlargement of original incisions or the creation of a new, large limbal incision for explantation. PCIOLs of more recent design may be removed through small incisions, even through the pars plana. Foldable IOLs present the surgeon with a few options for removal through a small, 3–4 mm incision. If the

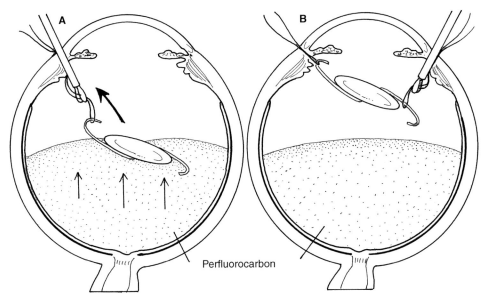

FIGURE 17.6. Technique for repositioning luxated PCIOL from the vitreous cavity. After pars plana incisions have been utilized for vitrectomy and other intraocular maneuvers, more anteriorly placed sclerotomies are made 1.0 mm posterior to the limbus for scleral suture fixation. *A,* Suture loop held by intraocular forceps. The suture loop is placed around the haptic of dislocated PCIOL in the vitreous cavity. *B,* The haptics are repositioned into the ciliary sulcus by maneuvering both haptics anteriorly.

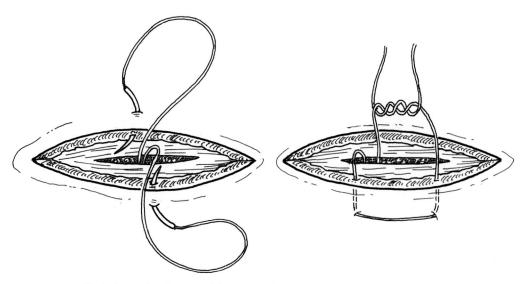

FIGURE 17.7. Techniques for closure of the suture site.

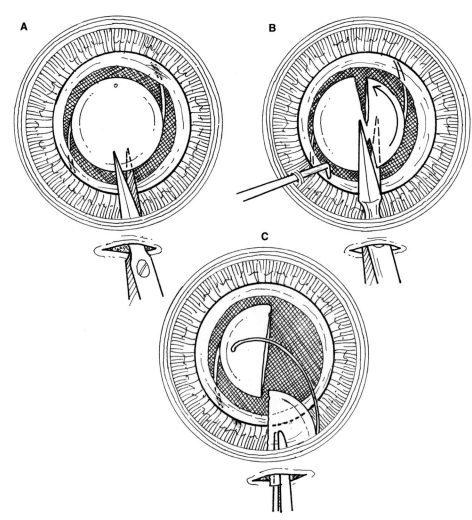

FIGURE 17.8. Bisection of a silicone PCIOL for removal. *A,* The first half of the IOL is bisected with Vanness scissors. *B,* The second half of the IOL is rotated 180 degrees with the Sinskey hook, then bisected. *C,* The bisected IOL segments are removed with forceps.

lens is acrylic, it may be folded prior to removal in one piece. Alternatively, it may be bisected and removed in two pieces.[5] If the lens is silicone, it may also be bisected for removal (Fig. 17.8).[6] Alternatively, the silicone optic is cut across approximately three-quarters of its diameter, and the IOL can then be manipulated longitudinally for removal in one piece.[7]

Removal of Phakic IOLs

Although any surgical intervention risks damage to the endothelial cells, the crystalline lens, the capsule, and the iris, the major advantage of phakic IOLs is the relative ease with which they can be removed or exchanged in comparison with aphakic lenses. The removal technique is relatively straightforward. An incision is made either in the previous wound or at a new site. The anterior chamber is filled with viscoelastic material and the lens is carefully released from its points of fixation and removed.[8,9]

IOL Exchange

In the absence of contraindications, some patients who require IOL removal may tolerate IOL exchange. Techniques for implanting new IOLs are described in other chapters.

■ Conclusions

Complications of IOLs, particularly IOL removal, are rare, but they present the ophthalmic surgeon with challenges regarding appropriate management. The development of a logical surgical plan may lead to improved visual outcome for the patient.

After IOL removal, patients should undergo a thorough ocular examination. Slit-lamp microscopy and gonioscopy should be performed to assess the cornea, iris, vitreous, and retina. If the IOL was repositioned or exchanged, the location of the lens and haptics should be noted. Best corrected visual acuity should be measured. Patients should be evaluated for postoperative resolution of refractive abnormality, visual distortion, uveitis, glaucoma, corneal edema, CME, or other IOL-associated complications. In cases of unexplained reduced visual acuity, specialized studies such as visual field testing and potential acuity meter testing and fluorescein angiography may be required.

■ References

1. Kraff MC, Sanders DR, Raanan MG. A survey of intraocular lens explantations. *J Cataract Refract Surg.* 1986;12: 644–650.
2. Sinskey RM, Amin P, Stoppel JO. Indications for and results of a large series of intraocular lens exchanges. *J Cataract Refract Surg.* 1993;19:68–71.
3. Mamalis N, Crandall AS, Pusipher MW, et al. Intraocular lens explantation and exchange: a review of lens styles, clinical indications, clinical results, and visual outcome. *J Cataract Refract Surg.* 1991;17:811–818.
4. Lindstrom RL. The polymethyl methacrylate (PMMA) intraocular lens. In: Steinert RF, ed. *Cataract Surgery: Technique, Complications, and Management.* Philadelphia: WB Saunders; 1995:271–279.
5. Koo EY, Lindsey PS, Soukiasian SH. Bisecting a foldable acrylic intraocular lens for explantation. *J Cataract Refract Surg.* 1996;22:1381–1382.
6. Koch HR. Lens bisector for silicone intraocular lens removal. *J Cataract Refract Surg.* 1996;22:1379–1380.
7. Batlan SJ, Dodick JM. Explantation of a foldable silicone intraocular lens. *Am J Ophthalmol.* 1996;122:270–272.
8. Garrana RMR, Azar DT. Phakic intraocular lenses for correction of high myopia. *Int Ophthalmol Clin.* 1999;39: 45–57.
9. Waring GO III. Phakic intraocular lenses. In: Fine IH, ed. *Clear Corneal Lens Surgery.* Thorofare, NJ: Slack; 1999: 360–362.
10. Visessook N, Peng Q, Apple DJ, et al. Pathological examination of an explanted phakic posterior chamber intraocular lens. *J Cataract Refract Surg.* 1999;25:216–222.
11. Osher RH, Cionni RJ, Blumenkranz MS. Surgical repositioning and explantation of intraocular lenses. In: Steinert RF, ed. *Cataract Surgery: Technique, Complications, and Management.* Philadelphia: WB Saunders; 1995:341–359.
12. Noecker RJ, Branner WA, Cohen KL. Intraocular lens explantation with and without penetrating keratoplasty. *Ophthalmic Surg.* 1989;20:849–854.
13. Mimouni F, Colin J, Koffi V. Damage to the corneal endothelium from anterior chamber intraocular lenses in phakic myopic eyes. *Refract Corneal Surg.* 1991;7: 277–281.
14. Seymour RG, Ramsey MS. Causes of intraocular lens removal. *Can J Ophthalmol.* 1989; 24:152–154.
15. Sawada T, Kimura W, Kimura T, et al. Long-term follow-up of primary anterior chamber intraocular lens implantation. *J Cataract Refract Surg.* 1998;24:1515–1520.
16. Smiddy WE, Ibanez GV, Alfonso E, et al. Surgical management of dislocated intraocular lenses. *J Cataract Refract Surg.* 1995;21:64–69.
17. Busin M, Cusumano A, Spitznas M. Intraocular lens removal from eyes with chronic low-grade endophthalmitis. *J Cataract Refract Surg.* 1995;21:679–684.
18. Doren GS, Stern GA, Driebe WT. Indications for and results of intraocular lens explantation. *J Cataract Refract Surg.* 1992;18:79–85.
19. Smith SG, Lindquist TD, Lindstrom RL. Removal of intraocular lenses. *Ophthalmic Surg.* Looseleaf and Update Service; 1996:IH 0–11.
20. Winward KE, Pflugfelder SC, Flynn HW, et al. Postoperative *Propionibacterium* endophthalmitis: treatment strategies and long-term results. *Ophthalmology.* 1993;100: 447–451.

21. Chien AM, Raber IM, Fischer DH, et al. *Propionibacterium acnes* endophthalmitis after intracapsular cataract extraction. *Ophthalmology.* 1992;99:487–490.

22. Gimbel HV. Endophthalmitis: immediate management using posterior capsulorhexis and anterior vitrectomy through reopened cataract surgery incision. *J Cataract Refract Surg.* 1997;23:27–31.

23. Teichmann KD. Propionibacterium acnes endophthalmitis requiring intraocular lens removal after failure of medical therapy. *J Cataract Refract Surg.* 2000;26(7):1085–1088.

24. Zimmerman PL, Mamalis N, Alder JB, et al. Chronic *Nocardia asteroides* endophthalmitis after extracapsular cataract extraction. *Arch Ophthalmol.* 1993;111:837–840.

25. Lane SS, Schwartz GS. IOL exchanges and secondary IOLs: surgical techniques. *Focal Points: Clinical Modules for Ophthalmologists.* 1998;16:1–14.

26. Assia EI, Blotnick CA, Powers TP, et al. Clinicopathologic study of ocular trauma in eyes with intraocular lenses. *Am J Ophthalmol.* 1994;117:30–36.

27. Parnes RE, Dailey JR, Aminlari A. Hypotonus cyclodialysis cleft following anterior chamber intraocular lens removal. *Ophthalmic Surg.* 1994;25:386–387.

28. Wiechens B, Winter M, Haigis W, et al. Bilateral cataract after phakic posterior chamber top hat-style silicone intraocular lens. *J Refract Surg.* 1997;13:392–397.

29. Insler MS, Benefield DW, Ross EV. Topical hyperosmolar solutions in the reduction of corneal edema. *CLAO J.* 1987;13:149–151.

30. Harbour JW, Rubsamen PE, Palmberg P. Pars plana vitrectomy in the management of phakic and pseudophakic malignant glaucoma. *Arch Ophthalmol.* 1996;114:1073–1078.

31. Endophthalmitis Vitrectomy Study Group. Results of Endophthalmitis Vitrectomy Study: a randomized trial of immediate vitrectomy and of intravenous antibiotics for the treatment of postoperative bacterial endophthalmitis. *Arch Ophthalmol.* 1995;113:1479–1496.

32. Anand R, Bowman RW. Simplified technique for suturing dislocated posterior chamber intraocular lens to the ciliary sulcus. *Arch Ophthalmol.* 1990;108:1205–1206.

33. Nabors G, Varley MP, Charles S. Ciliary sulcus suturing of a posterior chamber intraocular lens. *Ophthalmic Surg.* 1990;21:263–265.

34. Friedberg MA, Pilkerton AR. A new technique for repositioning and fixating a dislocated intraocular lens. *Arch Ophthalmol.* 1992;110:413–415.

35. Lewis H, Sanchez G. The use of perfluorocarbon liquids in the repositioning of posteriorly dislocated intraocular lenses. *Ophthalmology.* 1993;100:1055–1059.

36. Banker AS, Freeman WR, Vander JF, et al. Use of perflubron as a new temporary vitreous substitute and manipulation agent for vitreoretinal surgery. *Retina.* 1996;16:285–291.

37. Fanous MM, Friedman SM. Ciliary sulcus fixation of a dislocated posterior chamber intraocular lens using liquid perfluorophenanthrene. *Ophthalmic Surg.* 1992;23:551–552.

38. Chan CK. An improved technique for management of dislocated posterior chamber implants. *Ophthalmology.* 1992;99:51–57.

Chapter 18

Surgical Management
of Intraocular Lens Complications

Victor L. Perez and Roberto Pineda

Although cataract surgery is highly successful, IOL-related complications from surgery can be a source of major disappointment for both patient and surgeon. Despite improvements in surgical techniques and IOL design and quality, IOL complications can affect virtually any major structure of the eye. Prompt recognition and understanding of these potential complications is key to their management. In Chapters 11–17, the techniques of secondary IOL implantation, iris- and scleral-fixation, and IOL removal have been described in detail. Minor modifications of these techniques allow for adequate management of several IOL complications. This chapter outlines and classifies IOL complications, emphasizing the more commonly occurring clinical situations, and presents surgical techniques to manage these complications.

■ Deciding When to Perform Surgery

In most cases of IOL complications, the primary question for the surgeon is whether removal of the IOL is indicated. If so, will an IOL exchange be necessary, will IOL repositioning be sufficient, or should the patient be left aphakic? Furthermore, will the procedure improve the patient's symptoms without adding morbidity to that of the original surgery? The answers to these questions are often unclear, and decisions can be difficult to make. Once a decision has been made, a surgical strategy must be devised and thought through.

Although the indication for additional surgery is not always well defined, criteria have been established to help guide surgeons in objectively evaluating the risks and benefits of the proposed procedure. These criteria include the following:[1]

1. The clinical characteristics of the problem—its severity, duration and chronology
2. Results of nonsurgical treatment
3. Natural history of the IOL involved
4. Ease of performing surgery in the affected eye
5. The realistic complications of the procedure
6. The status of the fellow eye
7. Patient and family expectations and visual needs
8. The health needs and life expectancy of the patient

Careful evaluation of each criterion will aid in making the most appropriate decision. It is essential to cover these issues and decide whether surgical intervention would improve visual symptoms, augment the patient's quality of life, and achieve a level of visual rehabilitation consistent with the patient's expectations. Most patients are frustrated by problems from previous surgery and will welcome additional treatment options that could improve their visual function. A discussion among the physician, the patient, and relevant family members should be planned to provide a clear understanding of the treatment options and potential risks before a final decision is made. Open, frank communication is very important during this process.

■ IOL-Related Complications and Surgical Procedures

Optical Complications

Incorrect IOL Power Calculation
Poor postoperative vision due to an unsatisfactory refractive error can be a very disconcerting problem, especially after uneventful surgery. Two primary

preoperative factors affect lens power determination: keratometry and axial length (A-scan measurement). Errors in either the keratometry reading or the axial length will result in significant discrepancies in the IOL power. Additionally, the use of older IOL calculation formulas or insertion of the wrong IOL power can result in postoperative refractive error surprises. A 1-diopter error in the keratometry reading will result in an approximately equal error in the final prescription. A 1-mm error in the axial length will result in about a 2.5-diopter error in the desired outcome. Today, only advanced IOL power calculation formulas should be used. We recommend the Hoffer-Q or Holladay II IOL calculation formulas for short eyes (<22 mm), the SRK-T formula for long eyes (>26 mm), and the Holladay I formula for medium-long eyes (24.5–26 mm). Positional changes of the IOL (sulcus) can also produce unanticipated refractive errors postoperatively. A sulcus or iris-fixated lens will usually add −0.25 to −0.50 diopter of myopia to the final postoperative refraction (see Chapters 4 and 13).

As interest in refractive surgery continues to rise, with an estimated 1.8 million refractive surgery procedures predicted for the year 2002, special attention will be required for patients who need cataract surgery after refractive surgery in order to achieve satisfactory optical outcomes (see Chapters 1 and 4).

Anisometropia also creates a clinical dilemma for the patient when there is a discrepancy between the phakic eye and pseudophakic eye that does not allow simultaneous binocular vision owing to optical anieskonia. To maintain binocularity, a patient usually cannot tolerate a difference of more than 3 diopters between the phakic and the pseudophakic eye.[1] Moreover, anisometropia is the most common cause of aniseikonia, and 40% of pseudophakic patients have symptoms attributable to aniseikonia (Fig. 18.1).[2] One diopter of spectacle-corrected anisometropia introduces a 1% size difference, and as a general rule, patients cannot tolerate more than a 5% image size difference. When visual complaints are significant to the patient and cannot be addressed with spectacle or contact lens correction, the following surgical procedures can be considered.

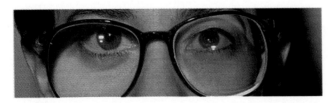

FIGURE 18.1. Myopic patient with aphakic correction (plus lens) in the right eye and a minus lens in the left eye. Anisometropia is the most common cause of aniseikonia.

Surgical Procedure—Cataract Extraction in the Fellow Eye

If the phakic eye has cataract changes that are clinically significant, cataract extraction with IOL implantation can be performed. Previous studies have shown that results in the first eye can be used to guide the power of the lens implanted in the second eye and reduce the risk of symptoms such as anisometropia.[3] Based on use of the appropriate advanced IOL power calculation formula (discussed in Chapter 4) and the surgeon's deciding with the patient the desired final outcome, emmetropia or the intended final refractive correction can be reasonably achieved.

Surgical Procedure—PCIOL Explantation and Exchange

Incorrect IOL power is one of the most common causes of posterior chamber IOL (PCIOL) explantation.[4,5] Several authors have suggested that IOL exchange should be considered the procedure of choice, particularly in the early postoperative period.[6] In a series review of 79 patients, Sinskey et al reported that IOL exchange could be performed with a relatively low risk of decreased visual acuity.[4] Murphy and Murphy felt that in patients with severe symptoms of anisometropia due to incorrect IOL power, IOL exchange is a viable option.[3]

Procedure: Explantation of a PCIOL for incorrect power is usually performed in cases in which the original procedure was uneventful, and is done early in the postoperative period. Therefore, factors such as intraocular adhesions and prolapsed vitreous are rarely encountered. However, if present, they should be managed appropriately, as described below. IOLs can be removed either through a limbal incision or through a clear corneal incision. The size of the wound can range from 3.0 mm to 6.0 mm, depending on the material of the IOL to be explanted. If the IOL is made of material that can easily be cut once the IOL is in the anterior chamber, a small incision can be used in combination with a newly implanted foldable IOL. If explantation is performed early in the postoperative period (<6 weeks), the original cataract incision (clear cornea or scleral tunnel) can be used without the need for an additional wound. If not, a paracentesis site is selected approximately 180 degrees away from the wound in the horizontal axis and viscoelastic material is injected into the anterior chamber. The PCIOL is then rotated out of the bag or sulcus into the anterior chamber using two Sinskey hooks. For nonfoldable IOLs, the haptic loops may require amputation, but this is not always necessary. Haptic excision can be performed using a specially designed haptic cutter or a McGills scissors. This allows the surgeon to freely

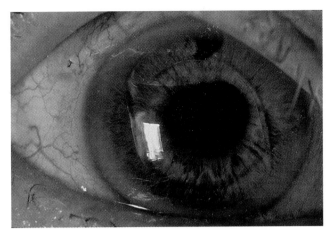

FIGURE 18.2. Kelman-style ACIOL. A PCIOL can be explanted and an ACIOL of appropriate power can be placed.

manipulate the optic in the anterior chamber and remove it through the wound (see Chapter 17 for a more detailed description of IOL explantation techniques).

Alternatively, if the IOL material can be cut (acrylic included), a McGills scissors or one of several snare-designed devices can be employed to divide the IOL and remove it through a smaller size wound (2.75–3.5 mm). The new IOL can then be appropriately placed in the bag or sulcus, depending on the integrity of the capsular bag and zonular support after IOL explantation. It is important to maintain the anterior chamber with viscoelastic material during the procedure to minimize trauma to surrounding intraocular structures. It may be necessary to use more than one syringe of viscoelastic medium to ensure an atraumatic procedure. Subsequent thorough removal of the viscoelastic medium at the completion of the IOL exchange is essential to prevent a postoperative intraocular pressure spike. If the posterior capsule or zonular support is compromised, then an alternative procedure for PCIOL fixation may be required (see Chapter 14) or an anterior chamber IOL (ACIOL) can be placed (Fig. 18.2; see also Chapter 11).

Surgical Procedure—Refractive Corneal Surgery

In cases of extensive tissue adhesion to the IOL and damage to the intraocular structures from the primary surgery, IOL exchange may be a poor choice of treatment. In these situations, refractive surgery may be an alternative. Both radial keratotomy and excimer laser photorefractive keratectomy have been found to be effective in the treatment of residual myopic error in pseudophakic eyes.[7,8] Newer refractive surgery techniques such as laser in situ keratomileusis (LASIK) and hyperopic and astigmatic laser correction are adding to the choice of alternative treatments. To date, no well-published studies exist addressing therapy in this subgroup of patients. (See Chapter 19 for details.)

Mechanical Malposition of IOL: Subluxation, Dislocation, and Tilt

IOL malposition is an indication for IOL explantation, especially for PCIOLs.[4] Malpositioning of the IOL can result from the original placement of the lens during surgery or may develop later as a result of several factors, such as the location of the haptics, capsular contraction forces, or subsequent eye injury. Although malposition can occur with both anterior and posterior chamber lenses, malposition of a PCIOL is more likely to cause optical complications such as unstable vision, monocular diplopia, decreased vision, halos, glare, optical aberrations, photosensitivity, and ghost images.[2,9] Significant decentration can also induce prism and decreased vergence leading to binocular diplopia, particularly if occurring in the vertical meridian. The amount of prism can be calculated using the Prentice equation: IOL power (in Diopters) multiplied by the magnitude of optic displacement (in cm).

ACIOLs have the least tendency toward malposition. However, when malposition of an ACIOL occurs, it is usually related to an error in IOL sizing. Migration of the haptic footplate through a peripheral iridectomy (particularly with three-point fixation lenses) can cause the implant to tilt and lead to corneal touch by the opposing haptic. IOL tilt usually does not require treatment because the optic portion of the lens rests close to the visual axis and the vision is unaffected. However, if there is obvious corneal contact with the ACIOL or localized edema in the peripheral cornea with confirmation of IOL touch by gonioscopy, then repositioning or removal is recommended. Decentration of the ACIOL is most commonly seen within the first 6 months postoperatively and can be caused by asymmetric adhesions around the haptics, residual capsulolenticular fibrosis, iris incarceration, and peripheral anterior synechiae (PAS). The most frequent cause of ACIOL decentration is vitreous fibroplasia from residual vitreous left in the anterior chamber at the time of surgery (see Chapter 11).

As with ACIOLs, dislocation or decentration of iris-supported implants is rarely encountered. However, as a general rule, with dislocation or decentration of an iris-supported IOL, lens explantation or exchange for an ACIOL or PCIOL should be performed.[10] Surgical repositioning can be considered if explantation or exchange would pose a risk of additional complications, such as corneal edema in an elderly patient with a low endothelial cell count.

Several situations can contribute to PCIOL decentration, including capsular or zonular rupture, capsular

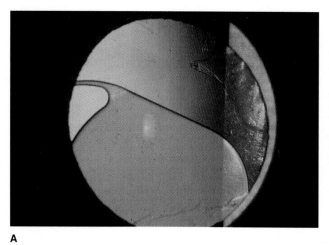
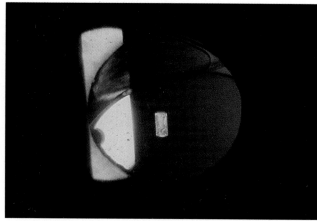

A

B

FIGURE 18.3. *A* and *B,* Inferior migration of the PCIOL occurs in cases of capsular or zonular disruption.

fibrosis, vitreous loss, asymmetric haptic fixation, haptic deformation, and cortical remnants with progressive PAS.[9] Subluxated PCIOLs are classified according to the anatomic cause and the migration of the lens within the posterior and anterior chambers. Lateral decentration of the PCIOL is commonly seen with the "capsular contraction syndrome," in which fibrosis and contraction of the anterior capsular opening causes capsular tension and differential forces induce lateral migration of the implant. This scenario is encountered in pseudoexfoliation, small capsulorrhexis (<4 mm), and when haptics are asymmetrically fixated. The "sunset syndrome" refers to inferior migration of the PCIOL and commonly occurs in cases of capsular or zonular disruption and vitreous loss (Fig. 18.3).[9] Superior PCIOL subluxation is known as the "sunrise syndrome" and has been ascribed to a number of mechanisms (see Chapter 13).[9]

Two additional types of PCIOL malposition complications can be encountered—IOL dislocation and IOL tilt. With PCIOL dislocation, violation of the vitreous cavity by the dislocated PCIOL occurs in the setting of inadequate zonular and capsular support. Although this most frequently happens intraoperatively, it has been reported up to 31 months after insertion.[11] In contrast, IOL tilt is primarily a complication of suture-fixated PCIOLs, but it also can be seen with ACIOLs and mispositioned PCIOLs in which one haptic is in the bag and the other haptic is in the sulcus. Pseudophakic IOL tilt can cause visually significant problems in up to 3.3% of patients with suture-fixated IOLs.[9]

Regardless of the type of subluxation, most cases can be addressed by nonsurgical intervention with initial reassurance and pharmacologic agents.[12] Miotics can reduce symptoms of glare and optical distortion by reducing the pupillary aperture, thereby minimizing the edge effect of the IOL optic.[13] If the symptoms are not relieved or if there is progression of subluxation, worsening of vision, excessive uveal touch, persistent uveitis, or retinal injury, surgical management is recommended.[14] Conceptually, the goal in correcting subluxations or dislocations is to convert the PCIOL from an in-the-bag position to an in-the-sulcus position without removing the lens.[15]

Surgical Procedures—PCIOL Rotation and Repositioning

This procedure should be used when the capsule is intact and the haptics of the IOL are not deformed.[9] IOL rotation should not be performed when the haptics have loops or positioning hooks (see Chapter 1) that could tear the capsule during the rotation.

Procedure: Two paracentesis incisions are made at the limbus approximately 180 degrees apart in the horizontal axis. Viscoelastic material is injected into the anterior chamber. It may be necessary to "visco-inflate" the capsular bag in order to free the IOL haptic and perform the rotation. Fused capsular leaflets can be separated using the viscoelastic cannula or with a Sinskey hook followed by the viscoelastic cannula. To manipulate the IOL, two Sinskey hooks are used to rotate the optic from its subluxated position into the pupillary space while the operator maneuvers the haptics into the ciliary sulcus. To achieve this, the Sinskey hooks must be placed into the optic-haptic junction or positioning holes of the IOL.[9] Alternatively, if there is concern for significant loss of capsular support, the pupil can be dilated and the IOL completely rotated out of the posterior chamber and into the anterior chamber. A Kuglen hook or Y-hook can then be used to inspect the peripheral capsule for integrity by manipulating the iris. Once the stability of the capsule has been determined, the IOL can be positioned in the safest location. Sinskey hooks are often used to perform this procedure. Once centered, the IOL is gently tapped to ensure stability. If movement of the capsular bag is observed during the rotation, another procedure will need to be considered, such as suture fixation of the current IOL or IOL exchange.

Surgical Procedure—Iris-Supported IOL Repositioning

Surgical reposition of iris-supported IOLs is considered in cases in which an exchange or explantation procedure may be risky. An example is an elderly patient with a low endothelial cell count.

Procedure: Little or no viscoelastic medium should be used, because it can be difficult to remove it at the end of the procedure without disturbing the vitreous. Similarly, the use of fluid may be undesirable because hydration of the vitreous body can collapse the anterior chamber and put the corneal endothelium at risk. Two limbal paracentesis incisions are made 180 degrees apart in strategically planned locations that will allow effective manipulation of the haptics. One Sinskey hook is used to retract and depress the iris while the other is used to elevate and decenter the optic in the opposite direction. Once the haptics have been carefully repositioned, the pupil is constricted with miotic agent to ensure proper fixation.[10]

Surgical Procedure—Modified McCannel Suture Technique

A suture technique is used when the capsule is significantly ruptured, the zonules are ruptured over more than 3 clock hours, or the haptics are deformed. It can also be performed when there is PCIOL instability after an IOL rotation procedure.[9,13] The procedure is described in detail in Chapter 13. Briefly, two paracentesis wounds are made near the limbus in the horizontal axis, and the anterior chamber is filled with viscoelastic medium. The optic of the IOL is centered with two Sinskey hooks and elevated to induce pupillary capture.[9] After injection of a miotic agent, constriction of the pupil over the PCIOL will indent the midperipheral iris to create an area of elevation over the optic-haptic junction. A single-armed 10-0 polypropylene (prolene) suture on a CIF-4 or CTC-6 needle (Ethicon, Somerville, NJ) is passed through a paracentesis wound into the anterior chamber, beneath the haptic, through the iris, and out through the peripheral cornea. The needle is cut after it passes through the peripheral cornea, and a Sinskey or Kuglen hook is used to capture the polypropylene suture intraocularly and pull it out

through the primary paracentesis wound. A collar-button or Y-hook can then be used to tie down the knot. The knot is trimmed and the iris redeposited to its normal position. The knot should be tied tightly and the knot ends should not be too short when polypropylene suture is used. Additional McCannel sutures may be required to stabilize the IOL. Finally, the optic is repositioned behind the iris and the viscoelastic medium is removed from the anterior chamber.[9] (see Figs. 13.1–13.6) However, if vitreous is present in the anterior chamber at the time of surgery, the IOL should be fixated first, followed by a mechanical anterior vitrectomy to prevent complete loss of the IOL into the vitreous cavity.

Surgical Procedure—PCIOL Exchange with Suture Fixation

IOL exchange with suture fixation is necessary in eyes with inadequate or no capsular support or with extensive zonular dehiscence, or when a major anterior vitrectomy is required. This procedure is also indicated when haptic amputation is required owing to fibrosis, adhesions, or the danger of capsular destablization (see Chapter 17).

Procedure: Partial-thickness triangular scleral flaps or a partial-thickness groove 3 mm in length are made in the oblique meridians (4 and 10, or 2 and 8) 1 mm posterior to the limbus. Through a limbal wound, the subluxated IOL is extracted from the eye and viscoelastic material is injected to push the vitreous posteriorly. Posterior synechiae, if present, are lysed, to provide access to the ciliary sulcus. A limited anterior mechanical vitrectomy is then performed to remove vitreous from the wound, anterior chamber, and areas adjacent to the oblique meridians. A one-piece PMMA PCIOL lens with a 7.0-mm optic and modified C-loops is suggested, such as the IOLAB model 6840B (Claremont, CA). A double-armed 10-0 polypropylene suture like the CIF-4 (Ethicon) or CTC-6 needle is tied or passed through each of the haptic loops. The inferior haptic sutures are then passed through the wound, into the anterior chamber, under the iris, and out through the ciliary sulcus beneath the scleral flap or in the groove. The superior haptic sutures are passed in similar fashion. The transscleral sutures are then buried under the half-thickness flaps or rotated in the groove to prevent suture erosion.[9] The IOL is assessed for proper positioning and stability, and the IOL wound is closed with interrupted 10-0 nylon sutures.

Surgical Procedure—Scleral Fixation Sutures for PCIOLs Dislocated into the Vitreous

This technique allows the repositioning and fixation of dislocated IOLs in the vitreous with no available capsular or zonular support. It is important to recognize that in certain situations, repositioning may not be a suitable option. The IOL structural stability, size, and haptic design are factors that will influence this decision.[10] For example, foldable silicone IOLs are less suitable for repositioning than PMMA IOLs, which have a more stable configuration. IOLs with smaller optical zones (<6-mm optics) are more likely to produce an optical edge effect and remain less stable when suspended from the scleral sutures.[10] Thin and short haptics (J-loops) do not provide the necessary support to achieve a stable IOL position after suturing.[10] Another important consideration in these cases is the benefit of performing a vitrectomy. When a vitrectomy is performed, vitreoretinal tractional forces induced by the IOL repositioning will be significantly reduced or eliminated, thereby minimizing the risk of cystoid macular edema (CME) and retinal detachment (RD).[11]

The surgical techniques are similar to many of those described in Chapter 14. Conjunctival incisions are made at 12 and 6 o'clock and two superior sclerotomies are made 3 mm posterior to the limbus for the purpose of vitrectomy and other intraoperative maneuvers. Two triangular scleral flaps are made in the oblique meridians 1.0 mm posterior to the limbus, and sclerostomy incisions are placed beneath the flap for suture fixation purposes. In cases of limited PCIOL dislocation with visualization of the peripheral aspect of the haptic, the cut end of a 9-0 or 10-0 polypropylene (prolene) suture can be wrapped around the mid-portion of the haptic and pulled back through the sclerotomy and secured. The second haptic can then be grasped with a second suture loop passed through the sclerostomy 180 degrees away and used to center and secure the lens.[10,16] Figure 18.4 describes the double-knot technique of trans-scleral–suture fixation for displaced IOLs.[16] In cases of decentered silicone plate IOLs, the double-knot technique may be more complex but may avoid explantation (Fig. 18.5).[17]

Alternatively, if the IOL has completely dislocated into the vitreous, the first haptic can initially be pulled into the ciliary sulcus region with the loop suture and then maneuvered as previously described. Once the lens is centered posterior to the iris, the sutures are tightened for permanent fixation. The edges of the prolene suture are then inverted at the sclerotomy wound and the flaps are oversewn with absorbable 8-0 Vicryl sutures (Ethicon).

Precipitates on the Lens Optic

IOL precipitates are composed of pigment, inflammatory cells, fibrin, blood breakdown products, and other elements (Fig. 18.6).[18] Precipitates usually occur early in the postoperative period and frequently clear spontaneously as the operate eye quiets down. However, in some cases the IOL precipitates persist and become visually significant.

Surgical Procedure — Nd:YAG Laser Therapy

The primary indication is visually significant precipitates on the surface of IOL optic that do not resolve despite appropriate anti-inflammatory therapy and that are not accompanied by intraocular inflammation. Patient complaints include glare and decreased vision.

Procedure: Precipitates can be removed from the IOL surface using a neodymium:yttrium-aluminum-garnet (Nd:YAG) laser. This laser has a wavelength of 1,064 nm and can disrupt tissue by achieving optical breakdown with a short, high-power pulse.[19] Optical breakdown results in the ionization or plasma formation of tissue, which then causes shock waves that disrupt tissue into the aqueous. The laser energy setting recommended for "IOL optic dusting" is 2–3 mJ.[10] After focusing the aiming beam of the laser on the anterior surface of the IOL, the operator slightly defocuses the laser anteriorly for anterior optic precipitates. When the laser is fired, the pressure generated by the optical breakdown in front of the target liberates the IOL precipitate into the aqueous, leaving the IOL optic clear in that area. This technique minimizes the risk of pitting or cracking the IOL optic. The lowest Nd:YAG power setting should be used initially and increased until the desired effect is achieved. It is not usually necessary to remove all precipitates from the IOL optic in order to improve the patient's symptoms.

Capsular Complications

Capsule Contraction Syndrome

The capsule contraction syndrome is an exaggerated reduction in the anterior capsulectomy opening and the equatorial bag diameter that occurs after extracapsular cataract extraction (ECCE).[18] The contraction of the capsular bag is caused by fibrous dysplasia of residual lens epithelial cells (LECs) countered by unopposed weak zonular support. This phenomenon is commonly seen in patients with pseudoexfoliation, or advanced age, or in association with uveitis, pars planitis, and muscular dystrophy.[20,21] By identifying this patient population preoperatively, the surgeon can modify certain steps during the initial surgery to minimize the risk that this complication will develop subsequently. It is recommended that the capsulorrhexis be well centered and more than 5.0 mm in diameter. Alternatively, a "can-opener" capsulectomy and a single-piece PMMA IOL can be used to maintain capsular bag size and shape stability.

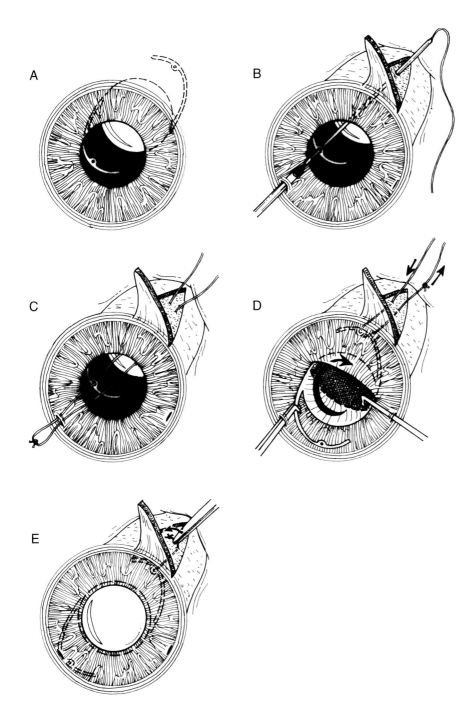

FIGURE 18.4. *A,* Sunset syndrome (LE) with inferior displacement of intraocular lens optic and haptics, surgeon's view. The intraocular lens is displaced inferonasally, and the superior haptic islet is visualized within the pupil. *B,* A straight needle is passed with a 10-0 Prolene suture from the inferonasal scleral flap, through the islet haptic, anterior to the iris, and then out the superotemporal paracentesis site with a 30-gauge needle as a guidewire. *C,* A second needle is passed as in *(B)* but enters the sclera 1 mm from the first suture and passes above, not through, the haptic islet. The two ends of the 10-0 Prolene sutures are tied outside the eye at the superotemporal paracentesis site. Thus the suture forms a semicircular loop beginning and ending at the scleral flap, traveling around the haptic (or through the islet of the IOL haptic, if present) and forming a loop through the diagonally opposite paracentesis. The technique for a haptic islet can be modified in the absence of a haptic islet, with one pass in front of the haptic and the second pass behind it. *D,* The IOL is brought up into the anterior chamber with an intraocular forceps and Sinskey hook through the paracentesis sites. Once in the anterior chamber, the IOL is rotated clockwise, to bring the suture-looped haptic inferiorly in line with the scleral flap incision and to bring the once-inferior haptic superiorly in line with the intact zonular support area. Once correctly aligned, the suture is rotated to externalize the knot. *E,* The IOL is dropped back down into the posterior chamber, and the suture is pulled to position the optic properly and then tied to the sclera to tether the haptic in place. The first knot is discarded when the second knot is trimmed. This second knot is then internalized with tying forceps. The other haptic is supported in the ciliary sulcus with capsule and zonular support. The IOL is now well positioned and stable. *(From Azar DT, Wiley WF. Double-knot transscleral suture fixation technique for displaced intraocular lenses. Am J Ophthalmol. 1999, 128(5):644–646, with permission from Elsevier Science.)*

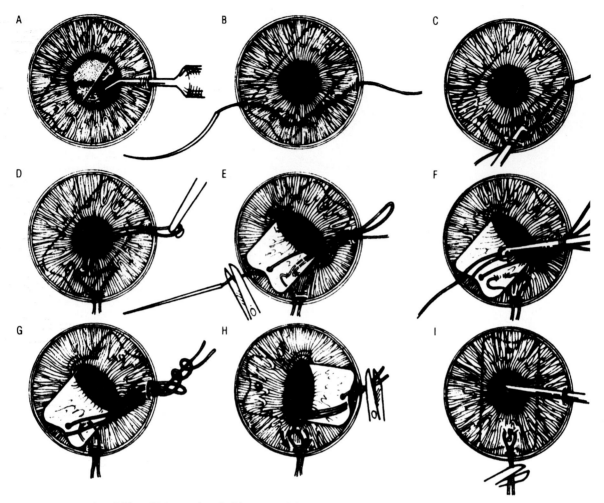

FIGURE 18.5. *A* to *I,* Two 10-0 nonabsorbable surgical (Prolene) sutures are used to preplace an iris loop and a loop around the intraocular lens eyelet. The loops are sutured together at the 9-o'clock position, and the intraocular lens is repositioned by anchoring the iris sutures at the 12-o'clock position. (The figures are drawn from the surgeon's perspective; *From Azar DT, Clamen LM. Iris fixation of a decentered silicone plate haptic intraocular lens double knot technique.* Arch Opthalmol. *1998;116(6):821–823, with permission. Copyright © 1998, American Medical Association.)*

Surgical Procedure—Nd:YAG Laser Therapy

When capsular contraction syndrome is recognized, Nd:YAG laser disruption of the anterior capsular margin should be performed.[22] This entity can occur as early as 2–3 weeks postoperatively and is most effectively treated when early contraction of the anterior capsule is noted.[20]

Procedure: With the Nd:YAG laser, pulses of 2–3 mJ are applied to the edge of the capsulorrhexis at least in four quadrants. The laser cuts are extended radially with one or two additional pulses. This will prevent further contraction because the margin of the anterior capsule will no longer have an integrity that can maintain the contractional forces. To prevent damage to the surface of the PCIOL, the aiming laser beams should be defocused slightly anteriorly, as described earlier. Re-currence of the capsule contraction is not uncommon if the anterior capsule laser cuts are poorly defined.

Posterior Capsule Opacification

Posterior capsule opacification (PCO) results from LECs that proliferate over the posterior capsule from the site of apposition of the anterior capsule flaps in patients who have undergone cataract extraction (Fig. 18.7). These cells eventually transform into fibroblasts with contractile capacity; the fibroblasts produce collagen deposits, which results in the formation of an opaque white fibrotic membrane behind the IOL.[23] The time of PCO formation varies from month to years in adults; however, in younger patients it occurs within 2 years after surgery.[24] Factors that may delay or prevent PCO formation include a wide anterior capsulotomy and the

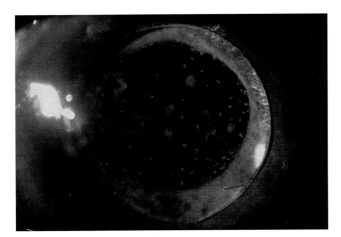

FIGURE 18.6. Intraocular lens precipitates are usually composed of pigment or inflammatory cells.

use of a convex PCIOL.[19] In addition, certain IOL materials and designs also seem to augment the rate of PCO formation (see Chapter 15).

Surgical Procedure—Nd:YAG Laser Capsulotomy

Nd:YAG laser capsulotomy is indicated for PCO that results in decreased visual acuity, marked glare, or impairment of the patient's ability to function. This procedure should not be done in patients with corneal scars, irregularities, or edema, which can interfere with visualization of the target and focusing of the laser. Potential complications include intraocular pressure spike, IOL pitting or cracking, decreased visual acuity, uveitis, IOL dislocation, CME, and RD.

Procedure: Dilation of the pupil with 2.5% phenylephrine and 1% tropicamide is recommended for good visualization of the capsule. A contact lens (Peyman or central Abraham) can be used to stabilize the eye and

improve laser focusing. The minimal amount of energy that causes tissue disruption should be used. The setting commonly used for Nd:YAG capsulotomies is 1–2 mJ/pulse.[19] To obtain the largest opening per pulse, areas of tension lines should be identified and laser shots used to cut across them. To perform a cruciate opening, laser pulses are initiated at the 12 o'clock position in the midperiphery, progressing toward the 6 o'clock position. By beginning at the superior and peripheral portion of the posterior capsule, the surgeon can check and modify the laser settings before treating the critical visual axis. Cuts are then made at the 3 and 9 o'clock positions and residual tags are cleaned up. The capsulotomy size should be as large as the pupil aperture in ambient light, usually 4 mm. To prevent an eccentric capsulotomy, pupil size must be determined before dilation is performed. Apraclonodine or a β-blocker should be administered immediately before, or after, the procedure or at both times to minimize an intraocular pressure increase. Retinal complications of Nd:YAG laser capsulotomy are discussed in Chapter 16.

Pupil and Iris Complications

Pupillary Capture

Pupillary capture occurs when a portion of the IOL optic passes anterior to the iris (Fig. 18.8). It is seen frequently with planar PCIOLs; however, anterior angulation of the haptics has decreased the prevalence of this phenomenon.[25,26] Although it is not considered a serious problem, patients with pupillary capture will have an irregular pupil, may have limited dilation of the pupil, and may develop inflammation. Minor decentration of the optic is also seen but will be asymptomatic, if the lens remains stable. Significant decentration is usually associated with the formation of irregular

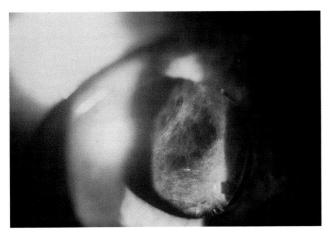

A

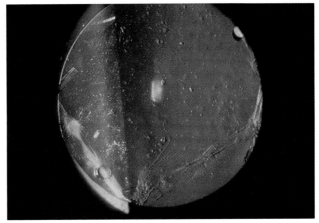

B

FIGURE 18.7. *A* and *B,* Migration of lens epithelial cells causes posterior capsule opacification.

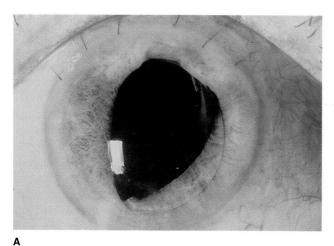
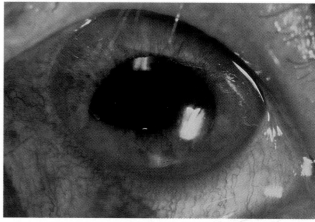

A   **B**

FIGURE 18.8. *A* and *B,* Pupillary capture occurs when a portion of the optic of a PCIOL passes anterior to the iris.

adhesions between the residual anterior capsule and the underlying posterior capsule. Pupillary capture must be corrected early, before these adhesions develop. Initially, dilation of the pupil should be attempted with the patient supine. When the optic falls back into the posterior chamber, the pupil is constricted with 2% pilocarpine or 0.25% echothiophate iodide.

Surgical Procedure—IOL Tapping
If the pupil cannot be dilated enough to allow the optic to fall back behind the iris in the posterior chamber or if recapture reoccurs with pupillary constriction, IOL tapping is necessary.

Procedure: After dilation of the pupil, a corneal stab wound is made at the limbus. Through this wound, the IOL can be tapped either with a spatula or with a sharp 27-gauge needle attached to a syringe. Topical anesthesia alone usually suffices for the tapping procedure. A sterile setting is required. There have also been reports of use of the Nd:YAG shock wave, similar to IOL dusting, to push the PCIOL into the posterior chamber.

Iris Tuck
In this condition, a segment or fold of the peripheral iris is trapped in the angle by the ACIOL haptic.[27] Iris tuck can occur during ACIOL placement if the lens is placed too posteriorly. It can also occur when the size of the ACIOL is incorrect. An oval pupil with the vertical axis parallel to the axis of the IOL is characteristic of iris tuck.[27] Minimal to moderate tuck may only be cosmetically problematic, but if it is accompanied by pain, chronic inflammation, or corneal or macular complications, surgical correction is necessary.

Surgical Procedure—ACIOL Repositioning
Repositioning can be performed when iris tuck is diagnosed early and the size of the ACIOL is correct and amenable to easy rotation in the anterior chamber. Repositioning should be performed with sterile technique.

Procedure: A paracentesis wound is made 180 degrees away from the site of the principal wound. Viscoelastic material is injected into the anterior chamber. A limbal incision is made near the sector where the haptic to be repositioned is located. The wound should be large enough that the haptic can be brought out of the eye to enable the ACIOL to be rotated. The ACIOL can be handled carefully with angled McPhearson forceps and viscoelastic assistance. Moving the IOL toward the distal part of the anterior chamber can cause a tear of the iris root and should be avoided. Once the implant is in place, the proximal haptic is placed in the angle of the anterior chamber by retracting the scleral lip of the incision. After viscoelastic has been removed from the eye, the wound is closed with interrupted 10-0 nylon sutures.

Surgical Procedure—ACIOL Explantation
ACIOLs should be explanted in the presence of significant pain, chronic inflammation, corneal complications, or CME. Oversized, rigid ACIOLs that tuck the iris most often require explantation.

Procedure: After a paracentesis wound has been made and the anterior chamber has been filled with viscoelastic medium, synechiolysis can be performed using viscoelastic and the attached cannula. If extensive adhesions are present, the haptics should be severed from the optic to avoid damage to the iris and angle and hemorrhage during manipulation of the optic. Several well-designed haptic cutters are available. A spatula is placed under the optic and used as a ramp to remove the ACIOL from the eye without damaging the posterior scleral lip of the wound. Once the optic has been explanted, the haptics are threaded back through the synechial tunnels and mobilized in the anterior chamber, where they can easily be removed with fine forceps.

Corneal Complications

Corneal Decompensation: IOL Syndromes

The use of an IOL implant has been associated with an increased risk of corneal edema years after cataract surgery (Fig. 18.9).[28] In fact, progressive loss of vision secondary to corneal edema was the leading cause of IOL explantation in several clinical studies.[29,30] Newer IOL designs, refinements in surgical technique, and placement of the implant in the posterior chamber have made this complication less common, and it is now most commonly seen after IOL dislocation.[2] Corneal edema is caused by excessive loss of endothelial cells at the time of surgery and by the type of implant used. The average loss of endothelial cells following routine cataract extraction has been reported to vary between 8% and 12%.[31] When an iris-supported IOL is inserted, endothelial cell loss is increased by 34%–72% as compared to PCIOL insertion, after which endothelial cell loss is minimal and the incidence of pseudophakic bullous keratopathy (PBK) is low, 1%–2%.[32,33]

Endothelial cell loss caused by an implant can be attributed to several mechanisms: IOL design, direct touch, and trauma due to IOL instability resulting in mechanical damage or inflammation. An increased incidence of PBK has been associated with use of semiflexible closed-loop IOLs.[34] Moreover, flexible, open, thin-loop ACIOLs with position holes or eyelets

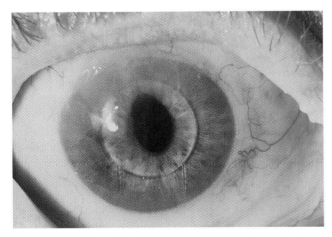

FIGURE 18.9. Corneal endothelial decompensation and edema occur due to IOL touch.

(Dubroff style), can erode into the angle, acting as a closed-loop IOL, and inducing corneal decompensation.[2,35,36] Excessive IOL mobility, pseudophakodonesis, can cause direct trauma to the cornea, a setup for chronic inflammation. This, in turn, can be detrimental to the endothelium. Unacceptable pseudophakodonesis can be evaluated on slit-lamp examination by noting "shimmering" of the anterior and posterior surfaces of the IOL with subtle eye movements.[2] Direct corneal touch can occur centrally or at the periphery. It is commonly associated with the use of ACIOLs and may be caused by improper positioning, migration, tilt, or excessive vaulting. Although patients initially may have no signs or symptoms of corneal decompensation, peripheral corneal IOL touch causes loss of endothelial cells locally and eventual migration of endothelial cells from the central cornea to the periphery. This process ultimately results in central corneal edema. Clinical recognition of these mechanisms is crucial and will help guide treatment. Objective indicators of poor endothelial reserve may include low cell density (<500 cells/mm^2), abnormal cell morphology (polymegathism or pleomorphism), or increased thickness on pachymetry.[2]

The decision to exchange an IOL in the presence of corneal complications can be controversial, especially in patients with good vision and intermittent evidence of IOL touch, pseudophakodonesis, or inflammation. Once a plan has been determined, the goal of surgery is to avoid the need for future procedures that could increase the risk of complications and compromise vision. A distinction must therefore be made between eyes that require only an IOL exchange or repositioning and eyes that would benefit from exchange and PK. This question requires serial examinations to determine a clinical trend of stability or decompensation. Evaluations should include cell density, cell morphology, corneal thickness, and assessment of IOL anomalies. Early exchange would be indicated in patients with good endothelial reserve but who demonstrate clinical progression of corneal decompensation. The IOL design also influences the decision. In patients with an ACIOL and clinical progression, explantation with or without PK would be recommended.[37] On the other hand, certain groups of patients are managed better with IOL explantation combined with PK after visually significant corneal decompensation.[2] This group includes patients with low endothelial cell counts (<500 cells/mm^2) or with preexisting corneal disorders, such as Fuchs' corneal endothelial dystrophy.

Surgical Procedures—IOL Exchange

Implant exchange should be considered in cases of documented clinical progression of peripheral corneal edema and good endothelial reserve. Other factors influencing the surgical decision include the type of implant (closed-loop ACIOL or iris-fixated IOL), the presence of malposition or tilt with corneal touch, and peripheral corneal contact by the haptic. The implant can be exchanged for either an open-loop ACIOL or a suture-fixated PCIOL. The surgical procedure involves removal of the IOL (see Chapter 17) followed by the insertion of another IOL (see Chapters 11 and 14).

Surgical Procedure—Penetrating Keratoplasty with IOL Exchange

PK is performed when there is clinical evidence of irreversible corneal decompensation (edema) responsible for poor visual function. In cases of cataract surgery, corneal transplantation should be delayed for at least 3–4 months, and intraocular inflammation must be well controlled. The decision of what implant is best to use varies with each case. Visual results after PK and IOL insertion vary considerably among different studies and are not conclusive regarding the style of IOL that would offer the patient a better outcome or fewer complications.[38]

A conjunctival peritomy is made and scleral flaps are raised at the site of suture fixation about 1 mm posterior to the limbus and 3 mm in length. The 1:30 and 7:30 o'clock limbal positions are preferred sites to minimize involvement of the long posterior ciliary arteries and nerves. The host cornea button is trephined and cut. If an ACIOL is present, it is carefully removed and an anterior vitrectomy is performed using an automated vitrectomy instrument. The anterior chamber is filled with viscoelastic medium, and synechialysis and/or iris reconstruction is performed in appropriate cases. A one-piece 7.0-mm biconvex PMMA lens is prepared using polypropylene suture to tie each haptic at the point of greatest spread. The needle of each polypropylene suture is passed transsclerally from inside to outside at the sites in the 1:30 and 7:30 o'clock positions, exiting the eye approximately 1 mm posterior to the corneoscleral limbus. After the PCIOL is properly positioned, the sutures are pulled taut and secured by taking a superficial scleral bite, then tied. The suture ends are cut short and covered by closing the scleral flaps with interrupted 10-0 Vicryl sutures. The PK is completed by suturing the donor corneal button with either interrupted or continuous running sutures. The surgical technique, indications, and outcomes are described in greater detail in Chapter 10.

Inflammatory Causes

Uveitis-Glaucoma-Hyphema Syndrome

Uveitis-glaucoma-hyphema (UGH) syndrome was a commonly observed complication of early-generation IOLs, especially ACIOLs (Choyce-style ACIOL).[27] The syndrome is thought to be due to mechanical irritation of the iris root and adjacent angle structures caused by the haptic footplate. This insult eventually results in uveitis, recurrent hyphema, and glaucoma. The incidence of this syndrome has declined steadily with refinements in IOL design and posterior chamber implantation. The condition usually subsides following removal of the implant (see Chapter 17).

Persistent Uveitis

Inflammation in the early postoperative period is in part related to surgical manipulation. The etiology of persistent iritis with or without hypopyon is complex and multifactorial. Among the various factors that may be involved, persistent iritis with various IOL types has been found to occur in an incidence of 0.4%–1.2% over a 1-year period.[4] Inflammatory reactions due to mechanical irritation of an IOL are a significant factor leading to breakdown of the blood–aqueous barrier by mechanical damage to intraocular tissues. In addition to the mechanical irritation caused by certain types of ACIOLs, ciliary sulcus–fixated PCIOLs can also produce chafing of the posterior surface of the iris and notable inflammation.

Infectious endophthalmitis is a devastating complication and should always be considered in patients with persistent inflammation without an obvious explanation. It usually arises early in the postoperative period and is associated with pain, chemosis, hypopyon, and corneal decompensation. The treatment of endophthalmitis depends on early diagnosis, which is aided by cultures of vitreous aspirate. Response to treatment and final visual acuity do not appear to be related to retention or removal of the IOL. The surgical procedures for persistent uveitis involve IOL repositioning and IOL explantation and exchange. Both procedures have been described earlier in this chapter and in Chapters 11, 14, and 17.

Vitreoretinal Complications

Cystoid Macular Edema

Cystoid macular edema (Irvine-Gass syndrome) is a well-known complication of cataract surgery that may occur with or without IOL implantation. Decreased visual acuity results from edema in the outer plexiform layer of the macula caused by an increased permeability of perifoveolar capillaries (see Chapter 16).[27] Most cases of CME are seen 4–12 weeks following cataract surgery. However, CME can also be seen as a complication of systemic disorders such as diabetes, hypertension, uveitis, and other conditions.

Many studies have examined the relation of IOL implantation to the incidence of CME. Studies in the 1970s by Binkhorst demonstrated a lower incidence of CME associated with cataract extraction combined with iris-fixated IOL implantation.[39] Several trends and conclusions have been followed by surgeons since then, based on the experience of many other studies.[27] The presence of an intact posterior capsule lowers the risk of developing CME. ECCE with PCIOL implantation is associated with a lower incidence of CME than iris-fixated IOL implantations. Finally, complications during surgery increase the incidence of CME, regardless of the IOL used. As a general rule, a patient in whom CME has developed and who has an additional IOL complication, such as malposition, iris tuck, corneal touch with edema, or persistent inflammation secondary to the implant position, should undergo surgical correction. The surgical procedures for vitreoretinal complications consist of IOL rotation and repositioning and IOL explantation and exchange. Both procedures have been described, earlier in this chapter.

Retinal Detachment

Patients who undergo cataract surgery are prone to RD if there is history of vitreous loss, high myopia, or previous RD in the fellow eye. The incidence of RD following IOL implantation has been reported to be between 0.55% and 1.65%.[40] Although IOL implantation does not seem to increase the risk of RD, certain IOL designs may make surgical reattachment more difficult.

Difficult Visualization of the Fundus

Visualization of the posterior segment was difficult with many of the older IOL styles, specifically iris-supported implants, where the pupil was often miotic and mydriasis difficult to obtain. With modern IOL designs visualization is less of a problem, but new complications are being encountered. In the evaluation of retinal tears, visualization of the fundus periphery can be difficult owing to glare and optical aberration of the IOL or PCO. Similarly, evaluation of certain areas of the fundus may be impossible if the IOL is decentered, tilted, or subluxated. This can be of importance in patients with diabetic proliferative retinopathy, where adequate photocoagulation of the retina would not be possible. For any patient population where visualization of the fundus is essential for diagnosis or treatment of a disease, surgical correction of the IOL can be considered a primary indication for intervention. Surgical procedures to improve visualization of the fundus include IOL rotation and repositioning, IOL removal and exchange, and Nd:YAG laser therapy. Each of these procedures has been described previously.

■ Surgical Complications

Proper surgical management of IOL complications can result in satisfactory visual outcomes. However, untoward effects may result from further intervention and must be considered in the equation. It is extremely important for surgeons to be familiar with complications, in order to recognize them promptly and manage them efficiently.

Postoperative complications after the management of dislocated IOLs include chronic CME, elevated intraocular pressure, RD, vitreous hemorrhage, monocular diplopia, and massive suprachoroidal hemorrhage (see Chapter 16).[41] Nonspecific retinal pigment epithelium macular changes are not uncommon in these patients and may represent retinal phototoxicity.[41] Suture-fixated PCIOLs with transscleral sutures are subject to suture exposure over the knot, scleral flap melt, endophthalmitis, intraocular hemorrhage, IOL torsion, and malposition due to suture breakage (see Chapter 14).

Although lens capsule complications following Nd:YAG laser therapy are infrequent, they can be significant. Elevated intraocular pressure after Nd:YAG laser treatment is a well-recognized but rare event today since the institution of α-agonists to blunt this response. However, when pressure elevation does occur, it is usually acute, occurring hours after the procedure, and transient, rarely remaining elevated chronically. The incidence of CME after Nd:YAG capsulotomy is similarly low (0.55%–2.5%) and may be further reduced if the interval between cataract extraction and laser capsulotomy is extended.[17,42] Other retinal complications of Nd:YAG capsulotomy include RD and macular holes. Furthermore, intraocular lens damage can occur in 15%–33% of eyes undergoing Nd:YAG capsulotomy. Lens pitting is usually not visually significant, and the extent of the damage largely depends on the material of the implant (glass fractures, PMMA cracks, and silicone leaves localized pits) (Fig. 18.10).

Finally, although PK with IOL exchange is safe and effective, patients can experience major complications with visual consequences detrimental to the desired outcome. In particular, these patients are at greater risk for suprachoroidal hemorrhage with possible expulsion due to prolonged hypotony following removal of the cornea. Other IOL complications include graft rejection, glaucoma, CME, and retrocorneal membrane formation.[27] These complications are discussed in greater detail in Chapter 10.

IOL complications can be very frustrating to the patient. A carefully planned approach to their management is strongly recommended. Three major factors will determine the final outcome of surgical management: (1) selection of the most appropriate surgical

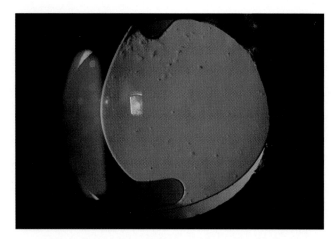

FIGURE 18.10. Lens implants can have localized pits.

technique, (2) proper recognition and management of postoperative complications, and (3) most important, the recognition of preexisting ocular pathology that may limit final visual potential. When these factors are clear to the patient and surgeon, a satisfactory outcome can be achieved.

■ References

1. Achiron L, Witkin N, Primo S, Broocker G. Contemporary management of anisekonia. *Surv Ophthalmol.* 1997;41(4): 321–330.
2. Carlson A, Stewart W, Tso P. Intraocular lens complications requiring removal or exchange. *Surv Ophthalmol.* 1998;42(5):417–440.
3. Murphy GE, Murphy CG. Minimizing anisometropia in bilateral pseudophakia. *J Cataract Refract Surg.* 1992;18(1): 95–99.
4. Sinskey R, Amin P, Stoppel J. Indications for and results of a large series of intraocular lens exchanges. *J Cataract Refract Surg.* 1993;19:68–71.
5. Lyle W, Jin J. An analysis of intraocular lens exchange. *Ophthalmic Surg.* 1992;23:453–458.
6. Allan B, Duguid G, Dart J. Intraocular lens exchange on day one after surgery [letter]. *J Cataract Refract Surg.* 1994;20:676–677.
7. Maloney RK, Chan WK, Steinert R, et al. A multicenter trial of photorefractive keratectomy for residual myopia after previous ocular surgery. Summit Therapeutic Refractive Study Group. *Ophthalmology.* 1995;102(7):1042–1052.
8. Oshika T, Yoshitomi F, Fukuyama M, et al. Radial keratotomy to treat myopic refractive error after cataract surgery. *J Cataract Refract Surg.* 1999;25(1):50–55.
9. Panton RW, Sulewski ME, Parker JS, et al. Surgical management of subluxed posterior-chamber intraocular lenses. *Arch Ophthalmol.* 1993;111:919–926.
10. Osher R, Cionni R, Blumenkranz M. Surgical repositioning and explantation of intraocular lenses. In: Steinert RF, ed. *Cataract Surgery: Technique, Complications, and Management.* Philadelphia: WB Saunders; 1995:341–352.
11. Smiddy W. Dislocated posterior chamber intraocular lens: a new technique of management. *Arch Ophthalmol.* 1989;107:1678–1680.
12. Panton RW, Stark WJ, Panton PJ. Malposition of posterior chamber intraocular lenses *Ophthalmol Clin North Am.* 1991;4:381–393.
13. Stark WJ, Bruner WE, Martin NF. Management of subluxed posterior-chamber intraocular lenses. *Ophthalmic Surg.* 1982;13:130–133.
14. Shepard DD. Indications for intraocular lens removal. *Ophthalmic Surg.* 1977;8:144–148.
15. Eifrig DE. Two principles for repositioning intraocular lenses. *Opthalmic Surg.* 1986;17(8):486–489.
16. Azar DT, Wiley WF. Double-knot transscleral suture fixation technique for displaced intraocular lenses. *Am J Ophthalmol.* 1999;128:644–646.
17. Azar DT, Clamen LM. Iris fixation of a decentered silicone plate haptic intraocular lens: double knot technique. *Arch Ophthalmol.* 1998;116:821–823.
18. Eifrig DE. Deposits on the surface of intraocular lenses: a pathological study. *South Med J.* 1980;73:6–8.
19. Ritcher C, Steinert R. Neodymium:yttrium-aluminum-garnet laser posterior capsulotomy. In Steinert RF, ed. *Cataract Surgery: Technique, Complications, and Management.* Philadelphia: WB Saunders; 1995:378–388.
20. Davison J. Capsule contraction syndrome. *J Cataract Refract Surg.* 1993;19:582–589.
21. Hansen SO, Crandall AS, Olson RJ. Progressive constriction of anterior capsular opening following intact capsulorhexis. *J Cataract Refract Surg.* 1993;19:77–82.
22. Steinert R. Neodymium:yttrium-aluminum-garnet laser in the management of postoperative complications of cataract surgery. In: Steinert RF, ed. *Cataract Surgery: Technique, Complications, and Management.* Philadelphia: WB Saunders; 1995:389–396.
23. McDonnell PJ, Zarbin MA, Green WR. Posterior capsule opacification in pseudophakic eyes. *Ophthalmology.* 1983;90:1548–1553.
24. Emery JM, Wilhelmus KA, Rosenberg S. Complications of phacoemulsification. *Ophthalmology.* 1978;85:141–150.
25. Jaffe G. Cataract surgery and its complications. St. Louis, MO: Mosby–Year Book; 1997.
26. Lindstrom RL, Herman WK. Pupil capture: prevention and management. *Am Intraocular Implant Soc J.* 1983;9: 201–204.
27. Apple DJ, Mamalis N, Loftfield K, et al. Complications of intraocular lenses: a historical and histopathological review. *Surv Ophthalmol.* 1984;29:1–54.
28. Steinert R. Corneal edema after cataract surgery. In Steinert RF, ed. *Cataract Surgery: Technique, Complications, and Management.* Philadelphia: WB Saunders; 1995: 358–363.
29. Kraff MC, Sanders DR, Raanan MG. A survey of intraocular lens explantations. *J Cataract Refract Surg.* 1986;12: 644–649.
30. Mamalis N, Crandall AS, Pulsipher MW, et al. Intraocular lens explantation and exchange. *J Cataract Refract Surg.* 1991;17:811–818.

31. Bourne WM, Kaufman HE. Cataract extraction and the corneal endothelium. *Am J Ophthalmol.* 1976;82:44–47.

32. Bourne WM, Kaufman HE. Endothelial damage associated with intraocular lenses. *Am J Ophthalmol.* 1976;81:482–485.

33. Stark WJ, Worthen DM, Holladay JT, et al. The FDA report on intraocular lemses. *Ophthalmology.* 1983;90:311–317.

34. Lim ES, Apple DJ, Tsai JC, et al. An analysis of flexible anterior chamber lenses with special reference to the normalized rate of lens explantation. *Ophthalmology.* 1991;98:243–246.

35. Cohen EJ, Brady SE, Leavitt K, et al. Pseudophakic bullous keratopathy. *Am J Ophthalmol.* 1988;106:264–269.

36. MacRae S. Positioning hole synechias with anterior chamber lenses. *J Cataract Refract Surg.* 1991;17:521.

37. Noecker RJ, Branner WA, Cohen KL. Intraocular lens explantation with and without penetrating keratoplasty. *Ophthalmic Surg.* 1989;20(12):849–854.

38. Holland EJ, Daya SM, Evangelista A, et al. Penetrating keratoplasty and transscleral fixation of posterior chamber lens. *Am J Ophthalmol.* 1992;114:182–187.

39. Binkhorst C. The iridocapsular (two-loop) lens and the iris-clip (four-loop) lens in pseudophakia. *Trans Am Acad Ophthalmol Otolaryngol.* 1973;77:589–617.

40. Binkhorst CD, Kats A, Tjan TT, Loones LH. Retinal accidents in pseudoaphakia: intraocular vs extracapsular surgery. *Trans Am Acad Ophthalmol Otolaryngol.* 1976; 81:120–127.

41. Mello MO Jr., Scott IU, Smiddy WE, et al. Surgical management and outcomes of dislocated intraocular lenses. *Ophthalmology.* 2000;107:62–67.

42. Stark W, Worthen D, Holladay JT, Murray G. Neodymium:YAG lasers. An FDA report. *Ophthalmology.* 1985;92:209–212.

Part V

Phakic Intraocular Lenses

Chapter 19

Phakic Intraocular Lens Implantation: Comparison with Keratorefractive Surgical Procedures

Sonia H. Yoo

A number of treatment options for the surgical correction of myopia and hyperopia exist. Excimer laser photorefractive keratectomy (PRK) and laser in situ keratomileusis (LASIK) are among the currently favored surgical options for treating myopia, hyperopia, and astigmatism. For cases of high myopia and hyperopia, however, the results of these procedures are less predictable. For this reason, there has been increasing interest in the use of phakic intraocular lenses (IOLs) to correct refractive errors, particularly for patients with high myopia and hyperopia. Phakic IOL implantation has the advantage of preserving the architecture of the cornea, arguably the healthiest part of a highly myopic eye, and may provide more predictable refractive results than surgical techniques that manipulate the corneal curvature. This chapter reviews the techniques and outcomes of currently favored keratorefractive surgical procedures and compares the results of these procedures with the results of phakic IOL implantation.

■ Keratorefractive Surgical Procedures

Long before the development of the excimer laser, Barraquer pioneered myopic keratomileusis to correct myopia.[1] A frozen corneal lenticule was carved with a lathe to the amount of desired corrected refractive error. In 1987, Krumeich and Swinger reported a procedure for preparing epikeratophakia tissue lenses for the correction of myopia using a microkeratome on unfrozen tissue.[2] Later, Ruiz developed the in situ version of this technique in which refractive keratectomy was performed on the corneal stromal bed. In 1983, Trokel et al reported using the excimer laser to make

submicron precision cuts in the cornea.[3] Several years after it began to be used in reshaping the corneal surface, the excimer laser was used to perform corneal stromal flattening in keratomileusis. Ten blind human eyes were treated in the United States with excimer laser photorefractive keratectomy (PRK) in 1989,[4] and in 1995 PRK was approved by the Food and Drug Administration (FDA) for the treatment of myopia. Subsequent studies led to approval of the excimer laser for toric ablations as well.

Although the results of PRK in patients with low myopia were excellent, the haze and regression often seen in patients with high myopia led to the development of LASIK. The earliest successes in LASIK resulted from the combination of two techniques that led to the development of the hinged corneal flap. Buratto et al introduced the technique of cutting a 300-μm-thick cap of cornea and applying the laser ablation to the back of the cap.[5] The development of the flap hinge is credited to Pallikaris and colleagues.[6] LASIK minimizes the risk of haze formation after laser ablation by preserving the relationship of the anterior structures of the cornea. Preservation of Bowman's layer is thought to only minimally stimulate new collagen and extracellular matrix deposition.[7]

The next frontier for the excimer laser was adapting its ablation pattern for the treatment of hyperopia. An annular ablation in the peripheral stroma defines an optical zone that effectively steepens the cornea.[8] The FDA study of 166 eyes at 12 months showed an uncorrected visual acuity of 20/40 or better in 95% of eyes with a preoperative refractive error of +1.0 to +6.0 diopters. Both hyperopic PRK and hyperopic LASIK currently are being performed, although the recovery

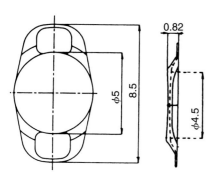 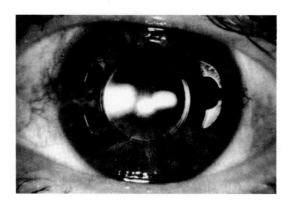

FIGURE 19.1. Worst iris claw lens.

time after both procedures is longer than with myopic laser ablations.

■ Phakic Lenses: Overview

Designs

The foundations of modern ophthalmology were laid in the second half of the 19th century. Refractive surgery also started during this period and was soon beset by many of the controversies that accompany it today. Clear lens extraction for the correction of myopia was introduced as a concept in the early 1800s, and the technique became increasingly popular from 1850 to 1900.[9] It was not until the end of the 19th century, however, that complications of this operation (e.g., retinal detachment [RD] and choroidal hemorrhage) began to be reported, and the technique largely fell out of favor.

The 1950s saw the emergence of the concept of correcting myopia by inserting a concave lens into the phakic eye. At this time, Strampelli,[10] Barraquer,[11] and Choyce[12] experimented with anterior chamber angle-fixed lenses, which were eventually abandoned because of the complications of corneal edema and chronic iritis. In 1988, Baikoff presented his version of an anterior chamber angle-fixed IOL.[13,14] The Baikoff IOL is a single-piece, biconcave ACIOL based on a multiflex Kelman ACIOL. It is made of polymethyl methacrylate (PMMA) containing an ultraviolet blocker. The lens is angled 20 degrees posteriorly and the optic is 5 mm in diameter. Complications of this lens included pupillary block, endothelial cell loss, halos/glare, iritis, implant rotation, RD, and iris retraction with pupillary ovalization.

Around the same time that the Baikoff lens was being developed, Worst and Fechner developed a biconcave anterior chamber lens fixed to the front of the iris[15] that stemmed from experience with the iris claw lens of Worst used for aphakic eyes (Fig. 19.1).[16] Com-

plications with this style of lens included iritis, cystic wounds, glaucoma, difficulty with fixation of the IOL, RD, cataract formation, and corneal decompensation from endothelial cell loss.[17] To minimize the possibility of IOL-cornea contact, in 1991 the biconcave design was changed to a convex-concave model with a lower shoulder and thinner periphery (Fig. 19.2).

In the mid-1980s, the implantation of posterior chamber IOLs (PCIOLs) in phakic eyes was reported by Fyodorov et al.[18] In 1987, the Moscow Research Institute of Eye Microsurgery reported favorably on PCIOL implantation in phakic eyes to correct high myopia.[18] The original lens design was a collar-button type with the optic located in the anterior chamber and the haptics behind the iris plane. Later, Chiron-Adatomed modified this design to produce a silicone elastomer PCIOL. The concave posterior optic curvature, which closely approximates the anterior crystalline lens curvature, has a radius of 9.9 mm. The anterior curvature is also concave. The optic diameter is 5.5 mm and the haptic thickness is 0.18 mm. This lens design has been reported to be associated with a high incidence of cataract formation after implantation.[19]

In 1993, Zaldivar et al began implanting a plate posterior chamber phakic IOL (Staar Surgical Implantable Contact Lens) (Fig. 19.3).[20] This lens design, modified from the one Fyodorov originated in 1986, is a one-piece silicone collar-button phakic IOL with a 500- to 600-nm Teflon coat. Incorporation of a porcine collagen/HEMA copolymer into the lens material has improved the biocompatibility of the newer lens. Phase I trials by the FDA were approved in February 1997 for

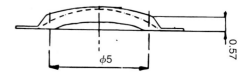

FIGURE 19.2. Ophtec Worst (Artisan) phakic IOL of − 10.00 diopters. This style has been in use since 1992.

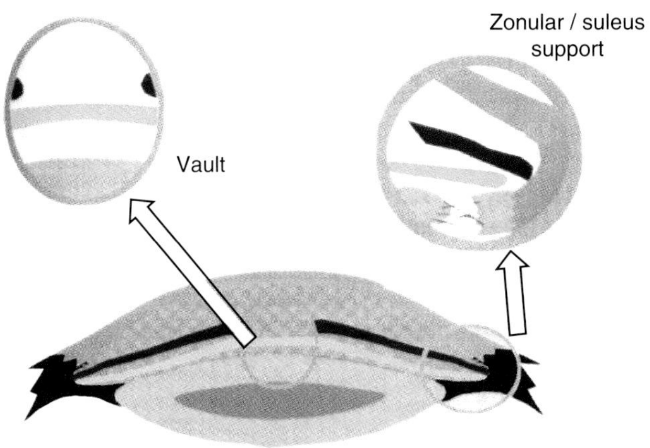

FIGURE 19.3. Staar posterior chamber phakic IOL. (*From Zaldivar R., Davidorf JM, Oscherow S., Ricur G., Piezzi V. Combined posterior chamber phakic intraocular lens and laser in situ keratomileusis: bioptics for extreme myopia.* J Refract Surg. *1999;15(3):299–308, with permission.*)

the treatment of hyperopia with this posterior chamber phakic IOL.[21]

Indications and Contraindications

Patients enrolled in the Phase I trials had a preoperative spherical equivalent (SE) ranging from −5.00 to −31.75 diopters.[14,17,20,22,23] The Staar posterior chamber phakic IOL was also implanted in hyperopic patients with an SE ranging from +2.50 to +10.875 diopters.[21] Inclusion criteria differed slightly from study to study; however, the basic tenets were similar: the endothelial cell count was normal (at least 2,500 cells/mm²) and the anterior chamber depth was adequate (3 mm or more). Exclusion criteria included inflammation of the anterior or posterior segment, chronic keratitis, corneal dystrophy, iris atrophy or rubeosis, aniridia, cataracts, vitreous pathology, retinal disease, microphthalmos, nanophthalmos, glaucoma, or previous intraocular surgery. For patients who received the posterior chamber phakic IOL, peripheral laser iridotomies were performed at least 4 days prior to surgery to decrease the incidence of postoperative pupillary block.

Results

Baikoff et al reported results in 121 patients (134 eyes) with myopia of −7.0 to −18.8 diopters in whom the ZB5M angle-fixated anterior chamber lens was implanted.[14] Postoperative follow-up ranged from 6 months to 3 years. The postoperative SE refraction averaged −1.0 diopter during the first 2 years, increasing to −1.3 diopters at 3 years. At 2 years, approximately 40% of eyes had an SE within 0.50 diopter and 65% had an SE within 1.0 diopter of the desired refractive

error. The uncorrected distance visual acuity (UCDVA) was 0.048 at baseline and 0.5 at 3 years. The uncorrected near visual acuity (UCNVA) was 0.65 at baseline and improved to 0.75. Spectacle-corrected visual acuity at baseline was 0.54; it improved to 0.7. Endothelial cell counts in the central and peripheral cornea were reduced by an average of 3.3% at 6 months and declined an additional 1%–2% over the remaining period of follow-up. Additional complications included halos/glare in 27.8% of eyes and iris retraction with pupillary ovalization in 22.6% of eyes. The IOL was exchanged in 3.0% of eyes and removed in 2.3% of eyes because of halos (1 eye) and a flat anterior chamber with severe inflammation (2 eyes).

Alio et al also performed a prospective clinical trial to determine the potential cumulative complications in patients implanted with angle-supported phakic IOLs for the correction of myopia.[24] Two hundred sixty-three eyes in 160 consecutive patients were included. Night halos and glare were reported by 20.2% of patients at 1 year and by 10% at 7-year follow-up. The rate of this complication was significantly lower in the larger optical zone phakic IOL (model ZSAL-4) group than in the ZB5M/ZB5MF group. The total cumulative loss of central endothelial cells after 7 years was 8.37%. Pupil ovalization was present in 5.9% of cases, although smaller degrees of ovalization were observed in another 10.3%. RD appeared in 3% of cases. Explantation was performed in 4.18% of cases because of cataract development (9 cases) and extreme pupillary ovalization associated with severe glare (2 cases).

Fechner et al reported the results of implanting of the Worst-Fechner iris claw phakic lens to correct high myopia in 127 eyes in 70 patients.[17] Postoperative follow-up ranged from 6 months to 8 years. At the 6-month examination, mean deviation of achieved from calculated refractive correction was +0.52 ± 1.46 diopters. In 62.1% of eyes the mean deviation was 1.0 diopter or less and in 12.1% it was more than 2.0 diopters (from the calculated correction). A refractive outcome of ± 1.0 diopter was attempted in 4% of eyes and achieved in 75% of these eyes. Mean spectacle-corrected visual acuity was 0.54 ± 0.27 preoperatively and 0.73 ± 0.3 6 months postoperatively. By the 8-year examination it had decreased to 0.65 ± 0.26. Endothelial cell counts revealed a significant correlation of cell loss with age (≥45 years), anterior chamber depth (≤3.4 mm), and IOL power (≥−11.0 diopters). In 13.4% of eyes, the endothelial cell density decreased; projection to 8-year follow-up indicated a decrease in 27% of eyes. In 8 eyes postoperative iritis developed, which diminished after surgeons began preoperative administration of high-dose prednisone; however, in 10 eyes a subconjunctival fistula developed that required wound resuturing after preop-

Table 19.1
LASIK for Myopia and Hyperopia: Pre- and Postoperative Data

Study	No. of Eyes	Preoperative Spherical Equivalent (D) Range	Follow-up Time (mo)	Postoperative Spherical Equivalent (D) Mean	Postoperative Spherical Equivalent (D) Range	% of Eyes with UCDVA 20/40 or Better	% of Eyes Within 1.0 D
Bas [27]	97		3	− 0.38		50	46
Fiander and Tayfour[28]	124	− 3.75 to − 27.0	3	+ 0.27	− 2.75 to + 4.0		
Salah et al[29]	88	− 2.0 to − 20.0	5.2	+ 0.22	− 3.62 to + 6.76	71	72
Pallikaris and Siganos[30]	21	− 8.5 to − 14.0	12	− 1.49	− 4.75 to + 1.37		
High/very high myopes	18	− 15.0 to − 25.87		− 5.38	− 15.0 to − 1.75		
Perez-Santonja et al[31]	143	− 8.0 to − 20.0	6	+ 0.18		46	60
Kim and Jung[32]	18	− 10.50 to − 21.50	6	+ 0.14	− 2.0 to + 3.50		47
Guëll and Muller[33]	21	− 7.0 to − 12.0	6	− 0.80	0 to − 3.5	71	85
	22	− 12.3 to − 18.5		− 1.80	0 to − 5.25	45	41
Knorz et al[34]	51	− 6.0 to − 29.0	4	− 1.9	− 9.5 to + 2.25		47
Buratto et al[35]	30	− 11.2 to − 24.5	12	− 2.3		10	57
Durrie[36]	1,013	− 1.0 to − 14.7	6			92	84
Rosa and Febbraro[37]	26	+ 2.0 to + 6.25	6	+ 0.5			
Ditzen et al[38]	20	+ 1 to + 4	12	+ 0.3		95	85
(Low/high)	23	+ 4 to + 8		+ 1.9		90	58
Suarez et al[39]	154	+ 1.0 to + 6.50	3	+ 0.1		72	>87
Goker et al[40]	54	+ 4.25 to + 8.0	18	+ 0.4		66	76

Abbreviation: UCDVA, uncorrected distance visual activity.

erative administration of the prednisone. Four eyes needed a penetrating keratoplasty.

Sanders et al reported the short-term safety and efficacy variables of the FDA Phase I clinical study of a plate-haptic posterior chamber phakic IOL (Staar Surgical Implantable Contact Lens).[21] Ten eyes in 10 patients were studied. At 6 months postoperatively, uncorrected visual acuity was 20/20 or better in 7 eyes and 20/40 or better in all 10 eyes. The mean postoperative SE was + 0.20 ± 0.61 diopters. Eight of 10 eyes were within ± 0.50 diopters of emmetropia, 9 eyes were within ± 1.0 diopter, and all eyes were within ± 1.50 diopters. No operative or postoperative complications were observed.

■ Comparison with Keratorefractive Procedures

The argument has been made that for high degrees of myopia and hyperopia, the most currently popular keratorefractive procedures, LASIK and PRK, change the naturally prolate aspheric cornea to an abnormally oblate one, which ultimately degrades the quality of vision.[25] The potential advantages of phakic IOL implantation over current keratorefractive surgical techniques include preservation of the asphericity of the cornea, procedural compatibility with established methods of aphakic IOL implantation, and removability of the lens implant. Phakic IOL implantation has the advantage over clear lens extraction in that it may result in excellent refractive accuracy while preserving accommodation.

Table 19.1 gives data from 14 published studies of LASIK performed for myopia and hyperopia. Table 19.2 gives data from 7 published studies of phakic IOLs implanted to treat myopia and hyperopia. In general, the predictability of the refractive outcomes with LASIK was comparable to that of phakic IOL implantation in eyes with smaller amounts of myopia and hyperopia. For higher refractive errors, however, the predictability of refractive outcome and uncorrected visual acuity were worse with LASIK than with phakic IOL implantation.

Various complications were reported in both the LASIK and phakic IOL studies. Complications reported

Table 19.2
Phakic IOL Implantation for Myopia and Hyperopia: Pre- and Postoperative Data

Study	No. of Eyes	Preoperative Spherical Equivalent (D)		Follow-up Time (mo)	Postoperative Spherical Equivalent (D)		% of Eyes with UCDVA 20/40 or Better	% of Eyes Within 1.0 D
		Mean	Range		Mean	Range		
Baikoff et al[14]	134	−12.5	−7.0 to −18.8	35.8	−1.0	−4.0 to +1.0	37.8	51.4
Fechner et al[17]	127	−14.3	−5.0 to −31.8	6 to 96	−1.9	−9.25 to −1.25		62.1
Krumeich et al[22]	35	−12.5	−6.0 to −21.25	6				
Zaldivar et al[20]	124	−13.4	−8.5 to −18.6	11	−0.8	+1.6 to −3.50	68	69
Davidorf et al[23]	24	+6.5	+3.7 to +10.5	8.4	−0.4	+1.25 to −3.88	63	79
Sanders et al[21]	10	+6.3	+2.5 to +10.9	6	+0.2	−0.50 to +1.50	100	90
Rosen and Gore[41]	9	+4.4	+2.25 to +5.6	1 to 6	0		89	100

Abbreviation: UCDVA, uncorrected distance visual acuity.

in the LASIK studies included flap dislocation, epithelial ingrowth, damaged flap, irregular cut, free flap, central steep islands and decentered ablation, and corneal ectasia with symptoms of glare and monocular diplopia. Complications reported in the phakic IOL studies included iritis, pupil ovalization, a transient increase in intraocular pressure, cataract development, lens decentration, endothelial cell damage, and RD.[26]

In summary, phakic IOL implantation for the correction of myopia and hyperopia seems to be an efficacious and predictable alternative to keratorefractive surgery, particularly for eyes with high refractive errors. Longitudinal, controlled multicenter trials are needed to determine the long-term safety of phakic IOLs.

■ References

1. Barraquer JI. The history and evolution of keratomileusis. *Int Ophthalmol Clin.* 1996;36:1–7.
2. Krumeich JH, Swinger CA. Nonfreeze epikeratophakia for the correction of myopia. *Am J Ophthalmol.* 1987;103:397–403.
3. Trokel SL, Srinivasan R, Braren B. Excimer laser surgery of the cornea. *Am J Ophthalmol.* 1983;96:710–715.
4. Taylor DM, L'Esperance FAJ, Del Pero RA, et al. Human excimer laser lamellar keratectomy: a clinical study. *Ophthalmology.* 1989;96:654–664.
5. Buratto L, Ferrari M, Rama P. Excimer laser intrastromal keratomileusis. *Am J Ophthalmol.* 1992;113:291–295.
6. Pallikaris IG, Papatzanaki ME, Siganos DS, Tsilimbaris MK. A corneal flap technique for laser in situ keratomileusis: human studies. *Arch Ophthalmol.* 1991;109:1699–1702.
7. Taylor DM, L'Esperance FAJ, Warner JW, et al. Experimental corneal studies with the excimer laser. *J Cataract Refract Surg.* 1989;15:384–389.
8. L'Esperance FAJ, Warner JW, Telfair WB, et al. Excimer laser instrumentation and technique for human corneal surgery. *Arch Ophthalmol.* 1989;107:131–139.
9. Seiler T. Clear lens extraction in the 19th century: an early demonstration of premature dissemination. *J Refract Surg.* 1999;15:70–73.
10. Strampelli B. Sopportabilita di lenti acriliche in camera anteriore nella afachia e nei vizi di refrazione. *Ann Oftalmol Clin Oculistica.* 1954;80:5–82.
11. Barraquer JI. Anterior chamber plastic lenses: results of and conclusions from five years experience. *Trans Ophthalmol Soc UK.* 1959;79:393–424.
12. Choyce DP. In discussion of Barraquer JI: Anterior chamber plastic lenses: results of and conclusions from five years experience. *Trans Ophthalmol Soc UK.* 1959;79:393–424.
13. Baikoff G. Phakic anterior chamber intraocular lenses. *Int Ophthalmol Clin.* 1991;31:75–86.
14. Baikoff G, Arne JL, Bokobza Y, et al. Angle-fixated anterior chamber phakic intraocular lens for myopia of −7 to −19 diopters [see comments]. *J Refract Surg.* 1998;14:282–293.
15. Fechner PU, van der Heijde GL, Worst JG. The correction of myopia by lens implantation into phakic eyes [see comments]. *Am J Ophthalmol.* 1989;107:659–663.
16. Los LI, Worst JG. Implant surgery: something old and something new. *Doc Ophthalmol.* 1990;75:377–390.
17. Fechner PU, Haubitz I, Wichmann W, Wulff K. Worst-Fechner biconcave minus power phakic iris-claw lens. *J Refract Surg.* 1999;15:93–105.
18. Fyodorov SN, Zuev VK, Tumanyan ER. Modern approach to the stagewise complex surgical therapy of high myopia. In: *Transactions of the International Symposium on IOL Implantation and Refractive Surgery.* 1987:274–279.

19. Brauweiler PH, Wehler T, Busin M. High incidence of cataract formation after implantation of a silicone posterior chamber lens in phakic, highly myopic eyes. *Ophthalmology.* 1999;106:1651–1655.

20. Zaldivar R, Davidorf JM, Oscherow S. Posterior chamber phakic intraocular lens for myopia of −8 to −19 diopters [see comments]. *J Refract Surg.* 1998;14:294–305.

21. Sanders DR, Martin RG, Brown DC, et al. Posterior chamber phakic intraocular lens for hyperopia [in process citation]. *J Refract Surg.* 1999;15:309–315.

22. Krumeich JH, Daniel J, Gast R. Closed-system technique for implantation of iris-supported negative-power intraocular lens. *J Refract Surg.* 1996;12:334–340.

23. Davidorf JM, Zaldivar R, Oscherow S. Posterior chamber phakic intraocular lens for hyperopia of +4 to +11 diopters [see comments]. *J Refract Surg.* 1998;14:306–311.

24. Alio JL, de la Hoz F, Perez-Santonja JJ, et al. Phakic anterior chamber lenses for the correction of myopia: a 7-year cumulative analysis of complications in 263 cases. *Ophthalmology.* 1999;106:458–466.

25. Rosen ES. Considering corneal and lenticular techniques of refractive surgery [editorial; comment]. *J Cataract Refract Surg.* 1997;23:689–691.

26. Garrana RMR, Azar DT. Phakic intraocular lenses for correction of high myopia. *Int Ophthalmol Clin.* 1999;39: 45–57.

27. Bas AM. Excimer laser in situ keratomileusis for myopia. *J Refract Surg.* 1995;11:S229–S233.

28. Fiander DC, Tayfour F. Excimer laser in situ keratomileusis in 124 myopic eyes. *J Refract Surg.* 1995;11:S234–S238.

29. Salah T, Waring GO, El-Maghraby A, et al. Excimer laser in-situ keratomileusis (LASIK) under a corneal flap for myopia of 2 to 20 D. *Trans Am Ophthalmol Soc.* 1995;93:163–183.

30. Pallikaris IG, Siganos DS. Laser in situ keratomileusis to treat myopia: early experience. *J Cataract Refract Surg.* 1997;23:39–49.

31. Perez-Santonja JJ, Bellot J, Claramonte P, et al. Laser in situ keratomileusis to correct high myopia. *J Cataract Refract Surg.* 1997;23:372–385.

32. Kim HM, Jung HR. Laser assisted in situ keratomileusis for high myopia. *Ophthalmic Surg Lasers.* 1996;27:S508–S511.

33. Guëll JL, Muller A. Laser in situ keratomileusis (LASIK) for myopia from −7 to −18 diopters. *J Refract Surg.* 1996;12:222–228.

34. Knorz MC, Liermann A, Seiberth V, et al. Laser in situ keratomileusis to correct myopia of −6.00 to −29.00 diopters. *J Refract Surg.* 1996;12:575–584.

35. Buratto L, Ferrari M, Genisi C. Myopic keratomileusis with the excimer laser: one-year follow up. *Refract Corneal Surg.* 1993;9:12–19.

36. Durrie D. LASIK for high myopia with or without astigmatism: the CRS Multi-Site Study with the Summit SVS Apex Plus Excimer Laser. Unpublished; available from author.

37. Rosa DS, Febbraro JL. Laser in situ keratomileusis for hyperopia. *J Refract Surg.* 1999;15:S212–S215.

38. Ditzen K, Huschka H, Pieger S. Laser in situ keratomileusis for hyperopia. *J Cataract Refract Surg.* 1998;24:42–47.

39. Suarez E, Torres F, Duplessie M. LASIK for correction of hyperopia and hyperopia with astigmatism. *Int Ophthalmol Clin.* 1996;36:65–72.

40. Goker S, Er H, Kahvecioglu C. Laser in situ keratomileusis to correct hyperopia from +4.25 to +8.00 diopters. *J Refract Surg.* 1998;14:26–30.

41. Rosen E, Gore C. Staar collamer posterior chamber phakic intraocular lens to correct myopia and hyperopia. *J Cataract Refract Surg.* 1998;24:596–606.

Chapter 20

Anterior Chamber Phakic Intraocular Lenses

David J. Galarreta Mira, Sonia H. Yoo,
George Baikoff, and Dimitri T. Azar

There are several possibilities for correcting refraction in myopia. Spectacles are the oldest and best tolerated method for the eye, but patients are now demanding alternative methods to avoid wearing glasses and to prevent peripheral distortion and minification of the image in high myopia. Contact lenses give a better image without distortion, but not all patients can tolerate them. Surgical alternatives should be considered only if spectacles or contact lenses are unsatisfactory or intolerable for the patient. In these cases, the ophthalmologist must offer various options. We have many surgical techniques for myopia, but the choice is contracted for high myopia.[1,2]

To obtain a good result with high myopia surgery, corneal procedures are very limited, and the predictability of the results achieved with this kind of treatment goes down as the myopia increases. Therefore, when the refractive error is more than 12–16 diopters, intraocular surgery becomes the most predictable and stable technique.[1,2]

Patients who demand surgical solutions for high myopia are usually young, so they have accommodation and we must try to preserve it. Extraction of the crystalline lens proposed by Fukala,[3] or its replacement by an artificial lens, proposed by Verzella,[4] is not without risk and may condemn these young patients to wearing glasses for the rest of their lives.

Fortunately, improvements in phakic intraocular lenses (IOLs) during this decade have converted this technique into a good option for high myopia. It can offer superb refractive accuracy (high predictability and stability), compatibility with a posterior implant after development of a cataract, reversibility, and preservation of accommodation in younger patients while maintaining corneal integrity. Minor or serious complications can, of course, occur, but ongoing improvements in implant design should reduce their incidence. A longer follow-up in these patients will give us many of the answers that we do not yet know.

◾ Design History

Implantation of an anterior chamber IOL (ACIOL) in phakic eyes to correct high myopia was proposed in 1954 by Strampelli,[5,6] followed by Barraquer[7] in 1959 and Choyce[8,9] in 1964. They used different implant designs. The history of phakic IOL implant designs can be divided into two generations.

First-Generation Phakic IOLs

Strampelli began to implant lenses in the early 1950s. His lens had a radius of curvature of 13 mm of its nonoptical portion with an angle support (Fig. 20.1).

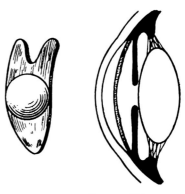

FIGURE 20.1. Strampelli lens.

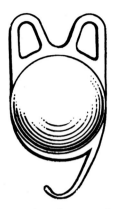

FIGURE 20.2. Cogan/Bomberg-Ans fenestrated lens.

The problem at that time was in manufacturing. The implants were rigid and thick, and the length was not always the most appropriate. These problems caused corneal decompensation, iritis, hyphema, intraocular hypertension, and pupillary block in spite of iridectomy. To avoid pupillary block, Cogan and Bomberg modified the design and created a fenestrated lens (Fig. 20.2).[7] However, pupillary block still occurred, and problems secondary to improper length, weight, thickness, and rigidity were still common.

Danheim contributed another lens without most of these problems, but the length was still fixed and inaccurate (Fig. 20.3).[7]

Barraquer subsequently introduced a new model with flexible haptics to fit to the length of the anterior chamber (Fig. 20.4).[7] Early results were encouraging, but complications led to the abandonment of this lens model a few years later. It was necessary to improve the lens designs and manufacturing, as Drews later noted, as well as the surgical procedure.[10] The development of anterior chamber implants to correct aphakia and the good results achieved with these implants confirmed the possibility of an artificial lens remaining in the anterior chamber. With many years of surgical experience and the development of viscoelastic substances and better designs, a new attempt was made in the 1980s.

Second-Generation Phakic IOLs

Three phakic IOL designs for correcting high myopia appeared in the 1980s. Fechner and Worst in the 1970s had proposed the "lobster claw" lens attached to the iris to correct aphakia; a few years later they used their design as an implant in a phakic patient with high myopia.[11] Fyodorov offered a new option with a posterior chamber implant supported by the anterior surface of the lens; this model, too, was later improved.[1] The third design was an angle-fitted lens similar to the first-generation lenses.

Praeger and Momose implanted their first lens in Japan in 1987.[12–14] The polymethyl methacrylate (PMMA) lens had haptics made of polyamide with a chord diameter of 12.5–13.5 mm. The lens power was −8, −10, or −13 diopters, so the lens was not always the correct power for the patient. Praeger and Momose reported results in a small series of 23 eyes. At the same time, Baikoff presented his Z-shaped angle-supported ACIOL, derived from the Kelman implant (Fig. 20.5).[2,15] The footplates were large to avoid iris wrapping. This model had 25 degrees of vaulting, and it was estimated to be 2 mm behind the cornea and 1 mm in front of the pupil. An important point was to supply a wide range of power between −8 and −30 diopters and diameters of 12, 12.5, 13, and 13.5 mm to better fit the angle.[16] The total optic diameter was 4.5 mm and the real one was 4 mm. This size was supposed to provide sufficient distance to the endothelium, but endothelial damage did appear. In an attempt to minimize

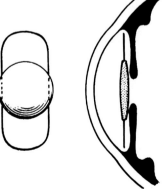

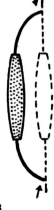

FIGURE 20.3. *A* and *B,* Danheim lens.　　　　**A**　　　　　　　　　　　　　　　　　　　　　　　**B**

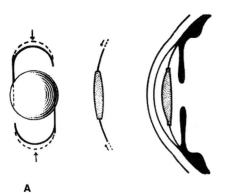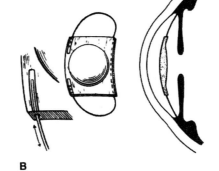

FIGURE 20.4. *A* and *B,* Barraquer lens.

the complications, Baikoff modified his original design and created a new lens called the ZB5M.[17]

In the ZB5M, the vaulting was lowered to 20 degrees and the optic edge was thinned to increase the distance from the endothelium by 0.6 mm (Fig. 20.6).[16] In other respects the ZB5M was similar to the first-generation Baikoff lenses. The optical results were as good as with the earlier lenses and the endothelial cell loss was less.[18] Later the surface was modified with fluorine to improve biocompatibility.[19,20]

At this point the anatomic and optical results of phakic IOLs were very good. However, halos, glare, and pupil distortion, previously considered minor side effects, had to be corrected, so Baikoff designed a new lens, called the NuVita MA20.[18] The real optic diameter was increased to 4.5 mm and the total diameter to 5 mm (Fig. 20.7). The thickness of the edge was decreased by 20% to increase the distance from the endothelium. The edge of the optical was modified with a special technique to decrease the incidence of halos. A new concave form was given to the posterior surface to increase the distance from the natural lens. The phakic IOL can have a power between −7 and −20 diopters and a length of 12, 12.5, or 13 mm. There are as yet no published reports on the use of this lens.

The ZSAL-4 lens, designed by Alio,[19] has features of haptic design similar to the ZB5M. The differences are that the ZSAL-4 lens has an angulation of 19 degrees, the anterior optic is flat, and the posterior optic is concave. This design increases the distance between the

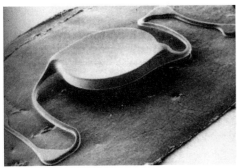

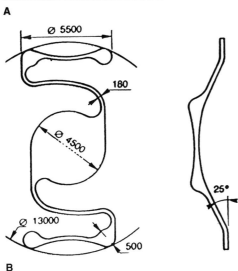

FIGURE 20.5. *A* and *B,* Baikoff Z-shaped phakic ACIOL.

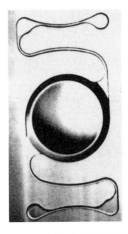

FIGURE 20.6. Baikoff ZB5M lens.

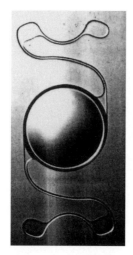

FIGURE 20.7. Baikoff NuVita MA20.

PIOL and the iris and endothelium. The optic diameter is increased to 5.5 mm and the real diameter to 5 mm in an effort to prevent halos. The phakic IOL is supplied in powers ranging from − 10 to − 23 diopters.

■ Admission Requirements

There is no fixed protocol for admission, but the common selection guidelines include (1) age approximately 20–50 years, (2) spherical equivalent greater than 8 diopters, (3) endothelial cell density at least 2,250–2,500 cells/mm², (4) stable myopia, (5) anterior chamber depth 3–3.4 mm or more, and (6) patient availability for close ophthalmologic supervision.[18,19,21] Exclusion criteria are inflammation of the anterior or posterior segment, chronic keratitis, corneal dystrophy, iris atrophy or rubeosis, aniridia, cataract, a history of vitreous pathology or retinal disease (prophylactic laser treatment needed in an unhealthy peripheral retina), microphthalmia, glaucoma, and diabetes mellitus.[2,18,19,21]

■ Preoperative Evaluation

A full ophthalmologic examination and prophylactic treatment, if necessary, are done preoperatively. Cycloplegic and subjective manifest refraction, gonioscopy, B-scan biometry, applanation tonometry, keratometry, anterior chamber depth, and systematic endothelial study should be done. Refraction of myopia greater than 20–25 diopters needs special care.[11,16]

Recently, the selection of lens power of the lens has improved, with newer and better formulas. Most frequently used is the formula of Van der Heijde:[22,23]

$$A = -(12 - 1,000)/R$$
$$E = K - (D + 1,336)/DC$$
$$F = K - (D + 1,336)/(DC + 1,000/A)$$
$$DI = 1,336 \times (1/F - 1/E)$$

A = patient's far point in mm
12 = distance from spectacle plane to cornea.
1,000 = conversion factor for meters to mm
R = spectacle correction in diopters
E = virtual object distance for phakic IOL in mm
K = 1 mm (distance from phakic IOL to crystalline lens)
D = anterior chamber axial depth in mm
1,336 = aqueous humor index multiplied by mm conversion factor
DC = power of cornea in diopters
F = phakic IOL image distance in mm
DI = implant power in diopters

The phakic IOL power can be modified depending on the desired refraction; the lenses are supplied in steps of 1 diopter. The lens length is selected by measuring the horizontal white-to-white diameter and adding 0.5–1 mm to this distance.[18]

■ Procedure

Phakic IOL implantation can be done under local or general anesthesia. If necessary, mild sedation can be used with local anesthesia. Pilocarpine is instilled in the eye 30 minutes before surgery.[1,16,18,19]

Two types of incision can be done. The classic one, proposed by Baikoff and Joly, is done temporally or nasally and parallel to the plane of the iris, avoiding contact with the eyelid speculum.[24] Alio et al chose a limbal superior incision with an additional 1-mm paracentesis for irrigation with acetylcholine.[19] In all cases the penetrating incision is 5–6 mm. Then the anterior chamber is filled with a viscoelastic substance (sodium hyaluronate or 2% hydroxypropyl methylcellulose).

A silicone slide sheet is introduced into the anterior chamber on the side opposite the incision. In the original procedure the lens is introduced horizontally, and once the distal haptic of the implant is in the angle, additional viscoelastic medium is injected, and then the proximal haptic is fitted in the opposite angle.

In the technique of Alio et al, the lens is introduced toward 6 o'clock from the superior incision.[19] Then the lens is rotated with a lens dialer to the meridian in which the pupil is best centered in relation to the phakic IOL optic. Careful maneuvers prevent damage to the structures of the angle.

Although iridectomy is not always necessary,[16] Alio et al always performed one.[19] It is advised in patients presumed to be at risk for pupillary block. The iridectomy should not interfere with the stability of the lens, and the lens should not touch the ciliary body. The incision is closed with a running or interrupted 10-0 nylon suture. To avoid postoperative IOP elevation, the anterior chamber is irrigated to remove viscoelastic medium. The iridocorneal angle is then examined for a possible improper position of the footplates. An antibiotic or antibiotic with corticoids is injected subconjunctivally. Topical corticosteroids and antibiotics are applied three times daily for 4–6 weeks. Topical nonsteroidal anti-inflammatory drugs may be applied three times daily for 3 months.[18,19]

■ Refractive and Visual Outcomes

Refraction

Phakic IOLs are the most predictable and stable of the refractive methods for preserving the crystalline lens in high myopia. The results reflect an excellent accuracy. In the multicenter French study which used the first generation of the Baikoff lenses, a mean deviation of − 0.2 diopter was achieved, with 95% of eyes between − 1.3 diopter and + 1.3 diopter of refractive error.[21] In

1998 Baikoff reported results of a new French multicenter study with the ZB5M lens.[18] The spherical equivalent (SE) averaged approximately − 1 diopter over 3 years, and no eye was overcorrected by more than + 1 diopter (Fig. 20.8). Refraction stability was 87%–91% (± 2 diopters) at 2 years and 80% at 3 years. In a small subset, the average change in SE between 6 months and 3 years was − 0.37 diopter. The mean error in refractive correction, measured as the difference between achieved and intended correction, was less than 1 diopter over the entire study.

The stability of this method is conditional upon the stability of the myopia, which is one of the requirements considered for this surgery. Myopia can progress in some cases, sometimes severely,[18] but the changes in refraction due to the evolution of the myopia are usually slow.

Distance Visual Acuity

Recovery of visual acuity is rapid; the preoperative level is attained by the second day postoperatively. Visual acuity in myopic eyes corrected with a phakic IOL increases by one Snellen line or more, owing to the retinal magnification induced by the phakic IOL; the results are better than with correction by other means.[25] In a small series, Praeger et al[13] reported 56.6% and 42% improvement of one or two Snellen lines, respectively. The first-generation Baikoff lenses obtained a mean of uncorrected visual acuity (UCVA) of 0.46–0.51 at 6

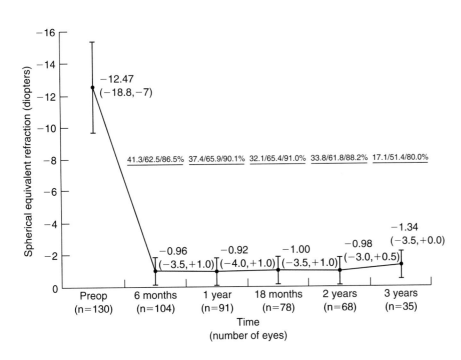

FIGURE 20.8. Mean (range) spherical equivalent manifest refraction over 3 years after implantation of the Baikoff ZB5M phakic IOL. Underlined figures are proportion of eyes within ± 0.50, ± 1.00, and ± 2.00 diopters of emmetropia.

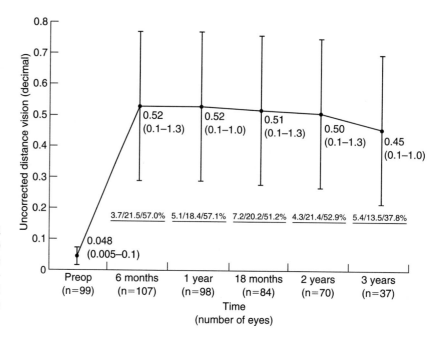

FIGURE 20.9. Mean (range) uncorrected distance visual acuity (Snellen/decimal) over 3 years after implantation of the Baikoff ZB5M phakic IOL. Underlined figures are proportion of eyes with visual acuity of 1.0, 0.8, and 0.5 or better. Results are from a French multicenter study.[18]

months[2,24,26–29] and 0.5–0.6 at 1 year.[2,24,29] The mean best corrected visual acuity (BCVA) was 0.4–0.56 before surgery,[2,16,24,26–30] 0.49–0.81 at 6 months,[2,16,24,26–29] and 0.6–0.8 at 1 year.[2,24,29,30]

In the French multicenter study, the intermediate (3-year) results with the ZB5M lens showed that distance UCVA averaged 0.048 at baseline, improved to 0.5–0.52 over the first 2 years, and then declined to 0.45 at 3 years (Fig. 20.9). Postoperative UCVA scores were as follows: 0.5 or better, 37.8%–57.1%; 0.8 or better, 13.5%–21.5%; and 1 or better, 3.7%–7.2%; the low-

est percentages for UCVA were recorded at the 3-year follow-up examination for 0.5 and 0.8 but not for 1. Distance BCVA improved from 0.54 to 0.69 at the 3-year examination (Fig. 20.10). Only 2.1%–8.3% of eyes lost two Snellen lines, and one eye (2.8%) lost three lines.

Near Visual Acuity

The conservation of accommodation is one of the most important advantages of the phakic IOL lens. The im-

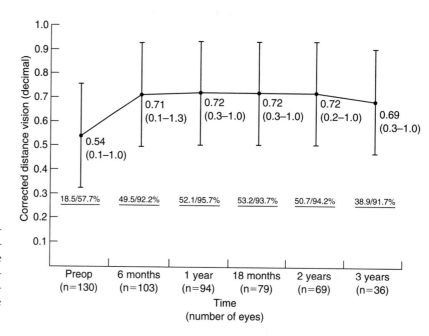

FIGURE 20.10. Mean (range) spectacle-corrected distance visual acuity (Snellen/decimal) over 3 years after implantation of the Baikoff ZB5M phakic IOL. Underlined figures are proportion of eyes with visual acuity of 1.0, 0.8, and 0.5 or better. Results are from a French multicenter study.[18]

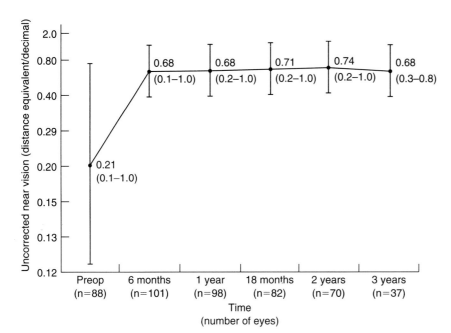

FIGURE 20.11. Mean (range) uncorrected near visual acuity (Snellen distance equivalent/decimal) over 3 years after implantation of the Baikoff ZB5M phakic IOL. Results are from a French multicenter study.[18]

provement was paralleled by increasing distance visual acuity in the French multicenter study with the ZB5M lens—from 0.21 to 0.68–0.77 (Fig. 20.11).[18]

Astigmatism

Mean postoperative refractive astigmatism is very low, and the surgery usually induces any change that occurs. Baikoff et al reported an increase of more than 1 diopter in approximately 15% of patients.[18] Continued improvement in phakic IOLs with flexible implants should reduce the size of the incision and decrease the astigmatism.

Visual Comfort

Visual comfort, an interesting new point, was evaluated by Baikoff et al.[18] Visual comfort at 6 months was judged to be good or very good by 98.2% of patients; at 12 months 97.9% considered visual comfort to be good or very good, and at 18 months more than 93.9% regarded visual comfort as good or very good.

■ Complications

Elevated Intraocular Pressure

Elevated IOP usually occurs during the early postoperative period and is transient. There are several causes. The most frequent, occurring with a reported incidence of 2.4%–29%,[2,16,18,19,26–29] is postoperative steroid application to eyes possibly sensitive to the medication. In one study the elevated IOP returned to normal when the steroid was stopped.[8] In patients who needed to take corticoids (such as patients with iritis), the addition of topical β-blockers controlled IOP.[6] The IOP can be controlled with anti-inflammatory and antihypertensive medication, and an elevated level returns to normal when the iritis has resolved. Inadequate removal of viscoelastic agent is an avoidable cause of elevated IOP; it should be prevented with a good cleaning of the anterior chamber at the end of the surgery.

Only a few cases of pupillary block secondary to phakic IOL implantation have been noted in the literature, but it is always a potential complication.[18] A previous thorough evaluation of the anterior chamber in every patient and an iridectomy in patients with suspicious findings can be helpful. If pupillary block occurs, a peripheral iridotomy should be performed.

Uveitis

Transient acute postoperative uveitis is usually secondary to iris trauma during surgery. The incidence of early postoperative uveitis is 2%–13.3% with first-generation Baikoff lenses[2,16,27–29] and 2.3%–4.56% with the ZB5M.[18,19] This condition is defined as an evident increase in the level of cell and flare counts above normal baseline observed on slit-lamp examination. The inflammation can be so severe as to cause sterile hypopyon or lens explantation.[18,19] An oversized lens has also been reported as a cause of uveitis.[20]

The condition usually responds quickly to topical steroid treatment, without late sequelae.[16,18,19] However, the presence of a phakic IOL in the anterior chamber altered blood–aqueous barrier permeability when tested with the laser flare cell meter[31,32] and fluorophotometry.[33] These changes can continue for several years as a consequence of the presence of the phakic IOL in the anterior chamber. The chronic inflammation may induce other complications such as glaucoma, cataract, or anterior synechiae.[32]

Delayed uveitis is less frequent but can occur; the treatment is the same as for early uveitis. The incidence is 0%–2.4% with Baikoff first-generation lenses[2,29] and 0%–0.8% with the ZB5M lens.[18]

Cataract

Care must be taken to avoid lens trauma during surgery. Miotics and viscoelastic agents help keep the distance from the lens, but the risk of cataract development remains after the surgery. The phakic IOL is a foreign body that modifies not only the blood–aqueous barrier but also the transmittance of the lens.[33] The decrease in lens transmittance could be the result of surgery or of changes in blood–aqueous barrier permeability. These changes cause metabolic disturbances that could decrease transmittance and speed cataract development.[33]

On short-term follow-up, the first-generation Baikoff lenses had a very low rate of cataract formation, 0%–0.7%.[2,16,24,27–29] Reducing the vaulting in the ZB5M did not cause a higher rate of cataract in the short term, but a long-term study by Alio et al[19] found an incidence of 4%. They reported a statistically significant difference in patient age at surgery between the group in which cataracts developed (42 ± 2.5 years) and the unaffected group. However, cataracts do develop earlier in patients with high myopia.[34] It is likely that development of the cataract only needs time. In all reported cases, cataract extraction followed by PCIOL implantation was successful.[19] The compatibility of this procedure is one of the most important advantages of the phakic IOL.

Pupillary Distortion

Pupil ovalization is one of the most common complications of phakic IOL implantation; the reported incidence is 4%–42%.[2,18,19,27–30] This wide range might reflect the subjective methods used to quantify whether or not this deformation is significant. Alio et al defined significant pupil ovalization as the observation of pupil deviation in the meridian of the placement of the phakic IOL haptic that reached the edge of the optic in at least one point.[19] They found pupil ovalization in 6.08% and lesser degrees of ovalization in 10.3%. The

cause of pupillary distortion was thought to be a lens that was too large and the force created by the haptics, but the possibility of a retractable fibrous membrane has also been proposed. The axis of the deviation usually coincides with the major axis of the lens.[19,35]

Another complication usually associated with pupil ovalization is iris atrophy; the reported incidence is 0%–4.8%.[2,19,29] The atrophy usually occurrs in the iris sector affected by ovalization. This atrophy can be severe and can lead to total sector iris atrophy.

Halos and Glare

Halos and glare can be very disturbing to the patient. Their prevalence is related to the diameter of the pupil and the diameter of the optic zone of the phakic IOL. In darkness, with a mid-dilated pupil, the optical zone can be smaller than the pupil,[26] and this difference creates halos. The reported incidence is 5%–60%,[16,18,19,24,27–30] but the percentage of patients in whom this disturbance interferes with normal daily activities is lower.[19] Pilocarpine 1% can be prescribed for patients who cannot tolerate the halos.[16]

Halos and glare were at first considered a minor side effect, but evolving phakic IOL design aims for new solutions. In the new phakic IOLs, NuVita MA20 and ZSAL-4, the real optic diameter was increased to 4.5 and 5 mm, respectively, to create less halo effect. Alio et al have reported a significant difference between the ZSAL-4 and the ZB5M lens, with a lower incidence for the new phakic IOL.[19] There are no reported results about halo effect with the NuVita MA20.

Pupil measurement in darkness with the Colvard test might be done prior to surgery. Patients should be informed of the probability of having postsurgical halos.

Endothelial Damage

The history of endothelial cell loss is linked to the history of lens design. With ongoing improvements in lens design and surgical technique, cell loss is now minor, and this trend will likely continue. Nevertheless, some degree of endothelial damage during surgery should always be assumed, as always happens when an eye is opened. This loss was estimated as 300 cells/mm² by Perez-Santonja et al for the ZB5M PIOL.[36] However, a permanent implant in the anterior chamber poses a continuous risk for progressive endothelial cell loss and marked pleomorphism.[28] Praeger et al noted a 5.5% nonprogressive endothelial cell loss with their lens after 3 years of follow-up, but the series was not very large.[13]

The largest studies were performed with the Baikoff lenses. The first-generation Baikoff lenses were associated with a large amount of cell loss. The 25-degree vaulting made the distance between the phakic IOL and the endothelium very narrow, and acellular zones corresponding to endothelial defects were probably due to contact between the cornea and phakic IOL.[28,37] The mean loss with these lenses in the first year was 9%–19%.[27,28,37–39] The range of the damage was very wide, with several patients experiencing severe cell loss.[30] Leroux et al reported results in a small series of 21 eyes with 8 years of follow-up; 19% of patients had severe endothelial damage with corneal decompensation.[30] Bour et al reported that the peripheral endothelial cell density was slightly lower than the central density owing to a smaller distance between the cornea and the phakic IOL.[37]

The problems with excessive vaulting led Baikoff to redesign his phakic IOL, and the result was the ZB5M. The new angle of 20 degrees was designed to decrease cell loss. Baikoff leads the French multicenter trial, which will follow patients for 5 years.[18] An interim report after 3 years noted a cumulative decrease in cell density in the central cornea of 4.5%, 5.6%, and 5.5% and in the peripheral cornea of 4.2%, 4.4%, and 3.9% during the first, second, and third year, respectively. Baikoff et al suggested that 3.8% of the observed reduction in the endothelial cell layer was attributable to the acute effects of surgery, and estimated a cell loss over time of 0.7% per year.[38]

Alio et al reported 7 years of data, with very similar results.[19] They did not report the difference in endothelial cell density between the peripheral and central cornea but reported the cumulative endothelial cell loss, which was 5.53%, 6.83%, 7.5%, 7.78%, 8.33%, 8.7%, and 9.26% at each successive year of follow-up. The authors showed caution about young age of implantation and the long-term relative risks young patients might face. According to the data, 20–30 years might pass before the lower limit of endothelial cell count (1,500 cells/mm^2) was reached, a situation in which the eye may have a decreased ability to sustain other types of surgery, including cataract extraction. The new ZSAL-4 lens was implanted in a small number of cases. The follow-up in these patients was only 2 years, but no differences were found between the ZSAL-4 lens and the ZB5M lens. No data are available for the NuVita MA20.

Benitez del Castillo et al, using endothelial fluorophotometry, found a continuously increasing endothelial transfer coefficient as a result of the presence of the phakic IOL in the anterior chamber, indicating that endothelial function was affected.[40] The cumulative damage provoked by an anterior chamber implant can lead to a definitive corneal insufficiency. The time required with the new phakic IOLs to evoke this damage is not known. Because most patients who receive these implants are young, further improvement in phakic IOL design could allow long life for these corneas.

Retinal Detachment

Retinal detachment (RD) is a potential hazard of the phakic IOL. The reported incidence is very low, but recently Ruiz-Moreno et al reported a rate of 4.8% in a large study with ZB5M lenses.[41] The incidence was significantly higher in patients who had undergone preoperative laser treatment for predisposing lesions in the retina than in those who had not undergone laser treatment (14.28% vs 3.94%). However, the lesions that caused RD were unrelated to the treated area. The higher incidence of RD in patients with predisposing lesions who received preoperative laser treatment underscored the doubtful efficacy of such prophylactic treatment in these patients. However, RD can appear in a zone previously treated.[18] It is very difficult to say whether this incidence was induced by the phakic IOL or by the myopia, because the incidence of RD is higher in myopic patients than in the emmetropic population.[41] The mean time to develop the RD was 17.4 months (range, 1–44 months).

These RDs were treated with classic procedures. The surgery was more difficult owing to poor visualization through the phakic IOL. In seven of eight cases reported by Ruiz Moreno et al the surgery was successful, and the visual acuities changed from 0.4 before RD to 0.27.[41] Obviously, with the scleral buckle, new myopia was induced with a mean of 1.7 diopters. In these seven cases it was not necessary to remove the lens to do the procedure. In one case a proliferative vitreoretinopathy (PVR) C3 developed after a recurrence of RD. The lens had to be removed, and silicone oil was injected. Visual acuity fell to light perception despite reattachment of the retina.

In other series as well, the reported incidence of RD has been very low, 0%–2.4%.[2,16,18,19,24,29,41] All cases were due to holes or retinal degeneration, except one with a combined rhegmatogenous-serous RD caused by severe fibrinoid uveitis.[42] This patient was managed with steroids, scleral buckle, vitrectomy, and silicone oil after developing PVR; final vision was very poor. Foss et al reported two cases, one bilateral.[43] In one eye PVR developed after three recurrences of RD; the result was very poor. The classic procedure of RD repair with the scleral buckle is usually but not always sufficient for a good result. Preoperative laser treatment of peripheral retinal lesions and careful handling of the globe during the IOL surgery are important preventative recommendations.

Replacement and Removal

Various causes can lead to explantation of the lens, the most common being endothelial damage and the resulting corneal insufficiency.[30] Severe inflammation,[18] cataract,[19] extreme halos and glare,[18,19] and PVR[41] have also been causes for lens removal. The reported incidence varies with the length of follow-up. Leroux-les-Jardins et al reported a 19% incidence at 8 years in a series of 21 eyes that sustained endothelial damage after implantation of the first-generation Baikoff lenses.[30] Alio et al reported a 4.18% incidence at 7 years with the ZB5M.[19] The better design of the ZB5M has been suggested as the reason for this difference.

Displacement or rotation of the lens as a result of inappropriate size and an error in calculating the power have been the most frequent causes for phakic IOL replacement. The reported incidence is 0%–4%.[2,16,18,27–29]

Other Complications

Other complications of phakic IOLs such as corneal edema,[18] expulsive choroidal hemorrhage,[21] flat anterior chamber,[18] and endophthalmitis[44] have been reported in a small number of eyes. Wound dehiscence, Urretz-Zavalia syndrome, and acute ischemic optic neuropathy have been reported as complications with the Fechner-Worst lenses but potentially can also occur with angle-fitted lenses.[1,21]

■ Summary

Phakic IOL implantation is the most predictable and most stable procedure in the treatment of high myopia. The simplicity and reversibility of the method permit it to be performed by most ophthalmologists. The optical results are excellent, and accommodation is preserved. However, complications are always possible. Endothelial cell damage is the main limitation to a long life of these ocular implants. The continuous improvement in phakic IOL design suggests an optimistic outlook for the future is warranted.

■ References

1. Garrana RMR, Azar DT. Phakic intraocular lenses for correction of high myopia. *Int Ophthalmol Clin.* 1999;39(1): 45–57.
2. Baikoff G, Joly P. Comparison of minus power anterior chamber lenses and myopic epikeratoplasty in phakic eyes. *Refract Corneal Surg.* 1990;6:252–260.
3. Fukala V. Operative Behandlung der hochstgradigen Myopie durch Ophakie. *Graefe Arch Ophthalmol.* 1890;36: 230–244.
4. Verzella F. Myopie forte: extraction du cristallin et implantation dans la chambre postérieure dans un but optique. *Bull Mem Soc Fr Ophtalmol.* 1986;97:347–350.
5. Strampelli B. Soppotabilita di lenti acriliche in camera anterior nell afachia e nei vizi refrazione. *Ann Otalomol Clin Oculist.* 1954;80:75–82.
6. Strampelli B. Anterior chamber lenses. *Arch Ophthalmol.* 1961;76:12–17.
7. Barraquer J. Anterior chamber plastic lenses: results and conclusions from five years' experience. *Trans Ophthalmol Soc UK.* 1959;79:393–424.
8. Choyce P. Intraocular lenses and implants. London, England: HK Lewis; 1964:153–155.
9. Choyce P. The present status of intra-cameral and intra-corneal implants. *Can J Ophthalmol.* 1968;3:295–311.
10. Drews RC. The Barraquer experience with intraocular lenses. *Ophthalmology.* 1982;89:386–393.
11. Baikoff G, Colin J. Intraocular lenses in phakic patients. *Ophthalmol Clin North Am.* 1992;5:789–795.
12. Praeger DL. Innovations and creativity in contemporary ophthalmology: preliminary experience with the phakic myopic intraocular lens. *Ann Ophthalmol.* 1988;20:456–462.
13. Praeger DL, Momose A, Muroff LL. Thirty-six month follow-up of a contemporary phakic intraocular lens for the surgical correction of myopia. *Ann Ophthalmol.* 1991;23: 6–10.
14. Praeger DL. Phakic myopic intraocular lens: an alternative to kerato-lenticulorefractive procedures. *Ann Ophthalmol.* 1988;20:246.
15. Baikoff G, Joly P. Utilisation d'une lentille intraoculaire de chambre antérieure pour corriger la myopie forte dans l'oeil phake. *Clin Ophtalmol Martinet.* 1989;2:99–103.
16. Baikoff G. Phakic anterior chamber intraocular lenses. *Int Ophthalmol.* 1991;31:75–86.
17. Baikoff G. The refractive IOL in the phakic eye. *Ophthalmic Pract.* 1991;9:58–61, 80.
18. Baikoff G, Arne JL, Bokobza Y, et al. Angle-fixated anterior chamber phakic intraocular lens for myopia of −7 to −19 diopters. *J Refract Surg.* 1998;14:282–293.
19. Alio JL, de la Hoz F, Pérez-Santonja JJ. Phakic anterior chamber lenses for the correction of myopia: a 7-year cumulative analysis of complications in 263 cases. *Ophthalmology.* 1999;106:458–466.
20. Eloy R, Parrat D, Tran Min Duc, et al. In vitro evaluation of inflammatory cell response after CF4 plasma surface modification of PMMA intraocular lenses. *J Cataract Refract Surg.* 1993;19:364–369.
21. Baikoff G, Samaha A. Phakic intraocular lenses. In: Azar DT, ed. *Refractive Surgery.* Stamford, CT: Appleton & Lange; 1997:545–560.
22. van der Heijde GL, Fechner PU, Worst JGF. Optische Konzequenzen der Implantation einen negativen Intraokularlinse bei myopen Patienten. *Klin Monatsbl Augenheilkd.* 1988;193:99–102.
23. van der Heijde GL. Some optical aspects of implantation of an IOL in a myopic eye. *Eur J Implant Refract Surg.* 1989;1:245–248.
24. Baikoff G, Joly P. Correction chirurgicale de la myopie forte par un implant de chambre antérieure dans l'oeil phak: concept—résultats. *Bull Soc Belge Ophtalmol.* 1989;233:109–125.

25. Garcia M, Gonzalez C, Pascual I, et al. Magnification and visual acuity in highly myopic phakic eyes corrected with an anterior chamber intraocular lens versus by other methods. *J Cataract Refract Surg.* 1996;22:1416–1422.

26. Joly P, Baikoff G, Bonnet P. Mise en place d'un implant négatif de chambre antérieure chez des sujets phaques. *Bull Soc Ophtalmol Fr.* 1989;89:727–733.

27. Colin J, Mimouni F, Robinet A, et al. The surgical treatment of high myopia: comparison of epikeratoplasty, keratomileusis and minus power anterior chamber lenses. *Refract Corneal Surg.* 1990;6:245–251.

28. Mimouni F, Colin J, Koff V, et al. Damage to the corneal endothelium from anterior chamber intraocular lenses in phakic myopic eyes. *Refract Corneal Surg.* 1991;7:277–281.

29. Baikoff G. Etude comparative des complications des epikeratoplasties myopiques et des lentilles intraoculaires de chambre antérieure pour le traitement des myopies fortes. *Ophtalmologie.* 1991;5:276–279.

30. Leroux-les-Jardins S, Ullern M, Werthel AL. Implants myopiques en PMMA de chambre antérieure: bilan à 8 ans. *J Fr Ophtalmol.* 1999;22:323–327.

31. Perez-Santonja JJ, Iradier MT, Benitez del Castillo JM, et al. Chronic subclinical inflammation in phakic eyes with intraocular lenses to correct myopia. *J Cataract Refract Surg.* 1996;22:183–187.

32. Alio JL, De la Hoz F, Ismail MM. Subclinical inflammatory reaction induced by phakic anterior chamber lenses for the correction of high myopia. *Ocul Immunol Inflamm.* 1993;1:219–223.

33. Benitez del Castillo JM, Hernandez JL, Iradier MT, et al. Fluorophotometry in phakic eyes with anterior chamber lens implantation to correct myopia. *J Cataract Refract Surg.* 1993;19:607–609.

34. Metge P, Pichot de Champfleury A. *La Cataracte du myopie forte.* Paris, France: Masson; 1994:447–465.

35. Saragoussi JJ, Othenin-Girard P, Pouliquen Y. Ocular damage after implantation of minus power anterior chamber intraocular lenses in myopic phakic eyes: case reports. *Refract Corneal Surg.* 1993;9:105–109.

36. Perez-Santonja JJ, Iradier MT, Sanz Iglesias L, et al. Endothelial changes in phakic eyes with anterior chamber intraocular lenses to correct high myopia. *J Cataract Refract Surg.* 1996;22:1017–1022.

37. Bour T, Piquot X, Pospisil A, et al. Repercussions endothéliales de l'implant myopique de chambre antérieure ZB au cours de la première année: étude prospective avec analyse statistique. *J Fr Ophtalmol.* 1991;14;633–641.

38. Baikoff G, Joly P, Bonnet PH. Evolution de l'endothelium corneen apres implant myopique. *Ophtalmologie.* 1991;5:525–526.

39. Saragoussi JJ, Cotinat J, Renard G, et al. Endothelium corneen et implants myopiques. *Ophtalmologie.* 1991;5:527–528.

40. Benitez del Castillo JM, Iradier MT, Hernandez JL, et al. Corneal endothelial permeability after implantation of angled fitted anterior chamber lenses in myopic phakic eyes. *Doc Ophthalmol.* 1996;91:201–206.

41. Ruiz-Moreno JM, Alio JL, Perez-Santonja JJ. Retinal detachment in phakic eyes with anterior chamber intraocular lenses to correct severe myopia. *Am J Ophthalmol.* 1999;127:270–275.

42. Alio JL, Ruiz-Moreno JM, Artola A. Retinal detachment as a potential hazard in surgical correction of severe myopia with phakic anterior chamber lenses. *Am J Ophthalmol.* 1993;115:145–148.

43. Foss AJE, Rosen PH, Cooling RJ. Retinal detachment following anterior chamber lens implantation for the correction of ultra-high myopia in phakic eyes. *Br J Ophthalmol.* 1993;77:212–213.

44. Perez-Santonja JJ, Ruiz-Moreno JM, Fernando de la Hoz. Endophthalmitis after phakic intraocular lens implantation to correct high myopia. *J Cataract Refract Surg.* 1999;25:1295–1298.

Chapter 21

Iris-Fixated Phakic Intraocular Lenses

Thanh Hoang-Xuan and François Malecaze

In the 1950s, Strampelli,[1] Barraquer,[2] and Choyce[3,4] were the pioneers of intraocular lens (IOL) implantation in phakic eyes to correct high myopia. The first phakic IOL was an angle-supported IOL that was coarse and of poor quality. Most phakic IOLs had to be removed because they induced complications, including hyphema, iridocyclitis, glaucoma, and corneal decompensation.[5,6] Phakic IOL quality has improved since the 1980s,[7] and excellent refractive results for correction of high myopia associated with a low complication rate have been obtained.[8]

Worst then decided to adopt a different approach, based on his long experience with the use of iris-fixated IOLs for pseudophakic patients. According to Worst et al, the first iris claw phakic IOL was an opaque lens implanted in 1980 to correct diplopia.[9] In 1986, Worst and Fechner changed this iris claw lens to a negative biconcave lens for the correction of high myopia.[10,11] Their concept of a midperipheral iris-supported phakic IOL to correct not only high myopia but also hyperopia[12] differed completely from the angle-supported Baikoff style phakic IOLs[8,13,14] and the posterior chamber phakic IOLs.[15,16] The iris claw phakic IOL also differs from the Binkhorst- and Medallion-type iris-supported lenses, which were based on pupil fixation, and used in the past as pseudophakic IOLs.

◼ Worst Iris-Fixated IOL (Artisan Lens)

Lens Designs

The first iris-fixated lenses were sutured to the iris stroma with a Perlon stitch or a stainless steel suture. The claw fixation method rendered iris stitching no longer necessary. Various lens designs with midperipheral fixation by a claw mechanism were tested before Worst in 1978 introduced his final conceptual model of the iris claw lens for secondary lens implantation or as a standby lens in cases of posterior capsule rupture. Because of the good tolerance and refractive results, the iris claw lens was then used as a primary implant after intracapsular and extracapsular cataract extraction (about 12,000 implantations in Holland up to 1990).[17,18] In 1986 the concept of the claw lens was applied to correct myopia in phakic patients. Initially, the iris claw phakic IOL for myopia was biconcave (Worst-Fechner biconcave lens. The iris claw lens is fixed to the anterior iris surface by enclavation of a fold of iris tissue into the two diametrically opposed "claws" of the lens. The fixation sites are located in the midperiphery of the iris, which is virtually immobile during pupillary movements.

In 1991, the design of this lens was modified into a convex-concave design to increase the distance between the phakic IOL and the corneal endothelium. Suppression of the prominent optical rim also reduced the prismatic effect possibly responsible for halos or glare. Initially called the Worst Myopia Claw lens, the iris claw phakic IOL is presently manufactured by Ophtec (Groningen, Netherlands) under the tradename of Artisan Myopia Lens. The vaulted design (0.5 mm) of the posterior face of the IOL ensures optimal space in front of the natural lens (about 0.8 mm) and prevents aqueous flow blockage. It also accounts for the forward displacement of the human lens during accommodation, which is at maximum about 0.6 mm.[19]

The optical part of the Artisan myopia lens comes in two diameters, 5.0 (Fig. 21.1) and 6.0 mm (Fig. 21.2), with a power range of −3.0 to −23.5 diopters

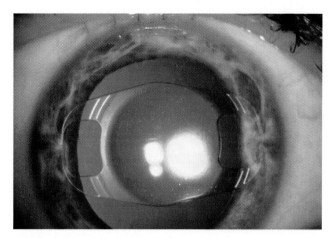

FIGURE 21.1. 5.0-mm diameter Artisan phakic IOL. Note that pupil dilation is not affected.

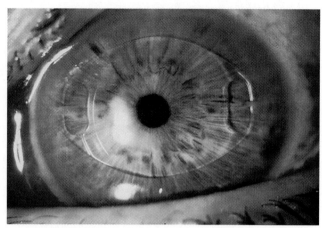

FIGURE 21.2. 6.0-mm diameter Artisan phakic IOL.

for the 5-mm-diameter lens and −3.0 to −15.5 diopters for the 6-mm-diameter lens, the power range increasing in 0.5-diopter increments. The thickness of the IOL in the optical axis is 0.2 mm. It is a one-piece, ultraviolet (UV) wavelength-absorbing, Perspex inch 1 CQ (polymethyl methacrylate, PMMA), compression-molded lens with an overall diameter of 8.5 mm and a total height of 0.9 mm. The weight is 10 mg in air (15.0-diopter lens).

In 1997 an iris claw lens specially designed for the correction of aphakia was introduced. Hyperopic iris claw lenses are also available (5 mm diameter, power range of +1.0 to +12.0 diopters).

Indications and Contraindications

The following conditions must be fulfilled for phakic iris claw lens implantation:

- Contact lens wear impossible and spectacle correction is contraindicated for occupational or psychological reasons
- Stable refraction
- Periphery of the retina is healthy or adequately treated
- No history of ocular disease, including glaucoma, cataract, uveitis, and macular disease
- Lifelong close ophthalmologic follow-up possible
- Endothelial cell density >2,000 cells/mm² (specular microscopic examination of the cornea should be performed preoperatively)
- A pupil smaller than 6 mm in scotopic luminance (but the reactivity of the pupil seems to be as important as pupil size)
- A deep anterior chamber: for high myopia, the minimal central depth of the anterior chamber as mea-

sured by ultrasound should not be less than 3.0 mm and 3.2 mm with a 5.0-mm and 6.0-mm-diameter optic of an Artisan Myopia Lens. To avoid any contact between the peripheral rim of the phakic IOL and the corneal endothelium, the critical distance between both is 1.5 mm for an average K-value of 43.0 diopters, according to the FDA guideline.

In 1986, Worst and Fechner recommended implantation of phakic IOLs for myopes of 5.0 diopters or more.[11,20] Today, with the successful results of LASIK for low and moderate myopia, there is a trend toward phakic IOL implantation only in high myopes (10 diopters or more), unless LASIK cannot be used safely because of unsatisfactory corneal thickness or corneal curvature. The indications for iris claw lenses have also been extended to high hyperopes.

Surgical Preparation

IOL Power Calculation. The power of the IOL is calculated on the basis of the corneal curvature (K), the anterior chamber depth measured by ultrasonography, and the spectacle correction, by applying a special mathematical formula (van der Heijde's tables).[21,22] Roughly, it will be about the same as the power of the spectacles at a vertex distance of 12 mm.

Medical Treatment. The vast majority of surgeons do not follow the recommendations of Fechner et al:[23] 1 hour preoperatively, 250 mL of 20% mannitol intravenously, and in some cases high doses of oral prednisone. They give no systemic medication at all.

Anesthesia. Most patients are operated on an outpatient basis. In this type of surgery—more than in phakoemulsification, for example—it is important to obtain full akinesia and analgesia. General anesthesia is recommended for less experienced surgeons or in circumstances where safety requires it. Once the surgical technique is mastered, local anesthesia (preferably parabulbar injection) can be used to achieve total immobility of the globe and eyelids.

Miosis. Preoperative application of topical pilocarpine results in miosis. Miosis is mandatory as it forms a protection shield for the natural lens during the insertion and fixation of the iris claw lens. A constricted pupil also facilitates proper centration of the lens.

Prevention of Pupil Block. There is theoretically no risk of pupil block glaucoma because the vaulted configuration of the Artisan Myopia Lens ensures normal aqueous outflow. However, a peripheral iridectomy during surgery, or argon or YAG laser iridotomy before surgery, particularly when a tunnel incision is performed, is recommended.

Guaranteeing Good IOL Centration. Using an argon laser, two marks can be made on the iris at diametrically opposite sites to facilitate proper IOL centration during surgery.

Operative Technique

Incision Techniques. Various incision techniques can be used: clear-corneal or scleral-tunnel incision superiorly, or clear-corneal incision temporally.

Incision Size. The incision should be at least 5.2 mm for the 5-mm lens and 6.2 mm for the 6-mm lens to avoid difficulties of IOL insertion.

Puncture Incisions. Two types of puncture incisions can be used depending on the entrapment technique of the iris: for a superior incision, (1) two small incisions of at least 1.1 mm at 10 o'clock and 2 o'clock, when iris entrapment needles are used, (2) two small incisions of at least 1.5 mm at 3 o'clock and 9 o'clock, when iris entrapment forceps are used (Fig. 21.3).

Viscoelastic Material. The viscoelastic substance is injected through one of the puncture incisions to create a deep anterior chamber. It is mandatory to use high-viscosity sodium hyaluronate to maintain working space in the anterior chamber. Materials of lower viscosity (e.g., methylcellulose, hydroxypropylmethylcellulose) should be avoided. If additional viscoelastic material needs to be injected during surgery, care should be taken not to let it slip under the IOL. It should be used as a stabilizing agent that presses the implant onto the iris surface. Before entrapment of the haptics, some viscoelastic should be injected on top of the implant to protect the endothelium.

Introduction of the Phakic IOL into the Anterior Chamber. The phakic IOL is introduced with the Artisan fixation forceps into the anterior chamber through its smaller diameter because of the size of the incision

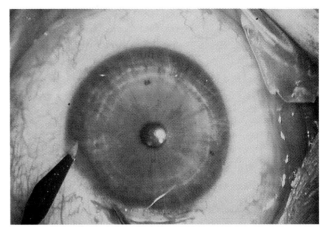

FIGURE 21.3. Corneal punctures are made to allow the iris entrapment needle or forceps to be passed.

and because, otherwise, the claws tend to interfere with the insertion (Fig. 21.4). Then the phakic IOL is rotated 90 degrees.

Guaranteeing Pupillary Miosis. Pupillary miosis should be guaranteed during the insertion and fixation procedure. The use of an intraocular miotic facilitates proper centration of the IOL and reduces the risk of lens touch.

IOL Centration and Fixation. Centration and fixation of the IOL is probably the most critical step of the procedure; its accuracy influences the postoperative results. Centration of the IOL involves determining the X and Y axes on the iris surface and consequently defining the two fixation spots. The pupil is used as a reference for centration. Correct axial centration of the operating microscope prevents postoperative parallactic errors. These errors are likely to occur when the eye fails to remain in a central position.

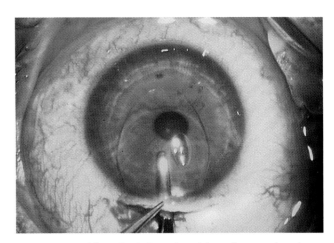

FIGURE 21.4. The IOL is introduced into the anterior chamber in a vertical position.

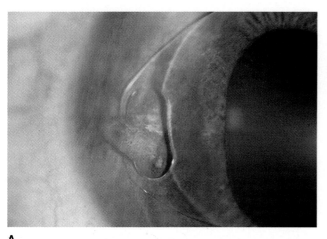
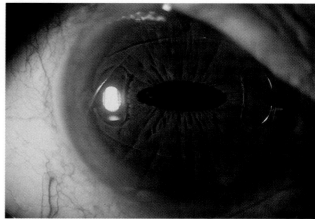

A   B

FIGURE 21.5. *A,* The Artisan lens claws enclave a fold of iris tissue to fixate the lens. *B,* The pupil is deformed because the enclavation sites are too central.

The enclavation spots can also be determined preoperatively, by making two marks on the iris surface with the argon laser. Fixation is performed by gently creating an iris fold under the claw and then entrapping the iris fold into the claw (Fig. 21.5). Two specially designed instruments can be used: (1) Artisan iris entrapment forceps, which allow one to grasp a 1-mm fold of midperipheral iris tissue and press the IOL claws over the forcep's tips (Fig. 21.6); (2) Artisan iris entrapment needles, which are blunt and allow one, through a vertical movement of the needle, to create a fold of midperipheral iris tissue. The IOL claws are then pressed over the fold (Fig. 21.7).

Iridectomy and Iridotomy. Although a prophylactic iridectomy or iridotomy as a standard procedure is theoretically unnecessary (the Artisan Myopia Lens is vaulted to encourage natural fluid flow), experience has shown that it can prevent pupil block glaucoma in certain cases (Fig. 21.8).

Wound Closure. Watertight wound closure is of paramount importance to prevent a shallow anterior chamber leading to IOL-endothelial contact in the immediate postoperative period.

Removal of Viscoelastic Material. Once the wound has been closed almost completely the viscoelastic material should be entirely removed to prevent a shallow anterior chamber and touch between the IOL and the cornea (Fig. 21.9).

Surgical Caveats

Anesthesia. Insufficient akinesia can lead to sudden eye movements, increasing the risk of lens or endothelium touch.

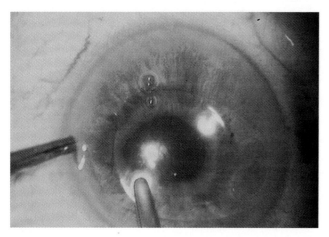

FIGURE 21.6. The Artisan iris entrapment forceps is used to grasp a 1-mm fold of midperipheral iris tissue, and then the iris claws are passed over the forcep tips.

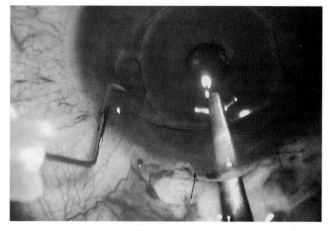

FIGURE 21.7. Blunt Artisan iris entrapment needles can also be used to create a fold of midperipheral iris tissue through a vertical movement of the needle.

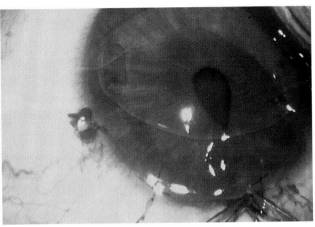
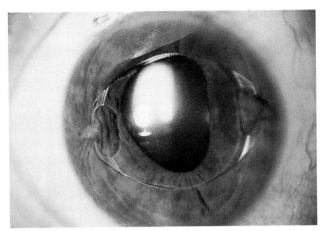

A   **B**

FIGURE 21.8. *A*, Prophylactic iridectomy is performed to prevent pupil block glaucoma. *B*, A reactive semi-mydriasis secondary to acute angle-closure glaucoma due to incomplete peripheral iridectomy.

Insufficient Pupil Constriction. Insufficient pupil constriction may cause the viscoelastic material to be trapped in the pupillary area under the implant and lead to difficulties in removing it completely at the end of the procedure. The implant also may touch the natural lens during implantation if miosis is insufficient. Centration of the implant is also more difficult under these circumstances.

Low-Viscosity Viscoelastic Material. Maneuvers during implantation or the implant itself can cause traumatic touch of the corneal endothelium or the natural lens. Touch can occur during collapse of the anterior chamber caused by external loss of the viscoelastic material. Therefore, a high-viscosity viscoelastic material is mandatory.

Incomplete Removal of Viscoelastic Material. Incomplete removal of the viscoelastic material can cause an early postoperative elevation in IOP.

Iris Prolapse. Because of the hydrostatic and hydrodynamic conditions during IOL insertion, there is greater risk of iris prolapse than in normal cataract surgery. Iris prolapse tends to occur more often with the use of direct corneoscleral incisions than with scleral-tunnel and clear-corneal incisions.

IOL Centration and Fixation. The most difficult step of iris claw surgery is entrapment of the iris fold into the slit of the haptics. The avoidance of possible postoperative problems, such as glare and halos, depends on perfect centration of the IOL at this step.

IOL Luxation. If the iris fold is too small, the IOL may dislocate into the anterior chamber and cause damage to the cornea.

Instrumentation. Inadequate surgical instruments such as homemade needles with sharp tips may damage the iris during entrapment.

Postoperative Management

Nonsteroidal and/or steroidal anti-inflammatory drugs are usually prescribed for 2–4 weeks after surgery. Glaucoma drugs are not used on a regular basis. Patients also must be instructed not to rub their eyes after surgery.

It is critical to inform the patient of the necessity for regular follow-up. In particular, long-term evaluation of the corneal endothelium density using specular microscopy is recommended.

Outcomes

Improvement of vision quality and enlargement of visual field are common outcomes. In the earlier series of Fechner et al (62 eyes, preoperative spherical equivalent

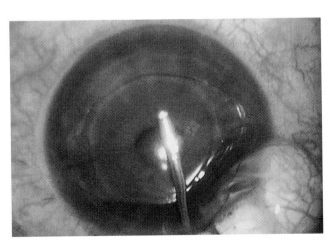

FIGURE 21.9. Viscoelastic material removed.

[SE] −7.0 diopters to −28.0 diopters), 63% of eyes were within 1.0 diopter correct.[20] None deviated more than 20% from the predicted correction. In the series of Worst et al including 18 eyes (range, −8.0 diopters to −18.0 diopters), predictability of outcome was good: seven eyes needed no spherical correction postoperatively, and only two eyes deviated more than 2.0 diopters from the aimed refraction.[9] In the series of Fechner et al including 109 implanted eyes (preoperative mean SE, −14.4 diopters, range, −5.0 diopters to −31.5 diopters), 75 eyes (68.8%) were corrected within 1.0 diopter of the desired refraction, and only 10 eyes (9.2%) deviated more than 2.0 diopters from the aimed result.[23] Landesz et al reported a 74.3% rate of postoperative SE refractive error within 1.0 diopter of emmetropia in a series of 35 eyes (range, −6.0 diopters to −28.0 diopters).[24] Menezo et al reported that 80.5% of eyes (90 eyes, range, −7.0 diopters to −24.0 diopters) were within 1.0 diopter of emmetropia.[25] Malecaze (personal data), in his series of 25 eyes (mean SE −13.43 diopters, range, −8.00 diopters to −17.25 diopters) implanted with the Artisan Myopia Lens, found 52% (13 eyes) and 84% (21 eyes) predictability values for 0.5 diopters or less and 1.0 diopter or less of aimed postoperative uncorrected visual acuity (UVA), respectively. Efficacy, as defined as the ratio between postoperative UVA and preoperative best corrected visual acuity (BCVA), was 0.80 in Malecaze's series. Comparatively, efficacy was 0.73 for LASIK in 41 myopic eyes (preoperative mean SE, −7.50 diopters) in the hands of the same surgeon. Mean UCA was 0.46, ±0.22 diopters, the first postoperative day so visual recovery was rapid.

There is a change in the retinal image size, which is increased by 20% compared with the image with spectacles.[21,22] Menezo et al found that 77 of 94 eyes (81.9%) gained two or more lines of BCVA compared to the preoperative values.[26] Malecaze (personal data) found that 16 of 25 eyes (64%) gained one line or more of BCVA postoperatively, and only one eye (4%) lost one line. He showed that induced-astigmatism was not a problem: It was 1.33 ± 0.88 diopters and 1.00 ± 0.73 diopters preoperativaly and postoperatively, respectively.

Very rarely, visual symptoms such as double contour are reported. Postoperative glare and halos usually disappear gradually.[24,26] The incidence of halos appeared unrelated to pupil size as measured with the Colvard Pupillometer (Malecaze, personal data).

Complications

Anterior Chamber Inflammation. There may be a correlation between the incidence of some complications and the experience of the surgeon. Rare cases of

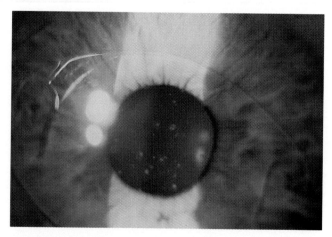

FIGURE 21.10. Pigments on the IOL indicate postoperative inflammation.

exudative iritis were described during the early period of the surgeon's learning curve, probably due to repeated traumatic attempts of iridic incarceration.[20,23,26] Most surgeons did not report any cases of postoperative iritis requiring systemic steroid therapy.[9,26] Early postoperative iridocyclitis has been reported in 6.4%[23] to 16%[27] of eyes. Late postoperative iridocyclitis also has been occasionally observed (Fig. 21.10).[28] Studies using a laser flare-cell meter showed contradictory results. Fechner et al reported no more inflammation than after a cataract extraction with posterior chamber implantation.[23] Also, iris angiography did not show vascular leaks in some studies.[23,26] Conversely, Pérez-Santonja et al, using a laser flare-cell meter, detected chronic subclinical inflammation between 1 and 2 years postoperatively.[28,29] Alio et al also reported elevated flare values 1 year following implantation of Worst-Fechner lenses, but their results were probably artifactual.[30] Finally fluorophotometry on 15 eyes implanted with the Worst-Fechner iris claw lens showed prolonged breakdown of the blood–aqueous barrier. This subclinical inflammation was attributed to the presence of the lens and not to the procedure itself.[31] Pigment deposition on the corneal endothelium also was observed, suggesting a release from the iris induced by the phakic lens.[28]

Glaucoma. Postoperative glaucoma can be corticosteroid-induced and usually resolves after discontinuation of steroidal therapy. Secondary glaucoma can also occur if the viscoelastic material has been inadequately removed. Only rare cases of temporary ocular hypertension have been reported.[26] In one case the pupil dilated and could not be constricted, and the phakic IOL had to be removed.[20] One case of anterior ischemic optic neuropathy occurred immediately after surgery, possibly due to increased IOP co-occurring with systemic hypertension.[32]

Iris Atrophy — Dislocation. Pérez-Santonja et al observed iris atrophy on both fixation sites in 81% of eyes, lens instability in 9.3%, and delayed implant displacement secondary to iris fold perforation or haptic disincarceration in 9.3%.[28] Mertens et al[33] and Risco and Cameron[34] also reported one case of delayed detachment of iris claw haptic and IOL dislocation. But no iris atrophy has been mentioned in most of the reports.

Decentration. Implant decentration can be measured using a slit-lamp beam or a digital imaging system.[28,35] Patients report halos that may be related to lens decentration in 23.4%–56% of cases, but this rarely requires reintervention.[26,28,36]

Endothelial Cell Loss. Some concerns exist with regard to the progressive decrease of corneal endothelial cell density. Various investigators found an acceptable mean endothelial loss (5.3%–8.9%) 1 year following iris claw phakic lens implantation,[24,37] which is similar to results of posterior chamber IOL implantation.[38] Menezo et al noted 7.63% and 17.9% of endothelial cell loss at 2 and 5 years, respectively, without morphometric changes.[26,36,39] They found no significant statistical differences between biconcave and convex–concave designed iris claw lenses, with respect to endothelium cell density. In a few cases, the endothelial cell count decreased because of corneal trauma during implantation.[20,40] Landesz et al implanted an opaque iris claw lens in a phakic eye to correct acquired diplopia, and found a 18.6% difference of mean endothelial cell density compared to the nonimplanted fellow eye 14 years after surgery.[41]

Several reports have shown that some eyes do develop unexplained endothelial cell loss following uncomplicated surgery.[23,28,42–44] Pérez-Santonja et al reported an endothelial cell loss of 17.6% at 2 years.[28] According to Fechner et al, significant progressive endothelial cell loss was observed in 13.4% of eyes implanted between 1986 and 1991, and a projected 8-year follow-up resulted in a decrease in 27% of eyes.[44] The loss may be related to eye rubbing or vaulting of the implant. This is a major factor motivating the design change of the implant to the convex–concave shape of the Artisan Myopia Lens. Menezo et al believe that the endothelial damage is due mainly to the surgical maneuvers since they found the most important changes during the first 6 months postoperatively.[36] According to these investigators, a shallower anterior chamber depth and a more powerful (and therefore thicker) minus implant are predictors of greater endothelial cell density decrease during this period. In addition, breakdown in the blood–aqueous barrier may lead to chronic inflammation that is directly toxic to the corneal endothelium.[28,45,46] Some surgeons advocate a poor implantation technique that results in higher endothelial cell loss.[47] In a multicenter study, Budo et al showed a mean endothelial density change of only 0.7% at 3 years in 129 eyes.[48]

Funduscopy. Cystoid macular edema is not observed, and the peripheral fundus is easily visualized through a dilated pupil. Only one case of flat retinal detachment was reported after iris claw phakic lens implantation.[23,42]

Miscellaneous. Cystic wounds associated with subconjunctival fistulas requiring resuturing have been reported.[23,28,42] Intraoperative hyphema due to the iridectomy or excessive iris manipulation can occur, but usually clears completely.[36] Pseudophakodonesis is not visible except in nystagmic patients.

Two cases of Urrets-Zavalia syndrome due to insufficient removal of the viscoelastic material associated with a frail iris were reported.[23] Viscoelastic injection associated with prolonged iris prolapse may damage the iris sphincter. Contact between the IOL and the natural lens has not been noted, and age-related cataract can be easily extracted in patients with an iris claw phakic lens.[49]

■ Advantages and Disadvantages of the Iris Claw Lens

The advantages of the iris claw lens are multiple:

- predictable postoperative refraction thanks to van der Heijde's tables,
- efficacy,
- excellent quality of vision,
- outpatient surgery,
- short recovery time,
- stable surgical results,
- reversible surgery, and
- low complication rate.

The main disadvantage of the iris claw lens is the surgeon's learning curve, which may be improved by training in wetlab courses before implanting patients. The intraoperative and postoperative risks inherent in iris claw phakic IOL implantation include induced astigmatism, increased permeability of blood–aqueous barrier, anterior chamber inflammation, and endophthalmitis. In Menezo and associates' experience in 111 cases, no intraoperative and postoperative complications were noted in 91.0% and 83.8% of eyes, respectively.[36] Long-term follow-up is mandatory with respect to the possibility of iris atrophy at the fixation sites and progressive endothelial cell loss.

■ References

1. Strampelli B. Sopportabilita di lenti acriliche in camera anteriore nella afachia o nei vizi di refrazione. *Ann Otamol Clin Oculist Parma.* 1954;80:75–82.

2. Barraquer J. Anterior chamber plastic lenses: results of and conclusions from five years' experience. *Trans Ophthalmol Soc UK.* 1959;79:393–424.

3. Choyce P. Discussion to Barraquer: anterior chamber plastic lenses—results of and conclusions from five years' experience. *Trans Ophthalmol Soc UK.* 1959;79:423.

4. Choyce P. Intraocular Lenses and Implants. London, England: HK Lewis; 1964:153–155.

5. Nordlohne MD. *The Intraocular Implant Lens: Developments and Results.* The Hague, Netherlands: W Junk; 1975:23.

6. Drews RC. The Barraquer experience with intraocular lenses, 20 years later. *Ophthalmology.* 1982;89:386–393.

7. Dvali MD. Intraocular correction of high myopia. *Vestnik Ophthalmol.* 1986;102:29–31.

8. Joly P, Baikoff G, Bonnet P. Mise en place d'un implant négatif de chambre antérieure chez des sujets phaques. *Bull Soc Ophtalmol Fr.* 1989;89:727–733.

9. Worst JGF, van der Veen G, Los LI. Refractive surgery for high myopia: the Worst-Fechner biconcave iris claw lens. *Doc Ophthalmol.* 1990;75:335–341.

10. Fechner PU, van der Heijde GL, Worst JGF. Intraokulare Linse zur Myopiekorrektion des phaquen Auges. *Klin Monatsbl Augenheilkd.* 1988;193:29–34.

11. Fechner PU, Worst JGF. A new concave intraocular lens for the correction of high myopia. *Eur J Implant Refract Surg.* 1989;1:41–43.

12. Fechner PU, Singh D, Wulff K. Iris claw lens in phakic eyes to correct hyperopia: preliminary study. *J Cataract Refract Surg.* 1998;24:48–56.

13. Alio JL, de la Hoz F, Pérez-Santonja JJ, et al. Phakic anterior chamber lenses for the correction of myopia: a 7-year cumulative analysis of complications in 263 cases. *Ophthalmology.* 1999;106:458–466.

14. Baikoff G, Arné JL, Bokobza Y, et al. Angle-fixated anterior chamber phakic intraocular lens for myopia of − 7 to − 19 diopters. *J Refract Surg.* 1998;14:282–293.

15. Marinho A, Neves MC, Pinto MC, et al. Posterior chamber silicone phakic intraocular lens. *J Refract Surg.* 1997;13:219–222.

16. Rosen E, Gore C. Staar Collamer posterior chamber phakic intraocular lens to correct myopia and hyperopia. *J Cataract Refract Surg.* 1998;24:596–606.

17. Fechner PU. Die Irisklauen-Linse. *Klin Monatsbl Augenheilkd.* 1987;191:26–29.

18. Singh D, Singh IR. Use of the Worst-Singh lobster claw intraocular lens in children. *Ophthalmic Pract.* 1987;5:18.

19. de Vries FR, van der Heijde GL, Goovaerts HG. A system for continuous high-resolution measurement of distances in the eye. *J Biomech Eng.* 1987;9:32–37.

20. Fechner PU, van der Heijde GL, Worst JGF. The correction of myopia by lens implantation into phakic eyes. *Am J Ophthalmol.* 1989;107:659–663.

21. van der Heijde GL, Fechner PU, Worst JGF. Optische Konsequenzen der Implantation einer negativen Intraokularlinse bei myopen Patienten. *Klin Monatsbl Augenheilkd.* 1988;193:99–102.

22. van der Heijde GL. Some optical aspects of implantation of an IOL in a myopic eye. *Eur J Implant Refract Surg.* 1989;1:245–248.

23. Fechner PU, Strobel J, Wichmann W. Correction of myopia by implantation of a concave Worst-iris claw lens into phakic eyes. *Refract Corneal Surg.* 1991;7:286–298.

24. Landesz M, Worst JGF, Siertsema JV, et al. Correction of high myopia with the Worst myopia claw intraocular lens. *J Refract Surg.* 1995;11:16–25.

25. Menezo JL, Cisneros A, Hueso JR, et al. Long-term results of surgical treatment of high myopia with Worst-Fechner intraocular lenses. *J Cataract Refract Surg.* 1995;21:93–98.

26. Menezo JL, Avino JA, Cisneros AL, et al. Iris claw phakic intraocular lens for high myopia. *J Refract Surg.* 1997;13:545–555.

27. Harto MA, Menezo JL, Pérez L, et al. Correccion de la alta miopia con lentes intraoculares (Worst-Fechner) en ojos faquicos. *Arch Soc Esp Oftalmol.* 1992;62:267–274.

28. Pérez-Santonja JJ, Bueno JL, Zato MA. Surgical correction of high myopia in phakic eyes with Worst-Fechner myopia intraocular lenses. *J Refract Surg.* 1997;13:268–284.

29. Pérez-Santonja JJ, Iradier MT, Benitez del Castillo JM, et al. Chronic subclinical inflammation in phakic eyes with intraocular lenses to correct myopia. *J Cataract Refract Surg.* 1996;22:183–187.

30. Alio JL, de la Hoz F, Ismail MM. Subclinical inflammatory reaction induced by phakic anterior chamber lenses for the correction of high myopia. *Ocul Immunol Inflamm.* 1993;1:219–223.

31. Pérez-Santonja JJ, Hernandez JL, Benitez del Castillo JM, et al. Fluorophotometry in myopic phakic eyes with anterior chamber intraocular lenses to correct severe myopia. *Am J Ophthalmol.* 1994;118:316–321.

32. Pérez-Santonja JJ, Bueno JL, Meza J, et al. Ischemic optic neuropathy after intraocular lens implantation to correct high myopia in a phakic patient. *J Cataract Refract Surg.* 1993;19:651–654.

33. Mertens E, Tassignon MJ. Detachment of iris claw haptic after implantation of phakic Worst anterior chamber lens: case report. *Bull Soc Belge Ophtalmol.* 1998;268:19–22.

34. Risco JM, Cameron JA. Dislocation of a phakic intraocular lens. *Am J Ophthalmol.* 1994;118:666–667.

35. Pérez-Torregrosa VT, Menezo JL, Harto MA, et al. Digital system measurement of decentration of Worst-Fechner iris claw myopia intraocular lens. *J Refract Surg.* 1995;11:26–30.

36. Menezo JL, Cisneros AL, Rodriguez-Salvador V. Endothelial study of iris claw phakic lenses: four year follow-up. *J Cataract Refract Surg.* 1998;24:1039–1049.

37. Mathys B, Zanen A, Schrooyen M. Lentille de chambre antérieure négative d'un nouveau type dans la myopie élevée. *Bull Soc Belge Ophtalmol.* 1991;242:19–26.

38. Werblin TP. Long-term endothelial cell loss following phacoemulsification: model for evaluating endothelial

damage after intraocular surgery. *J Refract Corneal Surg.* 1993;9:29–35.

39. Menezo JL, Cisneros AL, Cervera M, et al. Iris claw phakic lens: intermediate and long-term corneal endothelial changes. *Eur J Implant Refract Surg.* 1994;6:195–199.

40. Landesz M, Worst JGF, Siertsema JV, et al. Negative implant. *Doc Ophthalmol.* 1993;83:261–270.

41. Landesz M, Worst JGF, Van Rij G, et al. Opaque iris claw lens in a phakic eye to correct acquired diplopia. *J Cataract Refract Surg.* 1997;23:137–138.

42. Fechner PU, Wichmann W. Correction of myopia by implantation of minus optic (Worst iris claw) lenses into the anterior chamber of phakic eyes. *Eur J Implant Refract Surg.* 1993;5:55–59.

43. Pérez-Santonja JJ, Iradier MT, Sanz-Iglesias L, et al. Endothelial changes in phakic eyes with anterior chamber intraocular lenses to correct high myopia. *J Cataract Refract Surg.* 1996;22:1017–1022.

44. Fechner PU, Haubitz I, Wichmann W, et al. Worst-Fechner biconcave minus power phakic iris claw lens. *J Refract Surg.* 1999;15:93–105.

45. Miyake K, Asakura M, Kobayashi H. Effect of intraocular lens fixation on the blood-aqueous barrier. *Am J Ophthalmol.* 1984;98:451–455.

46. Apple DJ, Brems RN, Park RB, et al. Anterior chamber lenses. Part I. Complications and pathology and review of designs. *J Cataract Refract Surg.* 1987;13:157–174.

47. Krumeich JH, Daniel J, Gast R. Closed-system technique for implantation of iris-supported negative-power intraocular lens. *J Refract Surg.* 1996;12:334–340.

48. Budo C, Hesloehl JC, Izak M, et al. Multicenter study of the Artisan phakic intraocular lens. *J Cataract Refract Surg.* 2000;26:1163–1171.

49. Menezo JL, Cisneros AL, Rodriguez-Salvador V. Removal of age-related cataract and iris claw phakic intraocular lens. *J Refract Surg.* 1997;13:589–590.

Chapter 22

Posterior Chamber Phakic Intraocular Lenses

Jean-Louis Arné and Thanh Hoang-Xuan

The pioneers in phakic lens implantation to correct refractive errors, particularly high myopia, were Strampelli,[1] Barraquer,[2] and Choyce,[3] but the first-generation intraocular lenses (IOLs) were of poor quality and induced many complications.[4] In 1986, Fyodorov et al[5] originated the first plate posterior chamber phakic intraocular lens (IOL). They used a one-piece silicone collar-button phakic IOL with a Teflon coat. Encouraging initial results were achieved with different types of silicone phakic IOLs, but problems with cataract formation,[6,7] uveitis, glaucoma, and decentration[8] led to changes in lens design and type of material in order to improve biocompatibility. Chiron-Adatamed (Munich, Germany), under Fechner's guidance, improved the design of the silicone lens, but it still was unfoldable.[9] In contrast, the phakic IOL manufactured by Staar Surgical has collagen incorporated into acrylic material.

■ Lens Design

The current Staar Surgical implantable contact lens (ICL) (Fig. 22.1) is made of a collagen copolymer, a compound combining acrylic and porcine collagen (<0.1% collagen). Its refractive index is 1.45 at 35 degrees C. The material is soft, elastic, and hydrophilic.

The optical zone of the myopic lenses is 60 μm thick and the diameter is 4.5–5.5 mm, according to the power required. The optical zone diameter of the hyperopic lenses is 5.5 mm. Available powers are −3 to −21 diopters for myopic lenses and +3 to +17 diopters for hyperopic lenses. Several lengths are available, from 11.0 mm to 12.5 mm for hyperopic lenses and from 11.5 mm to 13 mm for myopic lenses. The posterior surface is concave, to vault over the anterior capsule.

■ Preoperative Evaluation

Exclusion criteria for phakic IOLs include previous intraocular surgery, endothelial dystrophy, opacities of the crystalline lens, glaucoma, pigment dispersion syndrome, diabetic retinopathy, preexisting systemic disease, and nonstable ametropia. The lens power is calculated with formulas that include manifest and cycloplegic refraction, keratometric power, anterior chamber depth, and corneal thickness.

The length of the lens is determined based on the horizontal corneal diameter. White-to-white measurement can be made by caliper, gauge, videokeratoscope, or photographic devices. The size of the phakic IOL chosen is in most cases white-to-white length + 0.5 mm, rounded to the nearest 0.5-mm increment.

■ Surgical Technique

Iridotomies

Two weeks before surgery, laser iridotomies are performed. Two peripheral superior iridotomies are placed 80 degrees apart to avoid the possibility of iridotomy occlusion by the haptics of the implant.

Preparation and Anesthesia

A combination of mydriatic topical medications (tropicamine 1%, phenylephrine 2.5%, or similar) is applied serially beginning 1 hour before surgery. The anesthesia method is based on patient and surgeon preferences and may be general anesthesia, peribulbar injection, or topical anesthesia.

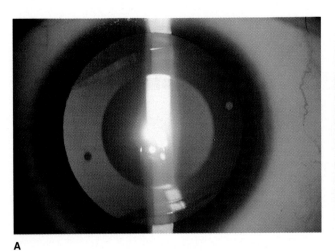
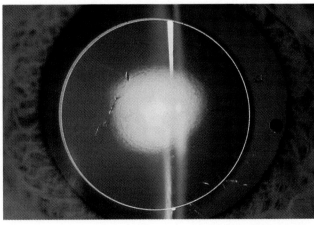

FIGURE 22.1. *A* and *B,* Staar Surgical posterior chamber phakic intraocular lens.

Surgical Procedure

A superior puncture incision is performed and aqueous humor is replaced by a viscoelastic gel. A temporal corneal tunnel (3.20 mm wide, 1.75–2.00 mm long) is created. A narrow diamond blade allows progressive opening of the anterior chamber. Viscoelastic material is injected. The implant can be inserted by two different techniques, with an injector or with forceps.

With an injector: The IOL is positioned into the lens insertion cartridge under direct vision through the operating microscope. In the absence of a soft tip injector, a small silicone sponge can be placed to protect the IOL from the hard injector arm. Because IOL insertion into the cartridge is complicated and time-consuming, it must be done before the incision is made. The injector tip is placed in the tunnel and the lens is injected into the anterior chamber. As the IOL unfolds slowly, its progression must be controlled to ensure proper orientation.

With forceps: The IOL is easy to fold between the jaws of a MacPherson forceps. The tip of the forceps, is introduced into the entrance of the tunnel. Then another MacPherson forceps, held in the operator's other hand, is used to grasp the sides of the implant. The first forceps is opened, regrasps the IOL a little further, and pushes it slowly. By repeating these maneuvers with the forceps, the operator moves the IOL into the tunnel and the IOL unfolds in a controlled manner. The tip of the forceps must not enter the anterior chamber, to avoid contact with the crystalline lens.

While the IOL unfolds, its proper orientation must be checked. Then each footplate is placed one after the other beneath the iris with a specially designed, flat, nonpolished manipulator without pressure being placed on the crystalline lens. It is important to avoid touching the optic of an ICL in the middle, as it is the thinnest part. Then the viscoelastic material is removed with gentle irrigation-aspiration and acetylcholine chloride is injected. Steroid or antibiotic eye drops are instilled. The patient receives 500 mg of intravenous acetazolamide at the conclusion of the surgery.

■ Functional Results

Predictability

Asseto et al implanted 15 lenses in 14 patients.[10] The average follow-up period was 7.00 ± 1.95 months. Mean spherical equivalent (SE) was − 15.3 ± 3.1 diopters preoperatively and − 2.0 ± 1.5 diopters postoperatively. Only 31% of the eyes had less than 1.0 diopter of residual myopia. However, an old model of lenses was used.

Rosen and Gore operated on 16 myopic eyes (preoperative SE, − 5.25 to − 14.50 diopters).[11] At 3 months after surgery, refraction ranged from − 1.25 to + 1.00 diopters; 56.2% of the eyes were within 0.50 diopter from emmetropia.

Zaldivar et al analyzed a cohort of 124 eyes.[12] The mean follow-up period was 11 months (range, 1–36 months). The mean preoperative SE was − 13.38 ± 2.23 diopters (range, − 8.50 to − 18.63 diopters). The target was emmetropia. The postoperative mean SE was − 0.78 ± 0.87 diopter (range, + 1.63 diopters to − 3.50 diopters); 69% of eyes were within 1.00 diopter and 44% within 0.50 diopter from emmetropia.

Arné and Lesueur implanted phakic IOLs in 58 eyes in 46 myopic patients.[13] Follow-up ranged from 9 months to 2 years. The mean SE was − 13.85 ± 4.61 diopters (range, − 8.00 diopters to − 19.21 diopters) preoperatively and -1.22 ± 0.58 diopter postoperatively; 56.9% of eyes were within 1.00 diopter of emmetropia. Residual myopia was more than 2.00 diopters in 15.5% of eyes.

There have been two studies on hyperopic posterior chamber phakic IOLs. Rosen et al operated on nine hyperopic eyes (preoperative SE range, $+2.25$ diopters to $+5.62$ diopters).[11] Three months postoperatively, the SE refraction ranged from -0.12 diopters to $+1.00$ diopter. Davidorf et al implanted a collamer phakic IOL into 24 eyes with hyperopia greater than 3.50 diopters.[14] The mean preoperative SE was $+6.51 \pm 2.08$ diopters (range, $+3.75$ diopters to $+10.50$ diopters). The mean postoperative SE was -0.39 ± 1.29 diopters (range, $+1.25$ diopters to -3.88 diopters). Postoperatively, 79% of eyes were within 1.00 diopter and 58% within 0.50 diopter from emmetropia. These results compare favorably with predicted results in the authors' series of highly myopic eyes.[12]

Visual Acuity

In the series of phakic IOL implantations in myopic eyes by Zaldivar et al, the preoperative best corrected visual acuity (BCVA) was 20/40 or better in 80% of eyes and 20/20 or better in 5% of eyes.[12] Postoperatively, uncorrected visual acuity (UCVA) was 20/40 or better in 93% of eyes and 20/20 or better in 19% of eyes. A gain of two or more lines of postoperative BCVA was attained in 36% of eyes; 7% lost one line and 0.8% lost two lines.[12]

In the series reported by Arné and Lesueur, the preoperative mean BCVA was 0.57 and the postoperative mean UCVA and BCVA were 0.40 and 0.71, respectively.[13] The postoperative UCVA was better than the preoperative BCVA in 15.5% of eyes, unchanged in 15.5%, and worse in 68.9%. Mean efficacy, the ratio of postoperative UCVA to preoperative BCVA, was 0.84; 20.6% of eyes preserved the same BCVA, 77% gained one or more lines, and 3.4% lost two lines. Safety, calculated as the ratio between postoperative and preoperative BCVA, was 1.46.

Good efficacy and predictability have been demonstrated in all studies on posterior chamber phakic IOL implantation for the treatment of high myopia. The marked gain in postoperative BCVA compared with preoperative spectacle-BCVA in high myopes is largely due to elimination of the spectacle-induced image reduction.

Conversely, only 8% of hyperopic eyes operated on by Davidorf et al demonstrated a gain in postoperative BCVA compared with the preoperative spectacle-BCVA.[14] In this series, 4% of eyes lost two or more lines of spectacle-BCVA due to postoperative glaucoma.

Stability

Excellent stability has been demonstrated in all series. On 51 eyes followed by Zaldivar et al, refraction was -0.90 diopter at 1 month, -0.91 diopter at 6 months, and -0.83 diopter 12 months postoperatively.[12]

Quality of Vision

The level of patient satisfaction is very high. In the study of Arné and Lesueur, 55.7% of the patients were very satisfied, 36.2% were satisfied, and 6.9% were moderately satisfied. No patient was dissatisfied. [13]

The rate of subjective complaints, including glare and halos, varies depending on the series: 2.4% for Zaldivar et al[12] and 55% for Arné and Lesueur.[13] The rate of halos was higher when the size of the optical zone of the ICL was small. Marinho et al had to remove a silicone phakic IOL because of excessive glare.[9]

In one study, contrast sensitivity was tested preoperatively in myopic patients corrected with their contact lenses and 6 months after implantation of an ICL.[13] The mean postoperative level without correction was higher than the mean preoperative level with correction, and the difference was statistically significant for each level of luminance.

■ Anatomic Outcome

Posterior chamber phakic IOL implantation between iris and natural lens is an original surgical procedure for which the potential hazards to the contiguous ocular structures must be assessed.

Endothelial Cell Damage

Although endothelial cell loss is a major concern with anterior chamber IOLs, it does not seem to be a problem with posterior chamber phakic IOLs. Fyodorov et al reported a mean decrease in endothelial cell density of 5% with their silicone posterior chamber phakic IOL,[5] and Asseto et al found a mean endothelial cell loss of 4% with the Staar IOL.[10] Arné and Lesueur, using the same phakic IOL, noted a mean endothelial cell loss of 2.1% 3 months after surgery.[13] It was 2.3% at 6 months, 2% at 1 year, and 2% at 2 years. In no case did endothelial cell loss exceed 3.8% at 1 year.

Inflammation

Subclinical inflammation has been reported as a frequent complication of the first model of silicone posterior chamber phakic IOLs. Two cases of postoperative

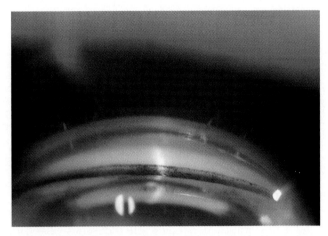

FIGURE 22.2. Pigmentary deposits are seen in the angle in an eye with posterior chamber phakic intraocular lens.

uveitis also were reported with the Chiron-Adatomed silicone phakic IOLs.[9] Conversely, no inflammation was found with the Staar collamer IOL on laser flare fluorophotometry.[13] Six months postoperatively, flare remained less than 8.1 ph/ms, even in an eye that had experienced an early but transient postoperative inflammatory reaction.

Pigment Dispersion

A pigmentary reaction was first reported by Asseto et al.[10] Pigment deposits on the periphery of the ICL optic are constant 1 year after surgery, but they have no visual consequence. In two cases, pigmentary deposits that were not present preoperatively were seen in the angle in association with elevated intraocular pressure (IOP) (Fig. 22.2).[13] For Zaldivar et al, this is a nonprogressive pigmentation.[12]

Although contact and rubbing of the optic shoulder against the posterior surface of the iris are the major logical sources of pigmentary dispersion,[15] the condition may also be partly surgically induced, by Nd:YAG iridotomies and trauma to the iris during implantation.[14] Pigmentary dispersion can be of concern, since highly myopic eyes are by nature at increased risk for glaucoma.

Elevated Intraocular Pressure

An elevated IOP can result from several mechanisms:

1. Pupillary block glaucoma. The incidence of elevated IOP is reduced if laser iridotomies are performed preoperatively. It is of particular concern in small hyperopic eyes. Postoperative pupillary block glaucoma occurred in 3 of 24 hyperopic eyes in the series of Davidorf et al[14] and in 2 of 124 myopic eyes in the study of Zaldivar et al.[12]

2. Glaucoma induced by postoperative topical corticosteroids.

3. Narrowing of the angle. This was demonstrated by ultrasound biomicroscopy studies and is a matter of concern in hyperopic eyes.[15]

4. Pigmentary deposits in the angle. They were associated with an increase in IOP in 14 of 124 eyes in the study of Zaldivar et al.[12]

Cataractogenesis

Cataract formation is one of the most crucial concerns for the future of posterior chamber phakic IOLs. Fechner et al implanted silicone posterior chamber phakic IOLs in 45 myopic eyes with clear crystalline lenses and found central subcapsular opacities in 8 eyes (17.8%) after 1–2 years.[6] Trindade and Pereira reported a case of significant cataract formation 6 months after uneventful implantation of an ICL.[16] Fink et al reported the occurrence of lens opacification in 3 eyes of 2 patients.[17] Arné and Lesueur observed 2 cases of anterior subcapsular opacities; one required removal of the ICL followed by phacoemulsification and posterior chamber IOL implantation.[13]

Several mechanisms have been advanced to explain cataractogenesis:

1. Trauma to the crystalline lens during the implantation procedure. However, in most reported cases the implantation was nontraumatic.

2. Contact between the ICL and the central area of the crystalline lens. This is considered the cause of cataract formation in several cases. Examination by ultrasound biomicroscopy[15] and Scheimpflug camera[13] can demonstrate this contact in cases of insufficient vault. A study using very high frequency ultrasound on 2 eyes implanted with a new posterior chamber phakic IOL failed to show any contact between the implant and the natural lens, even during accommodation and light reflex.[18] The choice of a large implant appears necessary to obtain a greater axial vault along with a larger space between the ICL and the central part of the crystalline lens. However, excessive vaulting will push the iris more forward and favor narrowing of the angle, increased contact between the ICL and the posterior surface of the iris, and consequently pigmentary dispersion. Excessive vaulting also may induce a contact between the haptics of the ICL and the periphery of the crystalline lens.

It is noteworthy and remarkable that anterior subcapsular opacification may develop in some

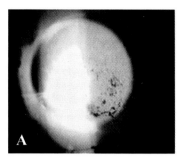 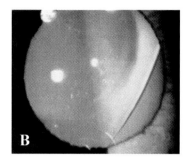 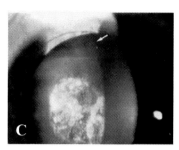

FIGURE 22.3. *A,* Pigment dispersion on the Staar lens 11 months after surgery, accompanied by anterior capsular fibrosis on the lens. *B,* Adatomed lens. Image shows a 2-mm decentration associated with highly diffuse anterior subcapsular opacification. Peripheral opacification of the anterior capsule of the lens, concentric to the optic zone of the lens was noted 16 months after surgery. *C,* Slit-lamp micrograph of a Staar lens 20 months after surgery. This intraocular lens type can be easily identified by the characteristic positioning holes in the haptic portion of the lens *(arrow).* Central middle dense speckled anterior subcapsular cataract and pharmacologically induced pupil dilation are noted. Histopathologic section of the anterior capsular natural lens following lens extraction in this patient showed a hyalinized laminate structure covered by a smooth epithelium with thickened hyaline areas and pigment deposits. (A *to* C, *From Menezo et al. Posterior chamber phakic intraocular lenses to correct high myopia: a comparative study between Staar and Adatomed models.* J Refact Surg. *2001;17: 32–42, with permission).*

eyes even after uneventful surgery and despite an absence of contact between the ICL and the natural lens.[16] Conversely, Trindade et al observed no cataract formation more than 2 years after surgery in an eye in which contact between the ICL and the natural lens at the level of the optic-haptic junction could be seen.[15]

3. Metabolic disturbances induced by the implant also may be more or less responsible for cataract formation, although the biocompatibility of HEMA collagen copolymers has proved excellent.

Menezo et al have observed a 33.3% rate of anterior subcapsukar cataract formation after Adatomed PCIOL implantation, as compared to 25% after Staar PCIOL implantation (Fig. 22.3).[19]

The treatment of cataract in patients implanted with posterior chamber phakic IOLs is not difficult. Explantation of the ICL is easily performed through the same unenlarged primary clear corneal incision. Phacoemulsification and posterior chamber IOL implantation can be done in routine fashion.

■ Advantages and Disadvantages

ICL implantation is an effective method for correcting extreme refractive errors. A gain in best corrected visual acuity is frequent for myopic eyes. However, improved power lens calculation formulas are needed to better predict the refractive outcome. Studies suggest good stability with regard to the refractive outcome. Tolerance also is excellent. Nevertheless, improvement in lens design is needed to avoid contact between the implant and the crystalline lens. Further evaluation of possible progressive pigmentary dispersion in the angle is mandatory, as glaucoma is a complication that causes concern in high myopic eyes.

■ References

1. Strampelli B. Sopportabilita di lenti acriliche in camera anteriore nella afachia o nei vizi di refrazione. *Ann Ottamol Clin Oculist Parma.* 1954;80:75–82.
2. Barraquer J. Anterior chamber plastic lenses: results of and conclusions from five years' experience. *Trans Ophthalmol Soc UK.* 1959;79:393–424.
3. Choyce P. In discussion of Barraquer: Anterior chamber plastic lenses: results of and conclusions from five years' experience. *Trans Ophthalmol Soc UK.* 1959;79: 393–424.
4. Drews RC. The Barraquer experience with intraocular lenses, 20 years later. *Ophthalmology.* 1982;89:386–393.
5. Fyodorov SN, Zuev VK, Aznabayev BM. Intraocular correction of high myopia with negative posterior chamber lens. *Ophthalmol Surg.* 1991;3:57–58.
6. Fechner PU, Haigis W, Wichmann W. Posterior chamber myopia lenses in phakic eyes. *J Cataract Refract Surg.* 1996;22:178–182.
7. Wiechens B, Winter M, Haigis W, et al. Bilateral cataract

after phakic posterior chamber top hat-style silicone intraocular lens. *J Refract Surg.* 1997;13:392–397.

8. Ertuk H, Ozcetin H. Phakic posterior chamber intraocular lenses for the correction of high myopia. *J Refract Surg.* 1995;11:388–391.

9. Marinho A, Neves MC, Pinto MC, et al. Posterior chamber silicone phakic intraocular lens. *J Refract Surg.* 1997;13:219–222.

10. Asseto V, Benedetti S, Pesando P. Collamer intraocular contact lens to correct high myopia. *J Cataract Refract Surg.* 1996;22:551–556.

11. Rosen E, Gore C. Staar collamer posterior chamber phakic intraocular lens to correct myopia and hyperopia. *J Cataract Refract Surg.* 1998;24:596–606.

12. Zaldivar R, Davidorf JM, Oscherow S. Posterior chamber phakic IOL for myopia of −8 to −19 diopters. *J Refract Surg.* 1998;14:294–305.

13. Arné JL, Lesueur LC. Phakic posterior chamber lenses for high myopia: functional and anatomical outcomes. *J Cataract Refract Surg.* 2000;26:369–374.

14. Davidorf JM, Zaldivar R, Oscherow S. Posterior chamber phakic intraocular lens for hyperopia of +4 to +11 diopters. *J Refract Surg.* 1998;14:306–311.

15. Trindade F, Pereira F, Cronemberger S. Ultrasound biomicroscopic imaging of posterior chamber phakic intraocular lens. *J Cataract Refract Surg.* 1998;14:497–503.

16. Trindade F, Pereira F. Cataract formation after posterior chamber phakic intraocular lens implantation. *J Cataract Refract Surg.* 1998;24:1661–1663.

17. Fink AM, Gore C, Rosen E. Cataract development after implantation of the Staar collamer posterior chamber phakic lens. *J Cataract Refract Surg.* 1999;25:278–282.

18. Kim DY, Reinstein DZ, Silverman RH, et al. Very high frequency ultrasound analysis of a new phakic posterior chamber intraocular lens in situ. *Am J Ophthalmol.* 1998;125:725–729.

19. Menezo JL, Martinez CP, Cisneros A, Costa RM. Posterior chamber phakic IOLs to correct high myopia. *J Refract Surg.* 2001; 17:32–42.

Chapter 23

Intracorneal Implants

Joseph Colin and Béatrice Cochener

In 1949, José Barraquer first proposed the use of alloplastic materials to correct refractive errors. Several intracorneal implants, or inlays, made of various materials (hydrogels, polysulfones) have been evaluated in animal and human eyes for the correction of myopia, aphakia, or presbyopia. However, none is currently used routinely.

Intrastromal corneal ring segments, or Intacs, are a new, nonlaser category of vision correction for the mild myope.[1-8] When placed in the peripheral stroma at approximately two-thirds depth, outside the central optical zone, the device reshapes the anterior corneal surface while maintaining the positive asphericity of the cornea.

The first-generation design of Intacs was referred to as the 360-degree ICR (intrastromal corneal ring). The current design, the ICRS (intrastromal corneal ring segments), consists of two segments, each with an arc length of 150 degrees (Fig. 23.1). Each Intacs segment has a hexagonal cross-section that lies along a conic section. With a fixed outer diameter of 8.1 mm and an inner diameter of 6.8 mm, Intacs leave a large, clear, central optic zone. Each segment has a small positioning hole at the superior end to aid with surgical manipulation once the segments have been inserted. The two segments are designated as clockwise (CW) and counterclockwise (CCW) to correspond to their orientation within the intrastromal tunnel.

Intacs act as passive spacing elements that change the arc length of the anterior corneal curvature. The refractive effect achieved is directly related to the thickness of the device. Placing the product in the periphery of the cornea causes local separation of the corneal lamellae, which results in a shortening of the corneal arc length. The net effect is a flattening of the cornea, thereby correcting for myopia by lowering the optical power of the eye. Increasing the thickness of Intacs causes greater degrees of local separation and increased corneal flattening. Thus, the degree of corneal flattening—or correction—achieved by Intacs is directly related to thickness.

The same effect can be observed by placing a pencil underneath a sheet of paper. With the added bulk of the pencil, the paper is no longer flat and is now shorter. In much the same way, when Intacs are placed within the stromal layers of the cornea, they shorten the arc length across the optical zone.

A nearly linear relationship has been established between the device thickness and the flattening achieved, with approximately an additional 0.70 diopter of flattening occurring for every 0.05-mm increase in device thickness. Intacs are available in the United States in three different thicknesses: 0.25, 0.30, and 0.35 mm. This selection of Intacs is intended for the reduction or elimination of mild myopia (−1.00 diopters to −3.00 diopters spherical equivalent at the spectacle plane) in patients

- who are 21 years of age or older,
- with documented stability of refraction, as demonstrated by a change of less than or equal to 0.50 diopter for at least 12 months prior to the preoperative examination, and
- in whom the astigmatic component is 1.00 diopter or less.

Based on laboratory and US clinical trial results, a continuous but nonoverlapping recommended prescribing range has been developed for each thickness (Table 23.1). Outside the United States, Intacs are also available in thicknesses of 0.40 and 0.45 mm to correct myopia up to −4.50 diopters.

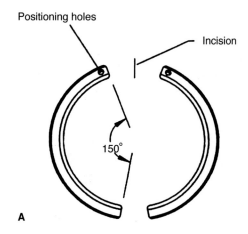

Positioning holes

Incision

150°

A

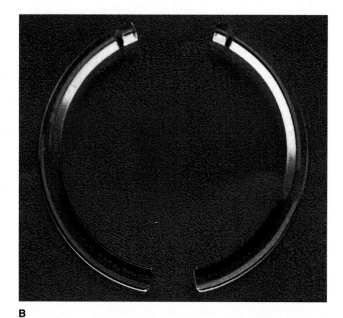

B

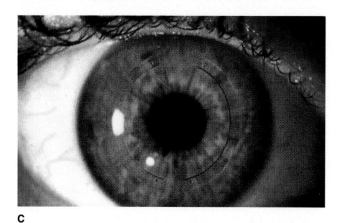

C

FIGURE 23.1. *A,* Intacs consist of two segments, each with an arch length of 150 degrees. *B,* KeraVision Intacs corneal ring segments. *C,* Intacs are placed outside the visual axis.

■ Surgical Technique

Marking the Center of the Cornea

The geometric center of the cornea is marked with a blunt instrument, using an operating microscope for fixation. An 11-mm zone marker can be used to aid in locating the center point. The marker is placed on the limbus and pressed down so that the crosshairs make a mild indentation mark at the geometric center of the cornea. A blunt Sinskey hook or other corneal marker is then used to mark the geometric center of the cornea, with the sterile marking pen used to ink the tip of the blunt Sinskey hook. Adequate marking (with gentian violet) should be done because this mark is later used for centration of the vacuum centering guide (VCG). The marked geometric center of the cornea should coincide with the entrance pupil and should be slightly inferior and temporal to the center of the entrance pupil in the undilated state. This center mark is used as the reference point throughout the surgical procedure. The use of pilocarpine to constrict the patient's pupil is not recommended because it may cause chemosis, which could lead to subsequent fixation problems with the VCG.

Making the Incision

A calibrated diamond knife is set to 0.430 m (430 mm), or 68% of the intraoperative pachometry reading taken at the incision site. The diamond should have an angled cutting edge of 15 degrees or less or a rectangular blade of 1 mm width or less. The operator makes a radial incision by tracing the entire length of the incision mark. Adequate pressure should be applied to the diamond knife footplate to ensure full depth of the incision.

To avoid neovascularization into the incision region, special care should be taken to ensure that the incision is kept approximately 1 mm away from the limbus. A lint-free surgical microsponge is used to remove any loose epithelial cells and excess balanced saline solution from the edges of the incision. The epithelium may be rolled away from the incision edges.

Creating Pockets at the Incision

A stromal spreader tip is inserted vertically down into the incision until it contacts the bottom of the incision. While maintaining contact at the incision base, the operator rotates the handle past the vertical until the blade is parallel to the stromal lamellae. Blunt dissection is done or a pocket is made on one side of the base of the incision by carefully rotating the blade of the instru-

Table 23.1
Prescribing Range of Intacs, by Thickness

Intacs Thickness (mm)	Predicted Nominal Correction (diopter)	Recommended Prescribing Range (diopter)
0.25	− 1.03	− 1.00 to − 1.63
0.30	− 2.00	− 1.75 to − 2.25
0.35	− 2.70	− 2.38 to − 3.00

ment within a single stromal plane. The procedure is then repeated on the other side of the incision base. These pockets should be at the same depth as the incision base, as wide as the full incision length (1.8 mm), and should extend the full length of the stromal spreader blade. When finished, the glide blades are test fitted by inserting them into the pockets. If the pockets cannot accommodate the glide blades, it may be necessary to reassess the incision to determine whether or not the incision length extends the full length (1.8 mm) of the incision mark. Once this has been confirmed, the pocketing technique is repeated to enlarge the pockets.

Alternative Techniques

The following alternative techniques can be used:

1. Using one hook to retract the edge of the wound, the operator inserts the base or foot of the second hook into the depth of the incision with the tip pointing centrally. The CW pocket is initiated under direct vision by rotating the hook to the left and moving the hook back and forth across the entire length of the incision. The same steps are repeated to the right for the CCW pocket. The hook *must not* be rotated from the left side to the right side across the base of the incision. The hook is exchanged for the stromal speader to complete the pocketing. The glide blades are test fitted in the completed pockets.

2. The footplate of the pocketing lever is placed flat onto the cornea with the tip extending down into the incision. The operator gently retracts along the incision face and rotates the handle up to, but *not past,* the vertical. Pockets are initiated by moving the pocketing lever along the entire incision on both sides. The lever is exchanged for the stromal spreader to complete the pocketing. The glide blades are test fitted in the completed pockets.

3. The base or foot of the pocketing hook is inserted to the base of the incision. The base of the hook should rest flat on the base of the incision. The hook *must not* contact the base of the incision. Under direct vision, the CW pocket is initiated by rotating the hook to the left and moving the hook back and forth in a single plane across the entire length of the incision. The hook is removed and the same steps are repeated on the right side for the CCW pocket. The hook *must not* be rotated from the left side to the right side across the base of the incision. The hook is exchanged for the stromal spreader to complete the pocketing. The glide blades are test fitted in the completed pockets.

4. The footplate of the pocketing lever is placed flat onto the cornea with the tip extending into the incision. The operator uses the lever to gently retract the incision face. The base or foot of the pocketing hook is inserted vertically until it rests flat at the base of the incision. The hook is rotated under the lever in a single plane to initiate the CW pocket. The hook is removed, and the same steps are repeated on the right side for the CCW pocket. The hook *must not* be rotated from the left side to the right side across the base of the incision. This technique helps to ensure that pockets are initiated at the proper depth. The lever and hook are exchanged for the stromal spreader to complete the pocketing. The glide blades are test fitted in the completed pockets.

Placing the Vacuum Centering Guide

A microsponge plagette or anesthesia ring or equivalent is saturated with topical anesthetic and placed on the sclera outside the cornea for approximately 1 minute prior to placement of the VCG. The anesthesia ring is removed before the VCG is applied.

The tubing from the VCG should be oriented to the temporal side, because this produces the most appropriate fixation. The VCG is oriented around the limbus, and final placement is arranged after the incision and placement marker is inserted into the VCG. If this technique is followed, the reticle of the incision and placement marker should fall very close to the geometric corneal center mark. Fine adjustment is achieved by gently raising the VCG and reapplying it. When the centration guide sight is centered on the geometric center mark, suction is applied, and gentle retropulsion of the globe will help to ensure adequate fixation.

The vacuum should start in the range of 400–500 mBar. Once a vacuum seal has been established, the operator confirms that the VCG is properly placed by checking centration. If the VCG is not properly positioned, the vacuum is released and the operator starts over from the beginning of this step. If the VCG is properly positioned, the vacuum is switched to high, 600–667 mBar. It is recommended that the vacuum not exceed 750 mBar. The incision and placement marker is removed.

Creating Intrastromal Tunnels

While maintaining the position of the VCG, the operator inserts the CW dissector into the VCG. The dissector body should be rotated until the dissector tip is adjacent to the incision site.

The CW glide tip is inserted vertically down into the incision until it contacts the bottom of the incision. The CW glide is inserted at least 1 mm into the pocket, and the dissector tip is rotated under the heel of the glide. CW rotation of the dissector body will allow the tip to enter the pocket. The tip should enter the pocket approximately 1–2 mm, no more. The glide is removed while leaving the dissector tip in position in the pocket.

While holding the VCG vertically with one hand, the operator rotates the dissector CW from the incision to create an intrastromal tunnel. The dissector is rotated CW until the support spoke of the dissector blade contacts the incision edge. In the event of an anterior chamber perforation or corneal surface perforation, the procedure is immediately discontinued.

The dissector is removed from the intrastromal tunnel by rotating the dissector body CCW until the dissector tip exits the tunnel. The dissector is removed from the VCG.

While maintaining the position of the VCG, the operator inserts the CCW dissector into the VCG. The dissector body should be rotated until the tip is adjacent to the incision site.

The CCW glide tip is inserted vertically down into the incision until it contacts the bottom of the incision. The CCW glide is inserted at least 1 mm into the pocket, and the dissector tip is rotated under the heel of the glide. CCW rotation of the dissector body will allow the dissector tip to enter the pocket underneath the glide. The tip is advanced approximately 1–2 mm,

no more. The glide is removed while leaving the dissector tip in position in the pocket.

Holding the VCG vertically with one hand, the operator rotates the dissector CCW from the incision to create a second intrastromal tunnel. The dissector is rotated CCW until the support spoke of the dissector blade contacts the incision edge. Breakthrough of the two intrastromal tunnels to create a continuous 360-degree tunnel is not required, as it may facilitate an inferior shift of the two segments.

The dissector is removed from the intrastromal tunnel by rotating the dissector body CW until the dissector tip exits the tunnel. The dissector is removed from the VCG. The vacuum is released, and the VCG is removed. Any stromal debris is removed from the incision site. The incision area is thoroughly irrigated with balanced saline solution prior to Intacs placement into the intrastromal tunnel.

Placing the Implants

The carrier is stabilized, with the rounded end etched with "KeraVision" face-up and pointing away from the operator. The cover back is slowly slid back with the thumb until the first segment is exposed and the cover snaps into its first position. With the free hand, the operator grasps the Intacs forceps so the prongs point straight down. The forceps are lowered over the carrier until the prongs contact the base of the cross-slot on each side of the segment. The operator gently grasps the segment at its midsection (the inner and outer edges of the segment should nest in the slots of the forceps) and lifts the segment out of the carrier.

The operator then inserts the segment directly through the incision and into the prepared intrastromal tunnel on the left (CW) side of the incision, as indicated by the package arrow (Fig. 23.2). If it is necessary to reposition the segment within the Intacs forceps, this is done by placing the segment back into the carrier, then regrasping the segment with the forceps. Once the segment is inserted approximately halfway into the intrastromal tunnel, the forceps are repositioned to complete insertion of the segment.

Intacs should not be placed on the surface of the cornea prior to insertion, as this may result in epithelial cell adherence or the introduction of bacteria into the intrastromal tunnel. Using forceps or a Sinskey hook, the operator manipulates the segment into the desired location within the intrastromal tunnel, aligning the outside edge of the segment with the ink markings created on the corneal surface by the incision and placement marker.

Using the technique just described, the operator removes the second segment from the carrier and in-

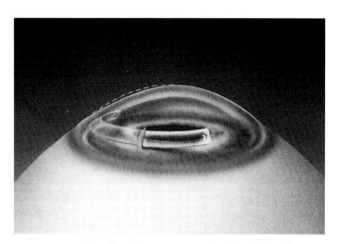

FIGURE 23.2. The first Intacs segment is placed into the prepared intrastromal tunnel. The dashed line indicates corneal flattening.

serts it into the second intrastromal tunnel on the right (CCW) side of the incision as indicated by the package arrow. Any stromal debris is removed from the incision area. The incision area is thoroughly irrigated with balanced saline solution.

Closing the Incision

The tissue edges are gently approximated to close the incision. If necessary, the incision may be irrigated to aid in approximating the tissue edges. If there is any difficulty approximating the incision edges, one or two interrupted sutures, 11-0 (recommended) or 10-0 nylon sutures or equivalent, are placed to close the incision. The suture depth should be to the level of the intrastromal pocket. Care should be taken to avoid microperforation by the suture needle. If two sutures are placed, they should trisect from the superior and inferior aspects of the incision to ensure apposition of the anterior edges of the incision. The suture knots are buried at the close of the procedure. Hydration of the incision at the close of the procedure can be beneficial in helping to approximate the tissue edges of the incision. The anterior incision edges must be apposed to prevent epithelial cells from entering the incision. Care should be taken to ensure that tension across the sutures is applied evenly. Overtightening of the sutures should be avoided as this may induce astigmatism.

■ Postoperative Care and Management

Immediately following surgery, an antibiotic-steroid combination ointment or solution (0.1% dexamethasone/0.3% tobramycin or equivalent is applied to the

operative eye. Any epithelial defect is treated with lubricating drops, for a small defect, or a bandage contact lens, for a large defect. Segment placement and incision closure are observed with slit-lamp examination. The operative eye is shielded with a clear shield, and the patient is given instructions for postoperative care.

Therapeutic Protocol

- Postoperative medications: antibiotic-steroid combination solution (0.1% dexamethasone/0.3% tobramycin or equivalent), four times daily for 1 week.
- Shields are used at night for 1 week.
- The patient is instructed to avoid rubbing the eye, as this may lead to segment migration or improper healing of the incision.
- An analgesic (acetaminophen, paracetamol, or equivalent) is prescribed for postoperative discomfort. Other pain medication may be prescribed at the surgeon's discretion.
- Typically patients experience mild to moderate discomfort or pain for a few hours after surgery. Surgeon should be contacted about more severe pain.
- The patient is informed that foreign body sensation or "scratchiness" is common during the immediate postoperative recovery period.
- Symptoms of *infection* include dull, aching pain or discomfort, with or without photophobia, any time in the postoperative period.
- During recovery, the eyes may feel dry the first 2–3 months. Expect vision to fluctuate during the first month.

Postoperative Visits

A typical schedule of postoperative visits may be 1 day, 1 week, 1 month, 3 months, and 6 months.

On the first postoperative day, visual acuity and intraocular pressure should be checked. A quick manifest refraction is useful, but in general it does not correlate with visual acuity. The size of the epithelial defects should be noted. Suture knots should be buried, and if they are not, an attempt to bury them should be made.

There may be mild subconjunctival hemorrhage and/or chemosis remaining from the VCG. Usually there is little to no intraocular inflammation. Visual acuity on day 1 is usually quite good, with the most patients seeing better than 20/40. If a patient does not see this well, he or she should be advised that refractive surgery procedures typically require some recovery time and the vision will most likely improve.

Therapy on the first day centers on managing the epithelial defects and initiating of postoperative topical medications. The patient is advised that over the next 3–6 weeks visual acuity will be good but may fluctuate from day to day and even during the course of a day.

Visual acuity on day 3 is usually slightly less than on day 1 secondary to superficial punctate keratitis from the topical medications and increased suture-induced astigmatism as the superior corneal edema in the incision region resolves.

By the end of the first postoperative week, the epithelium should be healed and any residual foreign body sensation resolved. Occasionally a "filament" develops at the incision site, causing foreign body sensation or pain. The filaments may be managed with hypertonic saline drops, debridement, or a bandage contact lens.

The use of a bandage contact lens to treat epithelial defects or filamentary keratitis should be monitored. Superficial neovascularization of the superior aspect of the incision may be aggravated by prolonged contact lens wear. The bandage contact lens should be discontinued as soon as the epithelial defect or filamentary keratitis resolves or at any time that limbal vascular buds form.

The uncorrected visual acuity typically remains better than 20/40 after week 1, but fluctuates from day to day and during the course of a day, usually in proportion to the induced astigmatism.

Suture-induced with-the-rule astigmatism may induce a "myopic shift" in the spherical equivalent since the concomitant flattening usually seen with suture-induced astigmatism may be blunted by the Intacs segments. Suture-induced astigmatism should be addressed early if the incision has healed and does not stain with fluorescein. Selective suture removal may be necessary if the induced astigmatism is greater than 1 diopter at 2 weeks. Sutures should be removed by 4 weeks. Clinical data suggest that with-the-rule astigmatism may be prolonged even after suture removal.

Between months 1 and 3, the surgeon begins assessing whether the patient is satisfied with his or her vision, or "20/happy." Options, including replacement, are discussed as appropriate. Prior to considering replacement, the surgeon should perform a cycloplegic refraction and evaluate topography.

By month 3, the visual acuity should have stabilized. Refractive stability is typically maintained from month 3, as less than 1 diopter of shift in the spherical equivalent between subsequent visits occurs for most patients. Astigmatism, if present, should be resolving gradually, and high degrees of cylinder should continue to resolve over time. In general, late complications of Intacs placement are rare. Patients should be followed on a normal routine basis after the 6-month examination.

■ References

1. Assil KK, Barrett AM, Fouraker BD, et al. One-year results of the intrastromal corneal ring in nonfunctional human eyes. *Arch Ophthalmol.* 1995;113:159–167.
2. Barraquer JI. Queratoplastia refractiva. *Ofthalmologicas.* 1949;2:10–30.
3. Burris TE, Ayer CT, Evensen DA, et al. Effects of intrastromal corneal ring size and thickness on corneal flattening in human eyes. *Refract Corneal Surg.* 1991;7:46–50.
4. Cochener B, Le Floch G, Colin J. Les anneaux intracorneens pour la correction des faibles myopies. *J Fr Ophtalmol.* 1998;21:191–208.
5. Fleming JF, Reynolds AE, Kilmer L, et al. The intrastromal corneal ring: two cases in rabbits. *J Refract Surg.* 1987;3:227–232.
6. Fleming JF, Wan WL, Schanzlin DJ. The theory of corneal curvature change with the intrastromal corneal ring. CLAO J 1989;15:146–150.
7. Nosé W, Neves RA, Burris TE, et al. Intrastromal corneal ring: 12-month sighted myopic eyes. *J Refract Surg.* 1996;12:20–28.
8. Schanzlin DJ, Asbell PA, Burris TE, et al. The intrastromal corneal ring segments: Phase II results for the correction of myopia. *Ophthalmology.* 1997;104:1067–1078.

Part VI

Refractive Intraocular Lenses and Future Developments

Chapter 24

Refractive Cataract Surgery: Prevention and Correction of Secondary Ametropia

Glenn C. Cockerham

Despite the increasing popularity of corneal reshaping procedures, cataract surgery remains the most common method of permanently altering refractive status. Ametropia can be corrected with placement of a properly chosen intraocular lens (IOL), freeing patients of the need for distance visual correction. Uncorrected astigmatism will degrade the visual image, through the circle of least confusion, despite attainment of the desired spherical equivalent with the IOL. Additionally, spectacle correction may cause distortion through meridional magnification. Consequently, visually significant postoperative astigmatism, either from surgically induced changes or from failure to significantly reduce existing astigmatism, will adversely affect the desired surgical outcome. With the large incisions necessary for intracapsular cataract extraction, postoperative astigmatism was historically viewed as a natural consequence of cataract surgery. Astigmatism of several diopters was not particularly noticeable in the spectacle-corrected aphake. However, thanks to advances in instrumentation and understanding of wound construction principles, surgically induced astigmatism can be minimized and preexisting astigmatism reduced or eliminated. This chapter presents current thinking on astigmatism modification in the setting of cataract surgery.

■ Principles of Wound Construction

The most important aspects of cataract wound construction affecting final postoperative astigmatism are incision length, incision location, and wound architecture. Experimental data suggest that incision length is the most important of these factors.[1] All incisions demonstrate against-the-wound (ATW) astigmatic changes over time (Fig. 24.1). This effect was noted well over 100 years

ago, and the large induced against-the-rule (ATR) astigmatism occurring after long superior incisions was called "classic" astigmatism. In cadaver eyes, Flaherty and Siepser noted that large incisions (10 mm at the limbus, 7 mm scleral pocket) produced twice as much immediate astigmatism as did smaller incisions (5 mm at the limbus, 3.5 mm scleral pocket).[2] Also in cadaver eyes, Samuelson and colleagues noted a linear increase in corneal flattening with larger incisions and observed that 3 mm is the maximum incision length that does not induce appreciable change (0.25 mm).[3]

Incision location relative to the corneal center appears to be important. One tenet of keratorefractive surgery holds that for a given incision length, more peripheral incisions produce less effect in inducing new astigmatism or correcting preexisting astigmatism.[4] The concept of the incisional funnel for scleral incisions as proposed by Koch integrates incision length and location.[5] The linear relationship between the cube of the incision and astigmatism, and the inverse relationship between astigmatism and the distance of the incision from the limbus, are incorporated into an astigmatically neutral space, or funnel (Fig. 24.2). Incisions placed into this funnel, regardless of length, should have equivalent stability.[5] The "frown" incision of Singer demonstrates these concepts, allowing placement of rigid IOLs through curved incisions that produce less astigmatism than do straight incisions of the same length.[6]

■ Astigmatically Neutral Wound Construction

The surgical goal in a patient without significant preoperative astigmatism is to maintain central corneal

281

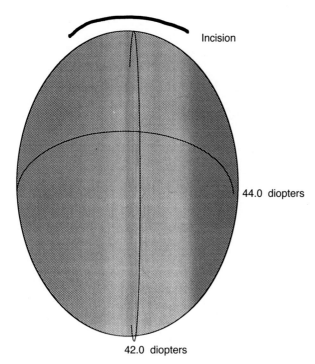

Incision

44.0 diopters

42.0 diopters

FIGURE 24.1. Corneal and scleral incisions produce some degree of against-the-wound astigmatism. In general, longer incisions induce more cylinder.

asphericity, inducing little or no astigmatism at surgery. As noted previously, wounds approach astigmatic neutrality at 3 mm length or less. Many clinical studies have shown that smaller incisions produce less ATW astigmatism and achieve stability faster than longer incisions (Tables 24.1 to 24.4).[7-32] Leen et al, however, demonstrated less initial surgically induced astigmatism (SIA) with shorter (4 mm) versus longer (6 mm and 11 mm) incisions, as well as faster stabilization, but no statistical difference at 3 months.[10] Self-sealing wounds 3.2 mm in length have achieved refractive stability by 2 weeks, while 5.5-mm self-sealing wounds do so at 1 month.[20] However, even with small incisions there is a gradual cylinder regression, or decay. Rainer and associates reported a mean induced ATW cylinder change of 0.41 diopters by vector analysis between 1 day and 4.4 years postoperatively in 63 eyes with a superior 4.0-mm scleral tunnel.[26] Other studies demonstrated a mean SIA of 0.2 diopter at 4 months with a 4.0-mm scleral incision[25] and of 0.92 diopter at 6 months with a 4.5-mm scleral incision.[16] A 3.5-mm scleral incision induced a mean SIA of 0.65 diopter at 6 months,[16] while a sutured 3.2-mm scleral incision produced a mean SIA of 0.66 diopter at 6 months.[29] Based on the keratorefractive principle that wounds closer to the corneal center produce more astigmatic effect, one would expect scleral tunnel incisions to induce less astigmatism than clear corneal incisions.[4] However, this is not universally true,

as shown in Tables 24.4 and 24.5.[33-36] Advances in phacoemulsification technology and in foldable and injectable IOLs allow the surgeon to routinely create wounds as small as 3.2 mm, thereby minimizing SIA.

■ Superior versus Temporal Incisions

Cataract wounds located superiorly (12 o'clock) induce more postoperative astigmatism than do otherwise identical wounds placed in a temporal (horizontal) meridian (Table 24.6).[29,30,33,37-45] This may be due in part to differences in vertical and horizontal corneal radii; the superior limbus is nearer than the temporal limbus to the corneal center. Cravy noted that a temporal 8.5- to 9.5-mm incision produced significantly less astigmatism than did a similar superior incision; this effect was attributed to the distractive force of eyelid closure on superior wounds.[37] Similar findings have been reported in scleral and limbal incisions.[33] Kawano noted that 6-mm corneoscleral incisions placed obliquely between 9 o'clock and 12 o'clock (BENT) were associated with significantly less induced astigmatism and faster stabilization than incisions placed superiorly, and were effective in reducing preexisting oblique astigmatism.[38]

This relationship has also been observed in corneal incisions. Long and Monica found that for corneal tunnel incisions placed on the steepest meridian, superior incisions induced slightly more astigmatism (0.9 diopter) at 12 months than horizontal incisions (0.6 diopter).[41] Similarly, Kammann and Dornbach reported that oblique 3.0- to 4.5-mm corneal incisions induced more astigmatism at 24 months than equal-length incisions in the temporal cornea.[39] Mueller-Jensen and Barlinn also noted significantly more astigmatism 2 years postoperatively with a superior 4.0-mm cataract incision than with a temporal incision.[40] However, Nielsen, comparing superior versus temporal 3.5-mm corneal incisions, found no significant differences in magnitude of astigmatism over 6 weeks.[42]

■ Reduction of Preexisting Astigmatism

Preoperative Considerations

Congenital astigmatism greater than 0.5 diopters has been reported in 44% of the population, and 8% have congenital astigmatism of 1.5 diopters or more.[46] Spectacle astigmatism must be vertexed to the corneal plane; compound myopic astigmatism is less at the corneal plane, while compound hyperopic astigmatism is greater. A reduction in cylinder magnitude at the

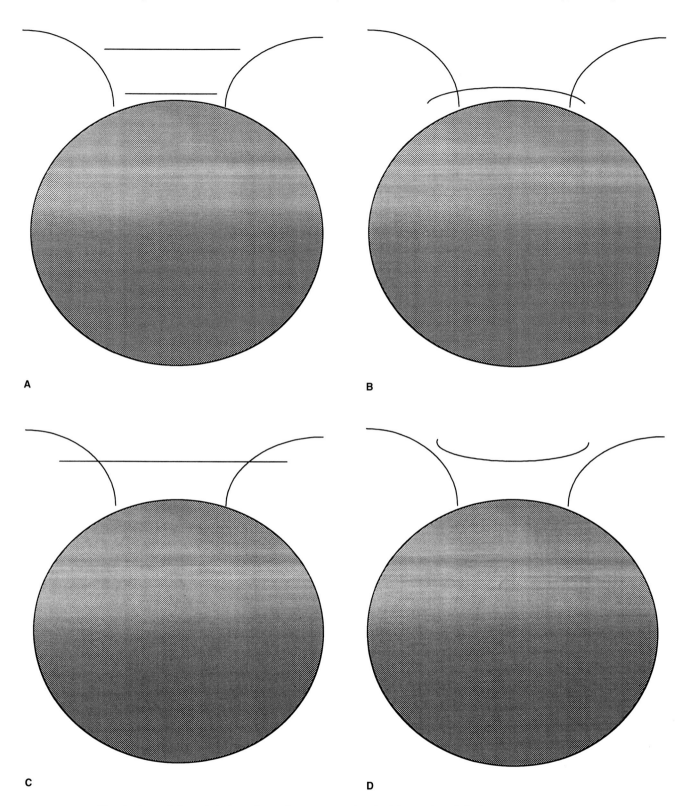

A

B

C

D

FIGURE 24.2. The incisional funnel is based on the concept that incisions placed farther away from the central cornea induce less postoperative astigmatic change. *A,* Incisions placed in the funnel have equivalent stability. A longer incision placed in a more posterior location may be as stable as a shorter incision placed more anterior in the funnel. *B,* A long perilimbal incision is unstable, extending beyond the boundaries of the incisional funnel. *C,* This straight incision located in the posterior funnel is somewhat more stable than the peril-imbal incision but is still relatively unstable. *D,* A frown-type incision located within the fun-nel is stable and allows introduction of a larger IOL compared with a straight incision.

Table 24.1
Surgically Induced Astigmatism (SIA) with Scleral Incisions 3–4.5 mm

Study	N	Inc.	Loc.	Closure	SIA Method	Mean SIA (SD) on Postop. Day 1 (or Week 1)	Mean SIA (SD) at Intermediate Follow-up	Mean SIA (SD) at Longest Follow-up
Davison[28]	130	4.0	ST/S 3 mm	× 10-0 (2)	Cravy	0.80 (0.94) WTR	0.49 (0.73) WTR 2 wk	0.34 (0.91) ATR 1 y
Gills & Sanders[21]	55	3.0	ST/S 3 mm	Horizontal	Naylor	NA	1.07 (0.11) 2–3 wk	0.67 (0.06) 3–4 mo
Leen et al[10]	26	4.0	ST/S 2 mm	Radial 10-0	Jaffe & Clayman	2.78 (2.01)	1.33 (1.04) 4–6 wk	0.99 (0.66) 2–3 mo
Martin et al[15]	55	3.5–4.0	ST/S 1.5 mm	Running, horizontal	Naylor	1.17 (1.29)	NA	0.78 (0.62) 3 mo
Neuman et al[12]	67	3.0–4.0	Limbal	Radial 10-0	Naylor	NA	1.29 (0.96) 3 mo	1.08 (0.69) 6 mo
Nouhuijs et al[29]	20	3.2	ST/S 1.5 mm	Cross	Jaffe & Clayman	—	—	0.66 (0.49) 6 mo
Olsen et al[32]	50	3.5	ST/A 2 mm	Sutureless	Olsen	0.55 (0.31)	—	0.36 (0.21) 6 mo
Oshika & Tsuboi[20]	52	3.2	ST/S 1.5 mm	Sutureless	Jaffe & Clayman	0.69 (1.19)	0.58 (1.04) 1 mo	0.45 (0.79) 3 mo
					Cravy	0.64 WTR	0.45 WTR 1 mo	0.44 WTR 3 mo
Pfleger et al[34]	56	3.5	ST/S 2.5 mm	Sutureless	Jaffe & Clayman	0.75 (0.50) 1 wk	0.73 (0.52) 1 mo	0.75 (0.58) 1 y
					Cravy	0.31 (1.02) ATR 1 wk	0.49 (0.91) ATR 1 mo	0.37 (1.0) ATR 1 y
					Naeser	0.26 (0.55) ATR 1 wk	0.39 (0.49) ATR 1 mo	0.50 (0.61) ATR 1 y
	51	4.5	ST/S 2.5 mm	Sutureless	Jaffe & Clayman	0.88 (0.62) 1 wk	0.90 (0.71) 1 mo	0.89 (0.61) 1 y
					Cravy	0.48 (0.94) ATR 1 wk	0.75 (0.90) ATR 1 mo	0.67 (0.93) ATR 1 y
					Naeser	0.46 (0.72) ATR 1 wk	0.68 (0.75) ATR 1 mo	0.66 (0.70) ATR 1 y
Rainer et al[26]	63	4.0	ST/S 3 mm	Sutureless	Jaffe & Clayman	0.85 (0.79)	0.60 (0.69) 1 mo	0.84 (0.50) 4.4 y
					Cravy	0.07 (0.71) ATR	0.17 (0.44) ATR 1 mo	0.48 (0.44) ATR 4.4 y
					Naeser	0.0 (0.89)	0.19 (0.48) ATR 1 mo	0.55 (0.48) ATR 4.4 y
Shepherd[67]	99	4.0	ST/S 2 mm	Horizontal	Cravy	0.13 (0.67) WTR 1 wk	0.02 (no SD) WTR 1 mo	0.22 (0.47) ATR 12 wk
Steinert et al[11]	65	4.0	ST/S 2–3 mm	Horizontal	Jaffe & Clayman	1.54 (1.32)	0.98 (0.68) 1 mo	0.82 (0.48) 3 mo
					Cravy	0.25 (2.29) WTR	0.05 (1.11) WTR 1 mo	0.21 (1.29) ATR 3 mo
Uusitalo et al[19]	10	4.0	ST/S 2mm	Horizontal	Cravy	0.02 (0.75) WTR	0.35 (0.79) ATR 1 mo	0.20 (0.38) ATR 6 mo
Uusitalo & Tarkkanen[25]	216	4.0	ST/S	Sutureless	Alpins			0.3 (1.0) 4 mo

Abbreviations: N, number of patients; Inc., incision length in mm; Loc., location of incision posterior to limbus in mm (ST, scleral tunnel; S, superior; A, on steep axis); SIA, surgically induced astigmatism; SD, standard deviation; Phaco, phacoemulsification; WTR, with-the-rule astigmatism; ATR, against-the-rule astigmatism.

Table 24.2
Surgically Induced Astigmatism (SIA) with Scleral Incisions 5.0 – 7.0 mm

Study	N	Inc.	Loc.	Closure	SIA Method	Mean SIA (SD) on Postop. Day 1	Mean SIA (SD) at Intermediate Follow-up	Mean SIA (SD) at Longest Follow-up
Azar et al[27]	50	5.5	ST/S 1 mm	Sutureless	Sinusoidal	1.28 (1.12)	1.10 (0.65) 8 wk	1.03 (0.65) 1 y
		5.5	ST/S 1 mm	1-radial 10-0	Sinusoidal	1.38 (1.07)	0.76 (0.61) 8 wk	0.81 (0.56) 1 y
		5.5	ST/S 1 mm	3-radial 10-0	Sinusoidal	1.85 (1.52)	1.02 (0.58) 8 wk	0.96 (0.48) 1 y
Davison[28]	146	5.5	ST/S 3 mm	2 × 10-0	Cravy	0.69 (1.07) WTR	0.41 (0.85) WTR 2 wk	0.23 (1.01) ATR 1 y
Gills & Sanders[21]	48	6.0–7.0	ST/S 3 mm	3-radial 10-0	Naylor	NA	2.27 (0.24) 2–3 wk	0.90 (0.10) 3–4 mo
Leen et al[10]	30	6.0	ST/S 2 mm	Radial 10-0	Jaffe & Clayman	2.44 (1.84)	2.28 (1.68) 4–6 wk	1.35 (1.10) 2–3 mo
Lyhne & Corydon[17]	26	5.2	ST/S 2 mm	Sutureless	Jaffe & Clayman	1.20	0.77 1 mo	0.68 6 mo
	25	5.2	ST/S 2 mm	1 cross (adj.)	Jaffe & Clayman	0.87	0.67 1 mo	0.67 6 mo
	24	5.2	ST/S 2 mm	1 cross	Jaffe & Clayman	1.10	0.61 1 mo	0.70 6 mo
Martin et al[15]	56	6.0	ST/S 1.5 mm	Run 10-0	Naylor	2.26 (1.87)	NA	0.80 (0.68) 3 mo
Neumann et al[12]	56	6.0	Limbal	Radial 10-0	Naylor	NA	1.06 (1.09) 3 mo	1.06 (1.15) 6 mo
Oshika & Tsuboi[20]	51	5.5	ST/S 2.5 mm	Sutureless	Jaffe & Clayman	0.84 (1.54)	0.50 (0.94) 1 mo	0.44 (0.88) 3 mo
Oshika & Tsuboi	46	6.5	ST/S 2.5 mm	Sutureless	Jaffe & Clayman	0.93 (1.85)	0.66 (1.73) 1 mo	0.33 (0.89) 3 mo
Singer[6]	34	6.0–7.0	ST/S 2 mm	Horizontal 10-0	Jaffe & Clayman	1.19 (0.91)	1.07 (0.63) 4 wk	1.30 (0.83) 1 y
Steinert et al[11]	65	6.0–6.50	ST/S 2–2.5	Various 10-0	Jaffe & Clayman	3.07 (1.78)	1.44 (0.92) 1 mo	1.03 (0.71) 3 mo
					Cravy	2.13 (3.40) WTR	0.30 (1.73) WTR 1 mo	0.20 (1.29) ATR 3 mo
Werblin[22]	102	6.5	ST/S 1.5 mm	Shoelace 10-0	Jaffe & Clayman	NA	1.0 (0.7) 2 mo	1.2 (0.6) 72 mo
Wirbelauer et al[30]	18	7.0		Sutureless	Vector	1.21 (0.73)	1.13 (0.52) 1 mo	1.16 (0.44) 5 mo

Abbreviations: N, number of patients; Inc., incision length in mm; Loc., location of incision posterior to limbus in mm (ST, scleral tunnel; S, superior); SIA, surgically induced astigmatism; adj., adjustable; SD, standard deviation; Phaco, phacoemulsification; WTR, with-the-rule astigmatism; ATR, against-the-rule astigmatism.

time of cataract surgery is probably indicated for astigmatism greater than 0.5–1.0 diopters. The condition of the fellow eye must be considered to avoid large differences in cylinder magnitude or axis, unless future cataract surgery is planned on the fellow eye also. The surgical goal should be reduction of astigmatism by 50%–75%, avoiding overcorrection. A small amount of residual myopic astigmatism may be beneficial by enhancing the depth of focus of the pseudophakic eye.[47]

Postoperative astigmatism in the horizontal axis (ATR) appears to allow better unaided near vision than cylinder in the vertical axis (with-the-rule [WTR]).[48]

Preoperative marking of the steepest axis with the patient seated is advocated by some surgeons for astigmatic corrections, including astigmatic keratotomy (AK) and photoastigmatic refractive keratectomy (PARK). The same principle applies to placement of cataract wounds for correction of astigmatism. Axial

Table 24.3
Surgically Induced Astigmatism (SIA) with Incisions Greater than 7.5 mm

Study	N	Inc.	Loc.	Closure	SIA Method	Mean SIA (SD) on Postop. Day 1	Mean SIA (SD) at Intermediate Follow-up	Mean SIA (SD) at Longest Follow-up
Leen et al[10]	31	11.0	Limbal	Radial 10-0	Jaffe & Clayman	2.47 (1.63)	2.59 (1.71) 4–6 wk	1.63 (1.31) 2–3 mo
Neuman et al[12]	59	10.0	Limbal	Running 10-0	Naylor	NA	2.27 (1.28) 3 mo	1.74 (1.16) 6 mo
Oshika & Tsuboi[20]	26	11.0	ST/S 1 mm	Running 10-0	Jaffe & Clayman	2.87 (3.12)	1.32 (2.66) 1 mo	0.69 (1.59) 3 mo
					Cravy	1.71 (4.78)	0.35 (1.72) 1 mo	0.25 (1.30) 3 mo
Uusitalo et al[19,25]	10	7.5	ST/S 2 mm	Horizontal, radial 10-0	Cravy	1.51 (2.20) WTR	0.19 (0.57) ATR 1 mo	0.10 (0.80) ATR 6 mo
Werblin[22]	36	12.0	ST/S 1.5 mm	Running 10-0	Jaffe & Clayman	NA	1.9 (1.2) 2 mo	2.2 (1.3) 72 mo

Abbreviations: N, number of patients; Inc., incision length in mm; Loc., location of incision posterior to limbus in mm (ST, scleral tunnel; S, superior); SIA, surgically induced astigmatism; SD, standard deviation; WTR, with-the-rule astigmatism; ATR, against-the-rule astigmatism.

misalignment with the patient supine may occur because of position-induced ocular torsion, head tilt during surgery, and eye distortion.[49,50] With the patient seated, the vertical or horizontal meridian can be marked preoperatively at the limbus with a surgical pen. In a study of 38 eyes, videokeratography performed on seated patients after the horizontal meridian had been marked with the patient supine demonstrated a mean axial misalignment of 4.4 degrees (SD 2.8), which could cause a 15% loss of surgical effect. The maximal misalignment was 14 degrees, corresponding to a 48% loss of astigmatic correction.[50] Alpins noted that treatment misalignment results in a shift in the orientation of existing astigmatism toward the axis of effective steepening.[51]

Incision Placement

Most ophthalmologists employ plus cylinder in measuring astigmatism. This convention has the advantage that the axis of plus cylinder is the steepest meridian with the most corneal power. Consequently, centering the surgical incision on the meridian with the greatest power in plus cylinder reduces astigmatic cylinder by exploiting the inevitable ATW changes from an incision. Cataract incisions function as keratotomy incisions, creating steepening 90 degrees away.

Incision Length

The magnitude of cylinder reduction is most directly affected by the incision length (Fig. 24.3). Although surgical reduction of astigmatism must be individualized by each surgeon according to his or her preferred cataract technique, some guidelines do apply. A 12.0-mm incision will induce twice as much ATW cylinder (or reduce twice as much cylinder in the same axis) as a 6.0-mm incision for a given technique. A 6-mm incision placed at the posterior limbus in the steep axis is estimated to reduce 2–3 diopters of cylinder.[52] This linear relationship probably ends at 3.0–4.0 mm.

Amigo and colleagues created clear corneal "preincision" grooves in the steepest meridian with arcs of 40, 45, or 55 degrees, depending on preoperative astigmatism.[53] These preincision grooves were set at 90% of ultrasonically determined corneal depth with an astigmatic keratotomy blade and combined with a 3.4-mm-wide corneal tunnel. Incision arcs were based on the corneal radius in the steepest meridian and varied in length; the 40-degree incision was approximately 3.4 mm long. The wounds were not sutured. The mean reduction in astigmatism by vector analysis at 6 months postoperatively was 0.03 diopters for incisions of 40 degrees, 0.35 diopters for incisions of 45 degrees, and 0.61 diopters for incisions of 55 degrees.[53]

Table 24.4
Surgically Induced Astigmatism (SIA) with Scleral Tunnel Incisions

Study	N	Inc.	Loc.	Closure	SIA Method	Mean SIA (SD) on Postop. Day 1 or Week 1	Mean SIA (SD) at Intermediate Follow-up	Mean SIA (SD) at Longest Follow-up
Anders et al[33]	NA	7.0	ST/S 1 mm	Sutureless	Jaffe & Clayman	0.69 (0.32) POD 1	0.93 (0.42) 4 wk	0.97 (0.41) 8 mo
	NA	7.0	ST/T 1 mm	Sutureless	Jaffe & Clayman	0.70 (0.39) POD 1	0.70 (0.35) 4 wk	0.65 (0.23) 8 mo
Gross & Miller[31]	93	4.0	ST/S 2.5 mm	Sutureless	Jaffe & Jaffe	1.26 (NA) POD 1	1.05 (NA) 1 wk	0.42 (NA) 6 wk
Nouhuijs et al[29]	20	3.2	ST/S 1.5 mm	Cross 10-0	Jaffe & Clayman	—	—	0.66 (0.49) 6 mo
Olsen et al[32]	50	3.5	ST/A 2 mm	Sutureless	Olsen	0.55 (0.31) POD 1	—	0.36 (0.21) 6 mo
Oshima et al[35]	40	3.0	ST/S 2 mm	Sutureless	Jaffe & Clayman	0.76 (0.41) 1 wk	0.65 (0.44) 4 wk	0.67 (0.37) 3 mo
Pfleger et al[34]	56	3.5	ST/S 2.5 mm	Sutureless	Jaffe & Clayman	0.75 (0.50) 1 wk	0.73 (0.52) 4 wk	0.75 (0.58) 1 y
					Cravy	0.31 (1.02) ATR 1 wk	0.49 (0.91) ATR 4 wk	0.37 (1.0) ATR 1 y
	51	4.5	ST/S 2.5 mm	Sutureless	Jaffe & Clayman	0.88 (0.62) 1 wk	0.90 (0.71) 4 wk	0.89 (0.61) 1 y
					Cravy	0.48 (0.94) ATR 1 wk	0.75 (0.90) ATR 4 wk	0.67 (0.93) ATR 1 y
Singer[6]	34	6.0–7	ST/S 2 mm	Horizontal 10-0	Jaffe & Clayman	1.19 (0.91) POD 1	1.07 (0.63) 4 wk	1.30 (0.83) 1 y
Wirbelauer et al[30]	18	7.0	ST/S 2 mm	Sutureless	Jaffe & Clayman	1.86 (1.03) POD 1	1.76 (0.79) 4 wk	1.82 (0.64) 5 mo
	15	7.0	ST/T 2 mm	Sutureless	Jaffe & Clayman	1.49 (0.67) POD 1	1.53 (0.60) 4 wk	1.53 (0.64) 5 mo
	22	7.0	ST/O 2 mm	Sutureless	Jaffe & Clayman	1.33 (0.73) POD 1	1.13 (0.71) 4 wk	1.01 (0.72) 5 mo

Abbreviations: N, number of patients; Inc., incision length in mm; Loc., location of incision posterior to limbus in mm (ST, scleral tunnel; S, superior; T, template; O, oblique; A, on steep axis); SD, standard deviation; ATR, against-the-rule astigmatism.

Wound Modification: Scleral Flap Recession

Modifying a cataract incision to reduce astigmatism avoids additional incisions and minimizes the number of surgical variables. Scleral flap recession in effect adds tissue to a wound, reducing cylinder in the steep axis more than would be expected with a normal incision. With this technique, 4–5 diopters of astigmatism reduction is possible. The scleral incision as described by Koch and Lindstrom is placed 2 mm posterior to the limbus.[54] The flap is secured in the recessed position with a running 9-0 nylon suture anchored at each end and tied centrally. Each 0.25 mm of recession reduces approximately 1 diopter of cylinder; recessions in excess of 1 mm are uncommon.

Sutures

Radial sutures induce astigmatism in the axis of suture placement owing to focal tissue compression (Fig. 24.4).[55] Generally, longer and tighter sutures produce more astigmatism.[56] Azar and associates studied the astigmatic effects of one-radial, three-radial, or no

Table 24.5
Surgically Induced Astigmatism (SIA) with Corneal Incisions

Study	N	Inc.	Loc.	Closure	SIA Method	Mean SIA (SD) on Postoperative Day 1 or Week 1	Mean SIA (SD) at Intermediate Follow-up	Mean SIA (SD) at Longest Follow-up
Gross & Miller[31]	105	3.2–3.5	CC/T	Sutureless	Jaffe & Jaffe	0.76 POD 1	0.74 1 wk	0.60 6 wk
Masket & Tennen[36]	45	3.0	CC/T	Sutureless	H-C-K	0.46 (0.31) 1 wk	0.52 (0.31) 2 wk	0.49 (0.23) 6 wk
Nouhuijs et al[29]	15	3.2	CC/T	Sutureless	Jaffe & Clayman	—	—	0.50 (0.36) 6 mo
Olsen et al[32]	50	3.5–4.0	CC/A	Sutureless	Olsen	1.41 (0.66) POD 1	—	0.72 (0.35) 6 mo
Oshima et al[35]	40	3.0	CC/T	Sutureless	Jaffe & Clayman	0.86 (0.66) 1 wk	0.53 (0.34) 1 mo	0.56 (0.38) 3 mo
		3.0		Sutureless	Cravy	0.31 (0.58) WTR 1 wk	0.22 (0.49) WTR 1 mo	0.19 (0.65) WTR 3 mo
Pfleger et al[34]	35	3.0	CC/T	Sutureless	Jaffe & Clayman	0.65 (0.41) 1 wk	0.71 (0.45) 1 mo	0.53 (0.42) 1 y
		3.0		Sutureless	Cravy	0.43 (0.76) WTR 1 wk	0.22 (0.75) WTR 1 mo	0.09 (0.66) WTR 1 y
		3.0		Sutureless	Naeser	0.30 (0.49) WTR 1 wk	0.21 (0.67) WTR 1 mo	0.09 (0.41) WTR 1 y
	31	5.2	CC/T	Sutureless	Jaffe & Clayman	1.27 (0.71) 1 wk	0.95 (0.51) 1 mo	0.84 (0.53) 1 y
		5.2		Sutureless	Cravy	1.30 (0.74) WTR 1 wk	0.90 (0.79) WTR 1 mo	0.54 (0.90) WTR 1 y
		5.2		Sutureless	Naeser	1.13 (0.74) WTR 1 wk	0.77 (0.65) WTR 1 mo	0.48 (0.75) WTR 1 y

Abbreviations: N, number of patients; Inc., incision length in mm; Loc., location of incision (CC, clear cornea; S, superior; T, temporal); SD, standard deviation; WTR, with-the-rule astigmatism.

suture closure of 5.5-mm superior cataract incisions. WTR astigmatism increased from baseline in the one- and three-suture groups and decreased in the sutureless group, and this relationship continued throughout the 12-month follow-up period.[27] With superior extracapsular cataract extraction (ECCE) incisions, surgeons have employed intraoperative keratometry to induce WTR astigmatism to counteract the ATW cylinder regression caused by the wound. However, regression, or suture decay, will occur over time, with the tempo of decay dependent on the suture material used.[57–64] Suture decay can continue over several years. In small-incision surgery, sutureless closure or a horizontal suture is often used to avoid the initial with-the-wound (WTW) changes caused by radial sutures.[65]

Limbal Relaxing Incisions

Another approach for astigmatism reduction is to combine a limbal relaxing incision (LRI) with cataract surgery. This technique utilizes a guarded diamond blade preset to 600 μm depth. No pachymetry or calibration microscope is necessary. LRIs of 6.0–8.0 mm are placed on the steepest meridian, based on preoperative keratometric or computerized videokeratography (Table 24.7). This nomogram aims for 50%–75% reduction in astigmatism, without overcorrection. Longer incisions are required than for standard arcuate or transverse keratotomies but may reduce induced irregular astigmatism and glare compared to more central incisions.[66]

Astigmatic Keratotomy with Cataract Surgery

Traditionally, with cataract techniques requiring longer incisions and the inherent cylinder regression, astigmatic keratotomy (AK) has been delayed until adequate corneal stabilization has been achieved. Some surgeons, recognizing the minimal astigmatic changes in small-incision surgery, have combined corneal relaxing incisions with phacoemulsification. Maloney et al

Table 24.6
Surgically Induced Astigmatism (SIA) in Superior versus Temporal Incisions

Study	N	Inc.	Loc.	Closure	SIA Method	Mean SIA (SD) at Initial Follow-up	Mean SIA (SD) at Intermediate Follow-up	Mean SIA (SD) at Final Follow-up
Anders et al[33]	90	7.0	ST/S	Sutureless	Jaffe & Clayman	0.69 (0.32) POD 1	0.93 (0.4) 1 mo	0.97 (0.41) 8 mo
	90	7.0	ST/T	Sutureless	Jaffe & Clayman	0.70 (0.39) POD 1	0.70 (0.35) 1 mo	0.65 (0.23) 8 mo
	90	7.0	L/S	Sutureless	Jaffe & Clayman	1.25 (0.76) POD 1	1.32 (0.64) 1 mo	1.33 (0.63) 8 mo
	90	7.0	L/T	Sutureless	Jaffe & Clayman	0.84 (0.59) POD 1	0.95 (0.54) 1 mo	0.86 (0.53) 8 mo
Cillino et al[45]	40	5.2	CS/S	Sutureless	Naeser	0.85 (1.02) ATR POD 1	0.71 (0.93) ATR 2 wk	0.86 (0.90) ATR 8 wk
	40	5.2	CC/T	Sutureless	Naeser	0.46 (0.85) WTR POD 1	0.55 (0.99) WTR 2 wk	0.51 (0.99) WTR 8 wk
Kammann & Dornback[39]	130	3–4.5	CC/O	Sutureless	Jaffe & Clayman	1.20 (0.79) 1 wk	1.21 (0.69) 1 mo	1.03 (0.44) 2 y
	65	3–4.5	CC/T	Sutureless	Jaffe & Clayman	0.85 (0.77) 1 wk	0.75 (0.52) 1 mo	0.51 (0.24) 6 mo
Long & Monica[41]	35	3–3.5	CC/S	0-1-radial	H-C-K	1.17 (0.56)	1.14 (0.63) 1 mo	0.90 (0.49) 1 y
	98	3–3.5	CC/T	0-1-radial	H-C-K	0.96 (0.62)	0.73 (0.49) 1 mo	0.62 (0.47) 1 y
Mueller-Jensen[40]	50	4.0	CC/S	Sutureless	Jaffe & Clayman	1.67 (1.22) 1 wk	1.18 (0.79) 1 yr	1.53 (0.95) 2 y
	50	4.0	CC/T	Sutureless	Jaffe & Clayman	0.89 (0.74) 1 wk	0.85 (0.69) 1 yr	0.64 (0.50) 2 y
Nielsen[42]	17	3.5	CC/S	Sutureless	Naeser	0.93 (0.89) ATR	0.56 (0.57) ATR 3 wk	0.55 (0.57) ATR 6 wk
	16	3.5	CC/T	Sutureless	Naeser	0.55 (0.45) WTR	0.59 (0.43) WTR 3 wk	0.46 (0.54) WTR 6 wk
	10	5.2	CC/S	Sutureless	Naeser	1.44 (9.6) ATR	1.47 (0.75) ATR 3 wk	1.24 (0.76) ATR 6 wk
	11	5.2	CC/T	Sutureless	Naeser	1.41 (1.13) WTR	1.20 (0.72) WTR 3 wk	0.82 (0.76) WTR 6 wk
Simsek et al[44]	20	4.0	CC/S	Sutureless	Jaffe & Clayman	1.76 (0.32) POD 1	1.31 (0.28) 1 mo	1.44 (0.31) 3 mo
	20	4.0	CC/T	Sutureless	Jaffe & Clayman	0.98 (0.26) POD 1	0.88 (0.27) 1 mo	0.62 (0.28) 3 mo
Wirbelauer et al[30]	18	7.0	ST/S	Sutureless	Vector	1.21 (0.73) POD 1	1.13 (0.52) 1mo	1.16 (0.44) 5 mo
	15	7.0	ST/T	Sutureless	Vector	0.70 (0.48) POD 1	0.65 (0.34) 1 mo	0.66 (0.32) 5 mo
	22	7.0	ST/A	Sutureless	Vector	0.88 (0.45) POD 1	0.86 (0.58) 1 mo	0.82 (0.50) 5 mo

Abbreviations: N, number of patients; Inc., incision length in mm; Loc., location of incision (ST, scleral tunnel; CC, clear cornea; S, superior; T, temporal; CS, corneoscleral; O, oblique; L, limbal; A, on steep axis); SD, standard deviation; WTR, with-the-rule astigmatism; ATR, against-the-rule astigmatism.

recommended AK with intraoperative keratometry for preoperative astigmatism greater than 2.5 diopters, followed by phacoemulsification.[52] Shepherd evaluated AK combined with phacoemulsification performed through a superior 4.0-mm scleral tunnel in 48 eyes.[67] The mean cylinder reduction was 39% in eyes with 1.00–1.25 diopters of preoperative astigmatism and 60% in eyes with 1.50–3.0 diopters, with 10 weeks to 14 months of follow-up. Kershner combined arcuate incisions with phacoemulsification in one operation (keratolenticuloplasty).[68] Phacoemulsification is performed through an arcuate incision placed just inside

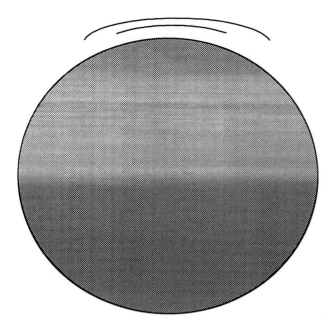

FIGURE 24.3. At a given location, a longer incision will produce more against-the-wound astigmatism than a shorter incision.

the limbus, and if necessary an additional arcuate incision is placed on the other side of the cornea at 7, 8, or 9 mm. As in routine astigmatic keratotomy, the incision length and distance from the corneal center are tailored to preexisting astigmatism (Table 24.8).

Toric Intraocular Lens

Shimizu and associates have developed an IOL with a toric curve on the back surface.[69] This lens, designed for reduction of horizontal, or ATR, astigmatism, was

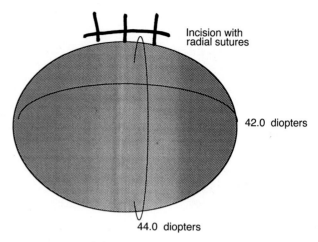

FIGURE 24.4. Radial sutures induce with-the-wound astigmatism. In general, more astigmatism is produced with longer and tighter sutures.

available in cylinder powers of 2.0 diopters and 3.0 diopters. In most cases the lenses were successful, with postoperative refractive astigmatism less than corneal astigmatism. However, undesired rotation of the IOL was noted in some patients, with diminution of the astigmatism correction. The appropriate role of toric IOLs in the management of astigmatism requires further study (see Chapter 25).

■ Intraoperative Measurement of Astigmatism

Various approaches have been employed to assess astigmatism intraoperatively. Qualitative devices reflect a circle or circles onto the corneal surface, allowing

---

Table 24.7
Modified Gills Nomogram for Limbal Relaxing Incisions (LRI) to Correct Astigmatism with Cataract Surgery

Astigmatism (D)	Incision Type	Length (mm)	Optical Zone
1	One LRI	6.0	At limbus
1–2	Two LRIs	6.0	At limbus
2–3	Two LRIs	8.0	At limbus
>3	Two LRIs + corneal relaxing incisions as indicated 3 months postoperatively	Based on arcuate keratotomy nomogram	7–8 mm at cornea

From Budak K, Friedman NJ, Koch DD. Limbal relaxing incisions with cataract surgery, *J Cataract Refract Surg.* 1998;24:503–508, with permission.

Table 24.8
Keratolenticuloplasty Nomograms

Correction (D)	Optical Zone (mm)	Arcuate Incision Length (mm)
< 1.0	10	2.5 (1)
1.0	9	2.5 (1)
1.5	9	3.0 (1)
2.0	8	2.5 (2)
2.5	9/7	2.5 (2)
3.0	9/7	3.0 (2)
3.5	8/7	3.0 (2)
4.0	6	2.0 (2)
4.5	6	2.5 (2)
5.0	6	3.0 (2)
5.5	5	2.0 (2)
6.0	5	2.5 (2)

Note: Values are corrected for age 60 +. Arcs are placed on the steepest axis of astigmatism (plus cylinder). Pachymetry is performed at the incision site, with a square diamond keratome set to 100% of pachymetry. Cataract keratotomy performed at 10 mm, 9 mm, or 8 mm only.
From Kershner RM. Keratolenticuloplasty. In: Kershner RM, ed. *Refractive Keratotomy for Cataract Surgery and the Correction of Astigmatism.* Thorofare, NJ: Slack; 1994:25–41, with permission.

estimation of cylindrical axis and power by the pattern produced. Examples include the handheld Placido disc and the Maloney keratoscope.[70] The Hyde astigmatic ruler is a handheld semiquantitative keratometer consisting of a flat aluminum rod with milled apertures; the first aperture is circular and the rest are elliptical, representing 2, 4, 6, and 8 diopters of cylinder.[71] The Hyde ruler has been reported to underestimate astigmatism.[72] Measurement error can arise from variance in distance to the cornea, from tilt, or from misinterpretation of the reflected image.[73] The Barrett keratoscope is a disposable qualitative keratoscope consisting of a toroidal lens on a handle capable of producing a bright reflected image. Morlet et al combined an astigmatic dial with the Barrett keratoscope; however, they noted some variance in readings, depending on the distance to the cornea.[73] Troutman et al designed a qualitative surgical keratometer by mounting a ring of fiberoptic lights onto a surgical microscope.[74] These instruments are useful for gross estimations, such as suture adjustment in penetrating keratoplasty, but cannot differentiate small amounts of cylinder.

Quantitative keratometry can measure changes in astigmatic magnitude of as little as 0.25 diopter.[75] An illuminated circle of known size is projected onto the apical cornea, and the radius of curvature of that sur-face is determined from the size of the reflected image. A few assumptions are inherent in keratometry. First, the cornea is assumed to be a spherical convex mirror with the center of curvature on the optical axis, and second, the refractive index is assumed to be 1.3375, to compensate for the negative power of the posterior corneal surface, although the true calculated refractive index is 1.375. The translation of corneal radius of curvature into dioptric power is based on the assumed refractive index. Quantitative keratometers may be mounted directly onto an operating microscope for intraoperative monitoring of astigmatism.

■ Corneal Topography

Corneal topography, or computerized videokeratography (CVK), has become an indispensable tool in refractive surgery. Most systems in current use are based on Placido disc technology, utilizing computer interpretation of alternating rings reflected from the anterior corneal surface. In earlier studies measuring astigmatic changes in cataract or refractive techniques, standard keratometry was the preferred method. CVK has proved accurate, reliable, and reproducible and is now often used with or in lieu of standard keratometry.[76–79] The ability to store, compare, and print longitudinal data is extremely helpful in understanding changes in astigmatism magnitude and axis over time. The use of color-coded scales in CVK has facilitated pattern recognition in regular and irregular astigmatism. Additionally, CVK provides valuable information on changes in the peripheral cornea, compared with the central 3 mm analyzed in keratometry. CVK allows evaluation of 70%–95% of the total corneal curvature versus the central 8% assessed with keratometry.[80] Preoperative and postoperative CVK can help the cataract surgeon appreciate astigmatic changes induced by his or her preferred technique (Figs. 24.5 and 24.6).

■ Measurement of Surgically Induced Astigmatism

Simple addition and subtraction of keratometric values does not adequately portray the changes created by a surgical incision of the eye. In 1975 Jaffe and Clayman introduced a way to find the resultant cylinder when two optical cylinders are crossed.[55] Astigmatic cylinders are depicted on a graph as vectors, representing force (magnitude) and direction (axis). If the preoperative and postoperative keratometry values are known, both the amount and axis of astigmatism induced by the surgery can be calculated from a modified parallelogram. Cravy

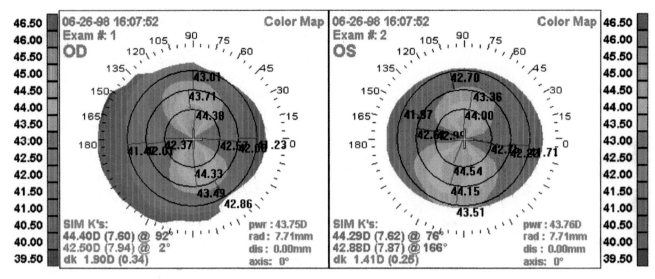

FIGURE 24.5. Computerized videokeratography. Native regular with-the-rule astigmatism is present bilaterally.

described the use of rectangular coordinates to calculate SIA.[81] Naeser reported a method to convert keratometric values to a polar value, allowing expression of corneal astigmatism as a single figure.[82] Alpins introduced a modification of the vector method that allows comparison of aggregate data.[83] Holladay et al reported a method of converting magnitude and axis of astigmatism to a Cartesian coordinate system, allowing comparison of data from different procedures and studies.[84] The use of standard methodology to determine SIA enables the surgeon to develop a nomogram and modify his or her technique accordingly, as well as to compare data from different surgeons and centers. Methods and examples are available in the literature.[27,51,55,81-88]

■ Management of Residual or Induced Astigmatism After Cataract Surgery

Many patients have undergone cataract surgery with large superior incisions and, as a consequence, have ATR astigmatism of greater than 1–2 diopters. Unilateral

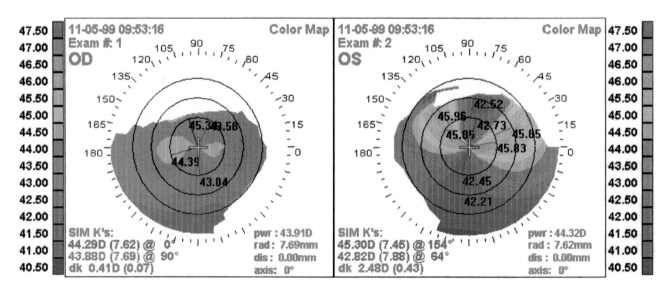

FIGURE 24.6. Computerized videokeratography. Right eye demonstrates native against-the-rule (ATR) astigmatism; left eye underwent uncomplicated cataract surgery with a superior scleral incision several years before, with a resultant increased ATR.

large-incision cataract surgery induces a disparity in cylinder magnitude and axis. Similarly, superior large-incision surgery in one eye, either elective or related to intraoperative complications, coupled with uncomplicated small-incision surgery in the fellow eye may create astigmatic asymmetry. In larger incisions, excessive ATR astigmatism may result from superior wound gape caused by inadvertently loose sutures, early removal of sutures, ingrowth of fibrous tissue, or poor wound healing.[89,90] Spectacle correction should be attempted; however, the distortions caused by meridional magnification of different cylinder axes and powers with spectacles may be disabling, especially in the older cataract patient. A soft contact lens may mask up to 1 diopter of corneal astigmatism; a toric soft lens will correct higher amounts of cylinder. A rigid contact lens will mask up to 4 diopters of regular astigmatism and will also correct irregular astigmatism.

Wound revision may be necessary for wound dehiscence with high astigmatism. Scar tissue and any filtering bleb are excised and the wound is securely closed with nonabsorbable sutures, aiming for an overcorrection of 2–3 diopters. Postoperative steroids should be used sparingly and tapered rapidly.[90] For large amounts of postoperative astigmatism caused by wound gape or very large incision surgery, Troutman introduced the concept of tissue removal, or wedge resection, to steepen the flat meridian.[91] Tissue removal can reduce very large amounts of astigmatism. Wedge resection, with suturing, reduced average keratoplasty astigmatism at 6 months from 11.4 diopters to 2.8 diopters in ten eyes.[91] Another approach is scleral flap resection, which removes tissue from the previous cataract incision and steepens the flat meridian. In cases of cataract wound dehiscence involving more than 10 diopters of ATW astigmatism, Gelender suggested a wound resection of 0.1 mm for each diopter of desired cylinder correction.[89] However, in a study of eye bank eyes, Koch et al found that the relationship between the amount of incision edge resected and the induced cylinder was unpredictable and statistically insignificant.[92]

A stable refraction, keratometry, and/or CVK are essential for predictability in astigmatic refractive procedures. Hettinger suggested that corneas achieve stability by 6 months after small-incision cataract surgery.[93] Indications for surgery include stable regular astigmatism greater than 0.5–1.0 diopters, usually with spectacle or contact lens intolerance. The surgical goal is reduction of astigmatism by 50%–75%.

Astigmatic keratotomy consists of corneal relaxing incisions to flatten the steep meridian through tissue addition. Tissue relaxation in the steep meridian is accompanied by steepening 90 degrees away, an effect known as coupling.[94] A coupling ratio of 1:1 does not change the spherical equivalent. Rowsey has summarized incisional refractive effects.[4] Incisions can be either arcuate (curved) or transverse (straight). Arcuate incisions, which follow the arc of the circular optical zone, have a potentially greater effect because they are 10% longer (following the curve) than straight incisions of equal chord length.[94] Arcuate incisions are placed on a 6- to 7-mm optical zone, transverse incisions on a 5- to 7-mm zone. The optical zone should not be smaller than 5 mm because of side effects such as glare and irregular astigmatism.[46] Incisions are made with a guarded diamond blade set at 100% of corneal depth as measured by ultrasonic pachymetry. The amount of astigmatism corrected depends on optical zone, incision length, number of incisions, and patient age. The effect of a given incision is greater in older patients. The technical details of astigmatic keratotomy are discussed elsewhere.[46,93]

Correction of astigmatism with the excimer laser is termed photoastigmatic refractive keratectomy (PARK). This can be accomplished with photorefractive keratectomy (PRK) or laser-assisted in situ keratomileusis (LASIK). Methods of toric ablation include an expanding slit, an elliptical ablation, use of an ablatable mask, and a scanning-beam laser.[95] With the VISX laser, cylinder amounts up to the level of myopia may be corrected in the elliptical mode. If the myopic cylinder exceeds the amount of myopia, a sequential ablation is performed. The amount of cylinder to be treated is represented in the minus cylinder notation. The manifest refraction is usually chosen as the basis for cylinder correction, although if there is disagreement between manifest refraction and keratometry or CVK readings, the treatment axis may be shifted according to surgeon preference and experience. Misalignment may cause a treatment undercorrection; an alignment error of 5% will reduce treatment effect by 17%.[96]

Piggyback Lenses for Correction of High Hyperopia and Secondary Ametropia

Gayton and Sanders described placing two IOLs into the capsular bag (piggyback lenses) for correction of high hyperopia.[97] The optical resolution of two lenses of lower power placed together is superior to that of a single IOL of high power because the steep surface curvature necessary for high power lenses creates aberration.[98] Because of this distortion, IOLs are generally not available in powers greater than 30–34 diopters.[98] Acrylic lenses, such as the Alcon 5.5-mm optic lens (AcrySof model MA30BA) are preferred. The center thickness of a 24-diopter acrylic lens is 0.72 mm.[99] Also, the index of refraction of an acrylic lens (1.54) is higher than that of a silicone lens (1.41), allowing acrylic lens to achieve a given power with less curvature.[99] Acrylic lenses are also reported to induce less postoperative capsular fibrotic change.[100] After standard capsulorrhexis and phacoemulsification through a small incision, the first lens is folded and placed into the capsular bag with viscoelastic material. The second lens is then folded and inserted such that the leading loop enters the incision and the capsular bag before the optic (longitudinal insertion); then the lens is unfolded in the bag.[99] Placement of the overlying haptics parallel with those of the first lens is recommended, as this configuration appears stable.[99,101] There have been unexpected hyperopic "surprises" with piggyback lenses, which may be due to a more posterior IOL location then anticipated.[98] IOL power formulas continue to be refined for better predictive ability.[98] Late hyperopic shifts have been reported as a result of Elschnig pearl formation in the peripheral interface between the two lenses that did not affect best-corrected visual acuity.[102] Piggyback lenses may also be useful in secondary ametropia due either to miscalculation of lens power or to inadvertent placement of the wrong lens at surgery. Adjustable optics may be available in the future, which would allow more precise correction of refractive error in pediatric cataract or after penetrating keratoplasty.[103]

■ Summary

Induced astigmatism of some degree is an inevitable consequence of any cataract incision. The advent of small-incision surgery permits routine cataract surgery to be performed with minimal induced astigmatism. An understanding of wound healing and wound dynamics allows the surgeon to modify the cataract incision length and placement to reduce existing astigmatism. Keratometry and CVK enable the surgeon to quantify changes in corneal astigmatism, and vector analysis informs the surgeon of the astigmatic effects of a particular technique. Adjunctive techniques, such as limbal relaxing incisions or astigmatic keratotomy, allow reduction of greater amounts of preoperative astigmatism. Laser or incisional refractive surgery is useful in the management of postoperative astigmatism, after corneal stability has been achieved. Piggyback lenses have proved useful in the correction of high hyperopia and of secondary ametropia after cataract surgery.

■ References

1. Armeniades CD, Borick A, Knolle GE. Effect of incision length, location and shape on local corneoscleral deformation during cataract surgery. *J Cataract Refract Surg.* 1990;16:83–87.

2. Flaherty PM, Siepser SB. Surgically-induced astigmatism in human cadaver eyes. *J Cataract Refract Surg.* 1989;15:19–24.

3. Samuelson SW, Koch DD, Kuglen CC. Determination of maximal incision length for true small-incision surgery. *Ophthalmic Surg.* 1991;22:204–207.

4. Rowsey JJ. Ten caveats in keratorefractive surgery. *Ophthalmology.* 1983;90:148–155.

5. Koch PS. Structural analysis of cataract incision construction. *J Cataract Refract Surg.* 1991;17:661–667.

6. Singer JA. Frown incision for minimizing induced astigmatism after small incision cataract surgery with rigid optic intraocular lens implantation. *J Cataract Refract Surg.* 1991;17:677–688.

7. Watson A, Sunderraj P. Comparison of small-incision phacoemulsification with standard extracapsular cataract surgery: post-operative astigmatism and visual recovery. *Eye.* 1992;6:626–629.

8. Hettinger ME. Astigmatism and cataract surgery. In: Krachmer JH, Mannis MJ, Holland EJ, eds. *Cornea: Surgery of the Cornea and Conjunctiva.* Vol 3. St. Louis, MO: Mosby–Year Book; 1997:2155–2164.

9. Brint SF, Ostrick M, Bryan JE. Keratometric cylinder and visual performance following phacoemulsification and implantation with silicone small-incision or poly (methyl methacrylate) intraocular lenses. *J Cataract Refract Surg.* 1991;17:32–36.

10. Leen MM, Ho CC, Yanoff M. Association between surgically-induced astigmatism and cataract incision size in the early postoperative period. *Ophthalmic Surg.* 1993;24:586–592.

11. Steinert RF, Brint SF, White SM, et al. Astigmatism after small incision cataract surgery. *Ophthalmology.* 1991;98:417–424.

12. Neumann AC, McCarty GR, Sanders DR, et al. Small incisions to control astigmatism during cataract surgery. *J Cataract Refract Surg.* 1989;15:78–84.

13. Shepherd JR. Induced astigmatism in small incision cataract surgery. *J Cataract Refract Surg.* 1989;15:85–88.

14. Lindstrom RL, Destro MA. Effect of incision size and Terry keratometer usage on postoperative astigmatism. *Am Intraocular Implant Soc J.* 1985;11:469–473.

15. Martin RG, Sanders DR, Van Der Karr MA, et al. Effect of small incision intraocular lens surgery on postoperative inflammation and astigmatism: a study of the AMO SI-18NB small incision lens. *J Cataract Refract Surg.* 1992;18:51–57.

16. Pfleger T, Scholz U, Skorpik C. Postoperative astigmatism after no-stitch, small incision cataract surgery with 3.5 mm and 4.5 mm incisions. *J Cataract Refract Surg.* 1994;20:400–405.

17. Lyhne N, Corydon L. Astigmatism after phacoemulsification with adjusted and unadjusted sutured versus sutureless 5.2 mm superior scleral incisions. *J Cataract Refract Surg.* 1996;22:1206–1210.

18. Reading VM. Astigmatism following cataract surgery. *Br J Ophthalmol.* 1984;68:97–104.

19. Uusitalo RJ, Ruusuvaara P, Järvinen E, et al. Early rehabilitation after small incision cataract surgery. *Refract Corneal Surg.* 1993;9:67–70.
20. Oshika T, Tsuboi S. Astigmatic and refractive stabilization after cataract surgery. *Ophthalmic Surg.* 1995;26: 309–315.
21. Gills JP, Sanders DR. Use of small incisions to control induced astigmatism and inflammation following cataract surgery. *J Cataract Refract Surg.* 1991;17:740–744.
22. Werblin TP. Astigmatism after cataract extraction: 6-year follow up of 6.5- and 12-millimeter incisions. *Refract Corneal Surg.* 1992;8:448–458.
23. El-Maghraby A, Anwar M, El-Sayyad F, et al. Effect of incision size on early postoperative visual rehabilitation after cataract surgery and intraocular lens implantation. *J Cataract Refract Surg.* 1993;19:494–498.
24. Mueller-Jensen K, Barlinn B, Zimmerman H. Astigmatism reduction: no-stitch 4.0 mm versus sutured 12.0 mm clear corneal incisions. *J Cataract Refract Surg.* 1996;22:1108–1112.
25. Uusitalo RJ, Tarkkanen A. Outcomes of small incision cataract surgery. *J Cataract Refract Surg.* 1998;24:212–221.
26. Rainer G, Menapace R, Vass C, et al. Surgically induced astigmatism following a 4.0 mm sclerocorneal valve incision. *J Cataract Refract Surg.* 1997;23:358–364.
27. Azar DT, Stark WJ, Dodick J, et al. Prospective, randomized vector analysis of astigmatism after three-, one-, and no-suture phacoemulsification. *J Cataract Refract Surg.* 1997;23:1164–1173.
28. Davison JA. Keratometric comparison of 4.0 mm and 5.5 mm scleral tunnel cataract incisions. *J Cataract Refract Surg.* 1993;19:3–8.
29. Nouhuijs HM, Hendrickx KH, van Marle WF, et al. Corneal astigmatism after clear corneal and corneoscleral incisions for cataract surgery. *J Cataract Refract Surg.* 1997;23:758–760.
30. Wirbelauer C, Anders N, Pham DT, et al. Effect of incision location on preoperative oblique astigmatism after scleral tunnel incision. *J Cataract Refract Surg.* 1997;23: 365–371.
31. Gross RH, Miller KM. Corneal astigmatism after phacoemulsification and lens implantation through unsutured scleral and corneal tunnel incisions. *Am J Ophthalmol.* 1996;121:57–64.
32. Olsen T, Dam-Johnson M, Bek T, et al. Corneal versus scleral tunnel incision in cataract surgery: a randomized study. *J Cataract Refract Surg.* 1997;23:337–341.
33. Anders N, Pham DT, Antoni HJ, et al. Postoperative astigmatism and relative strength of tunnel incisions: a prospective clinical trial. *J Cataract Refract Surg.* 1997; 23:332–336.
34. Pfleger T, Skorpik C, Menapace R, et al. Long-term course of induced astigmatism after clear corneal incision cataract surgery. *J Cataract Refract Surg.* 1996;22:72–77.
35. Oshima Y, Tsujikawa K, Oh A, et al. Comparative study of intraocular lens implantation through 3.0 mm temporal clear corneal and superior scleral tunnel self-sealing incisions. *J Cataract Refract Surg.* 1997;23:347–353.
36. Masket S, Tennen DG. Astigmatic stabilization of 3.0 mm temporal clear corneal cataract incisions. *J Cataract Refract Surg.* 1996;22:1451–1455.
37. Cravy TV. Routine use of a lateral approach to cataract extraction to achieve rapid and sustained stabilization of postoperative astigmatism. *J Cataract Refract Surg.* 1991; 17:415–423.
38. Kawano K. Modified corneoscleral incision to reduce postoperative astigmatism after 6 mm diameter intraocular lens implantation. *J Cataract Refract Surg.* 1993;19: 387–392.
39. Kammann JP, Dornbach G. Long-term results and indications for clear corneal surgery. *Eur J Implant Refract Surg.* 1995;7:97–100.
40. Mueller-Jensen K, Barlinn B. Long-term astigmatic changes after clear corneal cataract surgery. *J Cataract Refract Surg.* 1997;23:354–357.
41. Long DA, Monica ML. A prospective evaluation of corneal curvature changes with 3.0- to 3.5-mm corneal tunnel phacoemulsification. *Ophthalmology.* 1996;103: 226–232.
42. Nielsen PJ. Prospective evaluation of surgically induced astigmatism and astigmatic keratotomy effects of various self-sealing small incisions. *J Cataract Refract Surg.* 1995;21:43–48.
43. Edwards MG, Azar DT. Refractive cataract surgery. In: Azar DT, ed. *Refractive Surgery.* Stamford, CT: Appleton & Lange; 1997:527–533.
44. Simsek S, Yasar T, Demirok A, et al. Effect of superior and temporal clear corneal incisions on astigmatism after sutureless phacoemulsification. *J Cataract Refract Surg.* 1998;24:515–518.
45. Cillino S, Morreale D, Mauceri A, et al. Temporal versus superior approach phacoemulsification: short-term postoperative astigmatism. *J Cataract Refract Surg.* 1997:23: 267–271.
46. Lindstrom RL, Chu YR, Hardten DR, et al. Surgical techniques of incisional refractive surgery. In: Wu HK, Thompson VM, Steinert RF, et al, eds. *Refractive Surgery.* New York Thieme; 1999:135–168.
47. Sawusch MR, Guyton DL. Optimal astigmatism to enhance depth of focus after cataract surgery. *Ophthalmology.* 1991;98:1025–1029.
48. Trinidade F, Oliveira A, Frasson M. Benefit of against-the-rule astigmatism to uncorrected near acuity. *J Cataract Refract Surg.* 1997;23:82–85.
49. Smith EM, Talamo JH, Assil KK, et al. Comparison of astigmatic axis in the seated and supine positions. *J Cataract Refract Surg.* 1994;10:615–620.
50. Suzuki A, Maeda N, Watanabe H, et al. Using a reference point and videokeratography for intraoperative identification of astigmatism axis. *J Cataract Refract Surg.* 1997;23:1491–1495.
51. Alpins NA. Vector analysis of astigmatism changes by flattening, steeping, and torque. *J Cataract Refract Surg.* 1997;23:1503–1514.
52. Maloney WF, Grindle L, Sanders D, et al. Astigmatism control for the cataract surgeon: a comprehensive review of surgically tailored astigmatism reduction (STAR). *J Cataract Refract Surg.* 1989;15:45–54.
53. Amigo A, Giebel AW, Muinos JA. Astigmatic keratotomy effect of single-hinge, clear corneal incisions using various preincision lengths. *J Cataract Refract Surg.* 1998;24:765–771.

54. Koch DD, Lindstrom RL. Controlling astigmatism in cataract surgery. *Semin Ophthalmol.* 1992;4:224–233.

55. Jaffe NS, Clayman HM. The pathophysiology of corneal astigmatism after cataract extraction. *Trans Am Acad Ophthalmol Otolaryngol.* 1975;79:615–630.

56. Van Rij G, Waring GO III. Changes in corneal curvature induced by sutures and incisions. *Am J Ophthalmol.* 1984;98:773–783.

57. Cravy TV. Long-term corneal astigmatism related to selected elastic, monofilament, non-absorbable sutures. *J Cataract Refract Surg.* 1989;15:61–69.

58. Talamo JH, Stark WJ, Gottsch JD, et al. Natural history of corneal astigmatism after cataract surgery. *J Cataract Refract Surg.* 1991;17:313–318.

59. Storr-Paulsen A, Vangsted P, Perriard A. Long-term natural and modified course of surgically induced astigmatism after extracapsular cataract extraction. *Acta Ophthalmol.* 1994;72:617–621.

60. Richards SC, Brodstein RS, Richards WL, et al. Long-term course of surgically induced astigmatism. *J Cataract Refract Surg.* 1988;14:270–276.

61. Jampel HD, Thompson JR, Baker CC, et al. A computerized analysis of astigmatism after cataract surgery. *Ophthalmic Surg.* 1986;17:786–790.

62. Axt JC. Longitudinal study of postoperative astigmatism. *J Cataract Refract Surg.* 1987;13:381–388.

63. Parker WT, Clorfeine GS. Long-term evolution of astigmatism following planned extracapsular cataract extraction. *Arch Ophthalmol.* 1989;107:353–357.

64. Rowan PJ. Corneal astigmatism following cataract surgery. *Ann Ophthalmol.* 1978;10:231–234.

65. Masket S. Horizontal anchor suture closure method for small incision cataract surgery. *J Cataract Refract Surg.* 1991;17:689–695.

66. Budak K, Friedman NJ, Koch DD. Limbal relaxing incisions with cataract surgery. *J Cataract Refract Surg.* 1998;24:503–509.

67. Shepherd JR. Correction of preexisting astigmatism at the time of small incision cataract surgery. *J Cataract Refract Surg.* 1989;15:55–57.

68. Kershner RM. Keratolenticuloplasty. In: Kershner RM, ed. *Refractive Keratotomy for Cataract Surgery and the Correction of Astigmatism.* Thorofare, NJ: Slack; 1994:25–41.

69. Shimizu K, Misawa A, Suzuki Y. Toric intraocular lenses: correcting astigmatism while controlling axis shift. *J Cataract Refract Surg.* 1994;20:523–526.

70. Mandel MR. Instrumentation for corneal transplant surgery. In: Krachmer JH, Mannis MJ, Holland EJ, eds. *Cornea: Surgery of the Cornea and Conjunctiva.* Vol 3. St. Louis, MO:Mosby–Year Book; 1997:1571–1579.

71. Hyde LL. The surgical astigmatic ruler. *Am Intraocular Implant Soc J.* 1984;10:84–86.

72. House PH, Chauhan BC. An evaluation of the Hyde surgical astigmatic ruler. *Ophthalmic Surg.* 1988;19:554–558.

73. Morlet N, Lindsay P, Cooke P. A comparison of two semi-quantitative surgical keratometers: the modified Hyde ruler and Barrett keratoscope with "astigmatic dial." *Ophthalmic Surg.* 1994;25:144–149.

74. Troutman RC, Kelly S, Kaye D. The use and preliminary results of the Troutman surgical keratometer in cataract and corneal surgery. *Trans Am Acad Ophthalmol Otolaryngol.* 1977;83:232–238.

75. Swinger CA. Postoperative astigmatism. *Surv Ophthalmol.* 1987;31:219–248.

76. Davis LJ, Dresner MS. A comparison of the EH-270 Corneal Topographer with conventional keratometry. *CLAO J.* 1991;17:191–196.

77. Hannush SB, Crawford SL, Waring GO III, et al. Reproducibility of normal corneal power measurements with a keratometer, photokeratoscope, and video imaging system. *Arch Ophthalmol.* 1990;108:539–544.

78. Hannush SB, Crawford SL, Waring GO III, et al. Accuracy and precision of keratometry, photokeratoscopy, and corneal modeling on calibrated steel balls. *Arch Ophthalmol.* 1989;107:1235–1239.

79. Koch DD, Wakil JS, Samuelson SW, et al. Comparison of the accuracy and reproducibility of the keratometer and the EyeSys Corneal Analysis System Model 1. *J Cataract Refract Surg.* 1992;18:342–347.

80. Brody J, Waller S, Wagoner M. Corneal topography: history, technique, and clinical uses. *Int Ophthalmol Clin.* 1994;34(3):197–207.

81. Cravy TV. Calculation of the change in corneal astigmatism following cataract extraction. *Ophthalmic Surg.* 1979;10:38–49.

82. Naeser K. Conversion of keratometer readings to polar values. *J Cataract Refract Surg.* 1990;16:741–745.

83. Alpins NA. A new method of analyzing vectors for changes in astigmatism. *J Cataract Refract Surg.* 1993;19:524–533.

84. Holladay JT, Dudega DP, Koch DD. Evaluating and reporting astigmatism for individual and aggregate data. *J Cataract Refract Surg.* 1998;24:57–65.

85. Retzlaff J, Paden PY, Ferrell L. Vector analysis of astigmatism: adding and subtracting spherocylinders. *J Cataract Refract Surg.* 1993;19:393–399.

86. Holladay JT, Cravy TV, Koch DD. Calculating the surgically induced refractive change following ocular surgery. *J Cataract Refract Surg.* 1992;18:429–443.

87. Alpins NA. New method of targeting vectors to treat astigmatism. *J Cataract Refract Surg.* 1997;23:65–75.

88. Naeser K, Behrens JK. Correlation between polar values and vector analysis. *J Cataract Refract Surg.* 1997;23:76–81.

89. Gelender H. Management of corneal astigmatism after cataract surgery. *Refract Corneal Surg.* 1991;7:99–102.

90. Cravy TV. Modification of postcataract astigmatism by wound revision. *Int Ophthalmol Clin.* 1983;23(4):111–126.

91. Troutman RC. Microsurgical control of corneal astigmatism in cataract and keratoplasty. *Trans Am Acad Ophthalmol Otolaryngol.* 1973;77:563–572.

92. Koch DD, Del Pero RA, Wong TC, et al. Scleral flap surgery for modification of corneal astigmatism. *Am J Ophthalmol.* 1987;104:259–264.

93. Hettinger ME. Astigmatism and cataract surgery. In: Krachmer JH, Mannis MJ, Holland EJ, eds. *Cornea:*

Surgery of the Cornea and Conjunctiva. Vol 3. St. Louis, MO: Mosby–Year Book; 1997:2155–2164.

94. Thornton SP. Astigmatic keratotomy: a review of basic concepts with case reports. *J Cataract Refract Surg.* 1990;16:430–435.

95. Poon A, Taylor HR. Astigmatic photorefractive keratectomy. In: Wu HK, Thompson VM, Steinert RF, et al, eds. *Refractive Surgery.* New York: Thieme; 1999:307–318.

96. Khoury JM, Stark WJ, Azar DT. Photoastigmatic refractive keratectomy—PARK. In: Azar DT, ed. *Refractive Surgery.* Stamford, CT: Appleton & Lange; 1997:433–440.

97. Gayton JL, Sanders VN. Implanting two posterior chamber intraocular lenses in a case of microphthalmos. *J Cataract Refract Surg.* 1993;19:776–777.

98. Holladay JT, Gills JP, Leidlein J, et al. Achieving emmetropia in extremely short eyes with two piggyback posterior chamber intraocular lenses. *Ophthalmology.* 1996;103:1118–1123.

99. Masket S. Piggyback intraocular lens implantation. *J Cataract Refract Surg.* 1998;24:569–570.

100. Hayashi K, Hayashi H, Nakao F, et al. Reduction in the area of the anterior capsule opening after polymethylmethacrylate, silicon, and soft acrylic intraocular lens implantation. *Am J Ophthalmol.* 1997;123:441–447.

101. Shugar JK, Lewis C, Lee A. Implantation of multiple foldable acrylic posterior chamber lenses in the capsular bag for high hyperopia. *J Cataract Refract Surg.* 1996; 22(suppl 2):1386–1372.

102. Shugar JK, Schwarz T. Interpseudophakos Elschnig pearls associated with late hyperopic shift: a complication of piggyback posterior chamber intraocular lens implantation. *J Cataract Refract Surg.* 1999;25:863–867.

103. Mittelviefhaus H. Piggyback intraocular lens with exchangeable optic. *J Cataract Refract Surg.* 1996;22: 676–681.

Chapter 25

Astigmatic Intraocular Lenses, Multifocal Intraocular Lenses, and Other Specialized Intraocular Lenses

Rasik B. Vajpayee, Sandeep Jain, and Dimitri T. Azar

Since intraocular lenses (IOLs) were first implanted, the objective of ophthalmic researchers has generally been to develop an ideal prosthetic lens that would match the optical functions of a normal human crystalline lens. Every now and then new devices are developed including technologies that allow an IOL to vary its focus (like a normal lens), to eliminate the need for spectacle correction, or to provide best possible resolution (supervision). This chapter describes various types of newer IOLs that signify the beginning of the invention process in this field.

Toric IOLs

A number of devices and surgical therapies have been developed to pursue the objective of achieving emmetropia for ametropic cataractous eyes. Although various types of refractive surgeries are successful in correcting ametropia, the preexisting astigmatism in a patient with cataract remains problematic. Spectacle correction remains the most common method of astigmatic treatment in a pseudophakic patient, primarily because astigmatic keratotomy performed at the time of cataract removal results in relatively unpredictable outcomes. To overcome these problems, attempts have been to develop optimal toric IOLs that could simultaneously correct preexisting astigmatism and aphakia in a patient undergoing cataract surgery.[1,2]

Description of the Devices

Staar Surgical Toric IOL

The toric IOL developed by Staar Surgical is a single-piece silicone IOL. The haptics are plate haptics and the lens measures 10.8 mm in size. The plate haptic has large holes that allow the locking and stabilization of the IOL in the capsular bag by migrating epithelial cells. The IOL has been designed for placement in the capsular bag after phacoemulsification surgery. The lens has a 6-mm biconvex toric optic. Although the spherical power is incorporated in both anterior and the posterior surface of the lens, the toric component of the refractive power of the lens is incorporated only in the front surface of the lens. Thus, the anterior surface of the IOL carries a combination of spherical and cylindrical refracting powers. For correct and accurate alignment with the steep axis of the preexisting astigmatism of a patient, the IOL has linear marks on the peripheral part of the anterior surface of the optic (Fig. 25.1). These hash marks denote the axis of the cylindrical component of the refractive power of a toric IOL. The lens is available in a range of spherical powers, with cylindrical adds of 2 diopters and 3.5 diopters. The IOL offers protection against damage by ultraviolet (UV) light and can be injected through a 3-mm or smaller incision using an injector.

Nidek Toric IOL

The Nidek toric IOL is a three-piece posterior chamber lens of polymethyl methacrylate (PMMA) with Prolene haptics. The optic is oval and measures 6.5 × 5.5 mm in size. The overall length of the toric IOL is 13.5 mm. The cylindrical refractive power of the lens is incorporated on the concave back surface of the lens. The axis of the cylindrical power lies on the minor axis of the IOL. The line linking the two positioning holes present on the peripheral part of the optic denotes the axis of the toric power. The front curve has a convex surface, and for implantation in eyes with against-the-rule

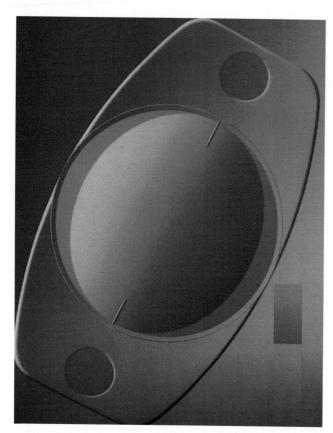

FIGURE 25.1. Staar Surgical toric IOL. The linear marks on the optic denote the axis of the cylindrical component of the refractive power of the toric IOL.

astigmatism, the lens must be positioned so that the line linking the positioning hole of the toric IOL lies horizontally. The IOL is available in two toric powers, 2.00 diopters and 3.00 diopters. When the lens is implanted, this is equivalent to a spectacle cylinder of 1.33 diopters and 1.98 diopters, respectively. The lens cannot be folded and requires a 5.6-mm corneal or corneoscleral incision.

Patient Selection for Toric IOL Implantation

Toric IOLs are valuable for the treatment of regular pre-existing astigmatism measuring 1.5–2.5 diopters. Ideal candidates for toric IOL implantation have regular and smooth keratoscopic mires with orthogonal steep and flat meridians. The amplitude and axes of the refractive and keratometric cylinder should be accurate and concordant. If there is a difference between the estimated values of refractive and keratometric astigmatism in a patient selected for a toric IOL implantation, lenticular astigmatism should be suspected and the choice of the toric IOL power and axis should be based on keratometric astigmatism. The cataract surgery would take care of any coexisting lenticular astigmatism. Staar Surgical has developed software that can calculate the overall spherocylindrical power required in a particular patient using the SRK-T formula.

Contraindications to Toric IOL Implantation

Contraindications to toric IOL implantation include the following:

• Irregular astigmatism
• Distorted keratometry
• Irregular topography pattern and nonorthogonal principal corneal meridians of astigmatism
• A lifelong patient history of satisfaction with spectacle cylindrical corrections
• Large eyes (white-to-white distance > 12 mm)

Results of Toric IOL Implantation

Shimazu et al evaluated the efficacy of the Nidek toric IOL in 47 patients with against-the-rule astigmatism.[1] Only 77% of eyes achieved a best corrected visual acuity of 20/25 or better at 3 months postoperatively. The 3.0-diopter toric IOLs offered better correction than the 2.0-diopter IOLs when the axis shift of the IOL was less than 30 degrees. The major problems observed were negative effects and the rotation of the lens axis during the postoperative period (Fig. 25.2).

In a randomized, prospective, controlled clinical trial conducted by Fine and co-workers, the patients implanted with Staar toric lenses were three times as likely to have a postoperative refractive cylinder of

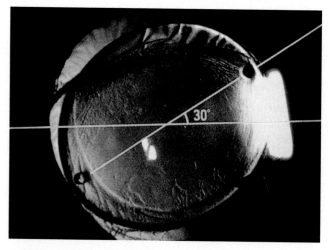

FIGURE 25.2. Toric intraocular lens. There is a postoperative axis shift of 30 degrees. *(From Shimuzu K, Misawa A, Suzuki Y. Toric intraocular lenses: correcting astigmatism while controlling axis shift. J Cataract Refract Surg. 1994;20:523–526, with permission.)*

0.50 or less as were control patients implanted with nontoric, plate-haptic IOLs.[2] The major problems observed were the presence of some postoperative residual cylinder, the difference between the axes of refractive and keratometric cylinders.

Complication and Problems with Toric IOLs

It is important to realize that none of the toric IOLs currently available can correct the full amplitude of the preexisting astigmatism in cataract patients. Also, it is important to correctly mark the steep meridian of the patient's cornea. Any inaccuracy of more than one-half clock hour will significantly reduce the impact of the IOL on the cylindrical component by at least 50%. If the error in marking or placement of IOL is greater than 1 clock hour, a new cylindrical error of greater magnitude would be created.

Postoperative rotation or decentration of a toric IOL can also lead to problems by altering its capability to correct the preexisting astigmatism. The impact would reduce the correction of astigmatism, and a negative effect can occur if the lens axis rotates by more than 30 degrees.

■ Multifocal IOLs

Although IOL implantation surgery has overcome the problem of visual rehabilitation of aphakia created after cataract surgery, the relative loss of accommodation remains a major concern, as most of the present generation IOLs are monofocal. The need to correct the resultant presbyopia has led to the introduction of several bifocal and multifocal IOLs that attempt to provide good vision at all distances. A multifocal IOL is a device that can provide good vision for both distance and near when implanted after the cataract surgery.[3] It eliminates the need for spectacle correction as routinely practiced after the implantation of commonly used monofocal IOLs.[4-7]

Types of Multifocal IOLs

Current multifocal IOLs incorporate either a refractive (Fig. 25.3A) or a diffractive (Fig. 25.3B) optical principle to achieve simultaneous optimal distance and near visual acuity.[3] The refractive multifocal IOLs can be further classified as spheric and aspheric designs, and the anterior and/or the posterior surface have been used for singular and combination designs.

Refractive Multifocal IOLs

Array Design Multifocal IOL

This device is the first multifocal lens to be approved by the Food and Drug Administration (FDA). It has an anterior spheric refractive surface and multiple posterior refractive surfaces. The front surface has a single zone and provides distance vision. The back surface of the array design has five zones (Fig. 25.4) with progressive addition from 0 to 5.0 diopters to the overall lens power. The device seems to focus several distances from infinity through the near point. Several studies have established the benefit of this lens after cataract surgery with regard to functional near and distance vision at the expense of contrast sensitivity.[7,8]

IOLAB Multifocal IOL

The device has two different spheric refractive surfaces on its anterior surface. There is a central 2-mm-diameter central optic for near vision. The central zone is surrounded by a lower-power ring-shaped zone for distance correction.

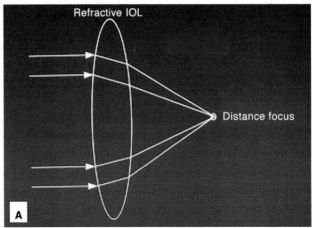

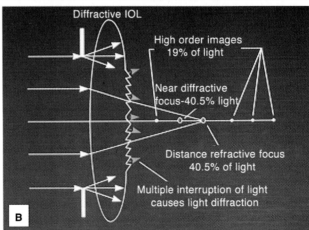

FIGURE 25.3. Types of multifocal IOLs. *A,* Refractive IOL. The back surface has multiple refractive zones. *B,* Diffractive IOL. The back surface has multiple diffractive zones.

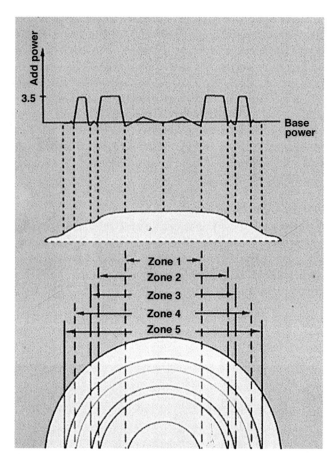

FIGURE 25.4. The AMO Array multifocal IOL. The anterior surface is spherical. The posterior surface has five zones with progressive addition from 0 to 5.0 diopters to the overall lens power.

Wright Medical Multifocal IOL

This lens has a combination of spheric and aspheric refractive designs on its anterior surface for distance and near vision. The spheric portion is meant for distance and the aspheric portion for near. The dioptric power of the aspheric portion is 3.0 diopters more than the power of the spheric distance vision surface.

Ioptex Multifocal IOL

A combination of spheric distance vision zones and aspheric near vision zones is used to provide simultaneous distance and near vision in this IOL. The aspheric zones meant for providing near vision are present in the midperiphery.

Pharmacia Ophthalmic Multifocal IOL

This multifocal IOL uses a combination of two or more different anterior spheric refractive surfaces for distance and near correction. The device has a central circular distance zone surrounded by a ring-shaped near zone that is further surrounded by another peripheral ring-shaped zone for distance correction.

Domilens Progress 3 Multifocal Lens

This device is a one-piece PMMA IOL with a biconvex 6.5-mm-diameter optic and an overall diameter of 12.5 mm. The anterior surface has aspheric longitudinal aberrations, providing near vision through the central portions of the lens, distance vision through the periphery of the aspheric portion, and intermediate vision in between. The diameter of the aspheric part is 4.7 mm, and all vision is obtained through this portion. The peripheral portion beyond the 4.7 mm and the posterior surface are spheric. The aspheric portion of the lens has no geometric interruption and yields a power of +4.75 diopters, which is equal to +3.0 diopters.

Diffractive Multifocal IOL

3M Multifocal IOL

The 3M multifocal IOL combines both refractive and diffractive optical principles to achieve simultaneous distance and near vision. Its anterior surface has a spheric refractive design and the posterior surface has multiple diffractive zones (Fig. 25.3B). With appropriate dimensions assigned for the 20–30 concentric zones on the posterior lens surface, the wave component of the incident light is controlled to form the required focal points for proper convergence of light from near and distant objects. Such diffractive construction of the lens allows balanced convergence of light at the focal points without dependency on optical apertures.

Chiron-Adatomed Multifocal IOL

This device is a one-piece bifocal diffractive silicone IOL. The near addition is 4.0 diopters, which corresponds to approximately 3.2 diopters in the spectacle plane. The lens is of a disc haptic design. The diffractive zone, consisting of 16 concentric rings, is situated on the posterior surface of the lens with an asymmetric light distribution for the far and near focus. There are two versions of this lens, distant-dominant and near-dominant. They employ the same optical principle of diffraction but differ in light distribution for the far and near focus. In the distant-dominant lens, 70% of the incident light is focused for distance vision and 30% for near vision. In the near-dominant lens the ratio is reversed.

Results of Multifocal IOL Implantation

Several investigators have evaluated the success of multifocal IOLs in clinical studies. The issues that have been examined include the frequency of spectacle use for distance and near vision, quality of the retinal image, extent of psychophysical performance, and acceptability of the multifocal lens by the patient. Although almost all of the studies report a significant near vision gain without spectacle correction, in a number of patients the multifocal IOLs result in poor retinal image quality as compared to monofocal lenses.

Vaquero et al compared the results of implanting the AMO Array multifocal lens with implanting a monofocal lens in a prospective study.[4] Although distance acuity and contrast sensitivity were similar in both groups, patients with the multifocal lens had significantly better near acuity. In a prospective, double-masked, comparative clinical trial, Steinert et al reported that significantly less correction was required in the multifocal group than in the monofocal group.[5] However, patients in the multifocal group sustained a small loss of contrast sensitivity.

Holliday et al evaluated the optical performances of several multifocal lenses, using laboratory and photographic studies.[6] They found a two- to threefold increase in depth of field for all multifocals, but they also found a 50% reduction in contrast in the retinal image and a one-line drop in best corrected acuity. Percival and Setty conducted several clinical trials of multifocal lenses and found multifocal lenses to provide better simultaneous distance and near acuities in a significantly higher number of patients.[7] Bleckman and co-authors found multifocal progressive IOLs to provide adequate visual performance at various distances only in optimal light conditions.[8]

In a small-sample retrospective study, Negishi et al demonstrated that eyes implanted with the five-zone refractive multifocal lenses had better near visual acuity than control eyes and compared favorably in other aspects of visual functions.[9] In a clinical trial, Wille reported better performance of monofocal lenses for distance vision when compared to multifocal lenses.[10] The mean postoperative acuity was 0.5 line higher in the monofocal group than in the multifocal group.

After testing contrast sensitivity and glare in patients implanted with diffractive multifocal IOLs, Winther-Nielsen and co-workers concluded that the most significant loss of contrast sensitivity is found with central glare under twilight conditions.[11]

In an FDA study update of multifocal lenses reported by Lindstrom, there was an uncorrected visual acuity of 20/40 or better and J3 or better in 50% of best case multifocal IOL patients, compared with 26% of the monofocal best case comparison group.[12] Although more patients in the monofocal group achieved a distance visual acuity of 20/20 or better, 92% of best case multifocal patients achieved functional near vision, compared with 37% of best case monofocal patients.

There was a small loss of contrast sensitivity that would be considered clinically insignificant under most conditions.

Goes compared the results with diffractive multifocal lenses versus monofocal lenses and reported 20/40 or better distance visual acuity in 98% of eyes in the best case group and functional reading capacity in 96% of best cases.[3] However, the contrast sensitivity was lower in eyes with multifocal lenses.

Gimbel et al evaluated and compared patients with bilateral multifocal IOLs with patients with bilateral monofocal IOLs in a retrospective analysis.[14] Although both the groups had a comparable uncorrected visual acuity of 20/40 or better, 63% of multifocal lens users needed no spectacle correction, compared to 4% of monofocal lens users. Fifty-four percent of multifocal lens users had near uncorrected vision of J1 to J3. However, multifocal lens users reported significantly more visual side effects of flare, glare, and halos. Also, a greater decrease in contrast sensitivity at low contrast levels was detected among multifocal lens users.

Vanderschueren and co-workers demonstrated that except for good uncorrected near visual acuity, multifocal IOLs can have several disadvantages, among them a lower initial acuity, a higher frequency of posterior synechiae, and slightly more difficult ophthalmoscopy than with conventional lenses.[15]

Akutsu et al evaluated visual performance through multifocal IOLs by measuring contrast sensitivity functions and reading speed for age-matched groups with multifocal and monofocal IOL and control groups.[16] Patients with multifocal lenses showed deficits in reading speed only for low-contrast text ($<30\%$) and small letters.

In a comparative study of monofocal versus multifocal lenses, Vaquero-Ruano et al reported a wider depth of focus and significantly better near vision without addition in patients with multifocal lenses.[17] The contrast sensitivity results at 96% and 50% were similar. Walkow et al prospectively evaluated a diffractive versus a refractive multifocal IOL and found similar and satisfactory functional results with both, except that near uncorrected vision was significantly better with the diffractive lens.[18]

In a case-control study, Javitt et al measured the functional status and quality of life after bilateral implantation of multifocal versus a monofocal IOLs.[19] The subjects with bilateral multifocal IOLs reported better overall vision, less limitation in visual function, and less spectacle usage than the control subjects with monofocal lenses. The difference was most significant in the rating of near vision without spectacles.

Steinert et al performed a prospective, double-masked, multicenter evaluation of zonal-progressive optic multifocal IOLs and a monofocal IOL.[5] Mean postoperative spherical equivalent (SE), astigmatism, and uncorrected and best corrected distance visual acuity were similar between the two groups. However, patients with multifocal IOLs achieved a significantly better uncorrected near visual acuity than patients with monofocal IOLs (J3+ versus J7). Regan contrast sensitivity was lower for the multifocal lenses at all contrast levels, and the difference achieved statistical significance at a very low (11%) contrast.

Jacobi et al developed a new concept of asymmetric bilateral multifocal IOL implantation.[20] This method uses two types of multifocal IOLs that differ from each other in the light distribution for the far and near focus.[20] A distant-dominant multifocal IOL with a light distribution of 70% for the far focus and 30% for the near focus is implanted in one eye, thus rendering this eye dominant for distance vision, enabling it to see a sharp and high-contrast image for far and a low-contrast image for near. The fellow eye receives a near-dominant multifocal IOL with a light distribution of 30% for the distance focus and 70% for the near focus. This eye sees a sharp and high-contrast image for near. In binocular viewing, both eyes receive a distinct image of objects at near and far, but image contrast differs between the eyes at respective distances. Jacobi et al found that the effect is additive and that the asymmetric model may be associated with improved contrast sensitivity compared with conventional multifocal IOLs.[20]

Problems and Complications of Multifocal IOLs

Compared to monofocal IOLs, multifocal lenses trade a certain amount of image clarity for an increased depth of focus. There is a quantifiable loss of contrast sensitivity with multifocal lenses. Also, pupillary apertures less than 2 mm could result in loss of distance visual acuity. Similarly, if the multifocal lens is decentered by more than 2 mm, a loss of near visual acuity can occur. The visual performance of diffractive multifocal IOLs is very minimally affected by decentration and changing pupillary size. Ghosting of images and glare from oncoming lights are some of the other complications reported after implantation of multifocal IOLs.

■ Accommodating IOLs

It is believed that some of the functions of the ciliary muscle, a key player in accommodation, are retained even after cataract surgery. Basing designs on this theory, ophthalmic researchers have developed an aphakic IOL that has been able to provide some accommodation in a clinical trial. The lens, known as

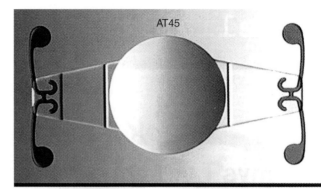

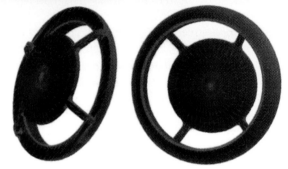

FIGURE 25.5. New intraocular lenses from C&C (*top*) and HumanOptics (*bottom*) are designed to move forward into the anterior chamber to accommodate, much like the natural lens. (*Courtesy of C&C Vision and HumanOptics.*)

the AT45 (C&C Vision, Aliso Viejo, CA), has been designed by Stuart Cumming of Aliso Viejo (Fig. 25.5, top).[21] Khalil Hanna has also designed an accommodating IOL (HumanOptics); it is three-dimensional and fills the capsular bag (Fig. 25.5, bottom).

Description

The accommodating AT45 lens is a conventional posterior chamber silicone lens. Its optic measures 4.5 mm in diameter. It does not have conventional plate or loop haptics but has two flexible arms located 180 degrees apart. These flexible arms allow the lens to move forward and backward in the posterior chamber on constriction and relaxation of the ciliary muscle. At the end of each arm is a T-shaped polyimide haptic that follows the curve of the capsular bag after implantation and maintains centration and stability by resting in the capsular bag.

Results of Implantation

The accommodating IOL is implanted after conventional phacoemulsification surgery through a 3-mm or 5-mm incision. The lens is maximally positioned against the vitreous face and is sealed in place, with 3 weeks of atropine treatment postoperatively. At the base of the arms of the lens are hinges that allow the lens to move forward, based on ciliary contraction and pressure from vitreous. Any forward movement of the lens allows for near vision, simulating natural accommodation.

The early results of Phase I clinical trial showed the lens to be safe, complication free, and well tolerated. The lens appeared to provide some accommodation. The lens is still in the evaluation stage, and further clinical trials are in progress.

■ Multicomponent IOL

Since their advent, refractive surgeries have attempted to produce ametropia that is comparable to what is achievable by spectacle and contact lens corrections. Although some of them are successful in certain ranges of refractive error, a multicomponent IOL is a new concept that allows fine tuning of an already fairly accurate refractive procedure.

Description of the Device

The multicomponent IOL is a three-component lens consisting of a base lens and two additional refractive attachments. The base lens has a planoconvex optical, and the overall mechanical design of the lens is similar to that of currently used posterior chamber lenses. The lens is made of PMMA and is one piece, with a diameter of 6.0 mm and an optical aperture of 5.5 mm. The basic lens looks much like a conventional PCIOL. The base lens has two machined slots whose thickness is approximately 1.2 mm. These slots accept the cap lens and hold the assembly together. The base lens is placed in and permanently heals into the posterior capsular bag. After implantation, it acts as a platform for the other two detachable refractive elements.

Attached to the base lens are two additional refractive elements. The middle lens, or sandwich lens, carries the astigmatic (4.00 diopter sphere and 0.00–4.00 diopter cylinder in 0.25-diopter increments) correction. This PMMA or silicone lens has an optical aperture of 5.5 mm. The other refractive attachment is a cap lens that has additional refractive power. This lens may be either monofocal or multifocal. This PMMA planoconvex lens has an optical clear aperture of 5.5 mm. It has a tab and two small haptics that, during the assembly, are set into slots in the base lens using a specially modified forceps.

The total central thickness of a multicomponent IOL is 1.88 mm for a 28.00-diopter lens. This is only slightly thicker than a standard silicone IOL of 20.00 diopters.

Results of Multicomponent IOL Implantation

The lens is still in the process of development, and results of clinical trials are awaited. Werblin has developed a hypothetical human surgical procedure that is analogous to routine phacoemulsification surgery with implantation of a PCIOL through a 7.00-mm incision (Fig. 25.6).[22] Once the base lens is implanted, the cap-and-lens assembly is intraoperatively affixed by the surgeon to the base lens. The sandwich lens is oriented at the appropriate astigmatic axis, based on the preoperative assessment of anticipated postoperative astigmatism.

Once refractive stability is achieved, the patient's refractive status is evaluated and the refractive attachments can be removed or changed, depending on the amplitude and type of residual refractive error or, in case of a multifocal attachment, if the patient is not satisfied with the quality of vision. Such change or removal involves a second operative procedure consisting of opening the original wound, detaching the cap and sandwich lens component, and replacing it with new attachments.

The lens has been used in a cat model, and at 6-month follow-up it was well tolerated. In two animals

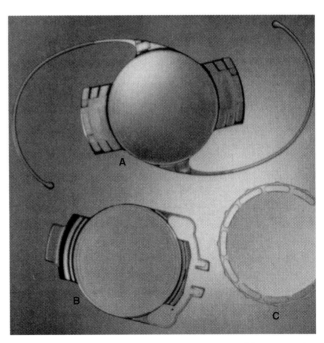

FIGURE 25.6. Multicomponent IOL. *(From Werblin TP. Multicomponent intraocular lens. J Refract Surg. 1996;12:187–189, with permission.)*

the cap-and-lens assembly was successfully exchanged 2 months after the original surgery.

■ Telescopic IOL

Patients with age-related macular degeneration (AMD) may suffer serious loss of vision in the advanced stages of the disease. The optical devices currently available, including various magnifiers, are of little use once vision is seriously compromised. Isaac Lipshitz has developed a new IOL for patients with AMD.[23] The lens combines a silicone lens with a Galilean telescope. This lens has been called the intraocular telescopic lens (IOTL). A fully implanted IOTL may be an effective optical solution for patients with AMD.

Description of the IOTL

Lipshitz's new IOTL is a regular silicone lens in which a Galilean telescope of 2 mm radius and 4.5 mm length has been blended. The implant is a single unit and goes in the posterior capsular bag after the cataract surgery. The IOTL can be upgraded externally by altering the patient's spectacle correction. The telescopic lens has a wider visual field than telescopic glasses or teledioptric lenses because the optical center of the lens is located near that of the eye. The Lipshitz telescopic lens has a focusing distance of 35 cm for the +2.5. At a magnification power of 6.0 mm, the focusing distance is between 17 cm and 18 cm.

Results of IOTL Implantation

The lens has been implanted in cadaver eyes, and clinical trials in humans are in progress. The implantation technique is simple. The test lenses were inserted in cadaver eyes through a 160-degree limbal incision in a procedure similar to the one used to perform routine extracapsular cataract extraction. Tests of the lens using a CCD camera and a US Air Force resolution chart revealed that the lens met the 50 line/mm requirement of the US Air Force when it conducts visual tests.

■ References

1. Shimizu K, Misawa A, Suzuki Y. Toric intraocular lenses: correcting astigmatism while controlling axis shift. *J Cataract Refract Surg.* 1994;20:523–526.
2. Staar Surgical. IOL update: turning on the cylinder. *Ophthalmology Management.* October 1999:3S–15S.
3. Duffey R, Zabel R, Lindstrom R. Multifocal intraocular lenses. *J Cataract Refract Surg.* 1990;16:123–129.
4. Vaquero M, Encinas JL, Jimenez F. Visual function with monofocal versus multifocal IOLs. *J Cataract Refract Surg.* 1996;22:1222–1225.
5. Steinert RF, Post CT, Brint SF, et al. A prospective, randomized, double-masked comparison of a zonal-progressive multifocal intraocular lens and a monofocal intraocular lens. *Ophthalmology.* 1992;99:853–861.
6. Holladay JT, van Dijk H, Lang A, et al. Optical performance of multifocal intraocular lenses. *J Cataract Refract Surg.* 1990;16:413–422.
7. Percival SPB, Setty SS. Prospectively randomized trial comparing the pseudoaccommodation of the AMO Array multifocal lens and a monofocal lens. *J Cataract Refract Surg.* 1993;19:26–31.
8. Bleckmann H, Schmidt O, Sunde T, Kaluzny J. Visual results of progressive multifocal posterior chamber intraocular lens implantation. *J Cataract Refract Surg.* 1996;22:1102–1107.
9. Negishi K, Nagamoto T, Hara E, et al. Clinical evaluation of a five-zone refractive multifocal intraocular lens. *J Cataract Refract Surg.* 1996;22:110–115.
10. Wille H. Distance visual acuity with diffractive multifocal and monofocal intraocular lenses. *J Cataract Refract Surg.* 1993;19:251–253.
11. Winther-Nielsen A, Corydon L, Olsen T. Contrast sensitivity and glare in patients with a diffractive multifocal intraocular lens. *J Cataract Refract Surg.* 1993;19:254–257.
12. Lindstrom R. Food and Drug Administration study update: one-year results from 671 patients with the 3M multifocal intraocular lens. *Ophthalmology.* 1993;100(1):91–97.
13. Goes F. Personal results with the 3M diffractive multifocal intraocular lens. *J Cataract Refract Surg.* 1991;17:577–582.
14. Gimbel HV, Snaders DR, Gold Raanan M. Visual and refractive results of multifocal intraocular lenses. *Ophthalmology.* 1991;98:881–888.
15. Vanderschueren I, Zeyen T, D'heer B. Multifocal IOL implantation: 16 cases. *Br J Ophthalmol.* 1991;75:88–91.
16. Akutsu H, Legge GE, Showalter M, et al. Contrast sensitivity and reading through multifocal intraocular lenses. *Arch Ophthalmol.* 1992;110:1076–1080.
17. Vaquero-Ruano M, Encinas JL, Millan I, et al. AMO Array multifocal versus monofocal intraocular lenses: long-term follow-up. *J Cataract Refract Surg.* 1998;24:118–123.
18. Walkow T, Liekfeld A, Anders N, et al. A prospective evaluation of a diffractive versus a refractive designed multifocal intraocular lens. *Ophthalmology.* 1997;104:1380–1386.
19. Javitt JC, Wang F, Trentacost DJ, et al. Outcomes of cataract extraction with multifocal intraocular lens implantation: functional status and quality of life. *Ophthalmology.* 1997;104:589–599.
20. Jacobi FK, Kammann J, Jacobi KW, et al. Bilateral implantation of asymmetrical diffractive multifocal intraocular lenses. *Arch Ophthalmol.* 1999;117:17–23.
21. New IOL restored some accommodation in trial. *Ocular Surgery News.* 1999.
22. Werblin TP. Multicomponent intraocular lens. *J Refract Surg.* 1996;12:187–189.
23. New IOL for AMD combines silicone lens with Galilean telescope. *Ocular Surgery News.* 1996.

Chapter 26

Clear Lens Extraction with Intraocular Lens Implantation

Nasrin A. Afshari and Dimitri T. Azar

Removal of the crystalline lens as a refractive measure to correct high myopia has been known conceptually as early as 1708, when Boerhaave of the Netherlands noted that high myopes can have good uncorrected vision after cataract extraction. After the introduction of sterilization techniques in 1889, Fukala in Austria and Vacher in France inaugurated a wave of interest in correcting myopia through clear lens extraction (CLE).[1] Another decade passed before the high complication rates after lens extraction surfaced, and then the procedure was abandoned for some time.

Since then, various surgical procedures have been developed to correct high myopia. Most of these procedures involve correction of myopia through modification of the corneal curvature. These procedures have included radial keratotomy (RK), epikeratoplasty, keratomileusis, and, more recently, photorefractive keratectomy, automated lamellar keratoplasty, and laser-assisted intrastromal keratomileusis.[2–8] Intraocular procedures such as intraocular lens (IOL) implantation in phakic eyes have also been employed to correct myopia. These IOLs may be placed in the anterior chamber as angle-supported (Baikoff) or iris-supported (Worst, Fechner) lenses, or in the posterior chamber.[8,9]

All of these procedures, however, have limitations related to the amount of the myopia. For example, RK would achieve the best result in eyes with myopia of less than 5.0 diopters, and the upper limit of correction is around 8.0 diopters.[10] Implantation of a minus power anterior chamber lens in a phakic eye has been associated with better accuracy and predictability than corneal refractive surgery in cases of high myopia.[5,8,9] However, this procedure may cause significant damage to the corneal endothelium.[11,12] Laser-assisted in situ keratomileusis (LASIK) is very promising in the treatment of both myopia and hyperopia, but pachymetry measures limit the correction of very high refractive errors.

Because of the limitations of other refractive surgical measures, CLE has been suggested to correct high refractive errors.[13] However, there is controversy concerning the risk-benefit ratio of this procedure because of the potential vitreoretinal complications. The new developments in cataract surgery—the use of small, self-sealing wounds, the advent of foldable IOLs, and the use of viscoelastic agents—have greatly reduced the risk and improved the outcome. The major risk in performing CLE in high myopes is the risk of retinal detachment (RD); however, advances in the preoperative retinal examination and treatment have improved the outcome in these patients.

■ Indications and Contraindications

Indications for CLE in high myopia or hyperopia are not well-defined. With the recent advances in LASIK technology, indications for CLE have become even more limited. LASIK not only preserves accommodation, it also nearly eliminates the risk of RD. Thus, one of the major considerations in performing CLE at this time includes inability to perform LASIK in a patient with a high refractive error who desires refractive surgery. These patients are typically selected on the basis of preoperative refractive error and intolerance of contact lenses, either because of inadequate functional wearing times or because contact lenses are inappropriate for their professional activities.

It is crucial to explain the risks and complications of the procedure at length to these patients, as the complications could occur a long time after the surgery. The importance of follow-up should also be emphasized, as funduscopic examinations at regular intervals are part of the routine postoperative care of these patients.

Many studies exclude patients with a prior history of RD, glaucoma, or previous anterior segment surgery. These conditions are commonly considered contraindications to CLE.

■ Surgical Techniques

The surgical techniques for CLE have followed the trend of the cataract extraction methods at the time. The best outcomes have been achieved with advances in phacoemulsification and foldable IOLs. Because a rapid recovery is of particular importance to refractive surgery patients, small-incision, self-sealing clear corneal wounds are desired. Astigmatism may be induced after clear corneal phacoemulsification. The location of the surgical incision should be carefully considered to decrease preexisting astigmatism and prevent the induction of astigmatism. By placing the clear corneal lens extraction incision on the steep axis, the surgeon can simultaneously correct preexisting astigmatism.

Because patients who undergo CLE are considerably younger than the usual cataract patients, the long-term complications should be of great concern. Minimal ultrasound energy should be used, as minimization of insult to the endothelial cells is essential for the long-term success of this procedure. The retina is diligently examined preoperatively and at regular intervals postoperatively. Intraoperatively, special attention is given to preserve the posterior capsule. Capsulotomy with the neodymium:yttrium-aluminum-garnet (Nd:YAG) laser is postponed until absolutely necessary. It is important to carefully measure the lens dioptric power in patients with high refractive errors. Measuring the axial length in these patients is difficult, and the resolution of ultrasound machine tends to decrease at extreme ends. Attention should also be given to the formula that is used to calculate the IOL dioptric power: the SRK-T formula, rather than the more frequently used SRK II formula, is more accurate in eyes with axial lengths of more than 28.4 mm.

■ Complications

Patients who undergo CLE for high refractive errors are subject to complications similar to those associated with cataract extraction. A tear in the posterior capsule, loss of vitreous, RD, cystoid macular edema (CME), and endophthalmitis are the most dreaded complications. A major concern in high myopes is RD. Baraquer and colleagues reported an RD rate of 7.3% among 165 eyes with pathologic myopia that were treated by CLE after an average follow-up of 31 months.[14] The technique involved intracapsular, aspiration, and extracapsular lens extraction. They reported a twofold increase in the rate of RD in patients who underwent capsulotomy. Also, in patients younger than 30 years, the risk of RD was 2.5 times greater than in patients older than 30 years. Seventy-five percent of RDs occurred at or after 18 months postoperatively, and the retina was reattached in 75% of all cases.

Extraction of the crystalline lens leads to mechanical and biochemical changes of the vitreous and can result in the development of posterior vitreous detachment. The ensuing traction on the retina may lead to RD at a higher rate in highly myopic patients, because they have some of the other predisposing factors such as lattice degeneration. Postoperative RD is not always a direct result of intraoperative surgical complications but can result from changes in ocular physiology. Ripandelli and co-authors, in a study of 41 eyes in 39 patients with high axial myopia and RD following CLE, reported that RD developed in 26 of these eyes despite a 360-degree prophylactic retinopexy on the pre-equatorial area.[15] Of the 26 eyes, 17 developed proliferative vitreoretinopathy. In this series RD occurred 1 month to 4 years postoperatively, except in two eyes with intraoperative choroidal hemorrhage. Although the retina was reattached in 36 eyes, only 9 eyes achieved a visual acuity of 20/60 or better. The authors concluded that blinding complications may occur following CLE despite prophylactic treatments.

Colin and colleagues, in a long-term follow-up of 52 myopic eyes in 32 patients with myopia greater than −12.00 diopters who had undergone phacoemulsification, reported the rate of RD to be 1.9% after 4 years and 8.1% after 7 years.[16,17] By comparison, the incidence of RD in individuals with a refractive error greater than −10.00 diopters who have not undergone ocular surgery is estimated to be 0.68% annually.[18] Thus, the incidence of RD in this long-term study was double the incidence of RD in individuals who have not undergone CLE.

The incidence of posterior capsular opacification (PCO) following phacoemulsification has been reported as 40%–60%.[13,19] The interval between surgery and opacification varies. Verzella reported PCO in 40%–60% of cases 5 years after CLE with phacoemulsification.[13] Lyle and Jin reported a similar incidence of 58% in myopic eyes, but the opacification occurred earlier, at an average of 10 months after operation.[20]

Patient age and the level of myopia were not predictors of PCO. The Nd:YAG laser has been commonly used for the treatment of PCO. Complications after Nd:YAG laser capsulotomy include CME and RD.[21] Axial myopia increases the incidence of RD following Nd:YAG capsulotomy. Koch et al reported the incidence of RD following Nd:YAG capsulotomy in eyes with an axial length of 25 mm or more to be 10%.[22] Lyle and Jin, however, reported no RD on mean follow-up of 15.6 months after Nd:YAG capsulotomy in 31 eyes with axial lengths greater than 25 mm.[20]

■ Clinical Outcomes After CLE for High Myopia

As the techniques of cataract extraction have evolved, the outcome of CLE has improved. Many studies report performing CLE with extracapsular techniques, but advances in phacoemulsification, foldable lenses, and clear corneal surgeries have helped to improve the results in more recent studies. In 1987 Goldberg reviewed the results of CLE in patients with axial myopia and reported significant complication rates following surgery in these patients.[23] Most of the patients had undergone intracapsular or extracapsular cataract surgery. Colin and Robinet reported on 52 eyes in which prophylactic retinal treatment, clear lensectomy, and PCIOL implantation had been done by phacoemulsification to treat high myopia (> 12 diopters).[24] They reported a mean postoperative spherical equivalent (SE) of − 0.86 diopters, with a corrected visual acuity of 20/40 or better in 88.5% of patients compared with 75% preoperatively. No CME, RD, or persistent corneal edema was observed after 1 year. A 4-year follow-up revealed a mean postoperative SE of − 0.92 diopter, with a corrected visual acuity of 20/40 or better in 82% of the eyes that had been treated by Nd:YAG capsulotomy.[16] (Nd:YAG capsulotomy had been performed in 36.7% of patients.) The incidence of RD during the 4-year follow-up period was 1.9%. A 7-year follow-up revealed stability in the SE, the Nd:YAG capsulotomy rate, and the rate of complications, including RD.[17]

Gris and colleagues retrospectively analyzed 46 CLE phacoemulsification procedures performed through large wounds.[25] Mean preoperative cycloplegic refraction was − 16.05 diopters and mean postoperative cycloplegic refraction was within 1.00 diopter in 48.4% of eyes and within 2.00 diopters in 92.5% of eyes. Capsular tear with vitreous loss occurred in one eye, and the mean endothelial cell loss was 2.6% during the first postoperative year.

Lee and Lee retrospectively studied 24 eyes in 16 patients who underwent CLE to treat myopia of greater than − 12.00 diopters.[26] The surgical technique was a scleral tunnel followed by phacoemulsification. The mean follow-up was 15 months. The mean preoperative SE was − 16.60 ± 3.75 diopters and the mean postoperative SE was − 1.53 ± 1.30 diopters. Best corrected visual acuity improved in 20 eyes (83.3%). Fifteen eyes (62%) were within 1.00 diopter of targeted refractive error postoperatively. PCO developed in one eye. Retinal breaks, RD, and CME were not observed in these patients during the follow-up period.

CLE in extreme myopia with negative power IOL implantation has also been found to be effective. Jiménez-Alfaro and colleagues studied 26 eyes in 17 highly myopic patients with a mean preoperative SE of − 20.85 ± 5.48 diopters.[27] The patients underwent clear lens phacoemulsification through a large scleral tunnel followed by implantation of a negative power PCIOL. The follow-up was at least 12 months, and the mean postoperative SE was − 0.50 diopter ± 0.67. In 88.4% of eyes there was an improvement in the best spectacle-corrected visual acuity. Intraoperatively, no complication occurred. Postoperatively, 11.5 % of eyes developed choroidal detachment, 19.2% of eyes had an intraocular pressure greater than 25 mm, and 15.3 % of eyes developed PCO, which was treated by Nd:YAG capsulotomy 6 months postoperatively. RD was not observed in any patient in this study.

The refractive outcome of simultaneously correcting myopia, hyperopia, and astigmatism in older patients undergoing cataract surgery has also been promising. Kershner reported results in 690 eyes in 538 patients who underwent clear corneal cataract surgery with the correction of myopia, hyperopia, and astigmatism.[28] The average age of the patients in this study was 72.6 years. Preoperatively, 58% of patients were myopic and 32% were hyperopic. SE was reduced to plano in 78% of patients postoperatively and to within 1 diopter in 17% of patients.

■ Clinical Outcomes After CLE for High Hyperopia

Lyle and Jin reported findings in six hyperopic eyes with a preoperative refraction of + 6.52 ± 1.44 (range, + 4.25 to + 7.87) that were treated by phacoemulsification and implantation of IOL in the capsular bag using the SRK-II formula.[29] The mean postoperative follow-up was 19.0 months and the mean postoperative SE was − 0.42 diopter. All six hyperopic eyes achieved a visual acuity of 20/40 or better. No complications occurred in this study. PCO developed in 33% of the hyperopic eyes.

Siganos and colleagues reported results in 35 hyperopic eyes in 21 patients treated by extracapsular CLE and PCIOL implantation.[30] The mean preoperative SE refraction was +9.19 diopters ± 0.34 (range, +6.75 to +13.75 diopters) and the mean follow-up was 5 years. The SRK II formula was used in 17 eyes and the SRK-T formula in 18 eyes. Mean postoperative correction was 0.8 diopter. Using the SRK II formula, 100% of eyes were within 1.00 diopter of emmetropia, and with the SRK-T formula, 83.3% were within 1.00 diopter of emmetropia. One eye required IOL exchange and another eye required photorefractive keratectomy for myopia secondary to IOL miscalculation. PCO developed in 54.2% of eyes and was treated by Nd:YAG capsulotomy.

More recently, Kolahdouz and colleagues reported results of phacoemulsification and IOL implantation in 18 eyes in 10 hyperopic patients.[31] The Hoffer-Q formula was used for IOL power calculation in 16 eyes and the Holladay-II formula was used for 2 nanophthalmic eyes. The mean preoperative SE in this series was +6.17 diopters and the mean postoperative SE was −0.21 diopter. All eyes achieved a visual acuity of 20/50 or better. Two patients lost two lines of spectacle-corrected visual acuity. In one patient PCO developed and was treated by Nd-YAG capsulotomy. Another patient developed malignant glaucoma. One IOL had to be exchanged in a nanophthalmic eye.

■ Conclusion

Despite its limitations, CLE to correct high refractive errors is an effective and relatively safe procedure in many patients. Advances in phacoemulsification have lowered the risks and improved the outcome of this procedure. The use of multifocal IOLs, toric IOLs, and accomodating IOLs makes CLE a viable alternative for a select group of patients with high myopic and hyperopic refractive errors. However, loss of accommodation and the risks of an intraocular procedure limit the indications for this procedure.

■ References

1. Seiler T. Clear lens extraction in the 19th century: an early demonstration of premature dissemination. *J Refract Surg*. 1999;15:70–73.
2. Waring GO III, Lynn MJ, Gelender H, et al. Results of the Prospective Evaluation of Radial Keratotomy (PERK) study one year after surgery. *Ophthalmology*. 1985;92:177–196.
3. McDonald MB, Kaufman HE, Aquavella JV, et al. The nationwide study of epikeratophakia for myopia. *Am J Ophthalmol*. 1987;103:375–383.
4. Nordon LT, Fallor MK. Myopic keratomileusis: 74 consecutive non-amblyopic cases with one year of follow-up. *J Refract Surg*. 1986;2:124–128.
5. Colin J, Mimouni F, Robinet A, et al. The surgical treatment of high myopia: comparison of epikeratoplasty, keratomileusis and minus power anterior chamber lenses. *Refract Corneal Surg*. 1990;6:245–251.
6. Shimizu K, Amano S, Tanaka S. Photorefractive keratotomy for myopia: one year follow-up in 97 eyes. *J Refract Corneal Surg*. 1994;10:S178–S187.
7. Rogers CM, Lawless MA, Cohen PR. Photorefractive keratectomy for myopia of more than −10 diopters. *J Refract Corneal Surg*. 1994;10:S171–S173.
8. Baikoff G, Joly P. Comparison of minus power anterior chamber intraocular lenses and myopic epikeratoplasty in phakic eyes. *Refract Corneal Surg*. 1990;6:252–260.
9. Fechner PU, Heijde GL, Worst JGF. The correction of myopia by lens implantation into phakic eyes. *Am J Ophthalmol*. 1989;107:659–663.
10. Waring GO III, Lynn MJ, Nizam A, et al. Results of the Prospective Evaluation of Radial Keratotomy (PERK) study five years after surgery. *Ophthalmology*. 1991;98:1164–1176.
11. Mimouni F, Colin J, Koffi V, Bonnet P. Damage to the corneal endothelium from anterior chamber intraocular lenses in phakic myopic eyes. *Refract Corneal Surg*. 1991;7:277–281.
12. Saragoussi J-J, Cotinat J, Renard G, et al. Damage to the corneal endothelium by minus power anterior chamber intraocular lenses. *Refract Corneal Surg*. 1991;7:282–285.
13. Verzella F. Refractive microsurgery of the lens in high myopia. *Refract Corneal Surg*. 1990;6:273–275.
14. Barraquer C, Cavelier C, Mejia LF. Incidence of retinal detachment following clear-lens extraction in myopic patients. *Arch Ophthalmol*. 1994;112:336–339.
15. Ripandelli G, Billi B, Fedeli R, et al. Retinal detachment after clear lens extraction in 41 eyes with high axial myopia. *Retina*. 1996;16:3–6.
16. Colin J, Robinet A. Clear lensectomy and implantation of a low-power posterior chamber intraocular lens for correction of high myopia: four-year follow-up. *Ophthalmology*. 1997;104:73–78.
17. Colin J, Robinet A, Cochener B. Retinal detachment after clear lens extraction for high myopia. *Ophthalmology*. 1999;106:2281–2285.
18. Perkins ES. Morbidity from myopia. *Sight Saving Rev*. 1979;49:11–19.
19. Wilhelmus KR, Emery JM. Posterior capsule opacification following phacoemulsification. *Ophthalmic Surg*. 1980;11:264–267.
20. Lyle WA, Jin GJC. Clear lens extraction for the correction of high refractive error. *J Cataract Refract Surg*. 1994;20:273–276.
21. Steinert RF, Puliafito CA, Kumar SR, et al. Cystoid macular edema, retinal detachment, and glaucoma after Nd:YAG laser posterior capsulotomy. *Am J Ophthalmol*. 1991;112:373–380.
22. Koch DD, Liu JF, Fill EP, et al. Axial myopia increases the risk of retinal complications after neodymium-YAG

laser posterior capsulotomy. *Arch Ophthalmol.* 1989;107:986–990.

23. Goldberg MF. Clear lens extraction for axial myopia: an appraisal. *Ophthalmology.* 1987;94:571–582.

24. Colin J, Robinet A. Clear lensectomy and implantation of low-power posterior chamber intraocular lens for the correction of high myopia. *Ophthalmology.* 1994;101:107–112.

25. Gris O, Güell JL, Manero F, et al. Clear lens extraction to correct high myopia. *J Cataract Refract Surg.* 1996;22:686–689.

26. Lee KH, Lee JH. Long-term results of clear lens extraction for severe myopia. *J Cataract Refract Surg.* 1996;22:1411–1415.

27. Jiménez-Alfaro I, Miguélez S, Bueno JL, et al. Clear lens extraction and implantation of negative-power posterior chamber intraocular lenses to correct extreme myopia. *J Cataract Refract Surg.* 1998;24:1310–1316.

28. Kershner RM. Clear corneal cataract surgery and the correction of myopia, hyperopia, and astigmatism. *Ophthalmology.* 1997;104:381–389.

29. Lyle WA, Jin GJC. Clear lens extraction to correct hyperopia. *J Cataract Refract Surg.* 1997;23:1051–1056.

30. Siganos DS, Pallikaris IG. Clear lensectomy and intraocular lens implantation for hyperopia from +7 to +14 diopters. *J Refract Surg.* 1998;14:105–113.

31. Kolahdouz-Isfahani AH, Rostamian K, Wallace D, et al. Clear lens extraction with intraocular lens implantation for hyperopia. *J Refract Surg.* 1999;15:316–323.

Chapter 27

Accommodating Intraocular Lenses and Lens Refilling to Restore Accommodation

Jean-Marie Parel and Brien A. Holden

■ Introduction

The surgical techniques proposed to restore accommodation past the onset of presbyopia can be categorized in two classes, those based on scleral expansion and those based on intraocular lens implantation and lens capsule refilling. This chapter describes and discusses the different techniques and summarizes the results of clinical and experimental animal trials. The restoration of accommodation has been demonstrated in nonhuman senile primates by at least two different teams using modifications of the lens capsule refilling technique originally described by Julius Kessler in the late fifties.[1-3] Recent advances in microsurgery, devices, and injectable polymers are very promising and human clinical trials are soon envisaged.

In young healthy human and nonhuman primates, accommodation allows for far and near vision and is caused by changes in the curvature and position of the crystalline lens. According to Helmholtz, during accommodation, the ciliary muscle contracts inwardly to some level, relaxing the zonular ligaments, which reduces the tension applied to the equatorial capsule.[4,5] As the capsular bag is always under positive tension (inner pressure greater then zero, calculated to be approximately 40 mm Hg, and greater than the physiologic intraocular pressure, 12–18 mm Hg), the capsule surface takes the shape of minimum energy and becomes more curved. The increase in anterior and posterior capsule radii of curvature accounts for the increase in refractive power of the crystalline lens. Controlled by the brain via a feedback loop, the ciliary muscle motion is dictated by the sharpness of the retinal image. The amplitude of accommodation is maximal in infants (10–16 diopters) and decreases with age, to approximately 2–6 diopters at 45 years, until it seizes completely at about 60 years.[6] The reduction in amplitude of accommodation is mainly attributed to the increase in hardness of the lens matter.[7,8] Since Julius Kessler's pioneering work, several surgical techniques have been proposed to remedy the loss of accommodation. These can be classified in two categories: extraocular (scleral shell expansion) and intraocular (IOLs and lens refilling).

■ Scleral Shell Expansion

Having observed an increase in the crystalline lens mass with age, Thornton, Fukasaku,[9] Schachar,[10] and others modified Helmholtz's theory. In the view of these researchers, the lens equatorial diameter increases with age, and because the scleral shell does not increase, the remaining annular space becomes insufficient to provide adequate tension on the zonules. Therefore, they proposed that surgically expanding the outer diameter of the scleral shell to give added space to the zonules will improve accommodation.

Fukasaku implemented Thornton's technique, which consists of making a 360-degree peritomy and 8 to 16 equidistant radial scleral incisions past the corneoscleral limbus using a guarded diamond knife equipped with a micrometer. The conjunctiva is then reposed and sutured to the limbus. Each incision is 3 mm long and approximately 90%–100% of scleral thickness as assessed by ultrasound pachymetry. Because the sclera is subjected to a constant outward tension produced by the intraocular pressure. They surmised that the sclera would increase in circumference with time.

Schachar's technique consists of implanting four 4-mm-long arc-shaped cylindrical rods of polymethylmethacrylate (PMMA) in four circumferential pockets delaminated in the sclera 1.5–2 mm below the limbus at the four quadrants of the globe. The pockets are about 4 mm long and 50% deep and made to receive the 4-mm-long by approximately 1-mm-diameter implant. The implant has two small pods at each end that are placed against the scleral wall and directed toward the center of the eyeball. The pods' function is to increase pressure against the scleral wall.

Both scleral expansion techniques are now in clinical trials in the United States. The inventors claim that they have been able to restore about 1.9 diopters of accommodation in several presbyopic patients in the early 3-month postoperative period. Both surgical techniques are the subject of multicenter clinical trials, although none are sponsored by the National Institutes of Health. No peer-reviewed scientific publications have been published to date. Also, no long-term data is available from the U.S. clinical studies. However, an independent European study using the Schachar implants has shown that improvement in accommodation is short lived. The study was conducted in 10 presbyopic patients who had lost accommodation (>0.5 diopters). In the immediate postoperative period, a few of the patients had regained about 1–1.5 diopters of accommodation, but all complained of some degree of eye irritation, photophobia, and pain. By the 3–6 months postoperatively all patients had lost accommodation, and the implants were removed (F. Malecaze, personal communication, 1999). In 1999, Mattews published results from an independent clinical pilot study involving three patients, which also confirms a lack of restored accommodation after implanting Schachar's devices.[11]

Scleral tissue is strong and not easily expansible. Tests performed by Duchesne and colleagues in human cadaver eyes at the Bascom Palmer Eye Institute have shown that expansion of the scleral shell requires intraocular pressure greater than 1,000 mm Hg.[12] Yet at that pressure, the increase in outer scleral diameter is less than 0.1 mm, far from the full 1 mm claimed by Schachar. In an experiment conducted by Nakagawa, an ophthalmic surgeon at the University of Fukuoka in Japan, Thornton's technique was performed in two 6-month-old adult rabbits.[13] Sixteen 3-mm-long radial incisions of 90%–95% depth were made (four between each of the four muscles), each starting at the limbus. Histologic studies performed 1 month postoperatively failed to show a single open scleral wound. All incisions had so tightly healed that they were barely identifiable in the histology slides. It is clear from these two experiments that neither Thornton's nor Schachar's sur-

gical technique restores accommodation by *expansion* of the scleral shell.

There are several concerns with Schachar's theory of accommodation. Weale attributed the increase in lens mass with age to an increase in the lens's anteroposterior thickness, not in its diameter.[7] Recent work by Glasser and Kaufman in iridectomized primates shows that zonular tension is produced by ciliary muscle contraction in both young and senile animals.[14] In these studies, contraction was provoked by electrical stimulation transmitted by an electrode implanted in the brain. In young primates, the lens equatorial diameter increased, while in senile primates it did not. The ciliary body to lens equator distance in both young and senile animals appeared identical and it was obvious from video recordings that the senile lens was too stiff to deform. All cataract surgeons, whom can easily aspirate the lens matter of young subjects but need to use powerful phacoemulsification devices in old patients, acknowledge this fact.

It is believed that incising the limbus in radial keratotomy (RK) procedures changes the refractive power of the cornea to a greater extent in comparison to where RK incisions do not transect the limbus. Because the annular limbus structure is composed of stiffer tissues that form the base of the corneal vault, might it be possible that transecting the limbus alters the corneal shape, producing a myopic-astigmatic or a multifocal cornea? Myopic astigmatism increases the depth of field at the expense of contrast sensitivity and could account for an increase in near vision acuity.[15] Where vision is concerned, a multifocal cornea would be equivalent to the multifocal contact lenses that are now prescribed for presbyopic patients. Corneal astigmatism and asphericity are easily quantifiable with the PAR-Sys,[16] a topography instrument designed to assess elevation and curvature with great precision (<0.2 diopters). We surmise that a well-planned Eye Bank eye study could elucidate the answers to this question.

■ Intraocular Lenses

Currently, several bifocal and multifocal IOLs are being implanted worldwide in cataract patients. All produce two or more discrete foci that give the patient two or more focal planes.[17] Far and near vision with these IOLs may not be acceptable to all patients, as they reduce visual acuity, decrease contrast sensitivity, and increase glare.[18] Also, none make use of the ciliary muscle-zonular framework accommodating mechanism. Recently, several authors have studied the accommodation potential of foldable IOLs implanted in the capsular bag, on the premise that when ciliary muscle is stimulated, the zonular framework would impose a force on the capsule which would then move the implant forward-backward along the optical axis of the eye. This phenomenon, called *pseudo*-accommodation, produces unreliable results, and in the best of cases, less than 0.9 diopters of accommodation.[19] Thus far, Hara and colleagues,[20] Cumming and Kammann,[21] and Hanna and Rol (personal communication, 1994) have proposed three types of IOLs to restore accommodation (see Chapter 25).

Hara's ingenious bi-IOL consists of two IOLs spaced by four thin helicoidal springs. Investigation of a prototype using PMMA for the optics and nylon wires for the springs was conducted in several in vivo experiments in rabbits. A large linear incision must be made in the capsule's periphery to insert the bulky implant, which then unbalances the elastic forces that the capsule applies to the IOLs. As a result, the IOLs tilt with respect to the optical axis and produce an unacceptable retinal image. Hara's proposed improvement, namely, the use of very high refractive index acrylics (n > 1.55) to reduce overall bulk and allow IOL folding, went unheard by the ophthalmic industry, and this research approach fizzled.

Cumming's device consists of a foldable IOL that has two Z-shaped cantilever haptics. The device is implanted via the usual 5-mm-diameter capsulorrhexis in the capsular bag. During the postoperative period, drugs are used to maintain the eye in its accommodated state until fibrosis secures the distal end of the haptic. Fibrosis may take less than 3 months in 45- to 60-year-olds, 6 months or longer in 60 to 75-year-olds, and may never occur in the very old (>90 years). Stopping medication allows the ciliary muscle to relax, placing full tension on the zonules, which pull on the bag and hence on the ends of the haptic. When the patient accommodates, the muscle constricts and liberates the cantilever, which moves the IOL optic toward the cornea. The cantilever is supposed to *amplify* the IOL forward motion. A recent study shows that with standard foldable acrylic IOLs (n ~ 1.57), the induced 0.2−1.1 mm forward motion of the IOL (assessed by ultrasound and optical pachymetry) produced an average of 1.1 ± 0.32 diopters (0.5−2.5 diopters, n = 20) of *pseudo*-accommodation in 60 ± 11-year-old patients whereas with PMMA IOLs, it was 0.81 ± 0.23 diopters (0.5−1.25 diopters, n = 18).[19] With cantilever haptics, the range should be greatly increased. One of Cumming's early prototypes was clinically tested at the Instituto Barraquer in Barcelona, but none of the patients regained measurable amounts of accommodation (< 1 diopter). Cumming attributed this to patient selection (age > 70) and noncompliance with medication.

Physicians were very concerned with the long-term effect of the sustained medication required with Cumming's implant.[22]

The implant of Hanna, Rol, and colleagues is medusa-shaped. It consists of a central optical element surrounded by a thin flexible skirt designed for endocapsular implantation through a central 4- to 5-mm-diameter capsulotomy. The central optical element is a very thin convex-concave meniscus made of a material with a very high index of refraction and a modulus of elasticity lower than that of the capsule. The optical element fits against the anterior capsule inner wall and is centered in the capsulorrhexis opening. The 360-degree skirt is designed to fit against the anteroequatorial walls of the capsular bag, its outside diameter fitting against the posterior capsule. Upon relaxation of the zonules, the equatorial diameter of the capsular bag diminishes and the medusa skirt comes under increasing tension. This tension translates as a forward motion of the optical element toward the cornea and an increase in the optical element's radius of curvature. For more details on the Hanna IOL please refer to Chapter 25.

■ Lens Refilling Techniques

Two techniques have been proposed (1) the endocapsular balloon and (2) direct refilling of the capsular bag with a soft synthetic material to replace the senile, stiffer nucleus. The premise of the two techniques is that accommodation will be restored if the content of the capsular bag has an elastic modulus similar to that of the newborn's crystalline lens. For these techniques to work, the capsule must remain as intact as possible; therefore, surgery must be performed through a very small capsule opening (minicapsulotomy). To avoid effects on the retinal image and on the fragile zonular ligaments, the minicapsulotomy is made at the periphery of the anterior capsule. Removal of lens matter and lens epithelial cells and implantation of the synthetic device is performed through the minicapsulotomy. Access to the crystalline lens is obtained via a small, under 3-mm-wide, corneal or cornea-limbal incision to minimize loss of the anterior chamber content and postoperative corneal astigmatism.

Although Treffers (personal communication, 1980) was first to propose the use of an endocapsular balloon in 1980, Nishi's group was the first to implant such a device.[23] This was after Nishi's attempt to refill a capsular bag after implanting a custom-made lens within a large capsulorrhexis.[24] They conceived a thin-wall cross-linked polydimethylsiloxane (PDMS) balloon having the dimensions of the crystalline lens and a thin umbilical tube located at the periphery. The

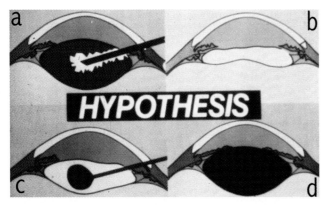

FIGURE 27.1. Phaco-ersatz concept. *A,* Cataract. *B,* Removal of lens matter via a small peripheral capsulotomy. *C,* Refilling the bag with a polymer having the same properties as a young child's lens. *D,* Filling lens until emmetropia is achieved.

balloon is evacuated of air and implanted in its collapsed form through a small, 1.2-mm capsulorrhexis made at the capsule periphery. A PDMS fluid is injected via the umbilical tube to reinsufflate the balloon. The wall of the umbilical tube near the balloon opening contains a PDMS adhesive that seals the bore when compression is applied to the tube's outer diameter with forceps. In this way, the umbilical cord can be cut close to the capsule surface. Following feasibility and biocompatibility studies in rabbits,[25] Nishi demonstrated that this method preserved accommodation in a small series of young primates.[26] However, the amplitude of accommodation decreased from 9 diopters in the early postoperative period to 1 diopter or less at 1 year. The decrease in amplitude was attributed partly to fibrosis, which encapsulated the bal-

loon, and partly to a change in the physical properties of the balloon, which allowed the PDMS fluid to permeate the balloon wall and ooze through the capsulorrhexis opening into the anterior chamber.[27] Control of the injected and remaining volume was found to be important.[28] For these reasons, Nishi et al adapted the valve device designed to pump air in bicycle tire tubes and made a self-sealing capsulotomy filling plug. It consists of a double washer with an umbilical cord similar to that described for the balloon. Cross-linked PDMS was used to make the device. The edge of the capsulorrhexis was sandwiched and permanently glued between the washers using a medical grade Silastic adhesive, and a polymeric fluid was injected through the tube to fill the evacuated capsular bag. The polymer takes a few hours to cross-link in situ to become a soft, pliable gel. After demonstrating that this device was safe and biocompatible in a rabbit model,[29] Nishi et al demonstrated effectiveness of the endocapsular balloon in senile primates.[30] Nishi had to perform a sectorial iridectomy in all the animals receiving either a balloon or the sealing washer to avoid postoperative iris inflammation caused by the protruding washer outer disc and tube stump.

Direct refilling of the capsular bag was introduced by Julius Kessler in the late 1950s. He showed the feasibility of this approach in Eye Bank eyes[1] and its biocompatibility in the rabbit model.[2] He also demonstrated the prolificacy of the rabbit to regenerate its lens matter.[3] Agarwal's group reproduced Kessler's techniques in the rabbit and attempted to assess accommodation in young primates.[31–34] Although they lacked modern microsurgical instrumentation and had to rely on "off-the-shelf" industrial polymers with inadequate physical properties, the work of these pioneers

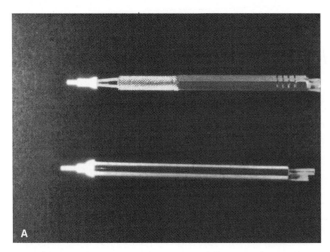

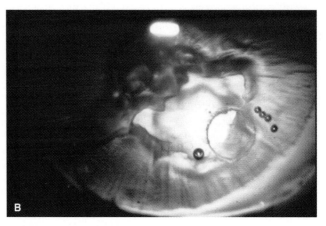

FIGURE 27.2. *A,* Instruments designed for the phaco-ersatz procedures. *B,* Thermal capsule trephine produces a uniform, >1-mm-diameter, opening.

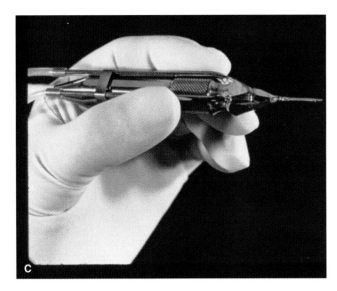

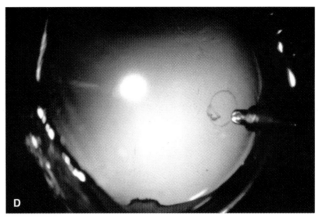

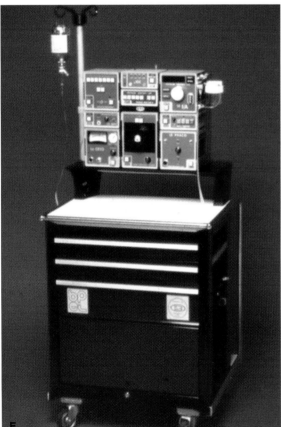

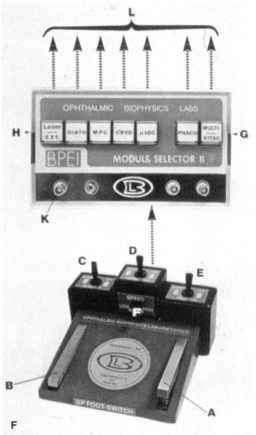

FIGURE 27.2. *(continued) C,* A mechanical phacoemulsifer. *D,* A mini infusion-aspiration probe, powered by a unitized console *(E)* and controlled by a multi-function foot-switch *(F).*

is extraordinary in its scope, ingenuity, and quality. Unaware of Kessler and Agarwal's past work, we introduced Phaco-Ersatz cataract surgery designed to preserve and restore accommodation in 1979 (Fig. 27.1) and applied modern technology to lens refilling (Fig. 27.2).[35] After demonstrating feasibility in cadaver eyes (Fig. 27.3) and safety in rabbits[36] (Fig. 27.4), we demonstrated the preservation of accommodation in young owl monkeys[37] and, later, restoration of accommodation in senile rhesus monkeys[38] (Fig. 27.5). Other

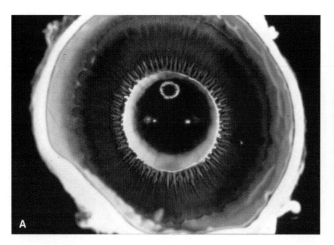

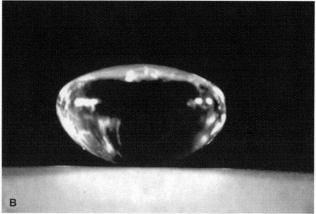

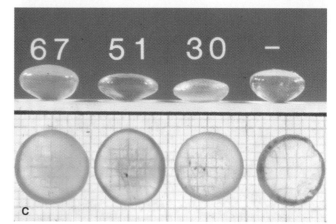

FIGURE 27.3. Surgical feasibility of the phaco-ersatz lens refilling procedure. Miyake view of the refilled human lens showing the capsulotomy opening (*A*) and the extracted lens shape (*B*) compared to human crystalline lenses of donors of different ages (*C*).

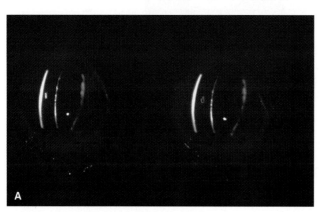

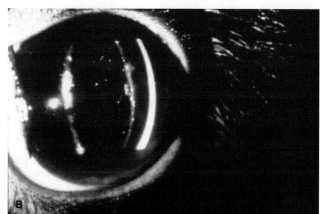

FIGURE 27.4. Safety study in the rabbit. Stereo photographs showing a clear cornea, anterior chamber, and lens refilled with a medical grade cross-linked polydimethylsiloxane gel. *A,* The 1 week postoperative visit. *B,* Apart from PCO, no changes occurred during the 6 months follow-up and no signs of foreign body reaction were noted.

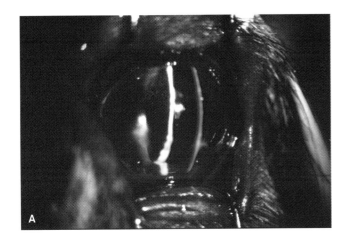

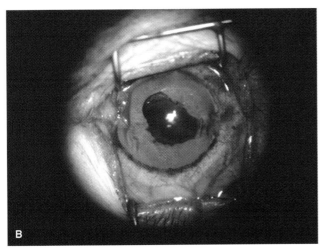

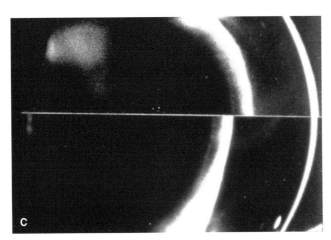

authors[39-47] have since modified Kessler's direct refilling technique as well as Hara and Nishi's balloon experiments and confirmed most of the preceding results.

Our team quickly came to the conclusion that the greatest barrier to the success of this procedure was the unwanted postoperative proliferation of lens epithelial cells (LEC) and subsequent fibrosis and opacification of the capsule (PCO) that obscures the visual axis. Previously, Kessler[3] and Agarwal et al[32] had observed secondary proliferation in all rabbits and monkeys, respectively that had undergone a lens-refilling procedure. PCO occurs in most human postcataract ECCE cases and is well described in the literature.[48,49] In our studies, PCO was observed 7–14 days after implantation in young adult rabbits (Fig. 27.6A), while in 2-year-old owl monkeys it took about 1 month, precluding adequate visualization of the fundus and refractometry at later postoperative visits (Fig. 27.6B). In the senile rhesus monkeys, PCO did not occur,

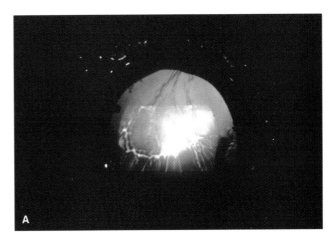

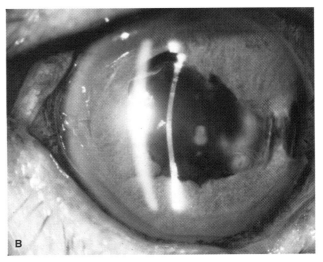

FIGURE 27.5. Efficacy study in the nonhuman primate using the same polysiloxane, optical, and ultrasound anterior segment depth measurements and a Scheimpflug camera. *A,* The preservation of accommodation was demonstrated in young animals. *B,* The restoration of accommodation in senile animals. *C,* Composite Scheimpflug view of the nonaccommodated and accommodated lens after phaco-ersatz surgery. An iridectomy had to be performed in the primates to measure accommodation amplitude using the Scheimpflug camera and the Zeiss Jena optical refractometer.

FIGURE 27.6. Posterior capsule opacification in refilled lenses at 1 week in the rabbit (*A*) and 1 month in the young monkey (*B*) precluded a clear visual view of the fundus.

although at the first postoperative year a Soemmering ring was clearly visible in every animal. It remained stable in size and density during the 4 years of the study and did not preclude observation of the fundus. We therefore launched several studies to assess methods and treatments designed to curb LEC proliferation. In the rabbit model, attempts at mechanical removal of LEC by brushing and ultrasonic and cryogenic treatments of the capsule did not prevent the development PCO, nor did lavage of the capsule with aqueous solutions containing the antimitotics methotrexate, 5-fluouracil (5-FU), and mitomycin C. Increasing the antimitotic concentration was effective, but also damaged surrounding tissues.[50] A 23-gauge C-shaped biodegradable controlled release implant containing 33% 5-FU by weight[51] inserted into the capsular bag equator appeared promising for ECCE cases (Fig. 27.7).[52] However, the physical presence of the implant may reduce the amplitude of accommodation of lens refilling techniques, because as the implant dissolves, the filled volume is reduced. Dihematoporphyrin ether photodynamic therapy (DHE-PDT) only worked with the DHE photosensitizer attached to polyclonal antibodies and high cw argon-ion 514-nm laser fluence (~ 60 J/cm²) was used (Fig. 27.8).[53–55] Recently the use of hypoosmotic solutions such as acetic acid, EDTA, and toxins has been investigated.[22,27,56] The common problem encountered in all of the various applications of antimitotics and toxic substances was leakage into the anterior chamber. This is a potential source of postoperative inflammation and toxicity to the delicate intraocular tissues, especially the corneal endothelium and the retina.

Underfilling of the capsular bag was another major problem because it resulted in hyperopia in all our animals. The PDMS polymers we used were partially cross-linked before injection, and were completely cured in situ at body temperature. Injecting a greater amount of polymer would have resulted in an increased endocapsular pressure, provoking the oozing of the polymer into the anterior chamber. When polymers of higher precured viscosity were used, correct filling was achieved but the resulting lens was too stiff and would either reduce the accommodation amplitude or negate it. Also, with such polymers, overfilling of the capsular bag occurred sometimes, producing myopia and, at times, capsule rupture.

These problems were solved recently by the use of polymers that are cross-linked in situ using light and the use of the minicapsulorrhexis valve (MCV; Fig. 27.9A). Both are fruits of the Restoring Accommodation project, an international effort to restore accommodation in presbyopes (approximately 20% of the world's population). The MCV is composed of a thin, round membrane (flap valve) bonded in its center to a thin crescent-shaped membrane (retainer). The MCV is foldable and can be introduced through the corneal incision into the minicapsulorrhexis,[57] so that its flap valve is positioned against the anterior capsule's inner surface and over the capsulorrhexis opening, while the retained member rests on the capsule's anterior surface. The MCV therefore seals the capsulorrhexis while allowing the introduction of small-diameter surgical instruments into the capsular bag (Fig. 27.9B). The device allows the bag to be filled with antiproliferating agents, lavage (infusion and aspiration) of the agents and cellular remnants, and the bag to be refilled with polymer to full capacity (Fig. 27.9C). The materials used to fabricate the device are transparent to the light required to cure the polymer. Therefore, curing can be done with the MCV in place, and the MCV can be removed after curing. After removal of the MCV, the polymer does not protrude, as its level remains below the edge of the capsulorrhexis and thus away from the posterior surface of the iris. In this way, the need for a mutilating iridectomy is avoided (Fig. 27.9D). The MCV and the new polymers also reduce the surgical time to a reasonable 20 minutes.

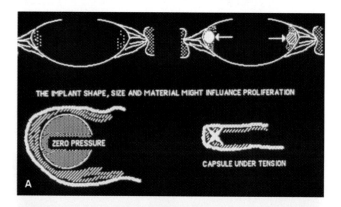

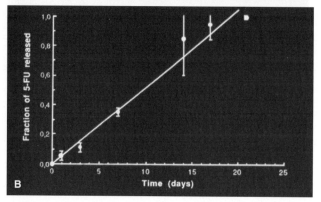

FIGURE 27.7. Endocapsular controlled drug release. *A,* Schematic showing the concept of the annular implant. *B,* Its release characteristics of 5-FU.

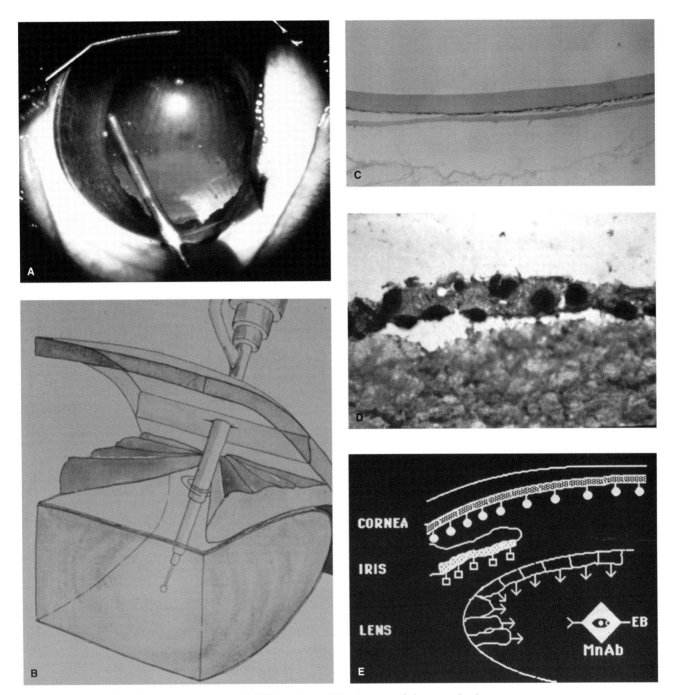

FIGURE 27.8. *A*, Photodynamic treatment of LEC consists of the lavage of the capsular bag with a photosensitizer solution. *B*, This is followed by endocapsular laser irradiation using a fiber equipped with a diffusing tip. *C*, This technique was found efficacious at killing LECs in rabbits that had underwent a phaco-ersatz procedure. *D*, Efficacy and safety are enhanced using monoclonal antibodies to LECs conjugated to DHE (*E*).

■ Conclusions

Recent studies have shown that accommodation can be preserved in young primates and restored in senile primates using lens-refilling techniques, whereas studies demonstrating scleral expansion techniques and modified IOLs have not. New technical developments have greatly improved the success rate of endocapsular surgery. Ex vivo and in vivo models have been developed to rapidly screen the efficacy of antiproliferating

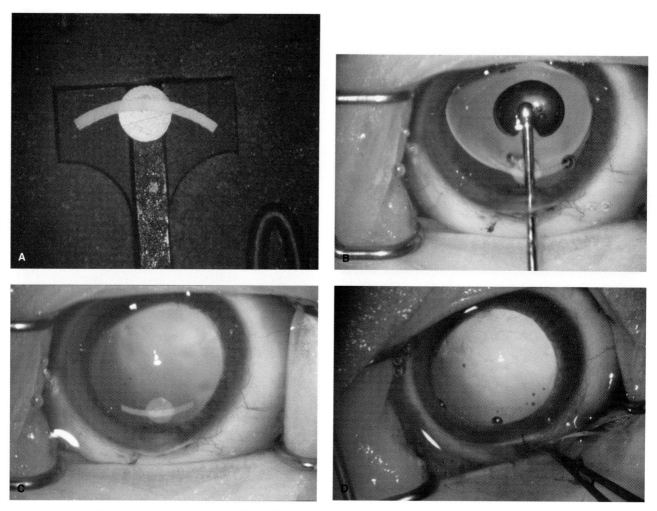

FIGURE 27.9. *A,* Minicapsulorrhexis valve. *B,* The MCV is folded with capsulorrhexis forceps. *C,* The MCV is placed in and on the bag's walls to close the capsulorrhexis opening. This allows safe filling of the bag. *D,* It is removed after the polymer is cured into a gel.

agents on LECs. The development of a monoclonal antibody photosensitizer and other anti-LEC agents is promising.

Several problems remain to be solved. Surgical instruments that make reproducible submillimeter capsule openings with uniform edges to resist tears[57–59] and submillimeter instruments to remove lens matter need to be developed. An efficacious anti-LEC agent that is safe for use on the delicate structures of the eye must be identified, because Nd:YAG laser capsulotomy will cause unwanted optical distortion of the refilled lens and potential retinal complications.[60,61] A microscope-mounted automated refractometer that can be used intraoperatively, and that is accurate, reliable, and simple to use has to be designed to enable the capsular bag to be refilled to the optically correct level. Current ophthalmic polymers do not satisfy the optical requirements of the eye and their injection is still problematic; thus, better materials need to be developed.[62] The geometry of the refilled capsule must be compared with that of the young crystalline lens to optimise the procedure.[63] An animal model of accommodation, other than nonhuman primates, should be identified to test the feasibility and the efficacy of the improved procedures. The optics of crystalline and ersatz lenses during accommodation must be studied to compare retinal image quality.[64] Finally, replacing a presbyopic but perfectly transparent human crystalline lens with a synthetic accommodating lens requires assurance that vision will be restored to at least the same preoperative level (20/20), and will occur with a success rate that approaches that of present-day cataract surgery.

■ Acknowledgments

The authors especially acknowledge Pascal O. Rol, recently deceased, for 17 years of continuous dedication to the Phaco-Ersatz project. Tony Clayton, Gordon Meij, and Juergen Vogt provided novel injectable polymers; Hassan Tahi further improved the Phaco-Ersatz surgical technique and participated to the creation of the MCV; Fabrice Manns, Arthur Ho, and Paul Erickson further developed the lens refilling optical model; Hassan Tahi and Marie Hamaoui helped develop the ex vivo capsule culture technique; William Lee, Izuru Nose, and David Denham designed and fabricated the surgical and laboratory instrumentation; the members of the Restoring Accommodation team and of the Accommodation Club, especially Professor Joaquin Barraquer, gave scientific advice and provided some of the information reported in this chapter.

Funding and materials were provided by the Cooperative Research Centre for Eye Research and Technology, Sydney, New South Wales, Australia; Professor Joaquin Barraquer, Instituto Barraquer, Barcelona, Spain; the Florida Lions Eye Bank, Miami, Florida; Research to Prevent Blindness, New York; and the Henri and Flore Lesieur Foundation, West Palm Beach, Florida.

■ References

1. Kessler J. Experiments in refilling the lens. *Arch Ophthalmol.* 1964;71:412–417.
2. Kessler J. Refilling the rabbit lens. Further experiments. *Arch Ophthalmol.* 1966;76(4):596–598.
3. Kessler J. Lens refilling and regrowth of lens substance in the rabbit eye. *Ann Ophthalmol.* 1975;7(8):1059–1062.
4. Southall JPC. *Helmholtz's Treatise on Physiological Optics.* New York: Dover Publications Inc; 1962:335–350.
5. Beers APA. *On the Mechanism of Accommodation: Ultrasonography Used to Investigate the Physiology and Pathophysiology of Human Accommodation in vivo* [dissertation]. Amsterdam, The Netherlands: Vrije Universiteit; 1996.
6. Alpen M. The eye in vision. In: Driscol WG, Vaughan W, eds. *Handbook of Optics.* New York: McGraw Hill; 1978:1–39.
7. Weale RA. *The Aging Eye.* London: HK Lewis; 1963.
8. Weale RA. *A Biography of the Eye.* London: HK Lewis; 1982.
9. Fukasaku H, Marron JA, Yamaguchi A. Anterior ciliary sclerectomy. The surgical cure for presbyopia [abstract]. Final Program of the 103rd Meeting of the American Academy of Ophthalmology, Orlando, FL; 1999:254; and Fukasaku H. Anterior ciliary sclerectomy: results in the treatment of presbyopia and glaucoma (abstract). Final program of the 104th meeting of the American Academy of Ophthalmology, Dallas, TX; 2000:104.
10. Schachar RA. Cause and treatment of presbyopia with a method for increasing the amplitude of accommodation. *Ann Ophthalmol.* 1992;24:445–452.
11. Mattews S. Scleral expansion surgery does not restore accommodation in human presbyopia. *Ophthalmology.* 1999; 106:873–877.
12. Duchesne B, Gautier S, Parel J-M, Lacombe E, Alfonso E. Endothelium-Descemet membrane strength after trephination. *Invest Ophthalmol Vis Sci.* 1996;37(3):S551.
13. Nakagawa N, Parel J-M. Data on file. Miami, FL: University of Miami School of Medicine.
14. Glasser A, Kaufman PL. The mechanism of accommodation in primates. *Ophthalmology.* 1999;106:863–872.
15. Huber C. Myopic astigmatism. A substitute for accommodation in pseudophakia. *Doc Ophthalmol.* 1981;52:123–178.
16. Belin MW, Cambier JL, Nabors JR, Ratliff CD. PAR Corneal Topography System (PAR CTS): the clinical application of close-range photogrammetry. *Optom Vis Sci.* 1995;72:828–837.
17. Rol PO. Design characteristics and point spread function evaluation of bifocal intraocular lenses. In: Parel J-M, ed. *Ophthalmic Technologies I.* Vol. 1423. Bellingham, WA; 1991:15–19.
18. Huber C, Haefliger E. Contrast sensitivity measured with square waves on the Macintosh II computer. Application to diffractive IOLs. *Eur J Implant Refract Surg.* 1991;3: 255–259.
19. Istanbul University study. Pseudo-accommodation with foldable intraocular lenses. *Refract Cataract Surg.* (in press).
20. Hara T, Hara T, Yasuda A, Yamada Y. Accommodative intraocular lens with spring action. Part 1. Design and placement in an excised animal eye. *Ophthalmic Surg.* 1990;21(2):128–133.
21. Cumming JS, Kammann J. Experience with an accommodating IOL [letter]. *Cataract Refract Surg.* 1996;22:1001.
22. Parel J-M. Summary and conclusions of the 3rd meeting of the Accommodation Club. *An Instituto Barraquer (Barc.).* 1998;27(3):327–331.
23. Nishi O, Hara T, Sakka Y, Hayashi H, Nakamae K, Yamada Y. Refilling the lens with inflatable endocapsular balloon. *Dev Ophthalmol.* 1991;22:122–125.
24. Nishi O, Sakka Y. Anterior capsule-supported intraocular lens. A new lens for small-incision surgery and for sealing the capsular opening. *Graefes Arch Clin Exp Ophthalmol.* 1990;228(6):582–588.
25. Nishi O, Hara T, Hara T, Sakka Y, Hayashi F, Nakamae K, Yamada Y. Refilling the lens with an inflatable endocapsular balloon: surgical procedure in animal eyes. *Graefe's Arch Clin Exp Ophthalmol.* 1992;230:47–55.
26. Nishi O, Nakai Y, Yamada Y, Mizumoto Y. Amplitudes of accommodation of primate lenses refilled with two types of inflatable endocapsular balloons. *Arch Ophthalmol.* 1993;111(12):1677–1684.
27. Hara T, Sakka Y, Sakanishi K, Yamamda Y, Nakamae K, Hayashi F. Complications associated with endocapsular balloon implantation in rabbit eyes. *Cataract Refract Surg.* 1994;20:507–512.
28. Nishi O, Nishi K, Mano C, Ichihara M, Honda T. Controlling the capsular shape in lens refilling. *Arch Ophthalmol.* 1997;115(4):507–510.

29. Nishi O, Nishi K, Mano C, Ichihara M, Honda T. Lens refilling with injectable silicone in rabbit eyes. *J Cataract Refract Surg.* 1998;24(7):975–982.

30. Nishi O, Nishi K. Accommodation amplitude after lens refilling with injectable silicone by sealing the capsule with a plug in primates. *Arch Ophthalmol.* 1998;116(10):1358–1361.

31. Agarwal LP, Angra SK, Khosla PK, Tandon HD. Lens regeneration in mammals. I. Rabbits (after extracapsular extraction). *Orient Arch Ophthalmol.* 1964;2:1–17.

32. Agarwal LP, Angra SK, Khosla PK, Tandon HD. Lens regeneration in mammals. II. Monkeys (after extracapsular extraction). *Orient Arch Ophthalmol.* 1964;2:47–59.

33. Agarwal LP, Angra SK, Tandon HD. Lens regeneration in mammals. III. Rabbits (after extracapsular extraction). *Orient Arch Ophthalmol.* 1964;2:95–100.

34. Agarwal LP, Narsimhan EC, Mohan M. Experimental lens refilling. *Orient Arch Ophthalmol.* 1967;5:205–212.

35. Parel JM, Treffers WF, Gelender H, Norton EWD. Phaco-ersatz: a new approach to cataract surgery. *Ophthalmology.* 1981;88(suppl 9):95.

36. Parel JM, Gelender H, Trefers WF, Norton EWD. Phaco-ersatz: cataract surgery designed to preserve accommodation. *Graefe's Arch Clin Exp Ophthalmol.* 1986;224:165–173.

37. Haefliger E, Parel J-M, Fantes F, et al. Accommodation of an endocapsular silicone lens (phaco-ersatz) in the non-human primate. *Ophthalmology.* 1987;94:471–477.

38. Haefliger E, Parel J-M. Accommodation of an endocapsular silicone lens (phaco-ersatz) in the old rhesus monkey. *Refract Corneal Surg.* 1994;10:550–555.

39. Barraquer J. Lentilles intraoculaires 1949–1994. Phaco-ersatz 2001. *An Inst Barraquer (Barc).* 1993–1994;24:27–36.

40. Gindi JJ, Wan WL, Schanzlin DJ. Endocapsular cataract surgery. I. Surgical technique. *Cataract.* 1985;2:6–10.

41. Stegmann R. Communication to the second meeting of the Accommodation Club, Barcelona, Spain; 1993.

42. Lucke K, Hettlich HJ, Kreiner CF. A method of lens extraction for the injection of liquid intraocular lenses. *Ger J Ophthalmol.* 1992;1(5):342–345.

43. Hettlich HJ, Lucke K, Kreiner CF. Light-induced endocapsular polymerization of injectable lens refilling materials. *Ger J Ophthalmol.* 1992;1(5):346–349.

44. Hettlich HJ, Lucke K, Asiyo-Vogel MN, Schulte M, Vogel A. Lens refilling and endocapsular polymerization of an injectable intraocular lens: in vitro and in vivo study of potential risks and benefits. *J Cataract Refract Surg.* 1994;20:115–123.

45. Hettlich HJ, Lucke K, Asiyo-Vogel M, Vogel A. Experimental studies of the risks of endocapsular polymerization of injectable intraocular lenses. *Ophthalmologe.* 1995;92(3):329–334.

46. Hettlich HJ, Asiyo-Vogel M. Experimental experiences with balloon-shaped capsular sac implantation with reference to accommodation outcome in intraocular lenses. *Ophthalmologe.* 1996;93(1):73–75.

47. Hettlich HJ. *Accommodative Lens Refilling: Principles and Experiments* [dissertation]. Goningen, The Netherlands: Pharmacia Upjohn; 1996.

48. Apple DJ, Solomon KD, Tetz MR, et al. Posterior capsule opacification. *Surv Ophthalmol.* 1992;37:73–116.

49. Kappelhof JP, Vrensen GFJM. The pathology of after-cataract. A minireview. *Acta Ophthalmol.* 1992;205 (suppl):13–24.

50. Parel J-M, Simon G. Phaco-ersatz 2001: update. *An Inst Barraquer (Barc).* 1995;25:143–151.

51. Hostyn P, Villain F, Kühne F, Malek N, Parrish RK, Parel J-M. Controlled drug release implant for 5-FU adjuvant therapy in glaucoma. *J Fr Ophthalmol.* 1996;19(2):133–139.

52. Duchesne B, Tahi H, Gautier S, Jallet V, Villain F, Parel J-M. Implant a relargage controle de 5-FU pour la prevention de la cataracte secondaire: étude preliminaire. *Bull Soc Belge Ophthalmol.* 1998;268:69–72.

53. Parel J-M, Cubeddu R, Ramponi R, Lingua R, Sacchi CA, Haefliger E. Endocapsular lavage with Photofrin II as a photodynamic therapy for lens epithelium proliferation. *Lasers Med Sci.* 1990;5:25–30.

54. Lingua RW, Parel J-M, Fliesler SJ, Fitzgerald P, Rodriguez IR, Hernandez E. Photodynamic therapy to retard lens epithelial proliferation after lensectomy. *Laser Light Ophthalmol.* 1988;2:103–113.

55. Takesue Y, Mui MM, Hachiya T, Parel J-M. Comparative photodynamic effect of Rose Bengal, erytrocin B and DHE on lens epithelial cells. In: Parel J-M, Ren Q, eds. *Ophthalmic Technologies III.* Vol. 2126. Bellingham, WA: SPIE; 1993:323–327.

56. Behar-Cohen F, David T, D'Hermies F, et al. In vivo inhibition of lens regrowth by fibroblast growth factor 2-saporin. *Invest Ophthalmol Vis Sci.* 1995;36:2434–2448.

57. Tahi H, Hamaoui M, Parel J-M, Fantes F. A technique for small peripheral capsulorhexis. *Cataract Refract Surg.* 1999;25:744–747.

58. Hettlich HJ, El-Hifnawi ES. Scanning electron microscopy studies of the human lens capsule after capsulorrhexis. *Ophthalmologe.* 1997;94(4):300–302.

59. Tahi H, Brenman K, Yu A, Parel J-M. Scanning electron microscopy of anterior capsule edges produced by different capsulotomy methods. *Invest Ophthalmol Vis Sci.* 2000;41(4):S5.

60. Parrish R, Parel J-M. Retinal detachment following Nd:YAG laser capsulotomy [letter]. *Am J Ophthalmol.* 1984;98:249.

61. Herzeel R, Belgrado G, Brihaye-Van Geertruyden M, Tassignon MJ. Complications of Nd:YAG laser capsulotomy: pathophysiology and prevention. In: Marshall J, ed. *Laser Technology in Ophthalmology.* Amsterdam: Kugler & Ghedini Publications; 1988:79–84.

62. Rol P, Parel J-M, Villain F. Optical transmission of implantable ophthalmic biopolymers. In: Parel J-M, Ren Q, eds. *Ophthalmic Technologies IV.* Vol. 2126. Bellingham, WA: SPIE; 1994:353–359.

63. Hamaoui M, Tahi H, Chapon P, et al. Ex vivo testing of crystalline lens substitutes. A pilot study. In: Rol PO, Joos KM, Manns F, eds. *Ophthalmic Technologies X.* Vol. 3908. Bellingham, WA: SPIE; 2000:15–19.

64. Parel J-M, Simon G, Ren Q, Rol P, Lee WE, Denham DB. In situ pre- and postoperative optical resolution of the lens, and pseudo-phacos: a preliminary report. In: Parel J-M, Ren Q, eds. *Ophthalmic Technologies III.* Vol. 1877. Bellingham, WA: SPIE; 1993:132–135.

Chapter 28

Future Developments

Herbert E. Kaufman

Although Ridley[1] was the first to insert IOLs in human eyes, the first widely used lenses in the United States were those of Binkhorst[2] (Fig. 28.1) and Worst[3] (the Medallion lens) (Fig. 28.2). Both were iris clip lenses and required significant anterior chamber depth for insertion. When we developed the clinical specular microscope,[4] we found that the endothelium was being damaged during the IOL insertion procedure.[5] Shortly thereafter we introduced the use of viscoelastics (methylcellulose and polyvinyl pyrrolidone),[6] which were later modified to include hyaluronic acid. In addition, lens design changed: lenses became relatively flat (uniplanar) and easier to insert without touching the endothelium. Also, Shearing discovered that the IOL could be inserted into the sulcus, eliminating the need for an iris clip.[7] Phacoemulsification and the technological modifications that made it practical, along with the widespread use of viscoelastics, IOL insertion into the intracapsular bag, capsulorrhexis, the modern techniques of "divide and conquer" cataract extraction, and the newer cracking techniques, have simplified and improved the safety of cataract surgery.

■ Current Perspectives

In the United States, the vast majority of cataract operations are now done with phacoemulsification. Extracapsular cataract extraction is becoming rare. The obligatory use of sutures, which distort the wound, is being replaced by clear corneal or at least small incision cataract surgery.

As we move to small incision, no-stitch surgery, performing phacoemulsification through a small incision and then enlarging the incision to insert an IOL

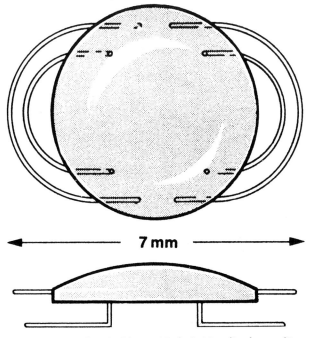

FIGURE 28.1. The Binkhorst Mark I iris clip lens. *(From Rosen, ES. The development and characterization of the intraocular lens. In: Rosen ES, Haining WM, Arnott EJ, eds. Intraocular Lens Implantation. St. Louis, MO: CV Mosby; 1984: 50–58, with permission.)*

makes little sense. Foldable lenses are the solution to this problem, and in the future higher refractive index lenses that are thin and easily folded and can pass through very small incisions will become more popular. Injectors will almost certainly be more user friendly and pass more easily through very small incisions. There will also be viscoelastics that break down by

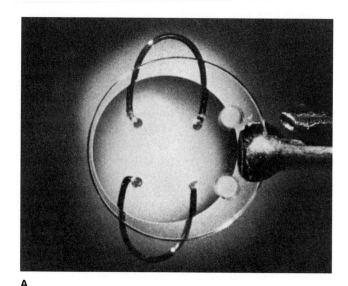

FIGURE 28.2. *A,* Haptic of medallion lens grasped by Shepard duckbill forceps with irrigating cannula. *B,* Medallion lens without haptic. *(From Williamson, DE. Medallion intraocular lens used in an outpatient setting. In: Engelstein JM, ed.* Cataract Surgery: Current Options and Problems. *Orlando, FL: Grune & Stratton; 1984:119–126, with permission.)*

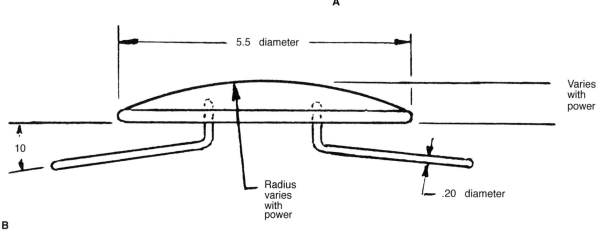

themselves making removal unnecessary and preventing postsurgery intraocular pressure rises. Recently, instruments that actually measure the wavefront of light as it emerges from its retinal reflection have been developed. This wavefront analysis permits the adjustment of refraction to create an ideal image on the retina. Use of this new technology will change the process of refraction from a subjective to a precise and objective procedure. Furthermore, it will be possible to couple wavefront analysis with machines that make intraocular lenses, intracorneal lenses, contact lenses, and excimer lasers to provide an ideal refractive surface, rather than the simple refractive surface now available.

The controversy over monofocal versus multifocal lenses continues, and the solution is not clear. Many surgeons who wish to give their patients freedom from glasses use monofocal lenses to provide monovision, typically with a + 2.00 add in the nondominant eye. This approach requires patients to switch back and forth between eyes, depending on the object of focus, but does not degrade contrast sensitivity, especially in dim light, the way multifocal lenses do. If a patient is very unhappy with monovision, bifocal spectacles can be prescribed. The anisometropia is not a serious problem; although the nonadapted patient must wear glasses, there is no significant permanent disability.

Multifocal lenses caused problems in the past. In many older series, a small number of patients could not adjust to the multifocal image, and the degradation of contrast sensitivity in dim light was disturbing.[8–10] In some series as many as 5% of patients who had otherwise good vision were dissatisfied and wanted the multifocal lenses removed. Some authorities believe that better patient selection could eliminate these problems, but to date there is no evidence that it is possible to select patients for multifocal lenses such that all selected patients will be happy. In addition, the use of multifocal lenses presupposes that there is no significant residual astigmatism and that the power correction is absolutely perfect.

The attempt to eliminate preexisting astigmatism, whether by the use of toric lenses or by small astigmatic incisions, has become a part of IOL surgery. At present, many surgeons prefer a simple astigmatic keratotomy made along the circumference of a 7-mm-diameter circle centered on the center of the cornea. Others prefer limbal incisions, although at this time these incisions are slightly less predictable than the corneal astigmatic incisions. In the future these approaches will be improved, and patients will not be left with significant astigmatism at the end of surgery.

At the time of cataract surgery it would be relatively easy to create a microkeratome corneal flap. After the cataract procedure, the precise needs of the cornea could be ascertained with a wave guide sensor to give perfect vision. An intracorneal lens could be tailored to the individual patient and slipped beneath the flap at any time after the surgery. Multifocal lenses can be tried and removed if the patient finds them objectionable; similarly, monofocal lenses can be tried—all by simply lifting the flap and placing a lens within the cornea. Such flaps can probably be lifted for years after the original surgery so that even if the refraction changes, an intracorneal lens could be adjusted to meet the precise needs of the patient.

■ A Glance at the Future

The Conduct of Cataract Surgery

Capsulorrhexis is a generally satisfactory, not overly complex maneuver. However, learning the technique and managing its occasional complications requires a significant effort, and even so, occasionally a capsulorrhexis may tear or extend toward the equator during surgery. A new approach using a high-frequency diathermy needle to make a capsulorrhexis does not rely on tearing perfect vectors and appears to give an adequate if somewhat less strong capsulorrhexis than that achieved with a continuous tear. In the future, we will almost certainly have an instrument that can be inserted into the eye to make a circular pattern on the lens surface and disrupt the capsule without the necessity and uncertainty of making a tear.

New picosecond lasers are being used to make corneal intralamellar cuts for LASIK flaps. These instruments can also be used to make a no-touch capsulorrhexis before cataract surgery to provide a perfect tear.

Phacoemulsification machines are becoming progressively more sophisticated so that probes are smaller, chambers no longer collapse, posterior capsules are not sucked into the machine, and inflow and outflow can be maintained independent of suction level. Still, improvements are possible. Kelman has suggested a rotating metallic "flea" controlled by a magnetic field to supplant ultrasound for breaking up the lens. A more likely approach involves making a small opening in the capsule and inserting a turbulence-producing suction mechanism into the hole to safely remove lens material without the risk of capsular damage. One such system currently in development, called the Catarex method, is fascinating, but as yet no data are available to demonstrate increased safety and ease of use. An erbium-YAG laser can be used to produce a lens-disrupting shock wave, but its superiority over mechanical techniques is not clear.

Intracapsular tension rings, used in Europe, permit the safer removal of cataracts in patients with dislocated zonules, Marfan's syndrome, pseudoexfoliation of the lens capsule, and other problems, and will probably be used more generally in the United States in the future.[11]

IOLs in Cataract Surgery

Astigmatism: Toric IOLs are available to correct astigmatism, but having the appropriate lens for each power at each level of astigmatism requires maintaining a large inventory. The possibility of shaping an existing IOL with an excimer laser to add the astigmatic component has been suggested, but this approach remains experimental. It is more likely that a corneal flap can be made, and a precise correction of both sphere and cylinder to "touch up" any error in the intraocular lens can be inserted. This would not only compensate for optical errors, but also treat presbyopia.

Accommodation: Adjustable IOLs remain an exciting possibility, especially the potential for lenses made of a soft material that could allow accommodation. Numerous studies have been done based on the idea of making a very small opening in the capsular bag and filling the bag with a viscous material such as a setting silicone to provide the necessary correction and still seal the opening. Equally appealing would be a balloon that could be inserted into the capsular bag, then filled to a predetermined calibrated level with a flexible or fluid material using a syringe. This approach would certainly permit accommodation if accommodation is really possible in these patients, and might even allow evaluation of the refraction at the end of the surgery and adjustment of the filled balloon to provide exactly the right correction.

The idea of adjustable IOLs is not new. Several patents have been granted for lenses whose power can be altered externally via electromechanical input, but the cost and practicality of such lenses is not yet clear. The need for conscious lens adjustment depending on focal distance seems too complex to make the development of such lenses practicable for common use.

In two new compressible lenses the optics move with accommodation, increasing the power and permitting some accommodation. It may be possible for compressible, haptic, intraocular lenses that will change position to provide sufficient accommodation, but these lenses are still under study.

High Refractive Errors: Many authors with considerable optical background have suggested the desirability of using two or more IOLs inserted either at the time of cataract surgery or in sequence later to correct for high refractive errors or to increase depth of focus. However, it seems likely that adequate optical correction can be incorporated into single lenses, and therefore it is unlikely that this double-lens approach will be necessary.

Appearance: A variety of lenses now available in Europe, such as large lenses with built-in "irises" for patients with aniridia or missing pieces of iris, will likely be available in the United States in the near future.

IOLs in Refractive Surgery

There is an increasing demand for permanent refractive correction. As refractive surgical procedures become safer and more predictable, it seems possible that eventually people will have their vision fixed as a matter of course, the way they now have their teeth fixed. How this will be accomplished, however, remains to be seen. Part of the current debate over the future of refractive surgery involves the question of where refractive correction is optimal: at the surface of or within the cornea, or in the anterior or posterior chamber.

Laser-assisted in situ keratomileusis (LASIK) is currently the most popular approach for refractive surgery. However, the need to have a half-million-dollar laser, patient, and doctor all in the same place limits the general use and desirability of this procedure. Additionally, excimer laser procedures are subtractive operations, so that problems, including decentered or imperfect ablations, are difficult to reverse or fix, and the resulting quality of vision is inferior to that of a normal cornea, especially for corrections larger than 10 diopters. We believe that in the future the excimer laser will be used less and less in the correction of refractive errors.

Implant- or "lens"-related corneal corrections have not achieved widespread acceptance. An early corneal surface procedure, epikeratophakia, involved machining a piece of frozen cornea and attaching it to the surface of the eye.[12] This operation, although relatively satisfactory, was expensive, difficult to do, and in high myopes showed about a 20% regression. The development of a synthetic epikeratophakia lens seemed to be a simple problem, but it has not been solved. The right polymer has not been found, nor has an ideal way to attach the lens so that it can remain a permanent part of the front of the cornea.

Much implant-related corneal refractive surgery has been limited by the fact that a lens inserted into the corneal stroma must be permeable to fluid and metabolites or allow sufficient flow around it from the aqueous to the epithelium. Choyce's intracorneal polysulfone implants, which had a high index of refraction and did not require deformation of the anterior corneal surface, were impermeable to fluid flow and caused stromal stress and opaque deposits.[13]

Synthetic intracorneal lenses with a refractive index close to that of the cornea are being implanted under microkeratome cuts identical to the LASIK flap. This procedure simulates Barraquer's keratophakia procedure using a tissue lens. The synthetic lens is made of a special biomaterial to transmit metabolites, and Stephen Kaufman has demonstrated that the microkeratome flap heals around such a lens and that the lens can be tolerated in animals for at least two years (personal communication). One advantage is that the flap can be lifted and the lens removed or exchanged, making the operation reversible, or potentially reversible or adjustable for a period of years. Similarly, these lenses can be tailor-made for each individual patient to correct high order wavefront abnormalities, and the procedure has the advantage of being reversible if the correction is not perfect. We think that such lenses will be popular for the correction of low and moderate hyperopia as well as astigmatism. They will permit trials of presbyopic correction such that if the patient finds them unpleasant, they can be removed. This surgery will be performed as an office procedure.

There is no doubt that the use of refractive IOLs will become more common. The use of IOLs in phakic eyes to correct refractive errors is gaining popularity in Europe and will likely be equally common in the United States when lenses with US Food and Drug Administration approval become available.

Lenses can be implanted in the anterior chamber of the phakic eye.[14] The Baikoff lens is basically a modification of the Kelman Multiflex design (Figs. 28.3 and 28.4). In the initial studies, corneal edema resulted from the lens edge being too close to the peripheral cornea. Subsequent designs caused both glare and pupillary ovaling in a significant number of patients, but in part at our suggestion the lens has been modified so that the area of iris contact is less and the area bearing the pressure of the lens seating in the angle is wider, so that contact is made over a larger circumference. In the new design, the optic is larger and the edges are treated to minimize glare; as a result, the incidence of pupillary ovaling, although still significant, is less, and glare is reduced. One inherent difficulty is that many pupils are not central, but because of the

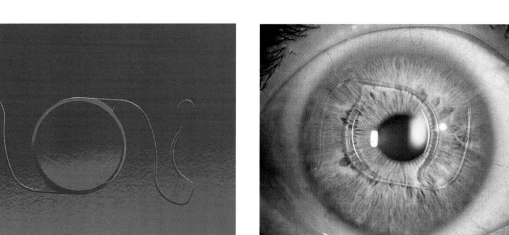

FIGURE 28.3. Baikoff III Nuvita phakic anterior chamber lens.

FIGURE 28.4. Baikoff-style phakic anterior chamber lens, implanted in a patient with high myopia.

haptic design, the lens itself centers on the geometric center of the eye. Some pupils are superonasal, and pupils in young people tend to be large, so this lens will never be perfect for all patients.

This type of lens will probably not achieve widespread use in the United States until a foldable design is developed and shown to be effective. A version having a soft optic and soft haptics is being tested. The design of the soft haptics is different from that of the Multiflex: it is possible that these haptics will not hold the lens firmly in the angle and the lens will ride up and down on the angle of the peripheral cornea, causing late cystoid macular edema and corneal edema, as did some of the previous anterior chamber lenses. Another design involves slightly narrower, Multiflex-design, methacrylate haptics that make contact with the angle and are connected by a methacrylate strip on one side of the optic. The optic is soft and foldable. Insufficient clinical results are available to evaluate this lens. It is possible that any lens which unfolds in the anterior chamber would have to be placed so far forward to avoid iris contact that it would have difficulty clearing the endothelium. No endothelial data are yet available on this lens.

The Artisan lens or iris claw lens is a Worst design that clips on the iris (Fig. 28.5). The lens can be centered precisely over the pupil. It seems well tolerated and effective and does not cause pupillary ovaling. It also seems less associated with glare. However, it is more difficult to insert. Occasionally the lens becomes loose and needs to be removed to avoid corneal edema, but in general this lens is very satisfactory.

It seems clear that an anterior chamber lens will be developed that is easy to insert and able to correct a variety of optical errors. At first the lenses will be designed to correct the large errors—high hyperopia and

myopia—but as the lenses improve, the anterior chamber IOL will gradually replace the laser for many refractive applications. Visual recovery is rapid, and the quality of vision is superb.

The intraocular contact lens, or ICL, is implanted behind the iris, where it rests on the sulcus, spanning from one side to the other and, ideally, just barely vaulting over the natural lens. Unfortunately, it is impossible to measure the sulcus-to-sulcus distance precisely. If the lens is too short, it rubs on the lens capsule, which may be the cause of a significant incidence of associated cataract formation. Also, short lenses tend to decenter. If the lens is too long, it pushes the iris structures up into the angle; in many series there has been a significant incidence of angle-closure glaucoma.

The early ICLs were made of silicone, which was not adequately biocompatible, but even the new HEMA-collagen copolymers have mechanical problems

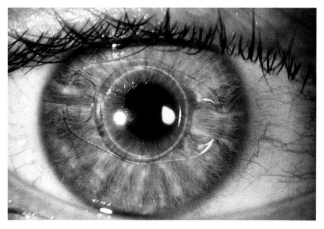

FIGURE 28.5. Artisan myopia lens, implanted in a patient with high myopia.

that have not yet been solved. The lens itself is relatively easy to insert, is optically effective, and is being used more frequently. However, the potential for cataract formation remains a concern.

A new posterior chamber design that "floats" in the pupil on secreted aqueous is being tested. The sizing of the lens is not critical, but long-term results are not yet available.

■ Summary

Cataract surgery has become a refractive procedure, and it is clear that patients appreciate their freedom from spectacles and are able to function in a superior way. Other refractive procedures involving either the cornea or the anterior or posterior chamber are also valuable and potentially very exciting ways to correct refractive errors. We believe that refractive surgery that is reversible and that can be performed without the cost and logistical problems of maintaining a laser will become more popular, just as refractive surgery itself will become progressively more accepted as risks decrease and benefits increase. As discussed in Chapter 25, combining wavefront technology with custom IOL manufacturing may be the next frontier in IOL technology for cataract and refractive error correction. Intracorneal lenses placed under a LASIK flap could be tailored to correct wavefront errors for the individual patient, and yet be removable if the result is imperfect. They could also offer advantages in the correction of presbyopia.

■ References

1. Ridley H. Intraocular acrylic lenses. *Trans Ophthalmol Soc UK.* 1951;71:617–621.
2. Binkhorst CD. Iris supported artificial pseudophakia: a new development in intraocular artificial lens surgery (iris clip lens). *Trans Ophthalmol Soc UK.* 1959;79: 569–584.
3. Worst JGF. L'implantation d'un cristallin artificiel (iris clip lens de Binkhorst). *Bull Mem Soc Fr Ophtalmol.* 1971; 84:547–562.
4. Bourne WM, Kaufman HE. Specular microscopy of human corneal endothelium in vivo. *Am J Ophthalmol.* 1976;81:319–323.
5. Kaufman HE, Katz J, Valenti J, et al. Corneal endothelium damage with intraocular lenses: contact adhesions between surgical materials and tissue. *Science.* 1977;198: 525–527.
6. Katz J, Kaufman HE, Goldberg EP, et al. Prevention of endothelial damage from intraocular lens insertion. *Trans Am Acad Ophthalmol Otolaryngol.* 1977;83:OP204–OP211.
7. Shearing SP. Posterior chamber lens implantation. *Int Ophthalmol Clin.* 1982;22:135–153.
8. Pieh S, Weghaupt H, Skorpik C. Contrast sensitivity and glare disability with diffractive and refractive multifocal intraocular lenses. *J Cataract Refract Surg.* 1998;24:659–662.
9. Bleckmann H, Schmidt O, Sunde T, et al. Visual results of progressive multifocal posterior chamber intraocular lens implantation. *J Cataract Refract Surg.* 1996;22: 1102–1107.
10. Winther-Nielsen A, Gyldenkerne G, Corydon L. Contrast sensitivity, glare, and visual function: diffractive multifocal versus bilateral monofocal intraocular lenses. *J Cataract Refract Surg.* 1995;21:202–207.
11. Gimbel HV, Sun R, Heston JP. Management of zonular dialysis in phacoemulsification and IOL implantation using the capsular tension ring. *Ophthalmic Surg Lasers.* 1997;28:273–281.
12. Kaufman HE. The correction of aphakia. *Am J Ophthalmol.* 1980;89:1–10.
13. Horgan SE, Fraser SG, Choyce DP, et al. Twelve year follow-up of unfenestrated polysulfone intracorneal lenses in human sighted eyes. *J Cataract Refract Surg.* 1996;22: 1045–1051.
14. Kaufman SC, Kaufman HE. Phakic intraocular lenses and clear lens extraction for high myopia: counterpoint. In: Elander R, Rich LF, Robin JB, eds. *Principles and Practice of Refractive Surgery.* Philadelphia: WB Saunders Co; 1997:459–471.

Index

Note: Page numbers in *italics* indicate illustrations; those followed by t indicate tables.

ISBN 0-7216-8699-0